Intravenous Therapy in Nursing Practice

Senior Commissioning Editor: Alex Mathieson
Project Editor: Mairi McCubbin
Project Controller: Derek Robertson
Designer: Judith Wright

Intravenous Therapy in Nursing Practice

Edited by

Lisa Dougherty MSc RGN RM ONCCert

Clinical Nurse Specialist/Manager, IV Services,
The Royal Marsden Hospital NHS Trust, London

Julie Lamb BSc(Hons) DPSN RGN

Haematology/Oncology Nurse Specialist/Manager,
King George Hospital, Ilford

Forewords by

George Castledine BA(Hons) MSc DipSocStud (Oxon) RGN RNT
Post-grad CertEd FRCN

Professor of Nursing and Community Health and Assistant Dean,
Faculty of Health and Community Care, University of Central England,
Birmingham, UK

Tom S. J. Elliott BM BS BMedSci BTech PhD FRMS FRCPath

Consultant Microbiologist, Director of Clinical Laboratory Services,
University Hospital Birmingham NHS Trust, Birmingham, UK

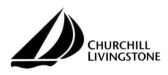

CHURCHILL LIVINGSTONE

EDINBURGH LONDON NEW YORK PHILADELPHIA ST LOUIS SYDNEY TORONTO 1999

CHURCHILL LIVINGSTONE
An imprint of Harcourt Publishers Limited

© Harcourt Publishers Limited 1999

ID is a registered trademark of Harcourt Publishers Limited

First published 1999   WB354 Intravenous therapy

ISBN 0 443 05983 7

British Library Cataloguing in Publication Data
A catalogue record for this book is available from the British Library

Library of Congress Cataloging in Publication Data
A catalog record for this book is available from the Library of Congress

Note
Medical knowledge is constantly changing. As new information becomes available, changes in treatment, procedures, equipment and the use of drugs become necessary. The editors, contributors and the publishers have, as far as it is possible, taken care to ensure that the information given in this text is accurate and up to date. However, readers are strongly advised to confirm that the information, especially with regard to drug usage, complies with the latest legislation and standards of practice.

The
publisher's
policy is to use
**paper manufactured
from sustainable forests**

Printed in China
NPCC/01

Contents

Contributors

Karen A. Bravery RGN RSCN ENB240, 998, 870, 934
Senior Sister, Great Ormond Street Hospital, London

15 Paediatric intravenous therapy in practice

S. Pearl Burnham RGN SCM
Nutrition Nurse Specialist, Havering Hospitals NHS Trust, Essex

14 Parenteral nutrition

Shelley Dolan BA MSc RGN ENB100, 237, 998
Clinical Nurse Specialist, The Royal Marsden NHS Trust, London

8 Intravenous flow control and infusion devices

Lisa Dougherty MSc RGN RM ONCCert ENB900, 995, 998
Clinical Nurse Specialist/Manager, IV Services, The Royal Marsden Hospital NHS Trust, London

9 Obtaining peripheral venous access
16 Safe handling and administration of intravenous cytotoxic drugs

Janice Gabriel PGD BSc RN FETC ONCCert MHS
Oncology Nurse Specialist/ Manager, St. Mary's Hospital, Portsmouth

11 Long-term central venous access

Sarah Hart MSc BSc(Hons) RGN FETC
Clinical Nurse Specialist – Infection Control, The Royal Marsden NHS Trust, Surrey and London

4 Infection control in intravenous therapy

Jill Kayley RGN DNCert
Community Specialist Nurse – HIV and IV Therapy, East Oxford Health Centre, Oxford

12 Intravenous therapy in the community

Julie Lamb BSc(Hons) DPSN RGN
Haematology/Oncology Nurse Specialist/Manager, King George Hospital, Ilford

1 Legal and professional aspects of intravenous therapy
7 Local and systemic complications of intravenous therapy

Michèle Malster BA(Hons) RGN
Lecturer, Nightingale Institute,
King's College London, London

3 Fluid and electrolyte balance

Maggie Nicol BSc(Hons) MSc RGN DN
PGDipEd
Senior Lecturer – Clinical Skills,
St Bartholomew School of Nursing
and Midwifery, London

*6 Safe administration and
management of peripheral intravenous
therapy*

Helen J. Porter RGN ONCCert MSc
Lead Cancer Nurse, University
Hospital Birmingham NHS Trust,
Birmingham

13 Blood transfusion therapy

Mojgan H. Sani BPharm
DipClinPharm MSc MBA MRPharmS
Consultant Pharmacist,
Pharmaceutical Adviser, Guy's &
St Thomas' NHS Trust, London

*5 Pharmacological aspects of
intravenous drug therapy*

Katie Scales BEd(Hons)
HDQCPhysiology DPSN RN RNT ENB100,
400
Assistant Nurse Director, Charing
Cross Hospital, London

*2 Anatomy and physiology related to
intravenous therapy*
*10 Vascular access in the acute care
setting*

Foreword

George Castledine

This is *the* textbook for every nurse, junior doctor and paramedic who has to deal with the administration of intravenous (i.v.) therapy. It contains a wealth of up-to-date, evidence-based information that is essential for high-quality care. The authors have brought together many key experts in the field to give us a truly comprehensive and essential guide to practice.

It says much about the development of the discipline of nursing that we now have nurse specialists who are not only competent in the core skills of nursing but the more-advanced technical aspects as well. This is a competent and thorough scientific account not only of what to do in i.v. situations but why we should do it.

There is no doubt that i.v. therapy has become more complex and intricate over the past few years, with various factors making life very difficult for the practitioner. This book gets to the root of many of these problems and helps bewildered practitioners with those they may encounter. This is not a book for those wishing to pick up a technique and then go off on their own without thinking of the consequences. There are sufficient warnings and essential guidelines to follow, which will protect not only the patient but also the practitioner.

Too often, i.v. therapy has been seen as something of a chore for junior medical staff. Good practice has never really developed and adequate in-service training and education has been lacking. I well remember being involved with an interdisciplinary working group set up to develop basic guidelines a few years ago. What appalled me so much from the evidence I heard was the ignorance and the blatant bad practice which was taking place. Simple things such as washing hands and explaining to the patient what was happening were being forgotten. Patients are now more sensitive and aware of the quality of care they should be receiving. It is not enough to ignore them or treat them as bodies to experiment on.

This is a very sensitive, as well as highly technical, account of how to behave with patients. All the latest guidelines from the various professional organisations and regulatory bodies are present. The occupational risk to health care workers is also covered in an excellent chapter on infection control. Calculating flow rates and understanding the pharmacological aspects and implications of drug interactions is something all health care professionals need to read up on. This book provides the ideal starting point and reference source. Not only are there essential chapters on all areas of i.v. work but detailed references to follow up on and reflect back into practice.

Although this is primarily a book for nurses I am sure it will be of use to junior doctors and paramedics. With the emphasis on more interprofessional working and understanding, this book is in an ideal position to lead the way. The guidelines, for example, on care of the peripheral i.v. site are as applicable, as is the rest of the book, to other health care professional who work in this area. Clear diagrams and illustrations help the reader to understand many of the practical implications for the practitioner. Simple boxes are used to cluster and collect essential information. In this way the book gives the reader a quick and easy information base. The use and dangers of various flow controls and infusion pumps is well presented to illustrate the difficulties around this topic. Throughout the book the accent is on safety and audit of practice. The psychological effects on patients are not ignored and the fears and phobias some patients experience are extensively covered.

From the very start of approaching the patient, to choosing the right vein, to monitoring progress and concluding the task, this book covers every angle and every aspect of care. There is so much information that I am sure this book will become a classic work in its field. It has been a privilege for me to have the pleasure of reading an advance copy and writing this Foreword. I would therefore strongly recommend it, especially to all those health care personnel concerned with i.v. infusion work. It captures not only the essentials of the subject but also manages to do it in a very readable and enjoyable way. It should be on the essential reading lists of all courses which cover the subject of i.v. therapy and nursing practice.

Foreword

Tom S. J. Elliott

There has been a requirement for a comprehensive text on all aspects of intravenous therapy for health care workers. This text meets such a need in a practical and easily accessible style. The book is divided into three main sections. The first describes the fundamentals of intravenous therapy including the associated anatomy and physiology, the pharmacological aspects of intravenous drug therapy and infection control. Of increasing importance is the legal and professional side of patient care, which is also comprehensively described. The second section deals with the practice of intravenous therapy, including the administration of intravenous therapy, and local and systemic complications. A practical review of intravenous flow control and infusion devices is presented. Methods for achieving vascular access are also clearly described. The use of long-term central venous access systems and intravenous therapy in the community, which is becoming increasingly common practice, complete this part of the book. The third and final section deals with specialities, including blood transfusion therapy, parenteral nutrition, paediatric intravenous therapy, and the safe handling and administration of intravenous cytotoxic drugs.

The anatomical and physiological aspects of vascular access are particularly well illustrated and there is a useful table summarising sites of vascular access. Electrolyte and fluid balance are described, taking the reader from basic physiology to more-complex aspects of everyday patient management. The pharmacological aspects of drug delivery via the intravenous route further presents details not only of the body's compartments but also metabolism, distribution and excretion, and therapeutic drug monitoring. The chapter on infections associated with catheters is comprehensive and reviews the literature in a practical manner. The avoidance of needlestick injury and the occupational aspects are also described.

The advantages and disadvantages of the intravenous route of administration are presented. Similarly, the safe administration and management of intravenous therapy, an essential component of this book, is presented in a practical format which should improve the use of intravascular devices. Local and systemic complications of intravenous therapy, including infection, extravasation, occlusion, and pulmonary and air embolisms, are all clearly outlined and methods of prevention listed. This is complemented by a useful section describing the available intravenous flow control and infusion devices with a discussion on selection and procurement.

The method for obtaining peripheral venous access is also comprehensively described. Interestingly this includes patients' fears and phobias, vasovagal reactions, pain relief and improvement to venous access, many of which are commonly overlooked in busy clinical practice. The preparation of the insertion site and approach to the patient, choice of the vein, together with other considerations such as length of treatment and device selection are described in detail. There is also a corresponding chapter on central venous cannulation in the acute care setting. The anatomical sites, types of catheters available and the methods of central venous catheter placement are well illustrated. The subsequent management and care of central venous catheters is also considered. Methods for long-term access, including the more recently introduced peripherally inserted central venous catheters, are reviewed in subsequent sections. The use of implantable injection ports with silastic membranes are also described. The practical management of complications associated with long-term central venous access is again well illustrated with a table and flowchart. With the increasing use of intravenous therapy in the community, a very useful chapter describes types of approaches to treatment of outpatients with the various access routes available.

In the third section of the book specialities including blood transfusion, parenteral nutrition, paediatric intravenous therapy and the application and administration of cytotoxic drugs are dealt with in detail. These provide a comprehensive, invaluable review for health care workers associated with these groups of patients.

The aims of this book to provide comprehensive and practical details of the fundamental principles associated with intravenous therapy and the associated procedures have been achieved. The text reflects the modern approaches to intravascular access therapy. It takes the reader from the basic understanding of the patient's anatomy to the practical applications of methods of placement and subsequent care of the devices. This text is essential reading for health care workers, including Nurse Practitioners, involved with intravascular catheterisation in patient management areas. This comprehensive text is a valuable source of information, bringing together all the facets of intravascular cannulation in a practical and elegantly presented manner.

Preface

The administration of intravenous (i.v.) therapy is now a common part of most nurses' roles. The profession has moved a long way since the Breckenridge report in 1976 which first outlined nurses' responsibilities regarding the addition of drugs to infusion bags and their hanging – the sum total of a nurse's involvement in i.v. therapy in the United Kingdom at the time. Since then, i.v. therapy has become increasingly more complex, and as technology has advanced, so too has the degree of nursing involvement.

Nurses now not only prepare and administer drugs, but also assess, insert and remove both peripheral and central venous access devices; evaluate, select and purchase access devices and infusion equipment; and provide education and training in the many facets of this challenging area of practice.

There has also been a move away from the hospital setting to the community, where i.v. therapy involves not only the health care professional, but also the patient and carer. As well as health care professionals in nursing and medicine, i.v. therapy also involves pharmacists, nutritionists and microbiologists. This has led to a demand for knowledge about i.v. therapy and its applications in all types of settings.

Unfortunately, there has been a lack of guidance in i.v. therapy in the UK, in spite of many excellent articles on the subject over the years. The Royal College of Nursing (RCN) IV Special Interest Group (formerly the British Intravenous Therapy Association, BITA) has recently produced guidance on practice, but the time is right for a definitive textbook written specifically for nurses in the UK. It was for these reasons that this book was written.

The aim of this book is to provide the fundamental principles which underpin i.v. therapy, and any associated procedures, in a comprehensive and practical way. The text is based on up-to-date research and includes practical procedures and problem-solving techniques.

Intravenous therapy is relevant to almost all areas of nursing, and features in specialities such as critical care and oncology. The book will help a wide range of health care professionals, including nurses and junior doctors. It will provide the student nurse with information on how to prepare and administer i.v. drugs for the first time, as well as informing the specialist nurse who wishes to expand her practice and insert peripherally inserted central catheters.

The book starts with the history of i.v. therapy and provides a comprehensive view of the development of the nurse's role and how practice has expanded. Professional and ethical issues, including accountability and training, are also covered. No textbook on i.v. therapy would be complete without foundation chapters on anatomy and physiology, fluid and electrolyte balance and infection control.

The chapters on the pharmacology and safe administration and management of i.v. therapy are preparatory chapters for those health care professionals starting out in i.v. therapy. They set out the practicalities of how to prepare and administer i.v. therapy safely, along with the factors which influence the methods of drug administration and the responsibilities of each health care professional involved in the process. Another vital chapter concerns local and systemic complications: each complication associated with i.v. therapy is discussed, covering the recognition, prevention and treatment of each type. The chapter on flow control takes the reader from the simple gravity drip to the various complex electronic infusion devices and includes recent Medical Devices Agency guidelines on intravenous equipment.

Venepuncture and cannulation are two of the most commonly performed invasive procedures and are now becoming an integral part of many nurses' roles. The chapter on obtaining vascular access provides step-by-step instructions for performing these tasks, along with the background of how these procedures impact on the patient. Vascular access has always been a feature in the acute care setting and the following chapter addresses common issues related to the care and maintenance of central venous catheters, as well as complications of insertion. This theme is continued in the chapter on long-term central venous access, which provides readers with a step-by-step guide to the insertion and removal of peripherally inserted central catheters, and addresses the quality-of-life issues for patients living with a central venous access device. Most of these patients will be cared for in their own houses – hence the chapter on i.v. therapy in the community, which focuses on the advantages and disadvantages for patients and emphasizes the requirements for good information and teaching.

Finally, the last four chapters of the book focus on more specialist subjects. Blood transfusion and parenteral nutrition therapy are short but comprehensive chapters which provide the reader with a broad overview of the subjects. Paediatric i.v. therapy provides a view of many of the subjects covered throughout the book (venepuncture sites, dose calculations and fluid balance) but from the paediatric perspective. The safe administration of cytotoxic drugs focuses specifically on the intravenous administration of these hazardous drugs and the problems associated with extravasation.

Many practices of i.v. therapy such as dressings and maintaining patency, remain controversial or lack sufficient scientific evidence to support them. The aim of this book is to provide a balanced view of the available research and opinions of experts, which should enable the reader to come to his/her own conclusions regarding i.v. practice.

The contributing authors were all selected for their expertise in the area covered in their chapters. They were felt to be clinically based practitioners with up-to-date knowledge and involvement in research and practice development in the field of i.v. therapy. The result is a book that will suit health care professionals, at every level and in almost every speciality, whose desire is to provide safe and evidence-based intravenous practice, with positive outcomes for the patient or client.

London, 1998

Lisa Dougherty
Julie Lamb

Acknowledgements

We were approached to write this book by Churchill Livingstone and would like to thank them and all their staff for their faith in our ability to produce this exciting and much needed text on i.v. therapy. We would especially like to thank Alex Mathieson for his encouragement, support and humour, which helped particularly when we despaired of ever pulling it all together. We would also like to thank all the contributors for putting up with our nagging and nit-picking – they all did a wonderful job and without all their hard work there would not be a book.

I would like to thank my colleagues Naim, Kate, Claire, and Carol, whose support was invaluable; my husband Mike whose patience was unending; and a special thanks to Lisa who took on the burden of editing while I was having my second baby.

Julie Lamb

Firstly, I would like to thank Val Speechley for inspiring me to become involved in i.v. therapy, Jane Mallett for all her guidance, particularly concerning my writing skills, as well as understanding the hard work that goes into editing a book. I would like to thank all my friends and colleagues at work for their support and belief in me, and finally I would like to thank Liz, who listened, advised and supported me throughout.

Lisa Dougherty

Fundamentals

Legal and professional aspects of intravenous therapy

Julie Lamb

INTRODUCTION

There are few areas in nursing where the role of the nurse has grown as fast and as effectively as in intravenous (i.v.) nursing. The development in this area reflects a general trend in the nursing profession. Nurses today monitor complex physiological data, operate sophisticated life-saving equipment and coordinate the delivery of patients' health care services. More importantly, nurses now have responsibility for exercising clinical judgement (Baldwin & Mantell 1995) (see Box 1.1 for a history of i.v. therapy).

The expanding responsibility of nurses practising in i.v. therapy has both advantages and disadvantages. The nurse's emerging role offers rewards such as intellectual stimulation and professional satisfaction. However, the increase in responsibility brings with it the increased capacity for liability and the added potential of legal risks.

Nurses employed in this area of practice require a working appreciation of their responsibilities and an understanding of the legal and professional implications which underpin their clinical nursing practice.

PROFESSIONAL GUIDELINES

The main codes for nurses practising in the UK are:

- The International Code for Nurses
- The UKCC *Code of Professional Conduct* for the Nurse, Midwife and Health Visitor.

The first code of ethics was adopted by the International Council of Nurses (ICN) in São Paulo, Brazil, in July 1953. This code was subsequently revised at the ICN meetings in Frankfurt, Germany, and again in Mexico City in 1973 (Tschudin 1992).

The first ICN code (1953) described the fundamental responsibility of the nurse as threefold:

- to conserve life
- to alleviate suffering
- to promote health.

Twenty years later, this duty was seen as fourfold:

- to promote health
- to prevent illness
- to restore health
- to alleviate suffering.

The ICN code is comprehensive in terms of an ethic of care. It acknowledges the universal need for nursing, the inherent respect for life and dignity, and the rights of humankind (Tschudin 1992).

■ **BOX 1.1**

History of intravenous therapy

The recorded history of i.v. therapy began in 1492 when a blood transfusion from two Romans to the dying Pope Innocent was attempted. All three died.

In 1628, Sir William Harvey's discovery of the blood circulatory system formed the basis for more scientific experimentation. Sir Christopher Wren in 1658 predicted the possibility of introducing medication directly into the bloodstream, although it was Dr Robert Boyle who, using a quill and bladder, injected opium into a dog in 1659, with JD Major in 1665 succeeding with the first injection into a human.

A 15-year-old Parisian boy successfully received a transfusion of lamb's blood in 1667; however, subsequent animal to human transfusions proved fatal and eventually, in 1687, the practice was made illegal.

In 1834, James Blundell proved that only human blood was suitable for transfusion, and later this century Pasteur and Lister stressed the necessity for asepsis during infusion procedures.

Karl Landsteiner, in 1900, led the way in identifying and classifying different blood groups, and in 1914 it was recognized that sodium citrate prevented clotting which opened the gate for the extensive use of blood transfusions.

Intravenous therapy was being used widely during World War II, and by the mid-1950s was being used mainly for the purpose of major surgery and rehydration only. Few medications were given via the i.v. route, with antibiotics more commonly being given intramuscularly.

Throughout the 1960s and 1970s, intermittent medications, filters, electronic infusion control devices and smaller plastic cannulae became available. Use of multiple electrolyte solutions and medications increased along with blood component therapy, and numerous i.v. drugs and antibiotics were being added to i.v. regimens.

The use of i.v. therapy has expanded dramatically over the last 30 years. This expansion continues to accelerate and can be attributed to the following factors:

- the understanding of hazards and complications
- improvement in i.v. equipment
- increased knowledge of physiological requirements
- increased knowledge of pharmacological and therapeutic implications
- increased availability of nutrients and drugs in i.v. solutions.

So much has changed in i.v. therapy over the years that we have now reached the point where it is considered to be an accepted component of medical care. New developments in treatments are occurring at an increasing rate and, with i.v. therapy permeating all clinical settings, the growth of 'high-tech' infusion therapy has followed.

Educational packs have expanded to include advanced studies in an effort to meet the needs of the advanced practitioner, and the growth of i.v. therapy has resulted in increased roles for nurses both nationally and internationally.

Each man and woman who, following appropriate education and training, becomes a registered nurse, midwife or health visitor also becomes a member of one of the regulated health professions. Their 'registration' since 1983 has been in the register maintained by the single statutory body established by Act of Parliament for these professions, the United Kingdom Central Council (UKCC) for Nursing, Midwifery and Health Visiting (Pyne 1996). It states that one of its principal functions is 'to establish and improve standards of training and professional conduct for nurses, midwives and health visitors'.

■ BOX 1.2

Exercising Accountability document (*UKCC 1989*)

- The interests of the patient or client are paramount
- Professional accountability must be exercised in such a manner
- The exercise of accountability requires the practitioner to seek to achieve and maintain high standards
- Advocacy on behalf of patients or clients is an essential feature of the exercise of accountability by a professional practitioner
- The role of other persons in the delivery of health care to patients or clients must be recognized and respected provided that the first principle above is honoured
- Public trust and confidence in the profession are dependent on its practitioners being seen to exercise their accountability responsibly
- Each registered nurse, midwife or health visitor must be able to justify any action or decision not to act taken in the course of her professional practice

In 1992, the UKCC issued the third edition of its *Code of Professional Conduct* which infers that the individual practitioner should be directed to recognizing and serving the interests of patients. This document is all about accountability (Pyne 1994). It begins with a core sentence from which all subsequent 16 clauses stem:

'As a registered nurse, midwife or health visitor, you are personally accountable for your practice and, in the exercise of your professional accountability, must...' (UKCC 1992a).

It leaves no room for uncertainty or ambiguity, stating clearly that nurses are personally responsible for their practice (Pyne 1994).

In response to developing practice, the UKCC felt it necessary to broaden the guidelines in some parts of the code. Its document *Exercising Accountability* (UKCC 1989) summarized a set of principles against which the nurse should exercise accountability (see Box 1.2). More recently, the UKCC has chosen to publish 'standards' documents to indicate the expectations it has of practitioners in respect of specific areas of practice (Pyne 1996).

One such document, the *Standards for the Administration of Medicines* (UKCC 1992b) states clearly that the Council has prepared these standards to assist practitioners to fulfil the expectations it has of them, to serve more effectively the interests of patients and clients, and to maintain and enhance standards of practice. It continues to list a number of principles in which the practitioner must exercise their professional judgement (see Box 1.3).

The Scope of Professional Practice

Another published document through which the Council has stated its expectations of practitioners is *The Scope of Professional Practice* (UKCC 1992c). The key messages to practitioners to be found in this document have their roots firmly in the *Code of Professional Conduct*, in particular the introductory paragraph and the first four clauses (see Box 1.4).

This document places the onus on nurses to recognize their own personal level of competence and moves nursing away from a system of post-registration certification of specified tasks. The intention is to create a greater flexibility and enhance the contribution of nurses to patient care (Lunn 1994).

Pyne (1992) suggests that this is an extremely important professional development, stating 'it is a sign of a profession coming to maturity and accepting that pro-

■ BOX 1.3

Standards for the Administration of Medicines (UKCC 1992b)

- Confirming the correctness of the prescription
- Judging the suitability of administration at the scheduled time of administration
- Reinforcing the positive effect of the treatment
- Enhancing the understanding of patients in respect of their prescribed medication and the avoidance of misuse of these and other medicines
- Assisting in assessing the efficacy of medicines and the identification of side-effects and interactions

■ BOX 1.4

Scope of Professional Practice (UKCC 1992c)

The registered nurse, midwife or health visitor:

- Must be satisfied that each aspect of practice is directed to meeting the needs and serving the interests of the patient or client
- Must endeavour always to achieve, maintain and develop knowledge, skill and competence to respond to the needs and interests of the patient or client
- Must honestly acknowledge any limits of personal knowledge and skill and take steps to remedy any relevant deficits in order to effectively and appropriately meet the needs of patients and clients
- Must ensure that any enlargement or adjustment of the scope of personal professional practice must be achieved without compromising or fragmenting existing aspects of professional practice and care and that the requirements of the Council's *Code of Professional Conduct* are satisfied throughout the whole area of practice
- Must recognize and honour the direct or indirect personal accountability borne for all aspects of professional practice
- Must, in serving the interests of patients and clients and the wider interests of society, avoid any inappropriate delegation to others which would compromise those interests

fessional practice must be based around those twin pillars of competence and accountability'.

The most recent professional publication issued by the UKCC is the *Guidelines for Professional Practice* (UKCC 1996). This has been produced to provide a guide for reflection on the statements within the *Code of Professional Conduct*. Their intention is that the booklet will assist nurses to:

- 'care' in a way that reflects your *Code of Professional Conduct*
- 'protect' patients and clients
- 'honour' your responsibilities as a registered practitioner.

The document aims to give clarification on a number of key issues such as consent, truthfulness, advocacy and autonomy, and gives guidance on all 16 clauses of the code.

The UKCC recognizes that professional practice and decision-making are not straightforward. The circumstances in which nurses work are always changing. The Council state that the way in which nurses work must be sensitive and relevant and must meet the needs of patients and clients. As a final point in their document, the UKCC stress that nurses must be able to adjust their practice to changing circumstances, taking into consideration local procedures, policies and cultural differences (UKCC 1996).

It is interesting to note that even today, whilst the practice of i.v. therapy is commonplace in most clinical settings, there is still no national i.v. training and competence programme. Reflected in practice, this means that when competent and expert practitioners change employers, whilst the *Scope of Professional Practice* might support the continuation of such practice, their employer's policy probably would not.

PROFESSIONAL REGISTRATION

At the heart of the UKCC's activities is the register. It is something which the law requires to be established and maintained. The professional register is a means of declaring, to all with an interest in knowing, that the men and women whose names feature within it are those from whom a reasonable standard of competence and conduct is expected. Additionally, it is stating that these are the people to whom the UKCC has declared its expectations, given its advice and presented its standards and whom it can call to account (Pyne 1996).

Removal from the register

Nurses are removed from the register for a variety of reasons (see Box 1.5), all of which constitute allegations of misconduct. This is defined in the rules as 'conduct unworthy of a nurse, midwife or health visitor' (Pyne 1996).

It is open to any person to make such allegations. If such a complaint is received by the UKCC about professional and not criminal behaviour, the UKCC will assemble evidence and present it in the first instance to the Preliminary Proceedings Committee for consideration. This committee has a range of decisions at its disposal. If it considers that the allegations or facts presented are of no great significance or are unlikely to be regarded as misconduct in a professional sense, the committee can choose to do nothing and decline to proceed.

■ **BOX 1.5**

Removal from the register

- Reckless and wilful unskilled practice
- Concealing untoward incidents
- Failure to keep essential records
- Failure to protect or promote the interests of patients or clients
- Failure to act, knowing that a colleague or subordinate is improperly treating or abusing patients
- Physical or verbal abuse of patients
- Abuse of patients by improperly withholding prescribed drugs or administering unprescribed drugs or an excess of prescribed drugs
- Theft from patients or employers
- Drug-related offences
- Sexual abuse of patients
- Breach of confidentiality

Conversely, if it concludes that the allegations or facts constitute a misconduct and raise questions about the practitioner's future registration status, it can refer the case for a formal public hearing by the Professional Conduct Committee (Pyne 1996). This committee has six options available to it:

- not to remove the name of the practitioner from the register
- to postpone a judgement for a fixed period
- to give a caution
- to refer to the Health Committee
- to suspend from the register
- to remove the name of the practitioner from the register.

The Professional Conduct Committee state that their intention is not to punish the nurse but to protect the public from irresponsible and harmful behaviour.

EXPANSION OF NURSING ROLES

The role of the nurse has developed in a far more fundamental way than simply taking on previously medical tasks (Rumbold 1993). Over the past two decades the nursing profession has begun to develop a knowledge base which is its own.

Nursing actions are no longer determined solely on the basis of the medical diagnosis, but also the nursing diagnosis. Clearly, in planning and giving nursing care, the nurse cannot ignore the medical condition of the patient, but it is only one factor among many which the nurse has to take into account (Rumbold 1993).

The development of specialist and advanced nursing should be seen as going hand in hand with the expansion of the nursing role in general. The UKCC makes the point in the *Scope of Professional Practice* that the terms 'extended' or 'extending' roles are no longer suitable since they limit rather than extend the parameters of practice (Castledine 1994).

The expanded role of the nurse is, of course, about much more than performing particular tasks – it is essentially about the interpretation of the role. 'Role' can be defined in terms of the rights and obligations accorded to the incumbent of a particular position. Although the DHSS regulations of 1977, *The Extending Role of the Clinical Nurse – Legal Implications and Training Requirements*, still stand at the time of writing, thinking within the profession has moved on. Emphasis now tends to be placed on the nurse's right to decide whether she is competent to do something, rather than on the possession of a certificate (Rumbold 1993).

In summary, the DHSS (1977) regulations state that the nurse's role may only be legally extended in the following circumstances:

- The nurse has been specifically and adequately trained for the performance of the new task and she agrees to undertake it.
- This training has been recognized as satisfactory by the employing authority.
- The new task has been recognized by the profession and by the employing authority as a task which may be properly delegated to a nurse.
- The delegating doctor has been assured of the competence of the individual nurse concerned.

In response to these guidelines and the rapid development of tasks previously performed by doctors but now delegated to nurses, the Royal College of Nursing (RCN) and the British Medical Association (BMA) issued a joint statement through a document entitled *The Duties and Position of the Nurse* (RCN 1978). This set out in formal terms guiding principles, recommending the setting up of special machinery through which it believed that questions relating to respective frontiers of professional responsibility could be effectively resolved at local level.

■ BOX 1.6

Intravenous drug therapy – BMA and RCN guiding principles

- Patients' interests are paramount
- Practitioners have a responsibility to draw attention to areas where local protocols conflict with the patient's best interests
- Intravenous therapy administration must be viewed as a partnership responsibility with standards consistent amongst the health care team
- The i.v. route is only to be used when there are no other alternatives
- All health care staff involved with i.v. therapy administration have a responsibility to ensure that they have attained the appropriate knowledge and skills to enable the delivery of safe and effective care
- Health care professionals should actively participate in minimizing the risks which are associated with i.v. therapy
- Policies and protocols should be developed at local level which should reflect the active contributions of experienced health care professionals
- Consistent standards must apply across the health care team
- Each practitioner is considered as responsible and personally accountable for their practice
- Intravenous therapy should be audited

The administration of i.v. drugs is probably the most well known area of medical to nurse delegation, it now being considered an integral part of nursing practice. With specific relevance to this area, Lord Breckenridge, in 1976, was asked to chair a working party to look at the addition of drugs to intravenous infusion fluids. Evidence presented to the working party, from the nursing viewpoint, identified that the addition and administration of drugs via i.v. infusion fluids was increasingly carried out by nurses (DHSS 1976). The working party recognized that nurses' authority and responsibility in this area of practice were not clearly defined and were made more confusing by local policies and standards of training which varied widely.

More recently, in 1993, a statement from the BMA and RCN on intravenous drug therapy (BMA/RCN 1993) set out principles and outlined policies to guide the health care team in developing i.v. practices that are appropriate and responsive to local health care needs (Box 1.6).

It could be argued that the expansion and development of nursing roles have been driven by a political force, in the main through the reduction of junior doctors' hours. Nurses would like to believe that they have exploited this directive to their professional advantage and satisfaction as well as to the benefit of patient care.

In November 1992, the Department of Health's Research & Development Division commissioned Greenhalgh & Company Ltd to undertake a 12 month research study into the interface between junior hospital doctors and ward nurses. The aim of the study was 'to contribute to the improvement in patient care' by examining the interface between junior hospital doctors and ward nurses with a view to enhancing the role of nurses and reducing the inappropriate workload of junior hospital doctors.

Within its terms of reference, three core questions were posed (Greenhalgh 1994):

- What do junior doctors and nurses currently do?

- What work is transferable between junior doctors and nurses for the benefit of patient care?
- What model or exemplars of good practice in this interface between junior doctors and nurses can be identified and disseminated for the benefit of patients and the service?

At the end of the study, the report identified key findings and recommendations (Box 1.7) which showed an obvious need to look at current nursing and medical practice based upon technological advances in medical/nursing treatments and to move forward in partnership to provide an environment of care in which 'good practice' can flourish.

LEGAL ASPECTS OF DRUGS

The main legislation controlling the supply, storage and administration of medicines is the Medicines Act 1968 and the Misuse of Drugs Act 1971. The law has very little interest in laying down detailed rules for nurses regarding the administration of medicines; however, guidance can be found in the UKCC (1992b) advisory document *Standards for the Administration of Medicines*.

Local policies may be drawn up which differ from the main guidelines and the advisory paper allows for this, but it sets out principles which should be taken into account in the setting up of these local policies (Dimond 1995). Prior to the administration of each drug, the nurse should complete the following checklist:

- Correct patient – consent, information
- Correct drug – side-effects, reconstitution, diluent
- Correct dose – ?first dose
- Correct site and method of administration – check patency of cannula if to be given intravenously
- Correct procedure – safe reconstitution, safe equipment, asepsis
- Correct documentation.

Nurse prescribing

Nurse prescribing is an acknowledgement and endorsement of the current contribution of nurses to patient care and a recognition of the need to supply items necessary for effective nursing treatment.

To prescribe effectively, nurses will need:

- an increased awareness of professional accountability
- a full understanding of the process of assessment and diagnosis that results in the act of prescribing
- a knowledge of therapeutics and practical prescribing (Andrews 1994).

It was the Cumberledge Report (1986) that first identified the need for limited nurse prescribing:

'The DHSS should agree a limited list of items and simple agents which may be prescribed by nurses as part of a nursing care programme and issue guidelines to enable nurses to control drug dosage in well defined circumstances.'

Following a number of subsequent reports which recommended that nurses should prescribe from a limited formulary, the Nurse Prescribing Advisory Group (DOH 1989) made 27 recommendations which were addressed to the Department of Health, the UKCC, health authorities and the professions. These recommendations relate to six core areas of practice:

■ **BOX 1.7**

The Greenhalgh Report

Key findings

Hospitals reported that the environment in which 'good practice' flourishes requires that:

- doctors and nurses work together as colleagues and partners in care
- doctors and nurses undertake activities 'appropriate' to their training and skills
- doctors and nurses are keen to accept change
- control mechanisms are placed to ensure an acceptable quality of care, i.e. joint education for practice and competency testing.

Doctors and nurses prefer activities to be described as being 'shared' rather than 'transferred' to them.

Key recommendations

- Availability of protocols to facilitate a team-based approach to patient care
- If research activities are to be performed by nurses, they should be shared with junior doctors as opposed to being transferred to nurses
- Nurses should undertake the six activities highlighted in the report which took up 11–16% of junior doctors' time:
  - taking a patient history
  - venous blood sampling
  - insertion of a peripheral i.v. cannula
  - referring a patient for an investigation
  - writing discharge letters to GPs and other doctors
  - administration of drugs (excluding cytotoxics and first doses) via a peripheral i.v. cannula

  (Additional activities were for negotiation at local level)
- The above activities should become an integral part of the registered nurse's role and not only performed by specialist nurses
- Initiatives in collaborative practice between junior doctors and nurses in joint planning of care should be pursued
- The use of integrated patient case notes should be encouraged to reduce duplication in obtaining patient details
- Joint training should be undertaken in at least the six activities identified for shared care and they should be included in the core curriculum for pre-registration nursing and undergraduate medical training
- Further research was required to test the results against those areas which were excluded from the research study parameters, i.e. obtaining patients' views; additionally, further work to be undertaken to define measurable outcomes for at least the six activities to support clinical audit and, utilizing the research databases, to examine junior doctors' non-clinical activities and the effects of consultant bed scatter on the ward team

- practice
- education
- administration
- legal issues
- communication
- public safeguards (Andrews 1994).

The report recommended that only those nurses with a UKCC recognized qualification in district nursing or health visiting should be authorized to undertake the independent activity of prescribing. The report also proposed that stoma care nurses, continence advisors, diabetic liaison nurses, palliative care nurses, community psychiatric nurses and community mental handicap nurses should not prescribe directly but could, in certain circumstances, alter the timing and dosage of drugs and supply items within predetermined protocols (Andrews 1994).

It seems likely that with acceptance and progression of the principles outlined by the UKCC in the *Code of Professional Conduct* (UKCC 1992a), *The Scope of Professional Practice* (UKCC 1992c) and the *Community Education and Practice Report* (UKCC 1991), combined with the broad remit of the Medicinal Products Prescription by Nurses etc. Bill (1992), the range and number of nurses empowered to prescribe will increase (Andrews 1994)

Presently there are four pieces of legislation which define the legal situation for nurses involved in the supply and administration of 'prescription-only medicines' (Elliott Pennels 1997):

- The Medicines Act 1968 – this is the starting point; Section 58 describes current requirements
- The Medicines Order 1983 – this legislation explains in further detail particular aspects of the Medicines Act 1968 and gives legal definitions of the terms used
- Medicinal Products: Prescribing for Nurses Act 1992 – this provides legal authorization to nurses to be involved in the supply and administration of 'prescription-only medicines' and states in Section 1 that 'registered nurses, midwives and health visitors … who comply with such conditions as may be specified' could become appropriate practitioners
- Medicines Order 1994 – this outlines the conditions to be met by nurses who were to be prescribing practitioners.

In summary, nurse prescribing in law and as a professional task applies only to some district nurses, health visitors and midwives working in the community. Only these nurses can lawfully prescribe, and they do so only in designated pilot sites, by use of the *Nurse Prescribers Formulary* (BMA/RPS/GB/RCN 1992, Luker et al 1997) and having undergone special training (Elliott Pennels 1997).

NURSING ACCOUNTABILITY

Accountability must be regarded as implicit within any area of practice where the professional practitioner delivers care. The practitioner has to make judgements and be answerable for those judgements – so states the UKCC in their document *Exercising Accountability* (UKCC 1989). However, nowhere in this document is a definition of accountability given, although the concept is seen as providing a 'central focus' of the code (Young 1991).

Sims (1967) defined accountability as 'being personally responsible for the outcome of professional acts'. The RCN widened the definition to link the degree of accountability to the degree of authority vested in the individual and stated that a nurse cannot be accountable without that authority.

Burnard & Chapman (1988) identified that, although a nurse can be responsible for an action, accountability means being able to explain why. Therefore, accountability requires knowledge (Young 1991)

Owing to its dependence on such issues as authority and autonomy, the concept of accountability is closely related to the concept of professionalism (Watson 1995). Watson (1992) concluded that 'accountability is the very essence of professionalism', with the justification that it sets professionals apart from other kinds of occupations. However, he states that it should be acknowledged that there are different ideas as to what constitutes a profession.

Nursing has some of the features of a profession in that training and a registered qualification are both required in order to practice (Thompson et al 1994). By virtue of this, nurses become accountable to the general public for their practice and this accountability is regulated by a statutory body, the UKCC, which governs the training of nurses and holds the authority to remove individuals from the register and thereby their right to practice (Watson 1995).

Thompson et al (1988) point out that nurses have a duty to the profession to behave in a manner which upholds codes of conduct, even though the organization within which they work gives more weight to doctors' opinions. They go on to say that nurses must be responsible. For example, if nurses think a prescription contains the wrong dose, they have a duty to question this and if there is still doubt they have a duty to refuse to give it. This, of course, requires knowledge and assertiveness (Orr 1995).

The UKCC (1992) states that 'as a registered nurse, midwife and health visitor you are personally accountable for your practice and in the exercise of your professional accountability must ...'. Accountability means being answerable for work and decisions about work, and being personally responsible for the standard of practice.

Legal accountability

Legal accountability is the principal form of accountability for every citizen, and nurses like all other professionals are personally accountable through the law for their actions or omissions (Tingle 1995).

There are four main arenas of accountability in law; when a patient suffers harm or when there is loss of, or damage to, property, the nurse may be called to account in four different courts and tribunals (Dimond 1995). However, not all actions will be heard in all four arenas (Tingle 1995; see Fig. 1.1):

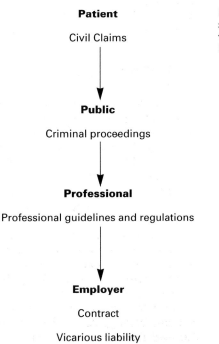

Patient

Civil Claims

Public

Criminal proceedings

Professional

Professional guidelines and regulations

Employer

Contract

Vicarious liability

Fig. 1.1 Arenas of accountability. (Reproduced with kind permission from Dimond 1995.)

- patient accountability – the UKCC (1989) states that the nurse is primarily accountable to the patient
- employee accountability – the nurse's employer will say that the nurse is accountable to them as an employee by virtue of her contract of employment
- UKCC accountability – the UKCC could view her conduct as being professional misconduct, and disciplinary proceedings could result
- society accountability – society has an interest in the situation, as safe hospitals are clearly in the public interest and furthermore public money from taxes funds the National Health Service.

NURSING RESPONSIBILITY

The increase in knowledge within all facets of i.v. therapy and the expanding use of toxic drugs have led to a growing appreciation of the need for accuracy and vigilance in the administration of i.v. drugs and fluids.

Recommendations for standards of practice began to appear in the 1980s following Lord Breckenridge's 1976 report (DHSS 1976), which found that the addition and administration of drugs via i.v. infusion was increasingly being performed by nurses. The report stated that 'doctors are frequently unaware of the special problems and hazards which frequently accompany the administration of drugs by their addition to intravenous fluids' and went on to say that consultants should ensure that junior medical staff, upon whom the responsibility for this aspect of care is delegated, should themselves possess adequate knowledge of its hazards. It concluded with the statement: 'education of all members of the medical profession in the practice of adding drugs to intravenous infusion fluid is of vital importance'.

With regard to the nurse's responsibilities, the report said that the legal position of the nurse who performs these duties must be clearly understood by the employing authority, the doctor and the nurse herself. The employing authority is vicariously liable for any negligence which may be committed by a nurse in the course of her employment and this applies to the addition of drugs to intravenous fluids as much as to any other duty. It is recommended that all nurses receive the training in order to effectively carry out the procedure related to this task, and suggested that the preparation of these responsibilities be included within the framework of basic training.

The report detailed the responsibilities of the doctor, nurse and pharmacist in the provision of i.v. therapy, highlighting that when considered in partnership, the delivery of i.v. therapy can achieve its optimum potential for a successful and complication-free outcome.

Responsibility is seen as being liable, able to be called to account, answerable for and accountable for (Dimond 1995). The concept of responsibility can be divided into:

- the personal aspect of being responsible
- legal aspect of having responsibility (Tschudin 1992).

There may be circumstances where a nurse could be held morally responsible but where there is no legal liability. For example, if a nurse fails to volunteer her services at the scene of a road accident, the law at present recognizes no legal duty to volunteer help and thus any legal action brought against the nurse would fail. However, many would hold that there is a moral duty to use her skills to help a fellow human being. Obviously the law and ethics overlap, but each is both wider and narrower than the other (Dimond 1995).

The fundamental responsibilities of the nurse are fourfold:

- to promote health
- to prevent illness
- to restore health
- to alleviate suffering (ICN 1973).

Nurses, however, have responsibilities not only to their patients, but also to the profession and to society as a whole. Nurses have a responsibility not just to ensure that their own knowledge and skills are constantly being improved, but also to contribute to the development of knowledge and skills within the profession as a whole (Rumbold 1993).

Responsibility is not complete without accountability. Many responsibilities and duties are only seen clearly when something goes wrong. Values are only discovered through challenges. The UKCC code is essentially a document outlining nurses' responsibilities. The way in which these are interpreted does depend upon the individual. The code is not a stick, nor are responsibilities heavy burdens. As usual, there is a balance to be achieved between both of them (Tschudin 1992).

STANDARDS OF CARE

All nurses owe their patients a duty of care. Liability is likely to follow if that duty is breached. A breach will consist of a failure to meet the requisite standard of care. That standard is determined by the Bolam test: 'the standard of the ordinary skilled man exercising and professing to have that special skill'. This standard is objective and is a well established principle (Lee 1996).

Lord Aitkin laid down the basis of the duty of care that we owe to others in Donaghue vs. Stevenson 1932 (Young 1996). A person must take reasonable care to avoid acts or omissions that he can reasonably foresee would be likely to injure a person directly affected by those acts. This concept forms a cornerstone of the civil wrong of negligence where a breach of duty with resultant harm constitutes liability, and later cases have only served to refine this (Young 1996).

For a successful litigation outcome, the plaintiff must establish three principles based on the balance of probabilities:

- that a duty of care is owed by the defendant to the plaintiff
- that there has been a breach of that duty
- that, as a result of that breach, the plaintiff has suffered harm of a kind recognized in law and which is not too remote.

For example, a litigation claim could be evoked if in the course of her duty, a nurse made a drug administration error which caused the patient distress and injury.

STANDARDS OF TRAINING

It is crucial in an area of clinical practice such as the administration of i.v. therapy that the practitioner has the appropriate knowledge base on which to underpin practice. Presently there is no national standard of i.v. training, and Trusts and employers are in the position of having to draw up local policies and education packs, the standard and content of which vary widely.

However, due to the emergence of dedicated i.v. nurses over the past two decades, and with i.v. therapy becoming more commonplace, recommendations for standards of practice appeared in the 1980s following the formation of the British Intravenous Therapy Association (BITA).

BITA was established in 1980 in response to a call from interested nurses who were concerned about the standards of i.v. practice and the preparation of nurses for this practice. The aim of the association was to promote, for the public benefit, investigation into i.v. practice, nurse education and research with concomitant dissemination of knowledge through publication.

In order to achieve these aims, the following objectives were identified:

- to establish codes of practice for nurses engaged in i.v. therapy
- to provide information and promote education related to i.v. therapy
- to establish and develop bursaries/grants for the pursuance of research into i.v. therapy.

In 1987, the *Guidelines for the Preparation of Nurses for the Intravenous Drug Administration and Associated Intravenous Therapy* were published (see Appendix). In 1988, BITA became allied to the RCN, and is now known as the Intravenous Therapy Special Interest Group. Today, it remains steadfast to the principles and objectives that were initially laid down in 1980.

If an i.v. training programme is to gain national recognition and acceptance, it is important that the content and standard of that programme are consistent and relevant to clinical practice, being coordinated and facilitated by clinical experts.

Recent developments have resulted in a guidance document for intravenous therapy being issued by the RCN Intravenous Therapy Special Interest Group in an attempt to steer training programmes and policy frameworks towards a national standard (RCN 1999).

All practitioners have a duty to provide safe standards of i.v. care to all patients. Health care staff involved in i.v. therapy must be able to demonstrate a sound knowledge of:

- fluid and electrolyte balance
- management of blood and blood product transfusion
- methods of i.v. drug administration
- pharmacology principles
- principles, practice and problems of i.v. therapy, including the psychological aspects of treatment.

Nurses who wish to expand their skills beyond drug administration, i.e. venepuncture and cannulation, need to attend additional competency and education programmes relevant to that area of practice. It is essential that practitioners keep abreast of clinical advances and changes in practice, and it is therefore recommended that training updates be attended at least every 2 years, or earlier if the practitioners deem it necessary.

VICARIOUS LIABILITY

NHS Trusts and other employers have two forms of liability: (1) direct liability, i.e. the Trust itself is at fault; and (2) vicarious or indirect liability, i.e. the Trust is responsible for the faults of others, mainly its employees (Dimond 1995). This has been established in a number of legal cases, but particularly clearly in the Roe and Woolly cases in 1954 (Young 1991):

> 'Hospital authorities are responsible for the whole of their staff, not only nurses and doctors, but also for anaesthetists and surgeons. It does not matter whether they are permanent or temporary, resident or visiting, whole time or part time. The reason is because even if they are not servants, they are agents of the hospital to give the treatment.'

Thus the employing authority can be sued instead of or as well as the negligent nurse. However, if damages are awarded, the Law Reform (Married Women & Tortfeasers) Act 1935 enables the employer to obtain a financial contribution from the staff involved (Young 1991).

RECORD-KEEPING

Under the Limitations Acts 1939–75, the period before an action for negligence can be initiated may be as long as 3 years from the time of damage occurring, or up to 21 years for a child. With the pressure on the courts, the case may not be heard for several more years. Thus the importance of nurses keeping accurate and thorough records can be understood. The UKCC (1993) has issued a standard document entitled *Standards for Records and Record Keeping* to assist nurses in making adequate and appropriate documentation (Young 1991). For example, if a drug is not administered at the prescribed time, it should be clearly documented on the prescription chart and in the patient's notes.

CONSENT TO TREATMENT

The notion of informed consent stems from the 1947 Nuremberg trials of 23 Nazi doctors accused of crimes involving human subjects. The Nuremberg Code (1947) laid down 10 standards to which doctors must conform when carrying out experiments on human subjects. Voluntary consent of the subject is the first of these standards. (The Nuremberg Code has now been replaced by the Declaration of Helsinki 1964.)

The idea of consent is based on the principle of respect for the person and thus on the concept of human rights of life and liberty (Tschudin 1992).

A patient's ability to understand and therefore reach an informed decision may be restricted by their intelligence, education or understanding of English. Problems with hearing and/or an awe of doctors may also limit ability (Young 1991).

Essentially, all nursing actions are invasions of a person's privacy. Most of these actions are considered necessary and consent is given implicitly by going into hospital. This, however, should never be taken for granted. Giving full explanations of what is being done, and why, how and when, is essential for the patient to remain a free agent and exercise the right to say no (Tschudin 1992).

Refusal of treatment

It is often difficult for nurses to accept a patient's refusal to give consent, particularly when the treatment being offered is life-saving. However, the nurse must remember that the patient has the right to choose and her role is to support the patient in this right (Young 1991). An action of battery may be brought if treatment is given in the face of an explicit refusal of consent (McHale 1996).

While a clear refusal should be respected, there are situations in which a patient's refusal may be overridden. General guidance for health care professionals was laid down in *Re T* (see Tingle & Cribb 1996). This case concerned a patient who refused a blood transfusion. This decision had been reached after she had spent some time alone with her mother, who was a Jehovah's Witness – *T* herself was not a Jehovah's Witness. The hospital caring for *T* sought an order authorizing them, if it became necessary, to administer a blood transfusion to *T* despite her refusal of consent.

In delivering judgement in this case, Lord Donaldson laid down a number of guidelines to assist health care professionals faced with patients who were refusing treatment (McHale 1996):

- If a patient had refused consent this could lead those treating him to ask whether he was capable of refusing consent to treatment.
- The implications of treatment refusal vary tremendously and the nurse should consider whether the refusal of treatment means that the patient will only suffer pain and discomfort at one extreme or whether refusal means almost certain death.
- The scope of the refusal should also be considered – whether it applies in all situations and whether it is based upon assumptions which have not been realized.
- In addition, the nurse should consider whether the patient's decision has been reached without undue influence being applied.

CONCLUSION

The practice of nursing, midwifery and health visiting today is the result of previous historical forces. Many of those forces have resulted in defensive and reactive changes rather than deliberate efforts to develop the potential of nursing practice and broaden the scope for practitioners to be more effective and efficient (Castledine 1994).

Nursing practice in the future is likely to become more autonomous and entrepreneurial. Professional barriers will continue to erode, with roles becoming more flexible. Advances in nursing knowledge have encouraged nurses to recognize their worth, expertise and ability to make informed decisions regarding patient care. With this increasing responsibility comes a need to improve the nurse's appreciation and understanding of expanding nursing practice.

REFERENCES

Andrews S 1994 Nurse prescribing. In: Hunt G, Wainwright P (eds) Expanding the role of the nurse. Blackwell Science, Oxford, ch 5, p 74–84

Baldwin D R, Mantell D L 1995 In: Legal aspects of nursing. Terry J, Baranowski L, Lonsway R A, Hedrick C (eds) Intravenous therapy: clinical principles and practice. WB Saunders, Philadelphia, ch 5, p 67–80

British Intravenous Therapy Association 1987 Guidelines for the preparation of nurses for intravenous drug administration and associated intravenous therapy. Travenol, UK

British Medical Association, Royal Pharmaceutical Society of Great Britain and Royal College of Nursing 1992 Draft nurse prescribers formulary. BMA/RPS/GB/RCN, London

Burnard P, Chapman C M 1988 Professional and ethical issues in nursing. John Wiley, Chichester

Castledine G 1994 Specialist and advanced nursing and the scope of practice. In: Hunt G, Wainwright P (eds) Expanding the role of the nurse. Blackwell Science, Oxford, ch 7, p 101–112

Cumberledge Report 1986 Neighbourhood nursing – a focus for care. DHSS, London

Department of Health (1989) Report of the Advisory Group on Nurse Prescribing (Crown Report). HMSO, London

Department of Health and Social Security 1976 Health service development addition of drugs to intravenous infusion fluids. HC(76) 9 (Breckenridge Report) HMSO, London

Department of Health and Social Security 1977 The extending role of the nurse – legal implications and training requirements HC(77)22. HMSO, London

Dimond B 1995 Legal aspects of nursing, 2nd edn. Prentice Hall, London

Elliott Pennels C 1997 Nurse prescribing. Professional Nurse 13(2): 114–117

Greenhalgh 1994 The interface between junior doctors and nurses: a research study for the Department of Health. Greenhalgh & Co, Macclesfield

Hunt G, Wainwright P 1994 Expanding the role of the nurse. Blackwell Science, Oxford

Hunt G 1995 Whistleblowing in the health service: accountability law and professional practice. Edward Arnold, London

International Council of Nurses (ICN) 1973 Code of nursing ethics. ICN, Geneva

Lee R 1996 Resources and professional accountability: the legal perspective. In: Tingle J, Cribb A (eds) Nursing law and ethics. Blackwell Science, Oxford, ch 7, p 130–148

Luker K A, Austin L, Hogg C et al 1997 Evaluation of nurse prescribing: final report and executive summary. University of Liverpool, Liverpool

Lunn J 1994 The scope of professional practice from a legal perspective. British Journal of Nursing 3 (15): 770–772

McHale J 1996 Consent and the adult patient. In: Tingle J, Cribb A (eds) Nursing law and ethics. Blackwell Science, Oxford, ch 6, p 100–117

Orr J 1995 In: Hunt G (ed) Whistleblowing in the health service: accountability, law and professional practice. Edward Arnold, London, ch 4, p 50–63

Pyne R 1992 Accountability in principle and in practice. British Journal of Nursing 1(6): 301–305

Pyne R 1994 Empowerment through the use of the code of professional conduct. British Journal of Nursing 3(12): 631–634

Pyne R 1996 In: Tingle J, Cribb A (eds) Nursing law and ethics. Blackwell Science, Oxford, ch 3, p 36–58

Royal College of Nursing 1978 The duties and position of the nurse. RCN, London

Royal College of Nursing/British Medical Association 1993 Intravenous drug therapy: a statement. RCN/BMA, London

Royal College of Nursing 1999 Guidance for nurses giving intravenous therapy. Johnson & Johnson Medical, London

Rumbold G 1993 Ethics in nursing practice, 2nd edn. Baillière Tindall, London

Sims L L 1967 Creating an educational climate for nursing practice. In: National League of Nursing in service education in public health nursing. The League, New York

Thompson I E, Melia K M, Boyd K M 1988 Nursing ethics. Churchill Livingstone, Edinburgh

Thompson I E, Melia K M, Boyd K M 1994 Nursing ethics, 3rd edn. Churchill Livingstone, Edinburgh

Tingle 1995 The legal accountability of the nurse. In: Watson R (ed) Accountability in nursing practice. Chapman and Hall, London, ch 10, p 163–177

Tingle J, Cribb A 1996 Nursing law and ethics. Blackwell Science, Oxford

Tschudin V 1992 Ethics in nursing, 2nd edn. Butterworth-Heinemann, Oxford

United Kingdom Central Council for Nursing, Midwifery and Health Visiting 1989 Exercising accountability. UKCC, London

United Kingdom Central Council for Nursing, Midwifery and Health Visiting 1991 Community education and practice report. UKCC, London

United Kingdom Central Council for Nursing, Midwifery and Health Visiting 1992a Code of professional conduct. UKCC, London

United Kingdom Central Council for Nursing, Midwifery and Health Visiting 1992b Standards for the administration of medicines. UKCC, London

United Kingdom Central Council for Nursing, Midwifery and Health Visiting 1992c The scope of professional practice. UKCC, London

United Kingdom Central Council for Nursing, Midwifery and Health Visiting 1993 Standards for records and record keeping. UKCC, London

United Kingdom Central Council for Nursing, Midwifery and Health Visiting 1996 Guidelines for professional practice. UKCC, London

Watson R 1992 Justifying your practice. Nursing 5(3): 11–13

Watson R 1995 Accountability in nursing practice. Chapman and Hall, London

Young A 1991 Law and professional conduct in nursing. Scutari, London

Young A 1996 In: Tingle J, Cribb A (eds) Nursing law and ethics. Blackwell Science, Oxford, ch 1, p 3–20

Anatomy and physiology related to intravenous therapy

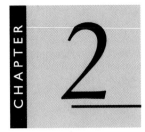

Katie Scales

INTRODUCTION

The circulation is a collective term used to describe movement of blood around the body by the heart and blood vessels.

The purpose of this chapter is to discuss the structure and function of the components that comprise the circulation, and some of the mechanisms which control blood flow. Physiology that underpins the practice of intravenous (i.v.) therapy will be explained and made relevant to clinical practice. The information is presented in an integrated manner, i.e. anatomy and physiology are combined to produce a more cohesive explanation of this complex science.

THE HEART

The heart is a hollow muscular organ lying slightly left of the midline within the thorax. The superior surface (where the vessels enter the heart) is called the base and is wider than the inferior surface, which is called the apex. The heart provides the force for the propulsion of blood through the arterial and capillary system and for its return through the venous system.

The heart is, in essence, a single organ containing two pumps that complement each other. The pump on the right side of the heart pumps blood through the lungs (the pulmonary circulation), while the pump on the left side pumps blood to all other parts of the body (the systemic circulation). Blood flow through the heart is unidirectional and the flow control is achieved by a series of valves that, in a healthy person, only allow blood to flow in a forward direction (Fig. 2.1).

From Figure 2.1, it can be seen that two major veins, the superior and inferior vena cava (SVC, IVC), enter the right atrium. These vessels contain the systemic venous return, i.e. the SVC conveys venous blood from the head, neck, arms and upper thorax, while the IVC conveys blood from the rest of the thorax, the abdomen and the lower limbs.

Venous return to the heart is passive and relies on negative pressure in the thorax to attract blood back to the heart, as well as local muscle activity in the limbs. Because there are no valves separating the SVC and IVC from the right atrium, the pressure is the same in the SVC/IVC as it is in the right atrium. When measuring central venous pressure, catheters are usually located in the subclavian vein or SVC. Mortality is increased when catheters are placed in the heart itself. Some catheters are designed for cardiac placement, e.g. pulmonary artery catheters.

Blood flows from the right atrium down into the right ventricle; it is then pumped into the pulmonary artery and pulmonary capillaries for gas exchange. Venous return from the lungs delivers oxygenated blood to the left atrium, and blood flows down into the left ventricle and is pumped out into the aorta for systemic distribution.

Fig. 2.1 The heart in vertical cross-section with blood flow indicated by arrows. (Reproduced with kind permission from Wilson & Waugh 1996.)

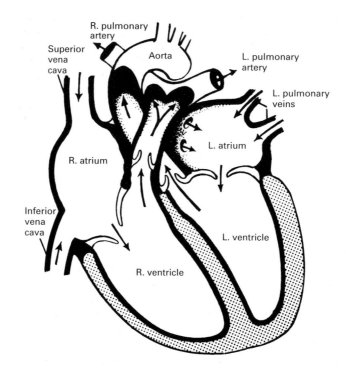

Closer inspection of the structure of the ventricle reveals finger-like projections of muscle arising from the apex of each ventricle; these are called papillary muscles. From the top of the papillary muscle, tendon-like cords connect with the cusps of the atrioventricular valves. These structures provide stability for the atrioventricular valves that might otherwise prolapse from the force of the ventricular contraction. There are reported cases of pulmonary artery catheters becoming entangled in these anatomical structures. This is often only discovered when the catheter fails to be removed by simple, gentle traction. Force should not be used as this will result in rupture of the structures within the ventricle. The management of an entangled pulmonary artery catheter is not easy and cardiac surgery to visually remove the device is not uncommon.

The rhythmical contraction and relaxation of the heart is termed the cardiac cycle, consisting of two phases: systole, when the heart contracts, and diastole, when the heart relaxes. Because of the systolic and diastolic activity of the heart, the cardiac output is intermittent, a pulsatile rather than a continuous flow. When the left ventricle contracts, it ejects its volume into the aorta. The resting arterial pressure of the aorta creates a resistance to ejection, which is termed afterload. The volume of blood returning to the heart to fill the ventricles is termed preload. Preload is affected by overall blood volume and the resting tone of the blood vessels. If peripheral vessels become excessively dilated, blood will begin to pool in the periphery, reducing venous return to the heart. The converse is also true: peripheral constriction inhibits pooling and increases venous return. Preload and afterload can both be controlled using vasodilating or vasoconstricting drugs. These drugs require haemodynamic monitoring and are usually restricted to critical care areas.

Serum levels

Correct serum levels of sodium, potassium and calcium are required for normal function of the heart. Too high a calcium level causes the heart to stop in systole, and too high a potassium level causes the heart to stop in diastole (Green 1985). This is of practical importance when undertaking intravenous therapy. If concentrated solutions containing potassium or calcium are infused rapidly via a central venous catheter directly into the heart, it is possible to cause cardiac arrest (Green 1985). This situation can occur unintentionally during the transfusion of cold, stored blood. When blood is cooled and stored, potassium leaches out of the red blood cells, causing a significant elevation in the serum potassium concentration. If this is transfused rapidly via a central venous catheter, asystole can be induced.

BLOOD VESSEL STRUCTURE

All blood vessels (with the exception of the capillary) have a similar construction. There are three layers to the vessel wall and the differences are determined by the location and function of each vessel.

The internal layer (tunica intima)

This is a layer of endothelium, a smooth layer of flattened pavement cells, arranged longitudinally along the vessel. The tunica intima also includes subendothelial connective tissue (Woodburne & Burkel 1994). Endothelium facilitates blood flow along the vessel, preventing the adhesion of blood cells to the vessel wall. Any trauma which roughens the lining encourages platelets to adhere to the vessel wall and may result in thrombus formation (Weinstein 1997) and the inflammatory process of phlebitis (Hadaway 1995). Endothelial cells can easily be damaged (Box 2.1).

The middle layer (tunica media)

This layer is composed of elastic tissue and smooth muscle fibres. The amount of smooth muscle found in the tunica media varies between vessels. The quantity and arrangement of smooth muscle fibres in arteries provide a relatively rigid structure. By comparison, veins have less smooth muscle and elastic tissue, and as a result are

---

■ BOX 2.1

Factors which may result in damage to endothelial cells

- Rapid advancement of a cannula
- Poor technique when advancing a cannula, i.e. not maintaining adequate traction on skin and vein
- Using a cannula which is too large for the lumen of the vein
- Using a cannula which remains relatively rigid after insertion
- Siting a cannula near to areas of flexion such as over joints
- Inadequate taping, which may result in movement of the cannula
- Poor skin preparation and incorrect use of dressings, which can lead to contamination of the site
- Infusion of any of the following irritant solutions
    — hypertonic
    — hypotonic
    — very low or high pH
- Infusion of particulate matter
- Rapid infusions of large quantities of fluid which may be too great for the vessel to accommodate

more prone to collapse if venous pressure is low (Green 1985). This layer is sensitive to changes in temperature, and mechanical or chemical irritation can cause spasm of the vessel. In veins, this can impede blood flow, resulting in pain which can often be relieved by heat. Arterial spasm from chemical irritation may have serious consequences; the artery can become damaged, leading to ischaemia, and this may cause necrosis and gangrene (Weinstein 1997).

Smooth muscle may also undergo what is called the stress relaxation phenomenon (Hadaway 1995). When a tourniquet is placed on the limb to aid distension of the peripheral veins, the muscle fibres elongate to accommodate the increased volume of blood in the veins. The pressure increases and then falls back to normal in spite of the increased volume. If the tourniquet is then removed, the volume and pressure suddenly fall, and within several minutes normal pressure is re-established. This can be helpful for deciding the length of time that a tourniquet is left in place, particularly when advancing long cannulae into veins, as obstruction may be encountered if not enough time has been left for the vein to return to normal (Hadaway 1995).

Smooth muscles can also react to excessive stretching. The muscles contract to resist the stretch; this is illustrated when a tourniquet has been left in place for a long period of time and the veins can no longer be palpated (Hadaway 1995).

The outer layer (tunica adventitia)

This layer is composed of connective tissue, collagen and nerve fibres. It surrounds and supports the vessel. The nerve fibres are mainly fibres of the sympathetic nervous system. Nerve impulses keep the vessel in a state of tonus – an increase in the rate of impulses will cause the vessel to constrict further, while a decrease will cause it to relax more. The amount of fibrous tissue varies between vessels. As a generalization, this layer is thicker in arteries than in veins; however, the vena cava and aorta have similar quantities.

DYNAMICS OF BLOOD FLOW

The movement of a fluid through a tube can occur in a turbulent or streamlined manner; the streamlined movement of a fluid is termed laminar flow. Blood flow around the circulation, in a healthy person, is considered to be laminar, i.e. non-turbulent flow that demonstrates a spearhead appearance when analysed. The blood in the centre of the vessel (around the axis of the vessel) travels faster than the blood which is in contact with the walls of the vessel. Friction forces cause the layer of blood in contact with the vessel wall to slow down; indeed, the velocity (speed) of blood in contact with the vessel is measured at zero (Berne & Levy 1993), while the blood in the centre of the vessel moves the fastest (Fig. 2.2). More pressure is required to move a turbulent fluid than is required to move a fluid whose flow is laminar.

In turbulent flow, the elements of the fluid move in all directions, flowing crosswise and lengthwise along the vessel (Hadaway 1995). This type of flow can occur when the inner surface of a vessel becomes roughened; if the diameter of a vessel changes abruptly (i.e. obstruction); or if the flow is greatly increased. In health, turbulent flow is only seen in the sinuses of Valsalva in the aorta and pulmonary artery. The sinuses of Valsalva are small outpocketings in the walls of the aorta and pulmonary artery adjacent to the aortic and pulmonary valves (Berne & Levy 1993).

Turbulence is usually accompanied by audible vibrations. Flow through diseased heart valves can be heard and is called a murmur. Profound anaemia causes a significant increase in cardiac output and a reduction in the viscosity of the blood; this can also produce audible turbulence. Turbulent flow can predispose patients to thrombus formation (Berne & Levy 1993).

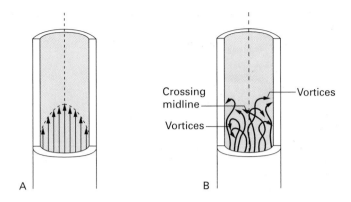

Fig. 2.2 A. Laminar blood flow. **B.** Turbulent blood flow.

Crossing midline

Vortices

Vortices

A

B

For the body tissues to survive, there must be adequate blood flow within the circulation. In order to maintain adequate flow, there must be an adequate head of pressure within the vessels that supply the tissues. Blood is like any other fluid – the only reason it will move from A to B is if the pressure at A is greater than the pressure at B (Green 1985). From the perspective of blood flow around the circulation, pressure in the aorta must be greater than the pressure in the right atrium if blood is to flow through the tissues and return to the heart.

The tone of the venous system is the most influential feature of venous return, because of the capacity that the venous system can hold. The average 70 kg man has 5 L of blood in circulation (Green 1994). At any given time, 1 L will be found in the pulmonary circulation, 1 L in the heart and arteries, and 3 L in the venous system (Green 1985). The veins are described as 'capacitance vessels' because of their ability to distend and accommodate greater volume (Berne & Levy 1993). In comparison, the arterial system has far less ability to change its capacity. The blood from the ventricles is ejected into the arterial system and it is arterial pressure that the ventricle has to overcome to eject the stroke volume. The arteries are therefore described as resistance vessels, because they produce resistance to blood flow (Berne & Levy 1993).

Despite cardiac output being intermittent (pulsatile), peripheral blood flow is continuous. This is due to aortic distension during ventricular contraction and elastic recoil of the aortic wall causing forward propulsion of blood during ventricular relaxation (Berne & Levy 1993). This is mainly due to the kinetic nature of the aorta. As blood is ejected from the left ventricle into the aorta, the aortic wall is stretched by the impact of the blood flow. As the heart enters the diastolic phase, the pressure wave in the aorta moves forwards down the artery. The aortic wall then recoils as the pressure lessens, and the volume of blood which is displaced by that recoil maintains the arterial diastolic pressure and ensures a continuous flow to the periphery even during the diastolic phase of the heart (Berne & Levy 1993; Fig. 2.3).

This ability of the aortic wall to distend and recoil is termed compliance. Compliance deteriorates with age and with diseases that reduce the elasticity of the aorta, e.g. atherosclerosis and calcification. As compliance reduces, systolic pressure rises because the pressure is not being absorbed by the wall of the aorta. At the same time, diastolic pressure appears to become lower because there is no recoil phase to maintain the flow during diastole. Hence the pulse pressure (the difference between systolic and diastolic blood pressures) appears to become progressively wider in the elderly and in atherosclerotic disease.

The section of the aorta which receives the stroke volume from the left ventricle suffers continual pressure, and the higher the blood pressure, the greater the shearing forces to which it is exposed. Local degeneration of the endothelium can occur,

Fig. 2.3 Distension and recoil of the aorta. (Reproduced with kind permission from Wilson & Waugh 1996.)

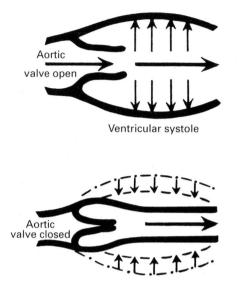

Aortic valve open

Ventricular systole

Aortic valve closed

Ventricular diastole

along with tearing of the arterial wall (Berne & Levy 1993). This is known as a dissecting aneurysm. Aneurysms can dissect upwards, causing dissection of the coronaries and tamponade, or downwards leading to dissection of the renal and hepatic arteries. The condition is potentially life-threatening and is a vascular emergency.

Blood moves rapidly through the aorta and its branches, which become narrower as they progress towards the periphery. The composition of the vessel wall also changes as the arteries become smaller. The aorta is predominantly an elastic structure – the property that facilitates distension and recoil and thus aids blood flow and pressure control. In contrast, small arteries are quite muscular. The pressure in the arteries is usually referred to as blood pressure, while the pressure in the great veins is usually referred to as venous pressure.

THE ARTERIAL SYSTEM

Blood leaves the left side of the heart via the ascending aorta. This is the largest arterial structure of the body, measuring 2.5 cm in diameter with a wall thickness of 2 mm (Berne & Levy 1993). The aorta curves to form an arch which passes behind the heart and descends vertically through the thorax and abdomen (Fig. 2.4). The aortic arch gives rise to three major arteries: the brachiocephalic trunk, the left common carotid artery and the left subclavian artery. The brachiocephalic trunk further divides to form the right subclavian artery and the right common carotid artery (Woodburne & Burkel 1994).

Each subclavian artery arches laterally, passing behind the clavicles and over the superior surface of the first ribs before entering the axilla area where they become known as the axillary arteries. The first part of the artery lies deeply; then it runs more superficially and becomes the brachial artery. The brachial artery runs down the medial aspect of the upper arm and passes to the front of the elbow. About 1 cm below the elbow, the brachial artery divides to form the radial and ulnar arteries (Wilson & Waugh 1996). The radial artery runs along the lateral (thumb side) of the forearm and produces the pulse commonly felt at the wrist, just in front of the radius bone.

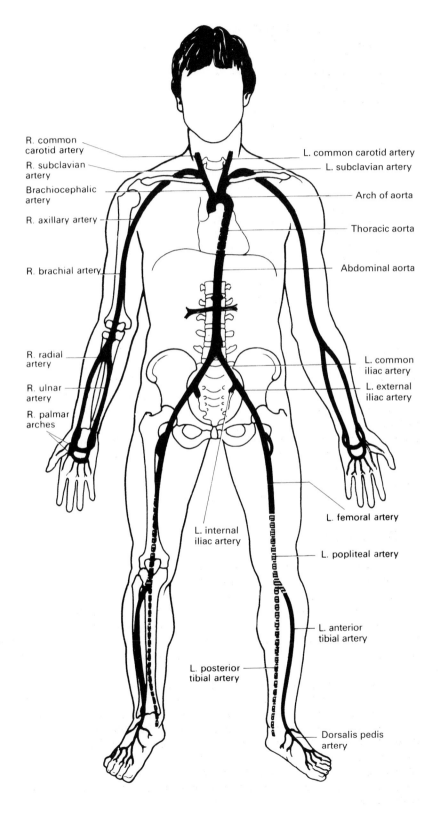

Fig. 2.4 Aorta and the main arteries of the limbs. (Reproduced with kind permission from Wilson & Waugh 1996.)

The ulnar artery runs along the opposite side of the forearm and passes across the palm of the hand. Anastomoses (connections) are found between the radial and ulnar arteries and are called the deep and superficial palmar arches. From these vessels arise the palmar metacarpal and palmar digital arteries which supply the structures of the hand and fingers (Wilson & Waugh 1996).

Because the brachial artery is the only arterial structure supplying the upper limbs, it is considered imprudent to site an intra-arterial device in the brachial artery unless no other access is available. Loss of brachial arterial supply would result in loss of blood flow in the entire limb. Use of a lower artery such as the radial is better practice, as collateral circulation to the lower limb can be provided by the ulnar artery. It is good practice to perform an Allen test prior to cannulating either the radial or the ulnar artery to ensure that collateral circulation exists (Soni 1989).

From the aortic arch, the aorta descends down through the thorax and abdomen, giving off branches to supply the organs and structures which surround it. The aorta bifurcates in the lumbar region to form the common iliac arteries before running down into the thigh where it becomes the femoral artery. The femoral artery continues to descend, running behind the knee where it becomes known as the popliteal artery. The popliteal artery divides just below the knee to form the anterior and posterior tibial arteries. The anterior tibial artery runs over the top of the foot, forming the dorsalis pedis artery, while the posterior tibial runs down the back of the leg and behind the ankle joint continuing along the sole of the foot.

Drug administration

It is rare to administer any drugs into the arterial system. The exception to this is the instillation of thrombolytic agents to thrombosed arteries. The most common occurrence is the direct instillation of streptokinase or a similar agent into the pulmonary artery for the treatment of massive and life-threatening pulmonary embolism. This is usually done via a pulmonary artery catheter.

Drug administration via arteries is contraindicated because it leads to arterial spasm and ischaemia of the distal limb. It most commonly occurs because a cannula has been incorrectly placed or because an arterial cannula has been inadequately labelled. In conscious patients, arterial drug administration can cause severe pain (but not always). In the unconscious patient, blanching of the limb is seen and there can be continued discoloration distal to the injection site (Soni 1989). This is a vascular emergency and a physician must be called to treat the situation as quickly as possible.

CAPILLARIES

As arterioles diverge into capillary structures, precapillary sphincters occur. Proportionally these structures have the most smooth muscle fibre of any vessel. This is the part of the vascular system that generates peripheral resistance. A single arteriole can divide into several capillaries, producing a rapid drop in pressure. As a result, flow through capillaries is continuous rather than pulsatile.

The capillary is responsible for blood flow to the cells and for nutrient and gas exchange. Capillary flow is sometimes termed nutritional flow (Berne & Levy 1993). The more highly active the tissue structure, the more extensive is the capillary network, e.g. cardiac and skeletal muscle have a higher capillary density than subcutaneous tissue or cartilage. Not all capillaries are the same diameter; in fact, some are smaller than the diameter of a red blood cell. The red cell is obliged to manipulate its shape to facilitate passage through the capillary (Berne & Levy 1993).

Capillaries are thin-walled vessels composed of a single layer of endothelial cells. The thin capillary walls allow the passage of nutrients and oxygen out of the blood and, in exchange, take up waste products of cell metabolism. Permeability of the capillary wall varies between tissue structures (capillaries of the gut and liver are more permeable than those of a skeletal muscle); it also varies along the length of the capillary (the venous end is more permeable than the arterial end). Capillary permeability can be altered by certain chemicals, e.g. histamine.

THE VENOUS SYSTEM

Veins convey the blood from the capillary bed back to the heart. Usually they are larger in diameter and thinner walled than their corresponding arteries. There are usually more veins than arteries, because the blood is travelling slower than it does in the arteries (Woodburne & Burkel 1994).

As the venous ends of the capillaries converge to form venules, the diameter of the vessels progressively increases. The cross-sectional area of a vein at low-to-moderate venous pressure is elliptical. Veins which are distended and under higher venous pressure demonstrate a more rounded cross-section (Green 1985; Fig. 2.5).

As the venules converge to form veins, the diameter of the vessels continues to increase. As the vessel diameter increases, the pressure continues to fall. Between the capillary and the right atrium, the venous pressure falls from 12 to 0 mmHg. The pressure of blood entering the right side of the heart is usually the same as atmospheric pressure (Green 1985).

When pressure is very low over long distances, there is little incentive for the blood to return to the heart. The venous return is assisted by two main mechanisms: negative pressure within the thorax and muscular activity in the limbs.

Fig. 2.5 Change in cross-sectional area of vein with increase in venous pressure.

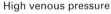

Low venous pressure High venous pressure

Valves

One feature of veins, not seen in the arterial system, is the presence of valves. A valve is a fold of the tunica intima, strengthened by connective tissue. Valves in veins are bicuspid and the cusps are crescentic in shape. The occurrence of valves is more plentiful in the veins of the limbs than in any other part of the venous system. Valves are sparse in the veins of the abdomen, thorax and neck (Woodburne & Burkel 1994). The head and neck have the advantage of gravity to assist the return of blood to the heart. Valves help to support the column of blood above the valve; the more frequent the valve, the smaller the column of blood it must support. This assists blood flow back to the heart and prevents pooling of blood in vessels most affected by gravity.

In a healthy person, the valves only allow blood flow in one direction and are effective in preventing venous distension from gravity. Blood in the saphenous vein, for example, is at a low pressure and a long way from the heart. Gravity is exerted on the vessel and its contents. Without skeletal muscle activity and the presence of valves, blood would pool in the periphery, veins would distend, and venous return would be reduced.

As an individual moves their limbs, the skeletal muscle contracts and relaxes. As the skeletal muscle contracts, it compresses the vein next to it and causes the blood in the vessel to be displaced. The valve below the muscle prevents the blood from

Fig. 2.6 Flow of blood through a vein aided by the contraction of skeletal muscle. (Reproduced with kind permission from Wilson & Waugh 1996.)

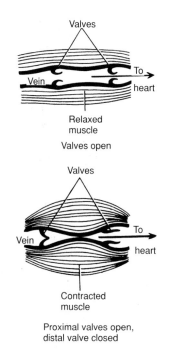

being displaced downwards; the valve above the muscle is forced open and the blood moves upwards into the next valve compartment (Fig. 2.6). As in the heart, blood flow through the valves is unidirectional in the healthy individual. When a person suffers from varicose veins, the veins have usually become distended, often due to persistently raised venous pressure, e.g. caused by pregnancy, obesity, hepatic or right heart failure. As the vessel diameter increases, the valve cusps no longer close correctly, the valves are rendered incompetent and blood flow ceases to be unidirectional. Individuals are at increased risk of venous thrombosis from stasis of blood in these distended veins.

Knowledge of the presence of valves in the hand and arm veins is important when considering cannulation or venepuncture.

Venous return

From the lower limbs

The lower limbs contain both deep and superficial veins. Communicating veins connect the superficial to the deep veins (Wilson & Waugh 1996). The deep veins run the same course as the arteries of the leg and have the same names.

There are two main superficial veins of the leg – the saphenous veins. The small saphenous vein begins at the ankle where the small veins which drain the top of the foot converge. It runs superficially up the back of the leg and enters the popliteal space where it joins the deep popliteal vein. The great popliteal vein begins on the inner aspect of the top of the foot and runs upwards along the inner aspect of the thigh. It joins the deep femoral vein just below the inguinal ligament (Fig. 2.7).

As the femoral vein reaches the level of the inguinal ligament, it becomes known as the external iliac vein and lies medially to the femoral artery. The femoral nerve lies lateral to the artery.

At the level of the sacroiliac joint, the external iliac vein is joined by the internal

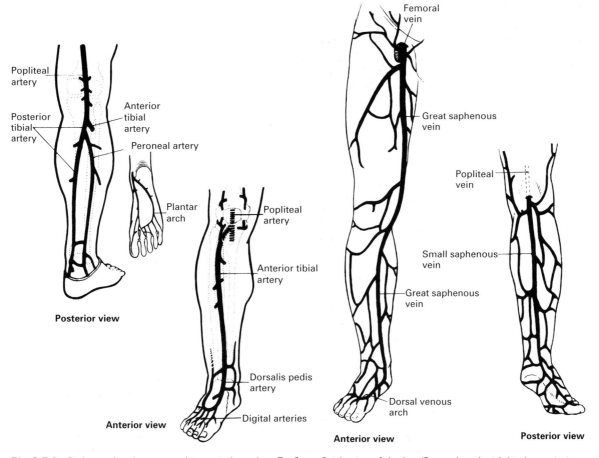

Fig. 2.7 A. Right popliteal artery and its main branches. **B**. Superficial veins of the leg. (Reproduced with kind permission from Wilson & Waugh 1996.)

iliac vein and forms the common iliac vein. The right and the left common iliac veins combine to form the inferior vena cava (Wilson & Waugh 1996; Fig. 2.8).

As small veins converge to form larger veins, the blood flow within the vessel increases. By the time the blood reaches the SVC or IVC, it will have a flow rate of approximately 2–3 L/min. (The circulation flows at 5 L/min and there are only two vessels entering the left side of the heart.)

The blood flow within the vessel is an important factor when selecting the vascular access for a patient. If the access is for an infrequent non-irritant drug then a vessel with a low blood flow in the periphery is quite appropriate. If the access is for parenteral nutrition (PN) or other irritant solutions, the access must be into a central vein with a high blood flow to ensure that the irritants are diluted and distributed rapidly before they can injure the vein.

From the upper limbs

Like the veins of the leg, arm veins are classified as deep or superficial. Deep veins follow the course of the major arteries, drain the areas supplied by the arteries and have similar names (Woodburne & Burkel 1994). The fingers are drained by the digital veins; these converge to form the dorsal metacarpal veins which end in the dor-

Fig. 2.8 Venae cavae and the main veins of the limbs. (Reproduced with kind permission from Wilson & Waugh 1996.)

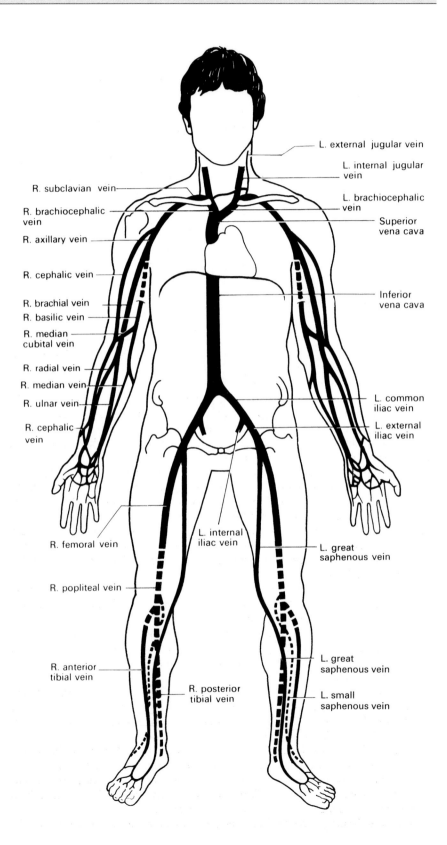

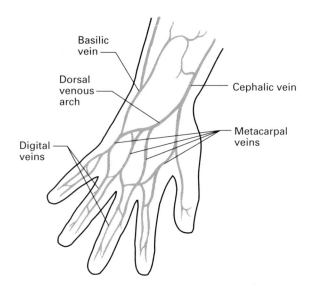

Fig. 2.9 Superficial veins of the dorsal aspect of the hand.

Basilic vein

Dorsal venous arch

Cephalic vein

Digital veins

Metacarpal veins

sal venous arch, a relatively prominent structure on the back of the hand (Woodburne & Burkel 1994).

The radial end of the dorsal venous arch continues to form the cephalic vein, also fed by the dorsal veins of the thumb, and ascends up the radial side of the wrist (Woodburne & Burkel 1994). The accessory cephalic vein emerges either from the dorsum of the forearm or from the ulnar end of the dorsal venous arch. It ascends diagonally across the dorsum of the forearm and joins the cephalic vein in the region of the elbow (Woodburne & Burkel 1994).

The ulnar end of the dorsal venous arch continues to form the basilic vein; it continues along the ulnar side of the forearm, being fed by tributaries from both the anterior and posterior surfaces of the forearm (Woodburne & Burkel 1994; Fig. 2.9).

The median cubital vein, a large branch of the cephalic vein, runs diagonally across the anterior aspect of the elbow, connecting the cephalic and basilic veins. The median cubital vein is only present in 70% of the population (Woodburne & Burkel 1994). All these veins are superficial, generally palpable and usually visible when the arm is inspected.

As the cephalic vein leaves the cubital fossa, it runs upward and turns inward, piercing the brachial fascia. It continues along the upper arm, finally emptying into the axillary vein (Woodburne & Burkel 1994).

Having been joined by the median cubital vein, the basilic vein continues upward and turns inward, piercing the brachial fascia midway between the elbow and the shoulder. At the level of the axilla, it joins with the brachial veins to form the axillary vein (Fig. 2.10).

The median antebrachial vein lies in the middle of the anterior forearm, beginning in the palmar venous arch and terminating in either the median cubital or basilic vein. The median cubital vein also connects with the deep veins in the cubital fossa (Woodburne & Burkel 1994).

The brachial veins are the deep veins of the arm. They run parallel to the arterial structures and are paired veins. The basilic vein joins with the brachial veins to form the distal part of the axillary vein. The cephalic vein empties into the proximal portion of the axillary vein. As the axillary vein ascends and passes over the first rib, it becomes the subclavian vein (Woodburne & Burkel 1994).

The venous drainage from the head and neck is via the internal jugular veins. The

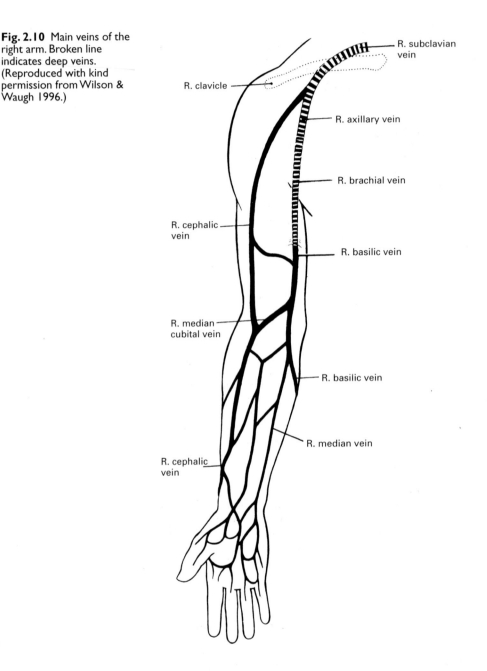

Fig. 2.10 Main veins of the right arm. Broken line indicates deep veins. (Reproduced with kind permission from Wilson & Waugh 1996.)

R. subclavian vein

R. clavicle

R. axillary vein

R. brachial vein

R. cephalic vein

R. basilic vein

R. median cubital vein

R. basilic vein

R. median vein

R. cephalic vein

internal jugular and subclavian veins merge to the brachiocephalic vein, and the right and left brachiocephalic veins merge to form the superior vena cava.

Veins are the routine source of vascular access for parenteral drug and fluid administration, and the locations of important veins for this purpose (as well as advantages and disadvantages of using them) are shown in Table 2.1.

Arrangement of the vasculature

Arteries and veins usually run in parallel to each other in the limbs. Core body temperature is 37°C and peripheral temperature is usually the same as the environment. If cold blood from the peripheries were to return to the heart, it could cause a fatal dysrhythmia. By veins being in parallel with the arteries, heat from the artery can pass across to the vein. Thus the venous blood warms up as it returns to the heart and arterial blood gradually cools as it flows out towards the periphery. This process is known as 'counter-current heat transfer' (Green 1985).

If blood is to be involved in temperature control, it has to flow close to the skin so that the heat can be radiated into the environment. Subcutaneous tissue, by

Table 2.1 Important veins for vascular access

Location	Advantages	Disadvantages
Peripheral veins of upper limb Dorsal venous network of the hand:		
● Digital veins	Last resort for fluid	Small
● Metacarpal veins	Well adapted for i.v. use Bones of hand provide a natural splint Enables successive venepuncture/cannulation sites above previous puncture site	May be fragile or poorly supported in elderly Restricts the use of the hand Extravasation of blood may readily occur May be more painful
Radial and ulnar veins	Very superficial	Nerves close to surface of skin make this a more painful area, especially at the inner aspect of the wrist
Cephalic vein	Large vein	Movement at the wrist may cause discomfort and restrict movement
Accessory cephalic	Easy to visualize, stabilize and palpate Excellent for transfusion administration Position makes it a natural splint	May be obscured by tendons controlling thumb
Basilic	Large vein Found by flexing the elbow and bending the arm Best route for midline and PICC insertion as straightest route to central veins	Often overlooked Site may make it more awkward to assess and observe Tends to have more valves, making advancement of cannula difficult May only be able to palpate a small segment Haematomas form easily on removal of devices
Peripheral veins of lower limb Dorsal venous network of foot	Easily accessible	More difficult to palpate Increased risk of complications due to impaired circulation prone to DVT Difficult to stabilize Restricts ability to walk
Medial and lateral marginal veins of the foot	Larger veins Easy to palpate and visualize	Increased risk of complications due to impaired circulation prone to DVT Difficult to stabilize Restricts ability to walk

Table 2.1 *(cont'd)*

Location	Advantages	Disadvantages
Central veins Subclavian Infraclavicular	Easily accessible Easier to maintain dressing (flatter surface) Preferred in children	May require a longer needle for insertion Associated with a number of complications such as pneumothorax, brachial nerve plexus damage, haemothorax, etc.
Supraclavicular	Short distance from skin to vein, therefore easily accessible	Dressing may be more difficult in hollow above clavicle Associated with a number of complications such as pneumothorax, brachial nerve plexus injury, haemothorax, etc.
Jugular	Associated with fewer complications than subclavian larger vein	Difficult to dress due to movement of neck and beard growth on male patients
Internal External	Easily accessible Superficial vein Usually visible and easy to palpate	May result in damage to carotid arteries Tip location in SVC not always as successful as internal
Femoral	Alternative site in emergency Tip location in IVC	Dressings difficult to maintain and associated with high infection risk, thrombosis

definition, lies under the skin and can sometimes obscure the visibility of veins. This may well contribute to poor temperature regulation in obese people as the superficial nature of veins is lost and the subcutaneous tissue becomes an insulation through which radiation of heat becomes progressively more difficult.

REGULATION OF THE VASCULAR SYSTEM

There are two key control mechanisms for the peripheral circulation – control by the nervous system and local control influenced by the tissues around the vessels. In the skin and splanchnic regions, nervous control is dominant, whereas in the heart and brain, environmental conditions are more influential (Berne & Levy 1993). Local control, known as autoregulation, is achieved by chemicals and levels of oxygen and carbon dioxide.

The arterioles are mainly responsible for regulating blood flow throughout the body. Smooth muscle fibres make up a large proportion of the vessel structure. The vessel lumen can be varied from complete occlusion to maximum dilation (Berne & Levy 1993). The vessel usually rests in a state of partial tone, i.e. it is neither fully relaxed nor fully contracted. It is therefore able to move in either direction in response to a stimulus.

Most of the body's arteries and veins are supplied solely by the fibres of the sympathetic nervous system (Berne & Levy 1993). Different vessels have different amounts of sympathetic supply. It is the sympathetic activity that maintains the resting tone of the blood vessel. Changes in sympathetic activity cause changes in vascular tone. Increased sympathetic stimulation of a blood vessel causes contraction, whilst decreased stimulation causes relaxation (Berne & Levy 1993). The alteration in lumen size creates a change in flow (or resistance). This mechanism is most highly active in the arteriole. A few vessels, mainly limited to the viscera and pelvic organs, have parasympathetic innervation. Increased parasympathetic activity in these regions causes relaxation of the blood vessels (Berne & Levy 1993).

The regulation of vascular tone by the sympathetic nervous system is termed 'vasomotor' control. This means that the vasomotor centre (VMC) of the brain is sending instructions to the blood vessels. This is done in response to information received by the brain about the state of the blood pressure, the cardiac output, the venous return, body temperature and stress stimuli (Green 1985).

One of the most important mechanisms for control of vascular tone is the baroreceptor mechanism. This is a rapid mechanism which quickly restores blood pressure, and is utilized, for example, when an individual decides to move from a lying to a standing position.

Baroreceptors are nerve endings which are stimulated by the degree of stretch of the blood vessel. High blood pressure causes significant stretch (distortion) of the vessel wall, and low blood pressure reduces the stretch (Berne & Levy 1993). The baroreceptors that influence the systemic circulation are located in the carotid sinuses and the aortic arch. The carotid sinus is the area of bifurcation of the common carotid artery (Berne & Levy 1993).

The baroreceptors send signals to the VMC, conveying information about arterial blood pressure. When arterial blood pressure is high, frequent impulses are sent to the VMC. The response of the VMC is to reduce the amount of sympathetic stimulation of the capacitance vessels (peripheral blood vessels), thus forcing peripheral pooling of blood to occur. At the same time, fewer signals are sent to the sinoatrial node and the heart rate subsequently slows. This has the effect of reducing venous return and cardiac output; blood pressure will subsequently be reduced. The opposite is also true. Low blood pressure reduces stimulation of the baroreceptors; they in turn send fewer impulses to the VMC. This is interpreted as low blood pressure and sympathetic stimulation of the blood vessels is increased, causing venoconstriction. This increases the venous return to the heart and, in conjunction with increased heart rate, brings about an increase in blood pressure.

This mechanism is invoked when physicians apply carotid sinus massage to the neck to aid diagnosis of tachycardias. Slowing the heart rate makes the complexes easier to diagnose.

Care must be taken when removing central venous catheters (CVA) from the internal jugular site because of its close proximity to the carotid artery. In sensitive patients, when pressure is applied to the puncture site, the carotid sinus can be unintentionally stimulated and the vasomotor centre will respond by slowing the heart rate and creating venodilation. The more continued the pressure, the slower the heart rate will become. This unfortunate side-effect of CVC removal is easier to notice in a monitored patient; the unmonitored patient may present with fainting (Berne & Levy 1993). Reducing the pressure on the neck will restore both the heart rate and blood pressure. Green (1985) reports that the mechanism can be evoked by wearing a tight shirt collar.

COMPOSITION AND FUNCTION OF BLOOD

Blood is a complex liquid which performs a number of essential functions:

- Transport
  — oxygen from the lungs to the tissues
  — carbon dioxide from the tissues to the lungs
  — nutrients from the gut to the tissues
  — wastes from the tissues to the liver and kidneys
  — hormones from their site of production to their target tissues.
- Homeostasis
  — regulation of blood pH by the use of buffers and proteins
  — regulation of body temperature by the distribution of heat
  — regulation of the composition and volume of the interstitial fluid compartment
  — control of blood loss by haemostatic mechanisms
  — immunity and control of infection.

Blood contains various chemicals in solution and a variety of cells in suspension (Table 2.2). The fluid component is termed plasma and makes up about 55% of the blood volume; blood cells make up the remaining 45% (Green 1985).

Blood is a viscous fluid. Viscosity is measured in relation to water, which is said to have a viscosity of 1.0. The viscosity of blood ranges from 4.5 to 5.5 (Tortora 1986). Viscosity relates to thickness and adhesiveness of a liquid. Blood feels 'sticky' or adhesive when touched, and is heavier than water when the same volumes are compared. Viscosity is an important feature of blood and heart function, and is affected by the haematocrit (percentage of cells in the blood) and plasma proteins. Many factors can influence viscosity, for example alteration in the concentration of cells, abnormalities of the red blood cell, hydrational state and nutritional imbalance. Vessel diameter also influences apparent viscosity.

Blood is usually 8% of total body weight. On average, women have 4–5 L of blood, while men have 5–6 L. This reflects the differences in physical size between men and women (Green 1985). If blood volume is taken to be 5 L, then 3 L of that volume is plasma. There are many dissolved substances in plasma, including proteins, electrolytes, vitamins, lipids, hormones, nitrogenous wastes and gases. The concentration of each of these will depend upon health, metabolic activity and diet (Berne & Levy 1993).

HAEMOSTASIS

The term haemostasis means the prevention of blood loss (Guyton 1986). Maintaining haemostasis is to balance the agents that cause blood to clot and the agents that inhibit the clotting of blood. For preservation of the human organism, any holes in the circulation must be quickly plugged, but the plug must not be so great as to obstruct the flow of blood along the vessel.

If a vessel is severed, the initial reaction is one of vascular spasm, partly from nervous reflexes and partly from spasm of the injured muscle in the vessel wall (Tortora 1986). The next phase in haemostasis is the formation of a platelet plug. When circulating platelets come into contact with the damaged surface of a blood vessel, they immediately undergo change. They change their shape by swelling and developing projections on their cell surfaces. Their surface becomes adhesive and they stick to the collagen fibres in the exposed wall of the blood vessel. The activated platelets release adenosine diphosphate (ADP) and an enzyme called thromboxane A into the blood (Guyton 1986). These agents act on nearby platelets and activate them too. This continues and a platelet plug is formed.

If the vascular damage is small, a platelet plug may suffice to prevent blood loss. If the damage is more significant then thrombus formation will be required to achieve haemostasis. Platelet plugs are constantly being manufactured to repair

Table 2.2 Cells present in blood

Name of cell	Type of cell	Produced by	Life span	Normal range	Function
Red blood cells (erythrocytes)	Aneuclear cell, i.e. no nucleus and no genetic material for reproduction	Bone marrow	120 days (Green 1985)	A normal haemoglobin level is 15 g/dl in men and 13.5 g/dl in women (Berne & Levy 1993)	Tissue oxygenation Raised Hb increases viscosity and impedes blood flow Neutrophils migrate to sites of tissue injury in response to chemical signals from other cells (chemotactic) 'phagocytic' behaviour, i.e. they ingest and destroy foreign material
White blood cells (leucocytes)	Neutrophils, eosinophils, basophils (granulocytes due to granular nature of their cytoplasm)	Bone marrow	4–5 days	A normal white cell count is 4000–10 000 cells/μl	Eosinophils travel rapidly to site of tissue injury (within 30 min) and appear to survive for weeks – phagocytic and chemotactic. Basophils are mobile phagocytic cells which can produce an anaphylactic response
	Monocytes	Mature in 24–48 hours and migrate to the liver, spleen and lymph nodes; remain for months or years – macrophages produced in the bone marrow, but T-lymphocytes mature in the thymus gland			Monocytes are the largest, mobile phagocytic cells capable of replication and have multiple functions – active in immune response
	Lymphocytes				Lymphocytes are non-granular cells – two main subgroups are the B- and T-lymphocytes. B-lymphocytes have immunoglobulins on their cell surfaces and can secrete specific immunoglobulin antibodies. There are several types of T-cell: (1) the helper cell which assists B-lymphocytes to produce antibodies; (2) the suppressor cell which inhibits B-lymphocytes from producing antibodies; (3) cytotoxic T-cells which cause cell destruction of identified antigens; (4) null cells which appear to be neither B- nor T-lymphocytes by characteristic; and (5) the natural killer cells which appear capable of destroying tumour cells, virus-infected cells or cells coated with antibody
Platelets	Aneuclear	Fragments of megakaryocyte cell in the bone marrow			Involved in clotting process

minor wear and tear of blood vessels. Individuals with a low platelet count are unable to perform this vital task and subsequently develop hundreds of minor haemorrhagic areas which are visible on the skin. These haemorrhages will also be occurring in the internal tissues and organs. This classic haemorrhagic picture is called a petechial rash.

Thrombus formation involves the manufacture of a blood clot. The rapidity of clot formation depends on the severity of the vascular injury. Clot formation is slower in minor injury than in major injury (Guyton 1986). In order to manufacture a thrombus, prothrombin must be converted to thrombin and fibrinogen must be converted to fibrin. The conversion of prothrombin can be achieved by both intrinsic and extrinsic pathways, and the formation of thrombin acts as a trigger for the conversion of fibrinogen. Calcium is needed during the conversion of both proteins.

The final clot is a network of fibrin strands running in every direction. The strands entrap red cells, platelets, white cells and plasma. Once the clot is formed, it begins to retract. The retracting clot draws the vessel walls together and compresses the fibrin network further.

The development of the blood clot is self-regulated. An important plasma protein exists called plasminogen. This is an inactive anti-clotting protein which, when triggered, converts to the active agent plasmin. Plasmin destroys the fibrin strands of the thrombus and has the ability to digest fibrinogen and several other clotting factors.

If plasmin were to develop unchecked, the entire blood clot could be dissolved and the risk of haemorrhage from the break in the vessel would recur. To combat plasmin a substance called alpha$_2$ antiplasmin exists, which binds with plasmin and neutralizes it (Guyton 1986). The balance between clotting and clot control is taking place all the time and involves a complex series of intrinsic and extrinsic pathways.

THE SKIN

The skin is made up of a surface layer (the epidermis) and an underlying thicker layer (the dermis). The epidermis is composed of stratified squamous epithelium. This layer is typically less than 1 mm deep and has many layers of cells (Woodburne & Burkel 1994). The epidermis contains no blood vessels but is penetrated by sensory nerve endings.

The dermis has several layers and is thicker than the epidermis. The deeper dermal layer, the reticular layer, is composed of a mass of collagenous and elastic connective tissue fibres. This accounts for the strength of the skin.

The dermis contains small quantities of fat, blood and lymph vessels, nerves and sensory nerve endings, hair follicles, sweat and sebaceous glands; smooth muscle fibres are also present (Woodburne & Burkel 1994; Fig. 2.11). The subcutaneous connective tissue is loose textured and is composed of fibrous connective tissue and elastic fibres; its correct name is the hypodermis (Woodburne & Burkel 1994). The distribution of subcutaneous fat varies in different parts of the body and is even absent in some regions, e.g. the eyelids. Where the fat layer is very prominent, it is termed adipose tissue. The hypodermis is generally thicker than the dermis (Woodburne & Burkel 1994).

The effects of ageing can alter the appearance and structure of the skin. The epidermis and dermis become thinner, loose and dry, with little subcutaneous tissue to support the vessels. This may account for the fragility and increased risk of bleeding at venepuncture sites, shearing of skin layers when tape and dressings are removed, and skin dryness which increases with the use of alcohol-based cleaning solutions (Hadaway 1995, Whitson 1996).

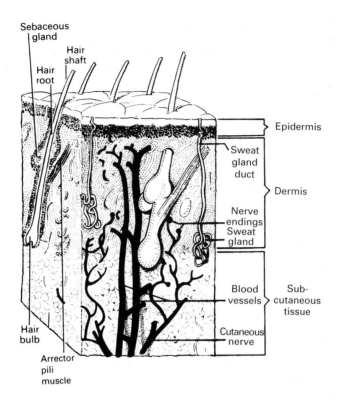

Sebaceous gland

Hair shaft

Hair root

Hair bulb

Arrector pili muscle

Epidermis

Sweat gland duct

Dermis

Nerve endings
Sweat gland

Blood vessels

Sub-cutaneous tissue

Cutaneous nerve

Fig. 2.11 The skin, showing the main structures in the dermis. (Reproduced with kind permission from Wilson & Waugh 1996.)

Perception of pain

The skin is a highly innervated structure. Any single point on the skin surface will have at least three different networks of nerve fibres running across it (Nathan 1988), making the skin a highly sensitive organ. The skin relays three types of information:

- the nature of the stimulus (is the skin pricked or pressed?)
- the intensity of the stimulus (is a pain mild or severe?)
- the location of the stimulus (is the hand or the arm being palpated?).

Nerve fibres in the skin are one of two types, large or small. Large nerve fibres are 'mechanoreceptors', which respond to changes in the skin surface, movement of the hairs on the surface of the skin, or anything touching or moving over the skin. The small fibres are thermoreceptors and nociceptors, and they respond to changes in temperature or any stimulus which can cause pain; the chemicals released by a nettle sting, for example, would be detected by a nociceptor. The skin of the hands and feet contains more nerve fibres than other parts of the limbs (Nathan 1988).

During cannulation or phlebotomy, the sensation of pain experienced is information from the skin rather than from the vessel. The stretching of the skin surface, local tapping of the skin, rubbing with alcohol and palpation of the vessel all trigger sensory pathways from the skin to the brain. In some cases, the sensations are also triggering memories of previous experiences (Nathan 1988). Preparation for cannulation, for example, may cause individuals to anticipate pain as a result of previous experiences.

Different types of nerves transmit different types of pain signal. Cutaneous nerves have different axons. A-beta nerves have large, heavily myelinated axons which respond to light touch. A-delta axons are smaller, less myelinated structures which respond to sharp pain and conduct rapidly. C-fibres are non-myelinated and slowly transmit sensations of an aching or burning nature (Hickey 1990).

If the cause of the pain also results in cell damage, then local chemicals will be released by the injured tissues and the awareness or sensitivity of the area will be 'heightened'. For example, skin which has been sunburned becomes highly touch-sensitive; taking off a shirt can cause immense pain if the back is sunburned.

There is a clearly identified pain pathway which goes from the periphery to the spinal cord, through the spinothalamic tract, to the thalamus and into the sensory cortex. There are differing theories on the perception of pain, the most widely accepted being that postulated by Melzack and Wall in the 1960s, known as 'the gate theory' (Melzack & Wall 1965).

According to the gate theory, the place where the pain is generated and the place where the pain is interpreted are linked by a nervous pathway which contains a gate. The pain message passes along the pathway by opening the gate. The more pain there is, the wider the gate is opened. The gate can be closed, and the pain pathway blocked, from either the proximal or distal side of the gate. The proximal (brain) side can close the gate by the use of diversional techniques such as relaxation or meditation. The distal (peripheral) side can close the gate by sending different signals, i.e. by rubbing the affected area or by transcutaneous nerve stimulation. Often, when we knock into something and experience pain, the first thing we do is to rub the affected area. By stimulating different nerve pathways, the original pain sensation can be prevented from passing through the gate and reaching the sensory cortex.

The kind of pain experienced by an individual depends mainly on two things: the type of tissue being damaged, and the agent that is causing the pain. Blood can cause pain when it is in the wrong place, e.g. when it leaks out of blood vessels. Equally, a lack of blood (ischaemia) can cause pain, as experienced by sufferers of intermittent claudication or angina (Nathan 1988).

Damage to peripheral nerves is painful; the pain of cancer is often due to the growth invading these nerves (Nathan 1988). The type of pain experienced when the skin is damaged will depend upon which layer of the skin is involved. Damage to the superficial layers causes itching or burning, while damage to the deeper layers causes an ache (Nathan 1988).

Pain reduction

When trying to reduce the pain of cannulation or phlebotomy, several techniques can be utilized. Assisting the individual to relax can lessen the awareness of pain. This can be done using meditation, breathing techniques (Nathan 1988) or other methods the individual may be familiar with. As little local stimulation of the area as possible prior to cannulation will reduce the hypersensitivity of the area.

Local anaesthetic agents may also be considered. These must be water-soluble, non-irritant, have a rapid onset of action, a suitable duration of action for the technique being performed, be non-toxic when absorbed into the circulation and have no lasting side-effects (Laurence 1975).

Local anaesthetics work by preventing the local nerve fibres from generating or conducting impulses, thereby interrupting the ascending pathways to the brain. This is achieved by preventing the cell membrane of the nerve from taking in sodium ions from its environment. Without the influx of sodium, a nerve cell cannot generate an action potential and a nerve impulse cannot be generated (Nathan 1988).

Local anaesthetic for cannulation varies depending on the nature and site of the cannula. Subcutaneous infiltration with lignocaine is usually used for central venous catheter insertion. This has the effect of inhibiting nerve transmission of the cutaneous and subcutaneous sensory nerves. Topical application of local anaesthetic creams is more common for peripheral cannulation.

CONCLUSION

A broad knowledge of the anatomy and physiology which underpins intravenous therapy is required by all practitioners who expand their practice to include this important skill. The range and depth of that knowledge will depend upon the specific area of practice and the role of the practitioner.

REFERENCES

Berne R M, Levy N L 1993 Physiology, 3rd edn. Mosby Year Book, St Louis, Missouri
Green J H 1985 An introduction to human physiology, 4th edn. Oxford University Press, Oxford
Green J H 1994 Basic clinical physiology, 3rd edn. Oxford University Press, Oxford
Guyton A C 1986 Textbook of medical physiology, 7th edn. WB Saunders, Philadelphia
Hadaway L R 1995 Anatomy and physiology related to intravenous therapy. In: Terry J, Baranowski L, Lonsway R A, Hedrick C (eds) Intravenous therapy: clinical principles and practices. WB Saunders, Philadelphia, ch 6, p 81–110
Hickey J 1990 The clinical practice of neurological and neurosurgical nursing, 3rd edn. JB Lippincott, Philadelphia
Hubbard J L, Mechan D J 1987 Physiology for health care students. Churchill Livingstone, Edinburgh
Laurence D R 1975 Clinical pharmacology, 4th edn. Churchill Livingstone, Edinburgh
Melzack R, Wall P D 1965 Pain mechanisms: a new theory. Science 150: 971–979
Nathan P 1988 The nervous system, 3rd edn. Oxford University Press, Oxford
Opie L 1990 Drugs for the heart. WB Saunders, Philadelphia
Soni N 1989 Anaesthesia and intensive care: practical procedures. Heinemann, London
Totora G J 1986 Principles of human anatomy, 4th edn. Harper & Row, London
Weinstein S M 1997 Anatomy and physiology applied to intravascular therapy. In: Weinstein S M (ed) Plumer's principles and practice of intravenous therapy, 6th edn. JB Lippincott, Philadelphia, ch 6, p 47–49
Whitson M 1996 Intravenous therapy in the older adult: special needs and considerations. Journal of Intravenous Nursing 19(5): 251–255
Wilson K J W, Waugh A 1996 Ross & Wilson: anatomy and physiology in health and illness, 8th edn. Churchill Livingstone, Edinburgh
Woodburne R T, Burkel W E 1994 Essentials of human anatomy, 9th edn. Oxford University Press, Oxford

Fluid and electrolyte balance

Michèle Malster

CHAPTER 3

INTRODUCTION

This chapter presents an overview of fluids and electrolytes, together with acid–base balance, and considers some of the common imbalances and their management. Each section starts by looking at normal balance and the homeostatic mechanisms which regulate it, before going on to describe the imbalances which can occur. The major imbalances of fluid, electrolytes and acid–base are presented in terms of their assessment and management. The more common causes of each imbalance are presented in tabular format, together with their physiological effects, in order to assist the reader's understanding of the rationale for interventions. The section on fluid and electrolyte replacement therapy gives details of the common crystalline and colloid solutions used in i.v. therapy, together with the indications for their use. The latter part of the chapter considers some of the more complex problems related to specific client groups.

FLUID BALANCE

Throughout the human life span, the water content and fluid compartments within the body alter. In infants, the fluid content represents 70–80% of their body weight, with the ratio of extracellular to intracellular fluid (ECF:ICF) being 3:2. This means that infants are particularly susceptible to dehydration, because extracellular fluid is more easily lost from the body than intracellular fluid. The percentage of total body water progressively decreases, reaching 60% of the body weight at 2 years of age. In the adult, the water content accounts for 60% of the body weight in males and 55% in females, and the ratio of ECF to ICF is approximately 1:2. From puberty there is evidence of sex differentiation in the total body water content; this occurs because of the greater percentage of body fat in females. Fat cells contain very little water and therefore the total body water (TBW) percentage decreases as the percentage body fat increases. It is important to remember this when managing i.v. therapy in obese patients.

For example, if the requisite amount of fluid replacement for a lean person weighing 100 kg (TBW = 70%) were to be given to an obese person weighing 100 kg (TBW = 35%), this would result in the latter receiving twice the required amount of fluid (Statland 1963; see Fig. 3.1).

Fluid compartments

There are two main fluid compartments in the body:

- intracellular fluid – fluid in the cells
- extracellular fluid
  — plasma, i.e. intravascular fluid (IVF)
  — interstitial fluid (ISF)
  — transcellular fluid (TCF).

Transcellular fluid refers to fluid contained in body cavities, e.g. cerebrospinal fluid, intraocular fluid, synovial fluid, etc.

Fig. 3.1 Body composition of a lean and an obese individual. (After Metheney 1992, with permission from Lippincott-Raven.)

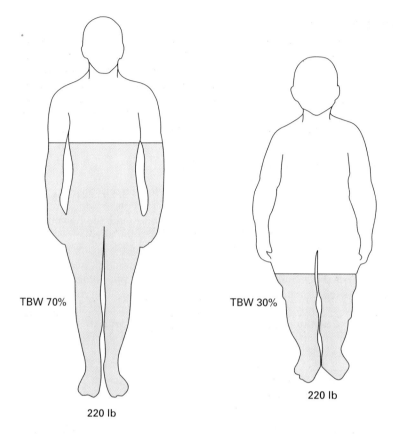

TBW 70%

220 lb

TBW 30%

220 lb

Composition

The body fluids are composed of water and dissolved particles (solutes). These solutes are referred to as electrolytes and non-electrolytes. When in solution, electrolytes can dissociate into either positively charged cations or negatively charged anions, which can conduct an electrical charge. In any solution, the number of cations must equal the number of anions; this is called electroneutrality. The major cations are:

- sodium (Na^+)
- potassium (K^+)
- calcium (Ca^{2+})
- magnesium (Mg^{2+}).

The major anions are:

- chloride (Cl^-)
- bicarbonate (HCO_3^-)
- phosphate (HPO_4^-)
- protein.

Within the ECF and ICF, there are large differences in the numbers of cations and anions. For example, within the cells potassium is the major cation, while outside the cells sodium predominates. The concentration of individual electrolytes is measured in millimoles per litre (mmol/L).

Non-electrolytes are substances which do not dissociate in solution, including urea, glucose, creatinine and bilirubin.

Transport mechanisms

The fluid compartments are separated from one another by semi-permeable membranes through which water and solutes may pass. While small solutes such as urea can pass easily through membranes, other large molecules such as proteins are confined to the intravascular fluid by the capillary membranes. The composition of each fluid compartment is maintained by the selectivity of its membrane. This ensures that nutrients can pass into the cells and waste products can pass out of the cells and ultimately to the plasma. The semi-permeable membranes involved include:

- capillary membranes which separate IVF from ISF
- cell membranes which separate ISF from ICF
- epithelial membranes which separate ISF and IVF from TCF (Horne & Swearingen 1993).

The means by which fluid moves from one compartment to another involves both passive and active transport mechanisms.

Passive transport

Simple diffusion Diffusion refers to the movement of solutes down a gradient from an area of high concentration (of solutes) to an area of low concentration until equilibrium is reached. Factors which affect the rate of diffusion include:

- concentration of solute
- size and molecular weight of solute
- surface area available for diffusion
- distance which the solute must diffuse
- temperature of the environment (Horne & Swearingen 1993).

Diffusion may also take place if there is a change in the electrical potential across the membrane. For example, anions will follow cations and the reverse will also happen. Movement of solutes will occur if they are lipid-soluble or if the substances are small enough to pass through the cell wall. However, large lipid-soluble substances, e.g. glucose, require a carrier to enable them to diffuse into the cell. This process is called facilitated diffusion.

Facilitated diffusion This method of diffusion also requires a concentration gradient, but the amount and rate of diffusion are dependent on the availability of carrier substance. After entering the cell, the carrier then releases itself and is available to aid diffusion of further substances. If the carrier becomes saturated (i.e. all the carrier is being used), even though a concentration gradient still exists, diffusion will be reduced.

Osmosis This is the movement of solvent (e.g. water) from an area of low concentration of solutes (particles) to an area of high concentration of solutes across a semi-permeable membrane. The forces involved relate to:

- oncotic pressure – the osmotic pressure exerted by proteins; for example, plasma proteins (albumin) exert pressure within the vasculature to hold fluid in the intravascular space
- osmotic pressure – the amount of hydrostatic pressure necessary to stop the osmotic flow of fluid
- hydrostatic pressure – the pressure exerted by the weight of the fluid (water) on the semi-permeable membrane; this provides the principal force by which fluid moves out of the arterial end of capillaries (Fig. 3.2).

Filtration Filtration is used to describe the movement of solutes (particles) and sol-

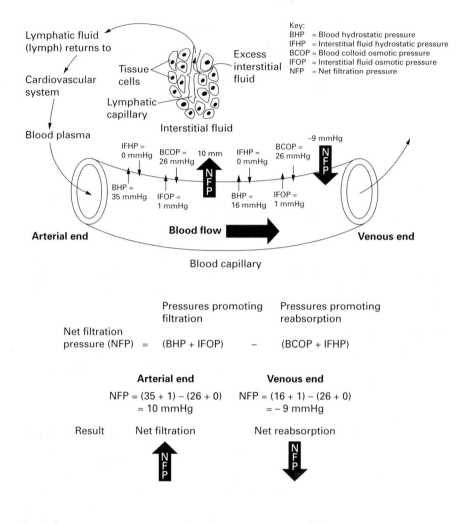

Fig. 3.2 Capillary bed dynamics – dynamics of capillary exchange. (From PRINCIPLES OF ANATOMY AND PHYSIOLOGY, 8th Edition, by General Tortora and Sandra Grabowski; Copyright © 1996 by Biological Sciences Textbooks, Inc., A C P Textbooks Inc. and Sandra Grabowski: Reprinted by permission.)

vent (fluid) from an area of high hydrostatic pressure to an area of low hydrostatic pressure.

Active transport

Where there is no electrical or concentration gradient, substances are unable to move by simple diffusion. Active transport, as its name suggests, requires the use of energy, in the form of adenosine triphosphate (ATP), to move substances against a pressure or concentration gradient. This form of transport may involve the simultaneous movement of different substances. For example, as sodium ions move into the cell, potassium ions move out simultaneously. This is more commonly referred to as the 'sodium–potassium pump'. This pump is responsible for maintaining the intracellular fluid volume, by ensuring that the osmotic pressure exerted by the intracellular proteins (to pull water into the cells) is counterbalanced by the output of sodium ions (Paradiso 1995). As well as these transport mechanisms, other factors, such as osmolality and tonicity, also influence the movement of fluid.

Osmolality

Osmolality is a measurement of the concentration of the body's fluids, or the ratio of solutes to solvent, and its unit of measurement is the milliosmole/kilogram of water (mOsm/kg). Osmolality reflects the ability of a solution to create osmotic pressure and hence affect the movement of water. For example, an increase in the osmolality of the ECF will cause water to move from the ICF to the ECF, while decreased osmolality will have the reverse effect. The osmolality of each compartment is governed:

- in the ECF by sodium
- in the ICF by potassium
- in the IVF by plasma proteins.

Tonicity

Molecules which affect the movement of water (e.g. sodium, glucose, etc.) are called effective osmoles, while smaller molecules which move easily across most membranes (e.g. urea) are called ineffective osmoles (Horne & Swearingen 1993). Effective osmolality is also termed tonicity. Solutions (e.g. sodium chloride 0.9%) which have the same tonicity as the body fluids are called isotonic. Those solutions (e.g. sodium chloride 0.45%) which have a lower tonicity are called hypotonic, while those with a greater tonicity (e.g. sodium chloride 1.8%) are called hypertonic.

Regulation of body fluids

The body systems involved in regulating the body fluids are renal, endocrine, cardiovascular, gastrointestinal (GI) and respiratory. They work interdependently to ensure that the homeostatic balance of fluid balance is maintained.

Renal system

The renal system is responsible for the regulation of sodium and water balance in the ECF. In response to a low serum sodium concentration, decreased plasma volume and increased sympathetic nervous stimulation, the cells in the juxtaglomerular apparatus in the glomerulus secrete a proteolytic enzyme called renin. Renin activates angiotensin 1, which is converted (by an enzyme from the lungs) to angiotension 2. Angiotensin 2 is a powerful vasoconstrictor and has two actions. Firstly, it causes vasoconstriction which increases peripheral resistance, thereby increasing arterial pressure. Secondly, it causes the release of a mineralocorticoid hormone called aldosterone from the adrenal cortex. Aldosterone acts on the distal convoluted tubule to increase the reabsorption of sodium; this retention of sodium leads to water retention and therefore the circulating volume is increased (see Fig. 3.3).

Changes in the serum levels of sodium and potassium also affect the release of aldosterone. A decreased serum sodium or increased serum potassium will increase the release of aldosterone. As a result, sodium absorption from the renal tubules is enhanced in exchange for potassium and hydrogen ions, which are excreted in the urine.

Endocrine system

The thirst centre in the hypothalamus is the initial regulator of water intake. The urge to drink is stimulated by a decrease in the ICF in the thirst centre cells, together with feedback from the gastrointestinal tract. Simultaneously, osmoreceptors in the hypothalamus detect changes in the osmolality of the ECF. When the osmolality of the plasma is increased, antidiuretic hormone (ADH) is released from the posterior pituitary gland. This hormone increases the permeability of the distal renal tubule to water and therefore more water is reabsorbed back into the circulation. As

Fig. 3.3 The renin–angiotensin–aldosterone system. (After Hinchliff et al 1997, with permission.)

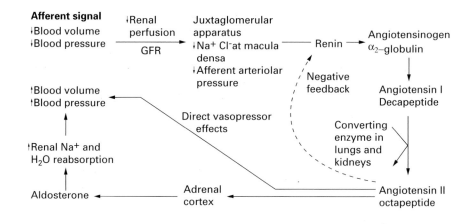

a result, only small amounts of concentrated urine are produced – sufficient to ensure the excretion of waste products. In contrast, if the osmoreceptors detect a decreased osmolality in the plasma, the secretion of ADH is inhibited, resulting in larger amounts of water being excreted as urine. At the same time, as the ICF volume in the thirst centre neurones increases, the thirst centre mechanism is inhibited (see Fig. 3.4).

Sensory receptors in the gastrointestinal tract provide feedback to the hypothalamus, so that ADH can be regulated to enhance water absorption from the intestines.

Cardiovascular system

Although large volume changes in the ECF interstitial fluid can occur with minimal change in body function, changes in the blood volume are less well tolerated. The function of the blood volume is to maintain tissue perfusion and therefore cell life. Approximately 25% of the cardiac output is pumped each minute to the kidneys at an optimal pressure, to maintain their perfusion, so that urine formation can occur. Changes in the blood volume have a direct effect on arterial blood pressure and therefore renal perfusion. This means that if the blood volume is increased, cardiac output and arterial pressure increase. An increase in renal arterial pressure leads to an increased glomerular filtration rate and ultimately increased urinary output.

Concurrently, baroreceptors and stretch receptors in the aorta and carotid arteries detect an increase in the arterial pressure and transmit inhibitory impulses to the sympathetic nervous system. This results in dilatation of the renal arterioles, which ultimately leads to an increase in urine formation.

Atrial natriuretic factor (ANF) is a polypeptide hormone secreted by the atria of the heart in response to an increased stretching of the atria, brought about by an increased blood volume. ANF causes a decrease in the tubular reabsorption of sodium ions so that the osmolality of the filtrate is increased, which draws water into the tubule and consequently increases the volume of urinary output. It should be noted that ANF is only effective in the short-term control of blood volume.

Gastrointestinal system

Within the gastrointestinal tract, the processes which help to regulate fluid volume are principally the processes of digestion and utilizing passive and active transport. Following digestive processes in the stomach, the chyme is mixed with gastrointestinal secretions and moves through the small intestine. Here, approximately 90% of the water and nutrients are absorbed. A further 500–1000 ml of water are absorbed from the large intestine, so that there is only a minimal loss in the faeces.

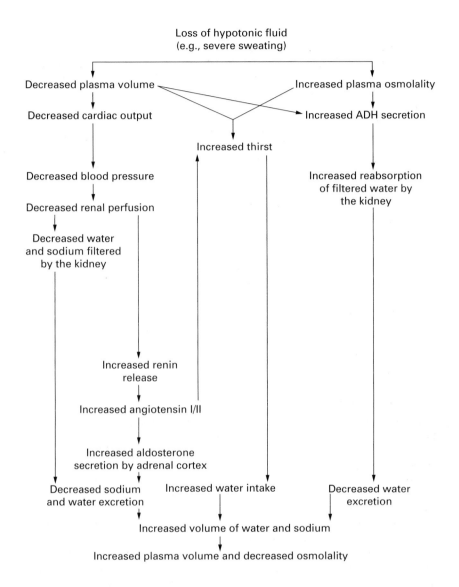

Fig. 3.4 Regulation of fluid volume and osmolality: a clinical example. (After Horne & Swearingen 1993, with permission.)

Respiratory system

Approximately 400 ml/day of fluid is lost as expired water vapour. This amount will vary with respiratory rate and environmental humidity.

FLUID VOLUME IMBALANCES

Hypovolaemia

Hypovolaemia refers to a decrease in the ECF volume and is caused by excessive fluid loss or decreased fluid intake. It occurs when the normal regulating mechanisms fail to cope adequately and may be accompanied by disturbances in osmolality, acid–base balance and electrolyte balance. If the hypovolaemia is very severe or prolonged, it may result in acute renal failure, because renal perfusion is not adequately maintained.

Assessment

History Severe fluid loss, e.g. diarrhoea, diaphoresis, vomiting, haemorrhage, etc. Decreased intake may be caused by starvation, unconsciousness, shock, etc.

Physical evidence Third space loss (e.g. ascites, bowel obstruction, etc.), diarrhoea, etc.

Clinical manifestations include evidence of compensation by the normal regulatory mechanisms, e.g. tachycardia, thirst, oliguria, etc. Reduced skin turgor, reduced jugular vein filling and furred tongue may be apparent. If hypovolaemic shock is present, the patient will appear pale with clammy skin and have a rapid, thready pulse and marked hypotension. As the dehydration progresses, the patient may exhibit signs of altered consciousness.

Tests include the following:

- Haematocrit
  — increased in dehydration
  — decreased in haemorrhage.
- Serum electrolytes – will vary according to the type of fluid loss, e.g. hypernatraemia will occur with excessive diaphoresis. Electrolyte imbalances which may occur include hypernatraemia, hyponatraemia and hyperkalaemia (see 'Electrolyte imbalances', p. 54).
- Blood urea nitrogen (BUN) – may be raised due to altered renal activity and reduced fluid intake.
- Arterial blood gas analysis
  — metabolic acidosis: pH < 7.35; bicarbonate < 22 mmol/L
  — metabolic alkalosis: pH > 7.45; bicarbonate > 28 mmol/L
  Metabolic acidosis is associated with shock, diabetic ketoacidosis, etc., while metabolic alkalosis results from diuretic therapy or excessive upper GI tract fluid loss.
- Urine specific gravity – increased to about 1.010, which indicates the action of ADH, trying to conserve fluid.

Management

If the patient is experiencing altered consciousness, measures to ensure safety are required. Monitoring of the level of consciousness may be indicated. The management of hypovolaemia aims to replace the fluid loss, correct any electrolyte imbalance and treat the underlying cause. The hypovolaemia in shock occurs either from a sudden major loss or from loss of more than 25% of the intravascular volume. The type of fluid lost will determine the replacement fluid, e.g. haemorrhage will require blood and blood products while water losses can be replaced with crystalline i.v. solutions such as sodium chloride 0.9% or dextrose 5%. The rate of i.v. infusion may need to be rapid in order to keep up with the loss and also to replace the deficit. The speed with which the replacement can be achieved will depend on the cardiac and renal function of the patient. For this reason, monitoring of the vital signs is essential and may require the insertion of a central venous catheter for haemodynamic monitoring. Other observations include skin colour, temperature and turgor.

Care is taken to ensure that the patient does not become overloaded, which could precipitate pulmonary oedema. Overloading can occur from infusing fluid too rapidly or infusing too much fluid.

Fluids used in replacement therapy include:

- compound sodium lactate

- human albumin, hetastarch or dextran solution
- fresh frozen plasma

(see 'Crystalline' and 'Colloid' solutions for details, pp. 66 and 68).

The ultimate aim of fluid replacement therapy is to restore adequate tissue perfusion, so observations of the patient's status will relate to this, e.g. level of consciousness (CNS perfusion), fluid intake and output (renal perfusion) and peripheral pulses (peripheral perfusion). Further management will depend on the cause, e.g. diabetic ketoacidosis, which is described in the relevant section of this chapter.

Hypervolaemia

Hypervolaemia refers to an increase in the ECF volume and is generally caused by an overload of i.v. fluid administration, abnormal renal function (causing increased reabsorption of sodium and water) or the movement of fluid from the interstitial space to the intravascular fluid. In susceptible patients, this may lead to pulmonary oedema and cardiac failure. However, usually the kidneys attempt to compensate by increasing the excretion of sodium and water and suppressing the release of aldosterone and ADH. Hypervolaemia is usually associated with alterations in acid–base balance, osmolality and electrolyte balance.

Assessment

History Intravenous fluid replacement therapy, cirrhosis, renal failure (oliguria), hypertonic i.v. fluid administration.

Physical evidence Oliguria, oedema, etc.

Clinical manifestations include bounding pulses, tachycardia, hypertension (compared to the patient's norm), neck vein distension and respiratory sounds associated with pulmonary oedema.

Tests include the following:

- Haematocrit – reduced because of haemodilution.
- Serum electrolytes – may reveal hyponatraemia due to excessive water retention.
- Serum osmolality – reduced.
- Blood urea nitrogen – decreased because the blood is diluted with excess water.
- Arterial blood gas analysis – may be altered in pulmonary oedema, showing a decreased P_{O_2} and alkalosis. A decreased P_{O_2} stimulates respiration causing a decrease in P_{CO_2}. The reduced ratio of P_{CO_2} to bicarbonate leads to an increased pH.
- Urine specific gravity – decreased, as the kidneys try to excrete the excess fluid.

Management

The main aim of treatment is to achieve a normal ECF volume. Management includes the use of diuretic therapy to aid excretion of the excess fluid, and restriction of sodium and water. The main risk is pulmonary oedema, so careful monitoring of respirations and breath sounds is necessary. Vital signs and fluid intake and output need to be monitored. Monitoring of blood gas analysis will facilitate correction of alkalosis, and hypoxaemia will require oxygen therapy. The underlying cause of the hypervolaemia needs to be treated. Haemodialysis is indicated if renal failure is present.

ELECTROLYTE REGULATION AND IMBALANCES

The concentration of individual electrolytes is measured in mmol/L. It should be noted that the normal ranges for serum electrolyte concentrations will vary slightly according to the method of laboratory assessment. Milliequivalents per litre (mEq/L), which are sometimes quoted in American texts as a measurement, are the same as mmol/L, but only for monovalent ions, e.g. Na^+ and K^+ (not for Ca^{2+} which is a divalent ion, i.e. 1 mmol = 2 mEq).

Sodium

Sodium is an important factor in maintaining the volume and osmolality of ECF. It influences the maintenance of potassium and chloride concentrations and is also essential for neuromuscular transmission (Innerarity & Stark 1990). It is regulated in relation to water and chloride and is the main cation that determines ECF osmolality. Changes in sodium concentration result in corresponding changes in the osmolality. As most of the sodium is outside the cells, its level can be measured by serum test, normal ranging between 136 and 145 mmol/L.

The natural means of sodium loss from the body are via sweat, urine and faeces. The kidneys and endocrine systems are the main regulators of sodium balance. Two contrasting mechanisms in the kidneys try to ensure that excess or lack of oral intake of sodium can be accommodated with minimal changes in serum sodium concentration. One mechanism ensures that excess sodium (together with water) passes via the glomerular filtrate into the urine, while the other mechanism endeavours to retain sodium, by encouraging its reabsorption (together with water) from the renal tubules when intake of sodium is low. This occurs in the presence of aldosterone, which is released in response to decreased plasma levels of sodium. As well as the production of aldosterone, the role of the endocrine system also involves the production of ADH. If the level of sodium in the ECF is increased, it increases the osmolality of the ECF which stimulates the secretion of ADH, thereby enhancing the reabsorption of water from the tubular filtrate. As a result, ECF osmolality is reduced.

Hyponatraemia

This is usually defined as a serum sodium below 135 mmol/L. However, it should be noted that in-patients may have a serum sodium of up to 5 mmol/L less than outpatients. The two basic mechanisms which result in hyponatraemia are concerned with either an increase in ECF water or a decrease in ECF sodium. The causes are listed in Table 3.1.

However, it should be noted that some conditions may give rise to a reduced serum sodium concentration, although there is no true hyponatraemia. One typical example is in hyperglycaemia, where the elevated glucose level exerts an osmotic 'pull' of water out of the cells into the ECF, thereby diluting the sodium in the ECF. Other examples are hyperproteinaemia and hyperlipidaemia, which reduce the percentage of water in the plasma. The ratio of sodium to water remains the same but, because the plasma water content is reduced, the serum sodium level is reduced (Horne & Swearingen 1993).

Assessment

History The medical history may identify the cause, e.g. history of diuretic therapy, adrenal impairment, syndrome of inappropriate antidiuretic hormone (SIADH), etc.

Physical evidence Vomiting, diarrhoea, etc.

Table 3.1 Causes of hyponatraemia

Cause	Physiological process
Prolonged diuretic use	Sodium reabsorption from the loop of Henle is impaired
Excessive diaphoresis	Large amounts of sodium are present in sweat
Prolonged vomiting, diarrhoea	Large ECF loss
Extensive burns	Large volumes of ECF (and therefore sodium) are lost
Renal disease	Excessive consumption or infusion of hypotonic solutions
Salt-losing nephritis	Loss of sodium
Nephrotic syndrome	Water retained in excess of sodium
Over-infusion of i.v. dextrose 5%	Excess water in the ECF will move into the cell to reduce the sodium/water ratio
Psychogenic polydipsia	Excessive water consumption
Anorexia, alcoholism, fasting	Inadequate oral intake
Syndrome of inappropriate ADH (SIADH)	Water is retained and sodium becomes overdiluted
Adrenal impairment	Reduced levels of aldosterone result in sodium excretion
Cirrhosis	Water retained in excess of sodium
Congestive cardiac failure	Water retained in excess of sodium
Drugs	
Intravenous cyclophosphamide	Increases renal sensitivity to ADH
carbamazepine	Induces ADH release
amitriptyline	Water retention
'Ecstasy'	Increased sodium loss
chlorpropramide	Increases action of ADH
Addison's disease	Increased sodium excretion

Clinical manifestations relating to impairment of the musculoskeletal system may be muscle cramps and twitching. Central nervous system impairment is due to the low ECF sodium causing water to move into the brain cells, which then swell. Symptoms may include headache, dizziness, convulsions and unconsciousness.

Diagnostic tests:

- Serum sodium level < 135 mmol/L (see text under 'Hyponatraemia', p. 54)
- Urine osmolality < 350 mOsm/kg (except SIADH)
- Serum osmolality < 285 mmol/kg, except in hyperglycaemia, etc.
- Urine sodium < 20 mmol/L, except in SIADH and adrenal impairment.

Management Patient safety is paramount both in terms of ensuring that no injury is sustained if the patient has neurological disturbances, and in relation to the correction of the hyponatraemia. Serum sodium levels <120 mmol/L require urgent treatment to remove the patient from danger, while sodium levels between 120 and 136 mmol/L need careful management to ensure that overcompensation does not occur. Generally the management falls into two categories: hyponatraemia with reduced ECF volume and hyponatraemia with increased ECF volume. The first is concerned with replacing the sodium and fluid losses, together with other electrolytes as necessary. In extreme cases, a hypertonic solution of sodium chloride (e.g. 2.7%) may be required, if the patient is severely depleted.

The second category of management is concerned with reducing the increased ECF volume. This will vary according to the cause, but may also include diuretic

Table 3.2 Causes of hypernatraemia

Condition	Physiological process
Inadequate water intake	Decreased ECF water volume
Watery diarrhoea	Excessive water loss
Severe insensible loss	Excessive water loss
Burns	Water and electrolyte loss
Osmotic diuretic therapy	Excessive water loss
Hyperglycaemia	Water loss due to osmotic diuresis
Diabetes insipidus	Excessive water loss due to lack of ADH
Near-drowning in salt water	Excessive sodium intake
Hypertonic i.v. saline	Increased sodium gain
Hyperaldosteronism (e.g. Conn's syndrome)	Sodium retention, due to excess aldosterone

therapy and water restriction. Serum electrolytes need to monitored, together with fluid intake and output, to ensure optimal management of this imbalance.

Hypernatraemia

This is defined as serum sodium greater than 145 mmol/L. As sodium is the main cation determinant of osmolality of the ECF, an increase in its concentration will cause hypertonicity which will result in water being 'drawn' out of the cells. This means that the ICF volume is decreased in hypernatraemia. The main causes of hypernatraemia are water loss, dehydration or sodium gain in excess of water, but it may also be a complication of aggressive treatment of hyponatraemia, as previously mentioned. The specific causes of hypernatraemia are presented in Table 3.2.

Assessment

History There may be a medical history of diabetes insipidus, osmotic diuretics, near-drowning, etc.

Physical evidence Water loss, e.g. major burns, diarrhoea, etc.

Clinical manifestations will include those relating to water loss (e.g. intense thirst, hypotension, dry mucous membranes) and sodium gain (e.g. flushed skin, peripheral oedema, low-grade fever). Hyperactive reflexes, lethargy and seizures may occur in severe hypernatraemia because of its effect on neuromuscular conduction and the central nervous system.

Diagnostic tests:

- Serum sodium > 145 mmol/L
- Serum osmolality > 295 mmol/kg because of the increased serum sodium level
- Urine osmolality > 525 mOsm/kg, except in diabetes insipidus when it is decreased.

Management If the patient shows signs of neurological impairment, care must be taken to ensure that there is no risk of injury. Correction of the hypernatraemia will depend on the cause and it centres around reducing the sodium level. Cautious administration of i.v. hypotonic solutions is recommended together with careful monitoring of vital signs, fluid intake and output, neurological status and serum sodium. The fluids of choice are dextrose 5% and hypotonic saline solutions. To minimize the risk of overcorrection and cerebral oedema (due to fluid overload and the shift of water into the cells, particularly in the brain), diuretics may also be given. Diabetes insipidus will require specific therapy using a vasopressin analogue.

Potassium

Potassium is the main cation in the ICF and is of vital importance in neuromuscular conduction, acid–base balance and cell function. It also has a direct effect on cardiac muscle conductivity. Although potassium ions continuously move in and out of the cells, most of the potassium is contained within the cells by the sodium–potassium pump, so that, by comparison with sodium, the serum level is low and ranges between 3.5 and 5.0 mmol/L. The distribution of potassium between the ICF and ECF is influenced by pH levels, aldosterone, adrenaline and insulin. In acidosis, when hydrogen ions move into the cells as part of the buffering mechanism, potassium ions move out in order to maintain electroneutrality: so one positive ion (H^+) is exchanged for another (K^+). As a result, serum potassium rises in acidosis. In alkalosis, the ions move in the opposite direction and so serum potassium falls. It can therefore be seen that changes in serum potassium levels may not always indicate a loss or increase in the total potassium level in the body, but only reflect changes in the ECF potassium levels.

Potassium levels in the body are regulated by the kidneys, which adjust the amount of potassium excreted in the urine. There is a reciprocal relationship between potassium and sodium, an illustration of which is provided by the action of aldosterone, which aids sodium reabsorption in exchange for the excretion of potassium.

Hypokalaemia

Hypokalaemia, defined as a serum level of potassium less than 3.5 mmol/L, occurs when there is loss of potassium from the body or a shift of potassium into the cells. Potassium is not stored in the body and serum levels are maintained within narrow limits. A low intake of potassium is rarely the cause of hypokalaemia, except for patients receiving parenteral nutrition who may have inadequate replacement of this electrolyte. The main loss of potassium is via the kidneys and a common cause is thiazide diuretic therapy. The main causes of hypokalaemia are presented in Table 3.3.

Table 3.3 Causes of hypokalaemia

Cause	Physiological process
Prolonged thiazide diuretic use	Increased loss in the urine
Parenteral nutrition	Inadequate potassium intake
Severe GI fluid loss	High potassium levels in gastric fluid, bile, etc.
Hyperaldosteronism	Increased loss in urine in exchange for sodium
Severe diaphoresis	Potassium loss in sweat
Severe stress	Corticoid release promotes sodium retention in exchange for potassium
Alkalosis	Potassium shift into the cells in exchange for hydrogen ions
Increased insulin secretion or therapy	Potassium shift from ECF into cells; also insulin is a carrier
Burns	Potassium loss
Hypomagnesaemia	Magnesium is important in activating sodium–potassium pump
Ectopic ACTH	Increased urine loss

Fig. 3.5 ECG changes associated with electrolyte imbalances. (Used with permission from *Fluid and Electrolytes*, 3rd edn, by S.A. Innerarity and J.L. Stark, 1990, © Springhouse Corporation, Springhouse, PA.)

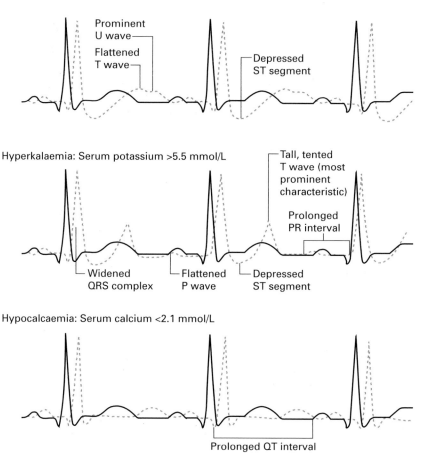

Hypokalaemia: Serum potassium <3.5 mmol/L

Prominent U wave
Flattened T wave
Depressed ST segment

Hyperkalaemia: Serum potassium >5.5 mmol/L

Tall, tented T wave (most prominent characteristic)
Prolonged PR interval
Widened QRS complex
Flattened P wave
Depressed ST segment

Hypocalcaemia: Serum calcium <2.1 mmol/L

Prolonged QT interval

Assessment

History There may be a medical history of thiazide diuretic therapy, congenital adrenal hyperplasia, pyloric stenosis, etc.

Physical evidence Major burns, gastrointestinal loss, etc.

Clinical manifestations of neuromuscular impairment such as muscle weakness, cramps, fatigue, paraesthesiae and diminished reflexes are typical signs. Paralytic ileus may occur due to decreased gut motility. Cardiac dysrhythmias may also occur due to impaired myocardial conduction.

Tests include:

- Serum potassium < 3.5 mmol/L
- ECG – may show ventricular dysrhythmias, S–T segment depression, flattened T-wave or presence of U-wave (see Fig. 3.5)
- Arterial blood gas analysis – may detect metabolic alkalosis, with pH > 7.45 and increased bicarbonate levels.

Management The aim of the management is to treat the underlying cause and to replace the potassium by oral or i.v. supplements. If the i.v. route is used for replace-

Fig. 3.5 *(cont'd)*

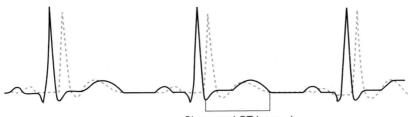

Shortened QT interval

Hypomagnesaemia: Serum magnesium <0.7 mmol/L

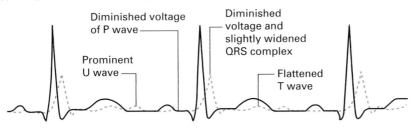

Diminished voltage of P wave

Prominent U wave

Diminished voltage and slightly widened QRS complex

Flattened T wave

Hypermagnesaemia: Serum magnesium >2.1 mmol/L

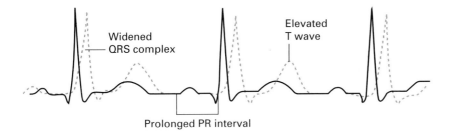

Widened QRS complex

Elevated T wave

Prolonged PR interval

Key: / Normal   Abnormal

ment therapy, the patient requires careful monitoring during administration of the estimated amount of potassium. The most frequently used preparation is potassium chloride diluted in an isotonic solution (which will also provide some hydration). Use of a burette infusion set or syringe pump will assist in a more accurate rate of administration. If peripheral veins are used, the rate of infusion will need to be reduced to avoid irritation of the veins by the potassium chloride. There is also a risk of damage to surrounding tissues if concentrated solutions extravasate, so delivery via a central venous catheter may be preferable. Care should be taken to avoid rapid infusion of potassium, which could lead to cardiac arrest as a result of hyperkalaemia. ECG monitoring is recommended to detect abnormal rhythms or the development of hyperkalaemia due to overcorrection.

Hyperkalaemia

Hyperkalaemia is defined as a serum potassium greater than 5.5 mmol/L. There are four mechanisms which contribute to an increase in ECF potassium. The first relates to an increased potassium intake resulting from potassium replacement therapy by

Table 3.4 Causes of hyperkalaemia

Cause	Physiological process
Potassium replacement therapy	Increased ECF potassium
Prolonged use of salt substitute	Increased potassium intake
Renal failure	Failure of tubules to balance potassium
Potassium-sparing diuretics	Retention of potassium
Bowel obstruction	Reduced potassium loss in faeces.
Burns, trauma, etc.	Cell damage releases potassium into ECF
Large volume blood transfusion	Cell lysis in donated blood increases with storage time
Hyponatraemia	Potassium ions move out of cell in exchange for sodium
Metabolic acidosis	Potassium ions move out of cell in exchange for hydrogen ions
Hyperglycaemia	Glucose osmotic diuresis causes potassium loss from cells
Hyperaldosteronism	Decreased potassium excretion
Addison's disease	Decreased potassium excretion
Chemotherapy	Cell lysis
Factors affecting accurate estimation:	
Prolonged tourniquet application during sampling	Haemolysis, releasing potassium from the cells
Fist clenching during blood sampling	May cause haemolysis
EDTA contamination	May lead to inaccurate reading
Haemolysed blood sample	Increased potassium estimation
Thrombocytosis	

the oral or i.v. routes. Occasionally, however, an increased intake may be due to use of salt substitutes (which are high in potassium) by patients on a low sodium diet. Secondly, if excretion of potassium is inhibited (as in renal failure) or if there is failure of the control mechanisms (e.g. adrenocortical insufficiency leading to reduced aldosterone and cortisol associated with Addison's disease), serum levels will rise. Thirdly, since potassium is mainly found inside the cells, any condition which results in their breakdown will release potassium into the ECF, as the sodium–potassium pump fails. Finally, electrolyte shifts requiring the movement of a cation (e.g. potassium) out of the cell may result in an increased ECF potassium level. This can occur during hyponatraemia and metabolic acidosis, where sodium and hydrogen ions, respectively, move into the cell and potassium moves out of the cell to maintain electroneutrality. The causes of hyperkalaemia are presented in Table 3.4.

Assessment

History There may be a medical history of prolonged or excessive salt substitute use, chemotherapy (cell lysis), hyponatraemia, diabetes mellitus, etc.

Physical evidence Crush injuries, burns, large-volume blood transfusion, diarrhoea, etc.

Clinical manifestations of neurological impairment may result in anxiety, irritability, muscle weakness, abdominal cramps and paraesthesiae. Cardiac dysrhythmias due to abnormal myocardial conduction will be accompanied by an irregular pulse.

It should be noted that cardiac output is usually decreased as potassium is a myocardial depressant.

Tests include:

- Serum potassium > 5.5 mmol/L
- ECG – may show dysrhythmias, elevated T-waves, depressed S–T segment, flattened or absent P-wave (which may lead to asystole if not treated), prolonged P–R interval and wide QRS complex (Fig. 3.5)
- Arterial blood gas analysis – may indicate metabolic acidosis with a low bicarbonate level.

Management Hyperkalaemia is a life-threatening condition and may lead to asystole. Prompt recognition of ECG changes is important and careful monitoring is necessary during treatment, which may need to be aggressive to prevent cardiac arrest.

Potassium tends to cause depolarization of the cell membranes, but increasing the serum calcium levels helps to antagonize this effect and this is the rationale for administering i.v. calcium. Calcium is generally administered in the form of calcium gluconate, although calcium chloride may be used as an alternative. However, it is important to note that these two preparations are not interchangeable, because calcium gluconate 10 ml contains 220 μmol/L (micromoles per litre) of calcium while the same volume of calcium chloride contains 680 μmol/L. A slow i.v. infusion of calcium gluconate will help to negate the depressant effects of potassium on the myocardium. It acts rapidly, but its duration of action is not sustained.

Acute symptomatic hyperkalaemia (serum level > 5.5 mmol/L) may require treatment on a temporary basis with an i.v. infusion of dextrose 50% with insulin, which will assist the movement of potassium back into the cells.

Other forms of treatment include haemodialysis if renal function is impaired, and an i.v. infusion of sodium bicarbonate to correct the metabolic acidosis, if present.

Calcium

Calcium helps to maintain the structure and function of cell membranes and is essential in neuromuscular conduction and contraction in the heart and skeletal muscles. It is also required for hormonal secretions, enzyme activation and blood coagulation.

The skeletal system contains almost 99% of the body's calcium, while 1% is within the ICF and 0.1% within the ECF. Approximately 50% of the calcium is chemically active, ionized calcium and this represents the serum level that is measured. Normal serum ionized calcium levels range from 1 to 1.25 mmol/L, but this is not routinely measured. The remainder is bound to protein, e.g. albumin, which means that albumin levels need to be considered when assessing calcium levels. This is important as laboratories normally measure total calcium only (range 2.2–2.6 mmol/L); the result may include compensation for albumin levels.

Calcium balance is maintained by parathyroid hormone (PTH), calcitonin and calcitriol (1,25-dihydroxycholecalciferol, an active form of vitamin D). Parathyroid hormone, released in response to a low ECF calcium, enhances calcium resorption (the movement of calcium from bone into the plasma) and promotes intestinal and renal absorption of calcium (via calcitriol), thereby increasing the serum calcium level. In contrast, a high ECF calcium stimulates the thyroid gland to release calcitonin, which acts as a physiological antagonist to parathyroid hormone, inhibiting calcium release from bone and resulting in a decreased serum calcium.

The pH level of the serum will affect the ionized calcium level as, in alkalosis, more calcium is bound to protein. Another factor affecting serum calcium is the reciprocal relationship between calcium and phosphorus. A raised serum calcium leads to a lowered serum phosphorus, while a lowered serum calcium leads to a raised phosphorus level.

Hypocalcaemia

This is defined as a serum calcium less than 2.1 mmol/L and usually represents a reduced level of circulating ionized calcium. Hypocalcaemia is usually associated with vitamin D deficiency, abnormal parathyroid secretion, reduced calcium intake or increased calcium loss. It may cause skeletal abnormalities, impaired neuromuscular activity and defective clotting mechanisms. The causes of hypocalcaemia are presented in Table 3.5.

Assessment

History Hypoparathyroidism (may also be a surgical complication of thyroid surgery), chronic alcoholism, malnutrition, etc.

Physical evidence Large-volume blood transfusion, etc.

Clinical manifestations of neuromuscular impairment may be found, such as tetany, increased reflex responses, circumoral and finger tingling, positive Trousseau's and Chvostek's signs (indicate latent tetany) (see Box 3.1 and Fig. 3.6). Other neurological signs include confusion, memory loss and seizures.

Table 3.5 The causes of hypocalcaemia

Cause	Physiological process
Inadequate intake	Reduced total body calcium
Vitamin D deficiency	Reduced calcium absorption
Hypoparathyroidism	Inability to release calcium from bone
Hyperphosphataemia	Reduced serum calcium
Hypomagnesaemia	Decreased action of parathyroid hormone (PTH)
Alkalosis	Increased binding of calcium to protein
Acute pancreatitis	Decreased PTH hypoalbuminaemia
Hypoalbuminaemia	Reduces bound calcium only
Large-volume blood transfusion	Increased citrate intake binds with calcium

■ BOX 3.1

Trousseau's sign

This is a sign of carpal spasm induced by ischaemia. It can be elicited by placing a blood pressure cuff around the patient's arm and leaving it inflated for 2 minutes, at a pressure greater than the patient's systolic pressure.

Chvostek's sign

This is typified by unilateral contraction of eyelid and facial muscles. It results from irritation of the facial nerve which can be provoked by tapping the side of the face, just in front of the ear.

Kussmaul's respirations

A typical slow, deep breathing associated with respiratory acidosis.

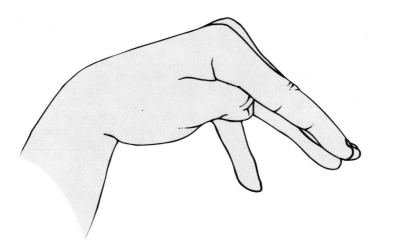

Fig. 3.6 Trousseau's sign. (After Ezrin et al 1979, with permission.)

Tests include:

- Serum calcium < 2.1 mmol/L
- Prolonged clotting times
- ECG – changes may include dysrhythmias and prolonged Q–T interval and S–T segment may be apparent (Fig. 3.5)
- Serum phosphate and magnesium concentrations – these may assist in identifying the cause.

Management The initial aim of management is to prevent injury to the patient (if there is evidence of central nervous system impairment), and monitoring of neurological status is indicated. Hypocalcaemia may reduce myocardial contractility, leading to heart failure and pulmonary oedema, so vital signs and ECG should be monitored. Correction of hypocalcaemia is achieved in the short term by the cautious administration of i.v. calcium gluconate as an infusion. It should be noted that i.v. administration of calcium is a particular risk in patients who are receiving digoxin therapy, as calcium can sensitize the heart to digoxin. Longer-term treatment will depend on the cause.

Hypercalcaemia

Hypercalcaemia is defined as a serum calcium greater than 2.6 mmol/L and is caused by either an increased intake and absorption of calcium or a decreased excretion. Decreased loss of calcium in the urine may occur due to conditions which cause increased secretion of parathyroid hormone and calcitonin. Other causes of hypercalcaemia are presented in Table 3.6.

Assessment

History Acute pancreatitis, bone deformity, hyperparathyroidism, etc.

Physical evidence Calcium substitute use, etc.

Clinical manifestations of neurological impairment of the central nervous system may be apparent, e.g. confusion, depression, etc. Hyperparathyroidism can lead to a reduced glomerular filtration rate (GFR) and renal stone formation due to precipitation of calcium. Calcification of soft tissue may also occur.

Tests include:

- Serum calcium > 2.6 mmol/L

Table 3.6 Causes of hypercalcaemia

Cause	Physiological process
Use of calcium supplements	Increased calcium intake
Increased vitamin D intake	Increased absorption of calcium
Medication	
antacids	Containing calcium
thiazides	Decreased calcium excretion
lithium	Inhibits action of ADH
Hyperthyroidism	Increased calcitonin release
Hyperparathyroidism	Increased parathyroid hormone secretion leads to increased calcium release from bone
Renal tubule disease	Increased renal loss of calcium
Hypophosphataemia	Inverse reciprocal relationship with calcium
Malignancy	Humoral factors increase calcium release from bone
Tuberculosis, sarcoidosis	Increased calcium release from bone

- Bone density – reduced on X-ray
- ECG – may show shortened S–T segment and Q–T interval (see Fig. 3.5).

Management Protecting the patient from injury is of prime importance if there is neurological impairment. Correction of the hypercalcaemia can be achieved by the administration of loop diuretics (e.g. frusemide) to encourage calcium excretion, together with i.v. infusion of sodium chloride 0.9% to enhance the diuresis (by increasing the ECF volume). Careful monitoring of electrolyte levels is required to assess optimal correction. Other forms of treatment relate to the causative factors, e.g. haemodialysis for renal failure, partial parathyroidectomy (for hyperparathyroidism) and the use of i.v. phosphates to correct hypophosphataemia.

Magnesium

Magnesium is mainly found in the ICF and bone and is related to calcium and phosphorus. Its concentration is largely regulated by the kidneys and ranges from 0.7 to 1.2 mmol/L. Magnesium influences neuromuscular irritability and is important in cardiac and skeletal muscle contraction. It also has an effect on peripheral vasodilatation and hence blood pressure and cardiac output.

Hypomagnesaemia

This is generally defined as a serum magnesium level less than 0.7 mmol/L and results from a loss of magnesium due to vomiting, diuretic therapy, etc. or from fluid and electrolyte changes associated with other imbalances, e.g. hypercalcaemia. The clinical presentation is usually one of altered neuronal activity similar to calcium disorders. Stridor is a major risk due to airway obstruction and ECG changes, and dysrhythmias may also occur (Fig. 3.5). Management aims to protect the patient from injury and to replace the magnesium very slowly.

Hypermagnesaemia

Hypermagnesaemia usually occurs with a serum magnesium greater than 1.2 mmol/L, due to dietary increase in magnesium (supplements, antacids, etc.), fluid and electrolyte shifts, or inadequate excretion. The clinical presentation may be similar to hyperkalaemia, including cardiac dysrhythmias. Management includes good monitoring and the administration of calcium gluconate to counteract the cardiac effects of the increased magnesium.

Phosphorus

Phosphorus is the major anion of ICF with a normal serum concentration of 0.8–1.5 mmol/L. As part of the phospholipid layer, it helps to maintain cell membrane integrity and is also an important component of teeth and bones. Phosphorus is essential for metabolism of fats, carbohydrates and protein, and for normal function of muscles, nervous system and red blood cells. It promotes energy transfer to cells (adenosine triphosphate) and acts as a urinary buffer to maintain acid–base balance.

Hypophosphataemia

This occurs when the serum phosphorus level falls below 0.8 mmol/L and may be caused by inadequate intake, excessive loss (GI tract loss or diuretics), cation exchange (e.g. hypokalaemia, etc.) or endocrine disorders (e.g. hyperparathyroidism, aldosteronism). Neurological manifestations include muscle weakness, fatigue, nystagmus and seizures. Platelet dysfunction may also occur. Impaired oxygen release, due to a reduction in 2,3-diphosphoglycerate (2,3-DPG) in erythrocytes, may lead to rapid, shallow breathing.

Management aims to replace the phosphate deficit. Monitoring for hypercalcaemia is indicated as this can be a concomitant problem.

Hyperphosphataemia

This exists when the serum phosphorus level exceeds 1.5 mmol/L. It should be noted that the reference range for children is higher. The main causes of hyperphosphataemia are renal failure, hypoparathyroidism, cellular destruction (with subsequent release of phosphates), vitamin D toxicity and enema use. Neuromuscular dysfunction may present as muscle spasms, tetany, circumoral paraesthesiae and positive Chvostek's and Trousseau's signs (Box 3.1). Soft tissue calcifications are associated with long-term hyperphosphataemia.

Care must be taken to protect the patient from harm, as seizures may occur. Aluminium hydroxide, a phosphate binding drug, may be administered to decrease serum levels. Calcium supplements may be required to raise serum calcium levels, thereby reducing the level of phosphate. Serum electrolyte concentrations need to be monitored.

FLUID AND ELECTROLYTE REPLACEMENT THERAPY

The aim of i.v. therapy is to restore or maintain normal fluid volume and electrolyte balance when the oral route is not possible. In this chapter, nutritional needs will not be considered and it should be noted that the normal i.v. crystalline fluids only provide sufficient kilocalories to limit starvation and catabolism. The infusion of i.v. fluids alters the composition of plasma by the addition of fluid and electrolytes and needs to be approached with caution, if fluid overload, fluid deficit, fluid shifts and unwanted alterations in electrolyte concentrations are to be avoided. The reader will appreciate that careful monitoring is essential, if the optimal outcome for the patient is to be achieved. While general guidelines are available for i.v. fluid and electrolyte replacement (e.g. Joint Formulary Committee 1997), it is essential that any regimen is tailored to the individual needs of the patient. The indications for i.v. fluid replacement include:

■ **BOX 3.2**

Assessment of need for intravenous fluid and electrolyte therapy

- Vital signs
- Fluid intake and output measurement
- Daily weighing
- Skin turgor
- Jugular vein filling
- Urinary specific gravity
- Central venous pressure measurement
- Serum electrolyte levels
- Arterial blood gas analysis

- replacement of abnormal fluid and electrolyte losses, some of which are described in this chapter
- maintenance of normal fluid and electrolyte balance, if the oral route cannot be used
- correction of fluid and electrolyte disorders
- promoting renal function.

Assessment of the patient's needs may involve visual observations of the patient, vital signs and laboratory tests as indicated in Box 3.2.

The fluids used for replacement therapy belong to two main types: crystalline and colloid.

Crystalline solutions

Crystalline solutions are electrolyte solutions and are categorized according to their tonicity (compared with plasma osmolar concentration). There are three types:

- isotonic
- hypotonic
- hypertonic.

The contents of selected i.v. replacement solutions are presented in Table 3.7.

Isotonic solutions

Isotonic solutions have the same osmolality as plasma and, when infused, expand both the ICF and ECF equally. Such fluids do not alter the osmolality of the vascular compartment. Examples of isotonic solutions are dextrose 5%, sodium chloride 0.9%, dextrose 4% with sodium chloride 0.18%, compound sodium lactate and Plasma–Lyte 148 (Baxter Healthcare 1989, Joint Formulary Committee 1997, Lund 1994, Royal Pharmaceutical Society 1996).

Dextrose 5% It should be noted that even though the patient may only require water replacement, it is not possible to infuse distilled water, because it would cause haemolysis of erythrocytes where it entered the vein. Dextrose 5% is therefore used instead, as it is metabolized to water and carbon dioxide. It is used to replace water deficits, because it moves into all fluid compartments. It should never be used as the sole means of expanding ECF, because it can cause dilution of the sodium concentration.

Sodium chloride 0.9% (normal saline) This solution contains 150 mmol/L of sodium and 150 mmol/L of chloride, but is not a physiological solution, because the amounts are not equal to those of ECF. Indeed, the chloride is considerably greater

Table 3.7 Contents of selected intravenous replacement solutions

Solution	Tonicity	Contents
Dextrose 5%	Isotonic	Glucose 50 g
Sodium chloride 0.9%	Isotonic	Na$^+$ 150 mmol/L
		Cl$^-$ 150 mmol/L
Dextrose 4% with sodium chloride 0.18%	Isotonic	Glucose 40 g
		Na$^+$ 30 mmol/L
		Cl$^-$ 30 mmol/L
Compound sodium lactate	Isotonic	Na$^+$ 131 mmol/L
		Ca^{2+} 2.0 mmol/L
		K$^+$ 5.0 mmol/L
		Cl$^-$ 111 mmol/L
		Lactate 29 mmol/L
Plasma-Lyte 148	Isotonic	Na$^+$ 140 mmol/L
		K$^+$ 5 mmol/L
		Mg^{2+} 1.5 mmol/L
		Cl$^-$ 98 mmol/L
		Gluconate 23 mmol/L
		Acetate 27 mmol/L
Sodium chloride 0.45%	Hypotonic	Na$^+$ 75 mmol/L
		Cl$^-$ 75 mmol/L
Sodium chloride 1.8%	Hypertonic	Na$^+$ 300 mmol/L
		Cl$^-$ 300 mmol/L
Dextrose 10%	Hypertonic	Dextrose 100 g
Sodium bicarbonate 1.26%		Na$^+$ 150 mmol/L
		HCO$_3^-$ 150 mmol/L
Sodium bicarbonate 4.2%		Na$^+$ 500 mmol/L
		HCO$_3^-$ 500 mmol/L
Sodium bicarbonate 8.4%		Na$^+$ 1000 mmol/L
		HCO$_3^-$ 1000 mmol/L

than that in the ECF (105 mmol/L) and may pose an increased burden on the kidneys, with a risk of hyperchloraemic acidosis if excretion is impaired (Metheney 1992). Sodium chloride 0.9% should be used with caution in patients with renal disorders. It is, however, the solution of choice for expanding the ECF volume, because it does not enter the ICF.

Dextrose 4% with sodium chloride 0.18% This solution is commonly used for postoperative fluid maintenance. It is used to infuse water with a reduced sodium content.

Compound sodium lactate (Ringer's lactate, Hartmann's solution) This solution is designed to be a near-physiological solution of balanced electrolytes. It contains less chloride than sodium chloride 0.9%, and provides bicarbonate (when the lactate is metabolized), which may be useful in treating metabolic acidosis. However, it is contraindicated in patients with lactic acidosis, if they are unable to convert the lactate (Metheney 1992).

Plasma-Lyte 148 This solution is another balanced electrolyte solution and the bicarbonate precursors are acetate and gluconate. It is used for fluid and electrolyte restoration.

Hypotonic solutions

These have a lower osmolality than plasma and contain less particles than plasma.

As a result, fluid shifts from the ECF into the ICF to achieve equilibrium. In excess, this may cause the cells to swell and they may even rupture. An example of these solutions is sodium chloride 0.45% (or less).

Sodium chloride 0.45% This is half-strength normal saline and is a useful solution for replacing water in patients who have hypovolaemia with hypernatraemia. However, excessive use may lead to hyponatraemia due to dilution of sodium, especially in patients who are prone to water retention.

Hypertonic solutions

When compared with plasma, these solutions have a higher concentration of particles. Hypertonic solutions cause fluid to move out of the cells into the ECF in order to equalize the concentration of particles between the two compartments. This has the effect of causing the cells to shrink, which may disrupt their function. Meanwhile, the ECF volume expands and care is required to ensure that this does not precipitate a fluid volume excess and overload. It should be remembered that hypertonic solutions tend to irritate peripheral veins. The common hypertonic solutions are Plasma-Lyte 148 with dextrose 5% (Baxter Healthcare 1989), sodium chloride and dextrose solutions.

Plasma-Lyte 148 with dextrose 5% This is a solution with the same electrolyte content as Plasma-Lyte 148, but which also contains dextrose. It is useful for intraoperative fluid replacement and may be indicated for use in babies and small children to minimize hyperglycaemia.

Sodium chloride 1.8% This solution is used to correct severe hyponatraemia. It needs to be infused very slowly to avoid the risk of overload, as previously mentioned, and some patients may require diuretic therapy to assist fluid excretion. Triple-strength saline (2.7%) is also available.

Dextrose 10% This may be used to provide kilocalories for the patient in the short term, but it is only sufficient to ward off the ketosis of starvation (Metheney 1992). One litre of dextrose 10% only provides 380 kcal. Hypertonic dextrose is also available in 20, 25 and 50% strengths, and the volume varies according to strength.

Colloid solutions

Colloid solutions are not electrolyte solutions, but rather fluids which contain solutes of a high molecular weight. They are hypertonic solutions which, when infused into the vascular compartment, exert an osmotic 'pull' on fluids from the interstitial and extracellular spaces. This means that they are particularly useful for expanding the intravascular volume and raising blood pressure. However, in susceptible patients this may lead to the risk of heart failure.

Colloid solutions are used to:

- correct hypotension
- expand intravascular volume
- mobilize third space fluids
- restore serum protein levels
- restore albumin levels.

The common colloid solutions include dextrans, hetastarch, gelatin, human albumin, plasma protein fraction and fresh frozen plasma. However, in view of the availability of other solutions, fresh frozen plasma should be reserved for specific situations other than intravascular fluid expansion. Its use is discussed in Chapter 13.

Dextrans These are polysaccharides which act as colloids and are available in two types: low-molecular-weight (LMW) dextrans and high-molecular-weight (HMW) dextrans. The molecular weight is denoted by the number, e.g. dextran 40 (LMW 40 000) and dextran 70 or 110 (HMW 70 000 or 110 000). Both types are available in a solution of either sodium chloride 0.9% or dextrose 5%. LMW dextrans are used to improve the microcirculation in patients with poor peripheral solution, while HMW dextrans are indicated in patients with hypovolaemia and hypotension. Patients require careful monitoring during infusion and incidences of urticarial and anaphylactoid reactions have been reported (Joint Formulary Committee 1997).

Hetastarch (Hespan) This is a synthetic colloid which, as its name suggests, is made from starch. It is used to increase the intravascular fluid, but may also interfere with coagulation. Haemodynamic monitoring is necessary to avoid the risk of circulatory overload. The incidence of anaphylaxis is less than that associated with dextrans. Hetastarch is excreted via the kidneys, so its use in patients with renal disease is contraindicated.

Gelatin (Haemaccel, Gelofusine) This has a lower molecular weight than the dextrans and therefore remains in the circulation for a shorter period. Its haemodynamic action is about 2–3 hours and excretion is via the kidneys.

Human albumin (Buminate) This solution is derived from plasma. There are two strengths: 4.5% (isotonic) and 20–25% (hypertonic: equivalent to five times the osmotic activity of plasma). The former is used to increase the circulating volume and restore protein levels (e.g. hypoproteinaemia and hypoalbuminaemia) in conditions such as burns, acute pancreatitis and acute plasma loss. The latter is used, together with sodium and water restriction, to reduce excessive oedema (Joint Formulary Committee 1997).

Plasma protein fraction (PPF) This is also prepared from plasma and, like albumin, is heat treated during preparation. It is recommended for slow infusion to increase the circulating volume.

ACID–BASE BALANCE

For cells to function at an optimal level, they require an environment with a stable pH. The maintenance of a stable pH level is achieved by the regulation of acids and bases in the body fluids, particularly in the ECF. Acids are substances which can release hydrogen ions, while bases can accept hydrogen ions. The pH is a measure of hydrogen ion concentration; the main determinant is the ratio of acid (carbonic acid) to base (bicarbonate), the normal ratio being 1:20. The pH level of blood, expressed as a numerical value, is inversely proportional to the number of hydrogen ions present. This means that the blood pH rises as the hydrogen ion concentration falls, and vice versa. Normal blood pH ranges from 7.35 to 7.45. If the pH falls below 6.8 or rises above 7.8, this is incompatible with life. A patient's acid–base balance can be determined by arterial blood gas analysis; in children, capillary blood may be used. Acidosis is defined as a blood pH < 7.35 and represents an increase in hydrogen ions or a decrease in bicarbonate ions. Alkalosis is defined as a blood pH > 7.45 and represents a decrease in hydrogen ions or an increase in bicarbonate ions. Changes in bicarbonate ion levels are associated with metabolic acid–base disturbances.

Acids

Most of the acids in the body result from metabolic processes (see Fig. 3.7). A metabolic process involves the conversion of either dietary or stored fuel to energy in the form of adenosine triphosphate (ATP) or an energy store such as glycogen and

Fig. 3.7 Production of acids. (From: HUMAN ANATOMY AND PHYSIOLOGY, by Elaine Marieb; Copyright © 1989 by Benjamin Cummings Publishing Company, Reprinted by permission.)

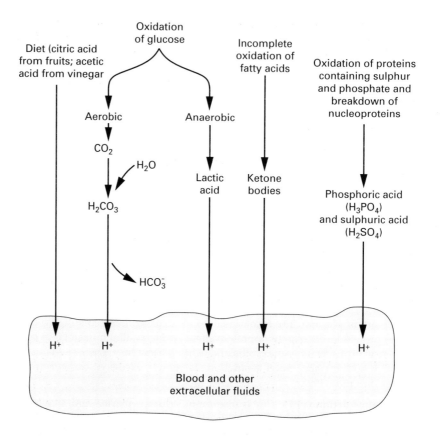

triglyceride (Halperin & Goldstein 1994). The increase in hydrogen ions generated by oxidation of fuel sources needs to be 'neutralized' in order to maintain the normal pH of body fluids. This is achieved when the excess hydrogen ions combine with either acids or bases, thereby forming substances which do not have an effect on the pH – this is otherwise known as 'buffering'.

Buffers

The main buffers include:

- protein
- bicarbonate
- phosphate
- ammonium.

Buffers occur in most body fluids and can respond immediately to changes in tissue fluid pH. The buffering systems involved include protein, bone, respiratory and renal systems.

Buffering systems

Protein buffer system

The protein buffer system is concerned with regulation of the pH in ICF. Haemoglobin is the major protein involved and acts as a buffer to carbonic acid, which is produced in large amounts as a result of metabolic activity in the tissues. In the lungs, the acid dissociates to carbon dioxide and water, which is excreted via respiration. Carbonic acid is important because, during the buffering process, haemoglobin loses its affinity for oxygen and therefore oxygen transport to the tissues is enhanced.

Phosphates are also important in maintaining the pH within erythrocytes, as well as renal tubular fluid.

Bone buffering system

Bone also takes part in buffering acids. However, prolonged acid loading causes an increased excretion of calcium from the bone, which may present in chronic renal failure due metabolic acidosis.

Respiratory system

The respiratory system provides the initial regulation of acid–base balance, by buffering and excreting carbonic acid (in the form of carbon dioxide and water). The lungs use carbon dioxide to regulate hydrogen ion concentration. Carbon dioxide combines with water to form carbonic acid; in the presence of carbonic anhydrase, this dissociates to carbon dioxide and water in the lungs, which can then be excreted during respiration. The following equation expresses this action:

$$CO_2 + H_2O \leftrightharpoons H_2CO_3 \leftrightharpoons H^+ + HCO_3^-$$

The free hydrogen ion, generated with carbonic acid, is buffered by haemoglobin.

The respiratory centre is directly affected by alterations in hydrogen ion concentration in the blood and within minutes can alter respiratory rate and depth to compensate. For example, an increase in hydrogen ions causes acidaemia, so respiration is increased to enhance carbon dioxide (acid) elimination. Conversely, if hydrogen ions are reduced (alkalosis), respiration is decreased to allow carbon dioxide (acid) retention. However, it should be noted that the respiratory system can only provide a short-term response; it is the renal system which provides longer term compensation.

Renal system

Bicarbonate buffering system The kidneys can provide a more permanent regulation of changes in acid–base balance, by adjusting the acidity or alkalinity of the urine, but the rate of response varies from hours to days. The primary buffering system is the use of bicarbonate ions, which involves the reabsorption of bicarbonate and secretion of hydrogen ions in response to acidosis, and the excretion of bicarbonate (together with sodium) when there is alkalosis.

Phosphate buffering system This occurs in body fluids and the tubules. It aids excretion of hydrogen ions in the urine and is important for maintaining the pH of urine.

Ammonium buffering system The metabolism of glutamine (an amino acid) in epithelial cells produces ammonia, which diffuses across the cell membrane into the tubule. Here it combines with actively secreted hydrogen ions to form ammonium sulphate, which is excreted in the urine. Hence hydrogen ions are excreted.

It is important to note that potassium can also be exchanged for hydrogen ions in order to alter pH. However, in renal disease this compensatory mechanism leads to hyperkalaemia, if oliguria or anuria are present.

Although the body's buffering systems are able to maintain optimal acid–base balance and therefore pH level in body fluids, following trauma or during the disease process imbalances can occur.

ACID–BASE IMBALANCES

Acid–base imbalances are usually referred to as respiratory or metabolic depending on the cause. Respiratory imbalances are caused by either inadequate or excessive respiration. Metabolic imbalances are usually caused by excessive hydrogen ion production from metabolic processes, or disorders of the GI and renal systems.

Acidosis refers to excessive increase in hydrogen ions or decrease in bicarbonate ions, while alkalosis is the reverse. The following imbalances will be considered:

- respiratory acidosis
- respiratory alkalosis
- metabolic acidosis
- metabolic alkalosis.

Respiratory acidosis

Respiratory acidosis is caused by decreased alveolar ventilation, which results in carbon dioxide retention. This increases carbonic acid and hydrogen ion levels with a concomitant drop in blood pH. Decreased alveolar ventilation may be due to inadequate respiration or intermittent positive pressure ventilation (IPPV), respiratory obstruction, inadequate respiratory effort or cardiovascular disorders. Specific causes are presented in Table 3.8.

Assessment

History Bronchospasm, pulmonary oedema, head injury, drug overdose, etc.

Physical evidence Agitation, airway obstruction, flail chest dyspnoea, etc.

Clinical manifestations include breathlessness, cyanosis and sweating. The increased carbon dioxide retention may lead to cerebral oedema and papilloedema; the patient may complain of headache and blurred vision.

Tests include:

- Arterial blood gas analysis – $P_aCO_2 > 40$ mmHg or 5.3 kpa, pH < 7.4
- Serum bicarbonate – in chronic acidosis, to assess level of compensation

Table 3.8 Causes of respiratory acidosis

Cause	Contributing factors
Inadequate respiration	Hypoventilation (spontaneous)
	Inadequate intermittent positive pressure ventilation (IPPV)
	Abdominal distension
	Chest injury
	Pneumonia
Inadequate respiratory effort	CNS depression
	Drug overdose
	Neuromuscular impairment
Respiratory obstruction	Laryngospasm
	Bronchospasm
	Chronic obstructive airways disease (COAD)
	Aspiration
Cardiovascular disorders	Cardiac arrest
	Pulmonary oedema

Fig. 3.8 Fowler's position.

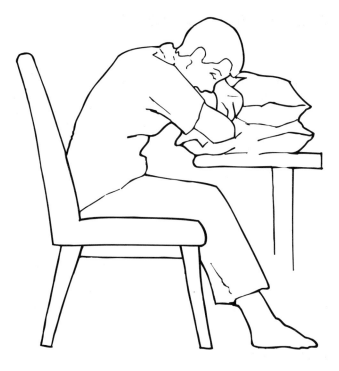

- Serum electrolytes – if hyperkalaemia is suspected
- Chest X-ray – to identify extent of the trauma, disease, aspiration, etc.

Management

This will vary depending on the cause, i.e. mechanical obstruction should be relieved, IPPV should be adjusted, etc. If breathlessness is severe or the patient is agitated, reassurance should be given. Vital signs (particularly respiration) and arterial blood gases should be monitored. In chronic acidosis, i.v. fluids may be administered if fluid intake is reduced, in order to loosen secretions. Optimal positioning, e.g. Fowler's position, may assist respiration (see Fig. 3.8). Physiotherapy and suction therapy may be required to manage impaired secretion removal. Oxygen therapy may be indicated if hypoxia is present. Caution is needed to avoid removing the hypoxic drive for respiration in chronic pulmonary disease.

Respiratory alkalosis

Respiratory alkalosis is caused by increased alveolar ventilation, leading to a reduction in serum carbon dioxide levels. Respiratory compensation is usually adequate, so the condition may have resolved in the time it takes for renal compensatory mechanisms to act. Acute respiratory alkalosis is often due to anxiety (with hyperventilation), but may result from pulmonary disorders or conditions leading to hypoxaemia. Chronic respiratory alkalosis may be caused by brain tumours, Gram-negative septicaemia and fever.

Assessment

History Anaemia, pneumonia, cardiac failure, hyperventilation (IPPV), high-altitude acclimatization, etc.

Physical evidence Anxiety with hyperventilation, fever, etc.

Clinical manifestations include confusion, fainting, tetany, paraesthesiae, etc.

Tests include:

- ECG – to detect cardiac dysrhythmias
- Arterial blood gases
  - $PaCO_2 < 40$ mmHg or < 5.3 kPa (acute)
  - $PaCO_2 < 35$ mmHg or < 4.6 kPa (chronic)
  - pH > 7.4
  - PaO_2 reduced, if hypoxia is present
- Serum electrolytes – to assess compensation, if the condition is chronic
- Serum phosphate – may drop, as phosphate moves into the ICF
- Serum bicarbonate – decreased, as renal compensation occurs (7–9 days).

Management

The patient will require reassurance, particularly if anxiety is the cause; sedation or tranquillizers may be indicated. Carbon dioxide levels may be increased by encouraging the patient to breathe in and out of a paper bag, which promotes rebreathing.

In chronic respiratory alkalosis, renal compensation results in a decreased serum bicarbonate. The underlying cause needs to be treated. However, oxygen therapy may be required if hypoxia is also present, e.g. heart disease associated with cyanosis. Monitoring of blood gas analysis is indicated.

Metabolic acidosis

Metabolic acidosis is caused by an excessive loss of alkali (base) or accumulation of acid. Loss of base in the form of bicarbonate occurs via the gastrointestinal tract or kidneys. Accumulation of acid is caused by anaerobic metabolism when cells are deprived of oxygen (e.g. burns, trauma, etc.), and also when increased energy utilization necessitates the metabolism of fat stores (e.g. in starvation and diabetes mellitus). The resultant acidosis leads to a drop in serum pH and an increase in hydrogen ion concentration; the latter stimulates chemoreceptors, and respiration is increased. The increase in respiration, which is the initial compensatory mechanism, enhances carbon dioxide elimination and lowers the plasma carbon dioxide level. The kidneys also help to eliminate hydrogen ions by means of the bicarbonate buffering system. Some of the specific causes of metabolic acidosis are presented in Table 3.9.

Table 3.9 Causes of metabolic acidosis

Cause	Physiological process
Salicylate, alcohol poisoning	Formation of non-carbonic acid
Diuretic therapy	Loss of bicarbonate, hyperkalaemia (if potassium-sparing drugs)
Diarrhoea	Loss of bicarbonate
Diabetic ketoacidosis	Increased fat metabolism
Hyperalimentation solutions	Increased acid, if lactate not given
Acute and chronic renal failure	Inability to excrete acids
Burns, trauma, shock	Increased lactic acid production
Glaucoma	Carbonic anhydrase inhibitor therapy causes bicarbonate diuresis (Willatts 1987)

It should also be noted that hydrogen ions enter the cell (to be buffered) in exchange for potassium, so alterations in potassium level are associated with acidosis.

Assessment

History Salicylate poisoning, diuretic therapy, etc.

Physical evidence Diarrhoea, burns, trauma, etc.

Clinical manifestations include Kussmaul's respirations (Box 3.1) and peripheral vasodilation with flushed, warm dry skin. Hypotension and cold, clammy skin is also seen in shock. Acidotic effects on the nervous system may cause confusion, headache and loss of consciousness. Cardiac dysrhythmias may occur in response to altered potassium levels. Patients with diabetes may have 'fruity' breath which is similar to the smell of 'pear drops'.

Tests include:

- Arterial blood gas analysis
  - pH < 7.35
  - (if compensated) $PaCO_2$ < 35 mmHg or < 4.6 kPa
- Serum bicarbonate < 22 mmol/L – also to assess metabolic compensation
- Serum electrolytes – to detect any imbalance, e.g. changes in potassium level are common, particularly hyperkalaemia (serum level > 5.5 mmol/L)
- ECG – to detect changes associated with alterations in potassium level (Fig. 3.5).

Management

Alterations in level of consciousness put the patient at risk of injury, so protection is necessary. The main aim of treatment is to reduce the acidosis. However, if hypokalaemia is present, this should be treated first, as correction of the acidosis with sodium bicarbonate could cause severe hypokalaemia when potassium moves back into the cells in exchange for hydrogen ions (see 'Hypokalaemia', p. 57). Close monitoring of ECG and vital signs is necessary.

Correction of the acidosis with sodium bicarbonate is indicated if the pH is less than 7.2, to avoid the threat of cardiac depression and dysrhythmias. The efficacy of treatment is monitored by arterial blood gas analysis, as there is no accurate means of estimating the dose required. It is important to ensure that, except in emergency situations, sodium bicarbonate is administered slowly to avoid over-compensation.

Interventions should also aim to treat the underlying cause. For example, the hyperglycaemic patient with metabolic acidosis will require the administration of insulin, which will also help to lower the concomitant hyperglycaemia associated with acidosis. The infusion of sodium chloride 0.9% will also enhance the reduction of potassium. In renal failure, haemodialysis will be required to correct any imbalance. Lactic acidosis in cardiovascular shock requires i.v. fluid replacement (to increase the blood volume and blood pressure) and management of tissue hypoxia. Treatment with sodium bicarbonate is controversial, because it may cause depression of the central nervous system (Eccles 1993). The reason is that, when the sodium bicarbonate buffers the lactic acid, carbon dioxide is released which easily passes across cell membranes. Carbon dioxide can therefore enter the cerebrospinal fluid and cause depression of the central nervous system.

Metabolic alkalosis

Metabolic alkalosis is caused by an excessive loss of hydrogen ions or excessive

Table 3.10 Causes of metabolic alkalosis

Cause	Physiological process
Vomiting, nasogastric suction	Loss of acid
Milk alkali syndrome	Excessive intake of alkali, hypercalcaemia
Diuretic therapy	Potassium loss
Cushing's syndrome	Potassium loss
Hyperaldosteronism	Potassium loss
Intravenous sodium bicarbonate	Overcompensation of acidosis
Large-volume blood transfusion	Citrate in donor blood is metabolized to bicarbonate

retention of bicarbonate ions. The main mechanisms involved are loss of hydrogen ions from the gastrointestinal tract, deficient bicarbonate excretion via the kidneys and diuretic therapy. The most common cause of hydrogen ion loss is from the gastrointestinal tract, via vomiting or nasogastric suction. Hydrochloric acid production in the stomach is associated with secretion of bicarbonate ions into the blood. These ions would then be used in the digestive juices to neutralize the chyme as it enters the duodenum. However, when gastric contents are expelled during vomiting, digestive juices are not stimulated, the bicarbonate ions are not utilized and so the serum bicarbonate level rises. Loss of acid increases the pH level in the blood and hydrogen ions are reduced. This inhibits chemoreceptor stimulation and reduces respiration. Hypoventilation allows carbon dioxide levels in the blood to rise in order to try to balance the excessive bicarbonate level. However, this compensation is limited, because a degree of hypoxia develops which then stimulates respiration (Eccles 1993).

Reduction of hydrogen ions also causes an increased dissociation rate of carbonic acid (in an effort to increase the hydrogen ion level) and more bicarbonate is produced and conserved by the kidneys. The conservation of bicarbonate results in an increased loss of hydrogen, potassium and chloride ions. Both bicarbonate and chloride compete to combine with sodium and, as chloride levels fall (during binding), bicarbonate levels rise in order to balance the sodium. Examples of specific causes of metabolic alkalosis are presented in Table 3.10.

Assessment

History Primary aldosteronism, diuretic therapy, etc.

Physical evidence Vomiting, nasogastric suction, etc.

Clinical manifestations relate to changes in mental function, e.g. apathy, confusion and seizures. With severe hypokalaemia, neuromuscular changes may be apparent, e.g. tetany, positive Trousseau's and Chvostek's signs (Box 3.1). The respiratory rate is decreased and the patient may experience dizziness.

Tests include:

- Arterial blood gases
  — pH = 7.45–7.6
  — $PaCO_2$ = 38–45 mmHg or 5.06–6.0 kPa
  — if acute: bicarbonate > 26 mmol/L
  — if chronic: bicarbonate > 45 mmol/L
    (Note: values vary with level of compensation)
- Serum levels of potassium and chloride – decreased (relative to sodium)
- ECG – may show changes related to hypokalaemia (Fig. 3.5).

Management

The patient's safety must be maintained if there are any signs of altered consciousness. Monitoring includes vital signs (particularly respiratory patterns), ECG, fluid intake and output, serum electrolyte levels and arterial blood gas analysis. The precipitating factors need to be addressed. For example, anti-emetics and fluid replacement for vomiting may be indicated, while review of diuretic therapy will reduce the risk for those patients with fluid retention problems.

FLUID, ELECTROLYTE AND ACID–BASE IMBALANCES

Overview

Imbalances occur when the normal homeostatic mechanisms of the body are unable to operate. The main processes involved in fluid and electrolyte imbalances relate to:

- decreased intake and increased excretion which lead to deficiency
- increased intake and decreased excretion which lead to excess.

Acid–base imbalances are caused by metabolic conditions which affect the normal mechanisms of regulation.

Gastrointestinal loss

Gastrointestinal loss of fluid and electrolytes commonly results from vomiting, diarrhoea, fistulae, gastric suctioning, infection, inflammatory disease, etc. In the upper GI tract, the fluids contain high levels of potassium, sodium, chloride and hydrogen ions. For this reason, loss of fluid from the stomach and upper intestine often results in hypokalaemia and metabolic alkalosis. In contrast, fluids from the lower GI tract tend to be alkaline due to a high level of bases, which means that excessive loss due to diarrhoea may result in metabolic acidosis.

Management

Monitoring of serum electrolyte levels, together with fluid intake and output, is necessary. Correction of any imbalance is generally achieved by administering i.v. fluids and electrolyte replacements, as indicated. Estimation of the degree of metabolic disturbance may be achieved by arterial blood gas analysis.

Renal disease

The kidneys are the main regulators of fluid, electrolyte and acid–base balance in the body. Imbalances are due to failure of the buffering systems. Renal failure is often categorized into two types: acute and chronic. Acute renal failure is generally regarded as a reversible condition with a sudden onset, while chronic renal failure is generally considered as irreversible with a longer, more insidious onset. Other renal disorders contributing to disordered buffering include glomerulonephritis, pyelonephritis, acute tubular necrosis, renal calculi and tumours.

The main contributing factors to renal damage are decreased renal perfusion (e.g. major trauma, shock, third space losses, etc.), infection, damage to the renal parenchyma and nephrotoxic agents (e.g. sulphonamides, frusemide, lead, etc.). The imbalances resulting from inadequate renal compensation depend on the type of renal damage:

- If the glomerulus is defective, filtration into the capsule is altered so that excess fluid and electrolytes can pass. The buffering systems fail, resulting in metabolic acidosis.

Table 3.11 Electrolyte imbalances in renal disease

Imbalance	Physiological process
Hyperkalaemia	Potassium excretion reduced
Hyperphosphataemia	Inability to excrete phosphorus
Hypocalcaemia	Reciprocal relationship between calcium and phosphorus
Hypermagnesaemia	Inability to excrete magnesium

- Tubular damage causes altered permeability, which results in abnormal excretion.
- Hormonal levels in the kidney are affected in renal disease. Low renal perfusion causes an increased renin release, which results in hypertension. Erythropoietin secretion is reduced and this leads to anaemia.
- High output of urine is associated with the polyuric phase of acute renal failure.
- Low output of urine is associated with electrolyte imbalance and uraemia. Oliguria and anuria result in hyperkalaemia, which may be asymptomatic up to a serum level of 6 mmol/L in acute renal failure and 7.5 mmol/L in chronic renal failure (Innerarity & Stark 1990).
- Hypervolaemia, due to oliguria, causes an excessive ECF volume which may precipitate peripheral and pulmonary oedema.
- Hypovolaemia may occur in the polyuric phase of acute renal failure, leading to hypotension.

The electrolyte imbalances which can occur in renal disease are presented in Table 3.11.

Management

The management will vary according to the type of renal disorder. Vital signs, fluid intake and output, and breathing (to detect the onset of pulmonary oedema) should be monitored. Haemodynamic monitoring may be indicated in some patients, and ECG monitoring will facilitate detection of changes due to hyperkalaemia and hypocalcaemia. Serum levels of urea and electrolytes need close monitoring. Arterial blood gas analysis is necessary to assess the level of metabolic acidosis and the degree to which correction is achieved. Intravenous sodium bicarbonate may be administered with caution, bearing in mind the risk of hypocalcaemia (caused by calcium binding with the bicarbonate) and possible hypernatraemia from repeat doses of sodium bicarbonate (due to increased sodium load, which may also precipitate pulmonary oedema).

Patients whose kidneys still respond to fluid excess may be given diuretics; others, in whom this is not possible, will require haemodialysis.

Syndrome of inappropriate antidiuretic hormone (SIADH)

SIADH is associated with excessive release of ADH, even when plasma osmolality is low. The condition may be caused by damage to the pituitary gland or its hypothalamic control (e.g. from head injury or during surgery) and some central nervous system disorders which raise intracranial pressure. Other causative factors include respiratory disorders and malignant tumours which, by various means, increase the secretion of ADH. The normal action of ADH is to increase the permeability of the renal tubule to water, in response to a reduced circulating volume, thus conserving water and increasing the blood volume. However, in SIADH, water conservation occurs regardless of the amount of circulating volume. As a result, the serum osmolality and serum sodium are reduced. An increased IVF volume leads to an increased glomerular filtration rate and inhibits the release of aldosterone, so sodium is lost in the urine, resulting in hyponatraemia. As sodium levels drop in the ECF, water moves into the cells down an osmotic gradient. In the brain, this increase in ICF can lead to neurological impairment due to cerebral oedema.

Management

Observation of the patient for signs of cerebral oedema is indicated, together with maintenance of the patient's safety. Monitoring of the patient's serum sodium levels and osmolality, weight, and fluid intake and output are indicated. Water intake should be restricted, while correction of the hyponatraemia with i.v. hypertonic saline can be achieved cautiously, using a volumetric control device to avoid overload.

Diabetes insipidus

This is caused by either a deficiency in the production or release of ADH, or a reduced renal response to ADH. It may have an idiopathic origin or be due to brain injury or tumour. The onset may be gradual or sudden depending on the cause. The condition is characterized by polydipsia and polyuria (with copious amounts of very dilute urine). The fluid balance may remain in equilibrium, if the fluid intake matches the output. Otherwise, there is rapid depletion of the ECF with a concomitant rise in serum sodium and osmolality. The resultant hypovolaemia may lead to shock and may also precipitate seizures or coma.

Management

Patient safety must be maintained. The hypovolaemia is corrected with hypotonic i.v. fluids and the underlying cause needs to be treated. The hypernatraemia may resolve with adequate fluid replacement. Diabetes insipidus of cerebral origin may be treated with a vasopressin analogue.

Diabetic ketoacidosis

This relates to either partial or total insulin deficiency in a patient with diabetes mellitus, but may also occur in patients with undiagnosed diabetes. The condition is associated with an inability to produce the necessary amount of insulin to cope with a crisis (e.g. stress, surgery or infection) or may result from a failure to administer an adequate amount of insulin (e.g. omission of a dose). If insufficient insulin is available, glucose cannot be utilized for the production of energy, so alternative sources have to be found, such as fat. Metabolism of fat leads to the production of ketone bodies (as an acid waste product) and results in metabolic acidosis. Both hyperglycaemia and ketosis lead to increased osmolality of ECF, causing a shift of fluid out of the cells. As a result of the increased osmolality, an osmotic diuresis occurs which is typified by the polyuria commonly seen in this condition. This resultant dehydration, when it occurs in the brain cells, can lead to neurological disturbances.

It should be noted that serum electrolytes may appear normal, because continuing catabolism (breakdown of the tissues) releases cations and water into the ECF. However, potassium levels may rise because insulin deficiency inhibits potassium movement into the cells, while acidosis encourages potassium to leave the cell. Dehydration tends to exacerbate the hyperkalaemia, as further sodium and potassium are excreted in response to the release of aldosterone. Dehydration may lead to lactic acidosis, if tissue perfusion is decreased. Failure to correct this situation leads to respiratory and renal compensation. Respiratory compensation results in Kussmaul's respirations, in order to correct the acidosis by excreting carbon dioxide, while the kidneys try to excrete excess acid in the form of ketonuria. Kussmaul's respirations are the typical slow, deep breaths associated with respiratory acidosis.

Concomitant electrolyte imbalances include hypokalaemia, hyponatraemia and hypophosphataemia.

Assessment

History Diabetes mellitus or signs and symptoms thereof, e.g. polyuria, etc.

Physical evidence Polyuria.

Clinical manifestations include fruity breath typically associated with ketosis. Neurological impairment may take the form of confusion and loss of consciousness. Loss of skin turgor may be apparent, if dehydration has occurred, and Kussmaul's respirations (see Box 3.1) denote a respiratory attempt to correct acidosis.

Tests include:

- Serum electrolytes – to determine extent of imbalance
- Arterial blood gases – to assess level of acidosis
- Blood glucose level – elevated
- Glycosuria and ketonuria are evident.

Management

The patient's safety is paramount. Correction of diabetic ketoacidosis is primarily concerned with correcting the dehydration and hyperglycaemia. Insulin needs to be titrated against blood glucose levels to ensure optimal correction. Intravenous sodium chloride 0.9% is often the solution of choice for rehydration, although hypotonic saline is useful to replace fluid loss, and compound sodium lactate may also be indicated to replace potassium 'loss' as it shifts from the ECF back into the cells. Fluid intake and output will need to be monitored, together with vital signs. Blood gas analysis is used to monitor the correction of the acidosis and to assess the need to administer i.v. sodium bicarbonate.

Hyperglycaemic hyperosmolar non-ketotic coma (HHNC)

This condition usually occurs with the onset of diabetes in middle-aged or elderly patients, but may occur in patients with non-insulin-dependent diabetes mellitus if there is a sudden progression in the disease state. It is a condition which is caused by an acute lack of insulin which results in hyperglycaemia, but is not severe enough to cause ketosis. As previously described, hyperglycaemia gives rise to an increased osmolality and osmotic diuresis, so there is risk of hypovolaemia, hyperkalaemia and hypophosphataemia. The water loss includes both ECF and ICF and, if severe, may cause the patient to lose up to 20% of the fluid volume. Depletion of the IVF volume causes increased viscosity of the blood, and in consequence the workload on the heart is increased. Increased blood viscosity, together with the patient's immobility, leads to the risk of blood stasis and the development of microemboli. Decreased perfusion of the kidneys and brain may lead to the possibility of fatal sequelae. The usual causes of this condition include inadequate secretion or action of insulin, excess dietary intake (i.e. inadequate insulin) and some drug therapies, e.g. phenytoin, thiazide diuretics, etc., which may suddenly be exacerbated by stress.

Assessment

History Diabetes mellitus.

Physical evidence Polyuria, loss of skin turgor, etc.

Clinical manifestations of neurological deficit due to dehydration of brain cells may be apparent. Warm, dry, flushed skin and possible fever are associated with dehydration, together with a rapid pulse and hypotension. Respirations are increased but, unlike Kussmaul's respirations, are not deep.

Tests include:

- Serum blood glucose level > 30 mmol/L
- Serum electrolytes – to assess imbalance
- Arterial blood gas analysis – to assess extent of metabolic acidosis
- Haematocrit – increased
- Urinalysis – glycosuria evident.

Management

Neurological deficit may place the patient at risk of injury, so this is a primary concern. Treatment is concentrated on rehydrating the patient, usually with i.v. sodium chloride 0.9%, but care must be taken not to overload the patient. Fluid intake and output need to be monitored and skin turgor noted, in order to assess efficacy of fluid replacement therapy. Insulin is administered and titrated to blood glucose levels. Serum electrolyte levels should be monitored, and potassium and phosphate replacements, if indicated, will require cautious administration (see 'Hypokalaemia', p. 57).

Burns

Burns may present one of the greatest challenges in terms of managing fluid, electrolyte and acid–base balances. This is because the extent and depth of burns vary greatly. The extent of burns is calculated by the 'rule of nines' (Fig. 3.9), while their severity is classified as first, second or third degree. The main problem is the rapid loss of circulating volume, and one of the challenges of management is to replace fluid loss without causing oedema. Imbalances are caused by disruption of skin integrity and cellular destruction. Within the first 8 hours following the burn, plasma leaks from the damaged capillaries into the interstitial space to form local oedema. It is suggested that the movement of protein (in the plasma) to the burned area causes oedema in non-burned tissue, because of the resulting hypoproteinaemia (Horne & Swearingen 1993). This shift of fluid may involve 10–50% of the circulating volume, resulting in severe hypovolaemia. Loss of skin also leads to fluid loss of up to 3 L/day via evaporation, depending on the environmental humidity. The increased capillary permeability gradually subsides over 48 hours.

Burns also decrease cell membrane potential, permitting sodium and water to enter the cell and potassium to leak out into the ECF and plasma. Tissue perfusion is decreased partly due to blood vessel damage, increased blood viscosity and erythrocyte aggregation, but also results from hypoxia caused by metabolic acidosis following increased anaerobic metabolism. Respiratory compensation for the acidosis will be limited following inhalational injury, because of the resultant tissue oedema in the lungs. If the lung injury is severe, mechanical ventilation will be required to manage the hypoxaemia and respiratory acidosis.

The initial stage of imbalance in burns is characterized by a fluid shift from the plasma to the ECF, together with oliguria as the kidneys attempt to conserve fluid. The next stage (48 hours after the burn) is characterized by a shift of fluid from the ECF (as the oedema fluid is reabsorbed) and a diuresis to remove the excess fluid. At this stage, hypervolaemia may occur, if i.v. fluid replacement is not adjusted or if renal damage has occurred. Electrolyte imbalances are common and the possible changes are presented in Table 3.12.

Fig. 3.9 'Rule of nines' for assessment of burns.
A. Anterior view.
B. Posterior view. (After Thompson et al 1989, with permission.)

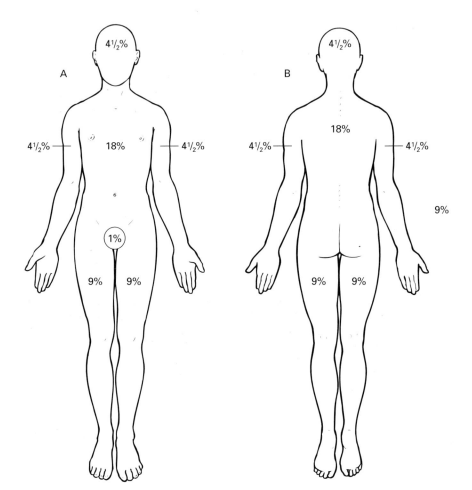

Table 3.12 Electrolyte imbalances associated with burns

Imbalance	Cause
Hyperkalaemia	Cell lysis in the initial stage leads to release of potassium into ECF
Hypokalaemia	Increased excretion due to aldosterone
Hypernatraemia	Inadequate water replacement
Hyponatraemia	Large amounts of sodium lost in oedema
Hypocalcaemia	Loss of ECF from burn and shift of calcium to the wound
Hypophosphataemia	Associated with respiratory alkalosis

Assessment

History Chemical, thermal or electrical burn.

Physical evidence of burn The extent and degree need to be assessed.

Clinical manifestation of tissue damage may include pain, hypoxia, etc. Evidence of fluid loss is characterized by shock, hypovolaemia, hypotension, oedema, blistering, etc.

Tests include:

- Serum electrolytes – to assess imbalances
- Arterial blood gas analysis – to assess level of acidosis or alkalosis, or optimal mechanical ventilation
- ECG – to monitor dysrhythmias associated with electrolyte imbalances
- Chest X-ray – to assess damage from inhalational injury.

Management

In the initial stage, aggressive treatment of the hypovolaemia must be instituted. There are various formulae which can be used, as cited by Horne & Swearingen (1993), Metheney (1992) and Willatts (1987). The usual fluids that are recommended are compound sodium lactate and colloid solutions, which need to be individualized for each patient. Compound sodium lactate is used to increase fluid levels (together with electrolytes), while colloid solutions are used to increase the circulating volume without increasing oedema. Optimal pain management will decrease the stress response and aid recovery. Monitoring includes haemodynamic monitoring, ECG, blood gas analysis, fluid intake and output, serum electrolytes and haematocrit. Acid–base and electrolyte imbalances will need to be corrected. Fluid replacement needs to be adjusted after the first 48 hours to avoid the risk of heart failure from hypervolaemia.

CONCLUSION

This chapter has reviewed the concepts of fluid, electrolyte and acid–base balance and considered some of the imbalances which can occur. These imbalances have been presented in terms of causes, assessment and management, which are designed to assist understanding of the rationale for interventions. The imbalances associated with specific client groups, towards the latter part of the chapter, give some indication of the complex nature of fluid, electrolyte and acid–base balance.

REFERENCES

Baxter Healthcare 1989 Product information sheet. Baxter Healthcare
Eccles R 1993 Electrolytes and body fluids and acid base balance. Edward Arnold, London
Ezrin C, Godden J O, Volpe R, Wilson R 1979 Systematic endocrinology, 2nd edn. Harper & Row, Hagerstown, MD
Halperin M L, Goldstein M B 1994 Fluid, electrolyte and acid–base physiology, 2nd edn. WB Saunders, Philadelphia
Hinchliff S M, Montague S E, Watson R 1997 Physiology for nursing practice, 2nd edn. Baillière Tindall, London
Horne M M, Swearingen P L 1993 Fluids, electrolytes and acid-base balance, 2nd edn. Mosby, St Louis
Innerarity S A, Stark J L 1990 Fluids and electrolytes. Springhouse, Pennsylvania

Joint Formulary Committee 1997 The national formulary, 33rd edn. The Pharmaceutical Press, Oxon

Lund W (ed) 1994 The pharmaceutical codex, 12th edn. The Pharmaceutical Press, London

Marieb E N 1989 Human anatomy and physiology. Benjamin Cummings, Redwood City

Metheney N M 1992 Fluid and electrolyte balance, 2nd edn. JB Lippincott, Philadelphia

Paradiso C 1995 Fluids and electrolytes. JB Lippincott, Philadelphia

Royal Pharmaceutical Society 1996 Martindale: the extra pharmacopoeia. Royal Pharmaceutical Society of Great Britain, London

Statland H 1963 Fluids and electrolytes in practice, 3rd edn. JB Lippincott, Philadelphia

Thompson J M et al 1989 Mosby's manual of clinical nursing, 2nd edn. Mosby-Year Book, St Louis, MI

Tortora G J, Grabowski S R 1996 Principles of anatomy and physiology, 8th edn. Harper Collins, New York

Willatts S 1987 Lecture notes on fluid and electrolyte balance. Blackwell Scientific Publications, Oxford

Infection control in intravenous therapy

Sarah Hart

CHAPTER

4

INTRODUCTION

Intravenous (i.v.) therapy is an integral part of patient care. Such patients are often seriously ill and immunocompromised, and they are therefore especially susceptible to infection. Nystrom et al's (1983) multicentre European study found that 63% of surgical patients had i.v. devices, and these patients were seen to develop a higher number of infections, septicaemias and bacteraemias than patients without i.v. catheters. This study also indicated that the risk of infection increased significantly with central venous catheters compared with peripheral cannulae.

Intravenous systems are invaluable in enabling direct access to the patient's vascular system for monitoring and administration of drugs, and in providing a convenient means of obtaining blood. Unfortunately these advantages are matched by the risk of the patient developing an i.v.-related infectious complication – seemingly, an i.v. catheter creates a pathway along which organisms that are normally excluded by the skin's defence mechanisms can enter.

Infection has been identified as a potentially life-threatening complication of i.v. therapy, causing phlebitis, wound infections, bacteraemia, septicaemia and even death (Elliott et al 1995). The care of patients with nosocomial catheter-related infections involves significant costs for both the hospital and the patients, including antibiotics, medical and surgical supplies, health care worker's time, delayed discharges, increased admission waiting times, as well as pain and anxiety for the patients and their families. These significant risks and costs associated with i.v. catheter-related infections mean that prevention of infection is an important concern and objective for all health care workers involved in the care of patients.

Many studies have tried to identify the incidence of catheter-related sepsis. Elliott (1993) reviewed the literature and suggested that the incidence ranged from 0 to 15%. He found that the numbers of i.v.-related bacteraemias reported to the Public Health Laboratory Service Communicable Disease Surveillance Centre had increased by 39% between 1989 to 1991. It can be argued that this escalation is, in fact, related to the increased use of i.v. catheters as well as to the improvement in the reporting and diagnosis of infection. Johnson & Oppenheim (1992) suggested a more conservative estimate of 3–7%, with the risk of infection increasing in neutropenic patients.

This wide variation in estimated infection rates reflects the lack of a consensus on the definition of catheter-related septicaemia and exit site infection. Nevertheless these figures do help to indicate the significant consequences of i.v.-related infections. When Elliott (1993) used a conservative estimate of 4% for the i.v.-related infection rate, he calculated that if in 1993 there were approximately 200 000 central venous catheters (CVCs) used in the UK, there would be a staggering 8000 cases of infection.

Box 4.1 provides a glossary of technical terms related to infection control.

RISK FACTORS FOR ACQUIRING INFECTIONS

A patient who has a decreased resistance to infection will have an increased suscep-

■ **BOX 4.1**

Glossary of technical terms related to infection control

Bacteraemia – bacteria present in blood as confirmed by culture with or without causing illness

Septicaemia – as 'Bacteraemia' but implies greater severity

Sepsis – clinical evidence of infection

Nosocomial infection – hospital-acquired infection not present or incubating at the time of admission

Colonization – persistent presence of microorganisms at a body site without causing infection

Endogenous – originating from on or within the body

Exogenous – originating from external causes

Immunocompromised patient – an individual with impairment of either or both natural and specific immunity to infection which increases the risk of infection by a variety of microorganisms

■ **BOX 4.2**

Factors that contribute to infection

- Age
- Immunosuppression
- Immunocompromised
- Loss of skin integrity
- Multiple invasive procedures
- Antibiotic therapy
- Presence of distant infection
- Poor nutrition

tibility to developing an i.v.-related infection. There are a number of reasons why patients are more vulnerable to infection (Box 4.2).

Age

Patients are more susceptible to infection at the extremes of age. In the elderly, there are many reasons for this increased risk, including changes in cell-mediated immunity and humoral immunity; physiological changes related to impaired circulation, cough reflex and poorer wound healing; and changes related to the absorption, distribution, metabolism and elimination of many antibiotics (Crossley & Peterson 1995). Young children also have an increased susceptibility to infection; although components of the immune system differentiate early in fetal life, functional maturity takes several years to complete. A baby's immature immune system is supported and augmented by maternal factors supplied by placental transfer, colostrum and breast milk. Premature babies have enhanced susceptibility to infection, not only because of their immunological immaturity but also because of the immaturity of many of their natural barriers to infection and because of the transgression of these barriers by the invasive monitoring and therapeutic techniques used in neonatal intensive care (Tristram & Pearay 1992).

Immunosuppression

A person may be immunosuppressed as a consequence of radiotherapy, chemotherapy or steroid therapy, and this subsequently causes granulocytopenia, cellular immune dysfunction and humoral immune dysfunction. A number of factors will determine the extent of the patient's immunosuppression, including the host defence defect caused by the disease itself and the dose and duration of immunosuppressive therapy, particularly corticosteroids.

The incidence of infection is directly related to the degree of immunosuppression; for example, the incidence of infection begins to rise once the granulocyte count falls below 500, with the most severe infections occurring when the count falls below 100 (De Jongh et al 1986).

Immunocompromised

A person may have a defect in the immune system as a result of an underlying disease, notably those affecting the bone marrow. Those patients with newly diagnosed leukaemia or myeloma are particularly susceptible to infection. In diseases such as chronic alcoholism or diabetes mellitus, the defect may not be so obvious as it is related to breaches in the first line of defence, such as injections, diabetic vascular disease or the high concentration of glucose in urine and secretions, which may promote the colonization by microorganisms. These factors will predispose the person to infection.

Loss of skin integrity

The intact skin forms a very effective barrier to invasion by microorganisms, as few organisms have a natural ability to penetrate it. Skin has the added advantage of being relatively dry and having a mild acidity, and the regular desquamation of skin scale also assists in the elimination of microorganisms. Inflamed skin is more permeable to water, which can lead to greater colonization by microorganisms. Damaged skin provides an entry for microorganisms, which can lead to inflammation, cellulitis, wound infections and septicaemia (Tramont & Hoover 1995).

Multiple invasive procedures

The skin and mucous membranes comprise the body's first line of defence against the entry of microorganisms. Breaches in these barriers, e.g. by surgical intervention or intravenous and urinary catheters, allows access to microorganisms which may cause infection. Each procedure undergone by an immunocompromised patient must be evaluated to ensure that every effort is made to reduce the extent of damage and that an aseptic technique is adopted at all times.

Invasive procedures can also lead to a shift in microbial flora (Wade 1994). For example, the minor trauma caused by shaving the skin prior to the insertion of a central catheter predisposes to invasion by the colonizing microorganisms of the skin and can be prevented by the use of hair clippers (Pettersson 1986).

When the skin is moist and hot, higher bacterial counts are found (Blank & Oawes 1958), which increases the risk of infection following invasive procedures.

Antibiotic therapy

The importance of effective antimicrobial therapy in the management of infection cannot be overemphasized. Unfortunately, antibiotics produce a shift in microbial flora. Alteration to normal microbial flora predisposes the patient to become colonized with organisms that are potentially more pathogenic. Such organisms may be acquired endogenously from the patient's own normal flora or exogenously from the hospital environment, visitors or health care workers, in particular from their hands. Henderson (1995) stated that alteration of the patient's skin flora as a result of antimicrobial therapy is a common event preceding catheter site infection.

Poor nutrition

The defence mechanisms of patients with severe underlying disease, who require intensive treatment, can be reduced further by inadequate nutrition. Besides the correlation between inadequate protein, vitamins and trace elements such as zinc and reduced production of the cells of the immune system, there is evidence that the skin and mucous membrane barriers may become impaired in cases of poor nutrition, due to thinning of the mucosa (Van Der Meer 1994).

Presence of distant infection

Recognizing the epidemiology of infection is important in establishing an approach to infection prevention. Colonization of the body by pathogenic microorganisms is a prerequisite for infection. Most patients with granulocytopenia who develop a *Staphylococcus aureus* infection carry this organism in their nose. Henderson (1995) suggested that most sporadic nosocomial bacteraemias are not device-related, but occur as a result of distant localized infection that goes on to seed the bloodstream; however, Elliott (1993) disagreed with this, stating that haematogenous seeding of organisms from a distant site onto a central venous catheter is thought to be rare.

All of these conditions depress the patient's immunological response to infection and may permit the invasion of organisms which can result in infection.

FACTORS INFLUENCING THE SURVIVAL OF MICROORGANISMS

The factors that can influence the survival of microorganisms include:

- the organism itself
- the number of organisms
- host resistance to infection
- environmental factors.

The organism itself may be pathogenic or non-pathogenic. Generally, only pathogenic organisms are capable of producing disease. This is related to the organism's natural capability to survive and proliferate in the environment; for example, Gram-negative bacteria such as *Klebsiella* and *Pseudomonas* thrive in damp conditions, which means they have the ability to contaminate and multiply in infusants. The rate of replication of the infecting organism is of central importance. Intravenous-related bacteraemias are usually caused by organisms that have the ability to multiply in 20–30 minutes. In a healthy person these organisms would be phagocytosed and removed, but in a neutropenic patient, uncontrolled replication can occur (Van Der Meer 1994).

The emergence of antibiotic-resistant pathogenic organisms has increased the risk of serious infection by changing the balance of survival in favour of the resistant organism. Many organisms, and the infections caused by them, respond to an antibiotic of proven efficacy and safety; however, a resistant organism will not be susceptible to the antibiotic of choice. *Staphylococcus aureus* is one of the most common causes of soft tissue infections, and infections caused by this organism are treated with flucloxacillin. Methicillin-resistant *S. aureus* (MRSA), however, is resistant to flucloxacillin and can easily colonize i.v. insertion sites, providing a reservoir of infection which may go on to cause serious disease (Wilson & Richardson 1996). There is a danger that MRSA will develop a resistance to other antibiotics, as recent reports of a vancomycin-resistant MRSA in Japan indicate (Williams et al 1997).

■ BOX 4.3

Organisms most commonly responsible for intravenous
bacteraemias in decreasing order of total isolates

- *Staphylococcus epidermidis*
- *Staphylococcus aureus*
- *Streptococcus* spp.
- *Pseudomonas aeruginosa*
- *Escherichia coli*
- *Enterobacter* spp.
- *Klebsiella* spp.
- *Candida* spp.
- *Corynebacterium* spp.
- *Acinetobacter* spp.

Effective infection control policies are essential if these resistant organisms are to be contained.

Elliott (1993) studied the organisms responsible for bacteraemias associated with i.v. devices in England and Wales, as reported to the Communicable Disease Surveillance Centre (see Box 4.3). *Staphylococcus epidermidis* is the most common cause of i.v.-related infection, mainly because it is a normal resident on the skin of both patients and health care workers. *S. epidermidis* also has the ability to grow and proliferate on catheters. Following attachment to a catheter surface the organism produces a glycocalyx slime-like substance which protects it from the patient's natural immune mechanisms and from antibiotics (Peters et al 1982).

Many patients in hospital have diminished resistance to infection, which means that organisms which are relatively harmless to healthy people may cause disease in such patients. The greater the number of organisms, the greater is the risk; however, even a small number of organisms contaminating i.v. fluids is extremely dangerous and can cause serious infection.

A wide variety of microorganisms, including virulent strains, can be found in the hospital environment (Koerner et al 1997). When a hospital department is physically clean, dust-free and dry, it is unlikely to be the main cause of exogenous infection. It is essential to maintain such an environment in order to provide the required surroundings for good hygiene and asepsis.

Microorganisms will easily proliferate at room temperature. This means that the longer an infusion container is in use, the greater the proliferation of bacteria will be. If contamination of the infusant has inadvertently occurred, the likelihood of infection will increase. The pH, temperature and presence of nutrients in the infusion will influence the rate at which organisms multiply (Sanderson & Deital 1973). Parenteral nutrition (PN) infusions, which are of a high nutritious value and are commonly left hanging for 24 hours, are of particular risk, which necessitates their production being undertaken in a controlled clean environment as near to the time of administration as possible. If PN containers have to be stored before use, this must be in a designated refrigerator at 4°C to reduce the risk of contamination and multiplication of organisms (Perceval 1981).

SOURCES OF MICROORGANISMS

Sources of microorganisms include air and skin. Microorganisms present in the air come from two basic sources: humans and the environment. Individuals with a chest infection will, when coughing, liberate many bacteria-containing particles into the air. Similarly, skin scales, which are constantly eliminated from the skin during desquamation, can be liberated into the air by movements such as bed-making and pulling the bed curtains.

The microorganisms on the skin are either resident or transient flora. Resident flora refers to permanent residents of the skin which are not readily removed by friction and includes *S. aureus* and *S. epidermidis*, both of which are major causes of i.v. infection. Resident flora play an important role in the prevention of colonization of the skin by other potentially pathogenic organisms. These organisms suppress the growth of many potentially pathogenic organisms by:

- the physical advantage of previous occupancy
- competing for essential nutrients
- producing inhibitory substances such as fatty acids which discourage other species of organisms from invading.

The disadvantage of resident flora found on the skin, and also in the gut, is that such flora can be spread into previously sterile parts of the body, e.g. when the skin is damaged or breached by an i.v. device. Resident flora can also be disturbed after administration of antibiotics and can lead to an overgrowth of potentially pathogenic organisms.

Transient flora are organisms that are not consistently found on the skin and that are loosely attached and easily removed when hands are properly washed. Unwashed hands, however, will readily transmit these organisms by direct contact onto whatever is being handled. This risk is particularly high during manipulation of the i.v. system.

ROUTES OF ACCESS OF MICROORGANISMS

Extraluminal

Extraluminal spread refers to the migration and entry of bacteria down the insertion site on the external surface of the catheter. The bacteria may originate from the air, the skin of the patient or health care workers, contaminated dressings and lotions. Prevention includes hand washing, aseptic technique, careful skin preparation, scrupulous hygiene by the patient and a clean environment.

Intraluminal

Intraluminal spread refers to the entry of organisms into the infusion system through contaminated fluids or additives into the infusion container or tubing. Similarly, if the catheter hub becomes contaminated, during manipulation of the hub, migration of bacteria can occur. Prevention includes the use of sterile equipment, aseptic technique, hand washing and keeping the number of i.v. catheter manipulations to a minimum.

Haematogenous spread

Haematogenous spread refers to the migration of organisms from a distant site of infection to the catheter, e.g. from the lungs, wound or bowel. This means that a catheter can be colonized from remote unrelated sites of infection. Prevention relies on fully evaluating the patient so that potential risks can be recognized and preventive measures commenced.

Contaminated infusants

The use of contaminated infusants can be avoided by careful inspection of the i.v.

Table 4.1 Examples of intrinsic sources of contamination

Problem	Cause
Infusion fluids	Cracked glass bottles
	Punctures in plastic containers
Administration equipment	Damaged packaging
Contaminated lotions	Damaged containers
Contaminated ointments, etc.	Misuse

fluid to make sure that it is clear and free from particulate matter and that the container is intact with no cracks in the bottle or holes in the plastic bag. The label must be checked to verify that the container is not out of date. All containers must be labelled to indicate the time and date that the container was opened; if it is not completed within 24 hours, the container must be removed and discarded.

TYPES OF INFECTION

Infections can be grouped into two categories: exogenous and endogenous. Exogenous infection refers to organisms originating outside the patient's body and implies cross-infection from staff, other patients, visitors or the environment. Endogenous infection arises from organisms or factors already present in or on the patient's body before the onset of infection. An example of endogenous infection is the haematogenous spread of bowel flora by translocation (Carter 1994), where viable bacteria move from the gut of immunocompromised patients to other organs.

Exogenous and endogenous contamination of the i.v. system may have intrinsic or extrinsic causes (see Table 4.1 and Box 4.4).

Intrinsic contamination

Intrinsic contamination of i.v. equipment occurs prior to administration, due to a breakdown of asepsis, and is generally attributed to faults in the manufacturing and sterilization process or, more commonly, to damage sustained by the product during transit or storage of the i.v. system. Fortunately, this type of contamination seldom occurs, but when incidents do take place there are significant consequences for the patients, so prevention is an important objective, which means that all equipment must be closely inspected before use.

If intrinsic contamination is suspected, the product must not be used, and if signs of intrinsically acquired infection occur, the system must be discontinued immediately and comparable products of the same batch investigated for a similar fault; they should not be used until a satisfactory explanation has been found for the intrinsic contamination.

Staff must always be aware of the risk of intrinsic contamination. Prevention is assisted by purchasers vigorously assessing products to ensure reliability and suitability for the task for which they are intended. A hospital product review committee can assist with this process.

The user of any product should be satisfied with the transportation and storage methods. This does not exclude the need to carefully examine all equipment before use to detect and eliminate any faulty items. Items that are found to be of an unacceptable standard must be investigated. It may be appropriate to refer the problem to the Medical Devices Agency (MDA) who will investigate the complaint. Passing

■ BOX 4.4

Examples of how extrinsic sources of contamination can occur

- Additives to the i.v. fluids
- Infusion container changes
- Contaminated air
- Injections/flushes/specimen collection
- Contaminated skin disinfectants
- Hands of staff
- Patient's normal flora

on complaints in this way allows the MDA to have an accurate picture of the standard of products throughout the country. The MDA can, if necessary, send out a hazard warning outlining the potential problem, which will help to prevent further incidents occurring.

Extrinsic contamination

Extrinsic contamination refers to contamination that occurs at any point during the use of the i.v. system and is generally due to improper operation, e.g. failure to maintain a sterile closed system. Hub-related contamination has been widely recognized as a precursor of catheter-related sepsis. Sitges-Serra et al (1995) discussed the fact that the microorganisms most commonly found on hubs are those varieties reflecting the hospital flora, with contamination occurring when a colonized hand is used to manipulate the catheter junction (Cicco et al 1989).

Contamination of i.v. equipment, including items such as lotions, ointments and dressing packs, is prevented by maintaining aseptic technique at all times (see Box 4.4).

An example of extrinsic contamination was highlighted by Bauer & Denson's (1979) survey, which found high i.v. infection rates associated with the use of non-sterile Elastoplast on venepuncture sites. Similarly, Chodoff et al (1995) reported seven cases of nosocomial Gram-negative infections as the result of the use of contaminated saline solutions.

Intravenous practice has to take into consideration the risks of infection, and all policies and procedures should be designed to reduce these risks. If, however, contamination does inadvertently occur, the potential problem should be recognized by skilled nurses before complications have had time to set in (Lundgren & Ek 1996).

The following guidelines should be included in i.v. procedures:

- The administration set must be changed every 24 hours (DHSS 1973). This guideline originated because of outbreaks of septicaemia associated with i.v. fluids (Goldmann et al 1973). Bryan (1987), however, suggested that these guidelines were outdated and discussed studies which indicate that changing administration sets after 48 and 72 hours does not compromise safety and has considerable cost savings.
- Infusion containers should not hang for more than 24 hours, except for blood and blood products which should be completed within 5 hours (Blood Transfusion Service of the United Kingdom 1996).
- Maintain a closed system whenever possible.
- Hub manipulation should be kept to a minimum. Prevention of contamination during connection and disconnection involves the use of an aseptic technique and

cleaning of the catheter and i.v. administration hub with an aseptic solution prior to disconnection.

• Use luer-lock connection fittings whenever possible to prevent accidental disconnection of the administration set.

• Limit the number of connections, e.g. three-way taps and stopcocks, in the i.v. system as these have been found to have a high contamination rate (Mehtar & Taylor 1981) due to the increased number of open ports which facilitate endoluminal contamination. These taps and stopcocks should be changed at the same time as the administration set (Goodinson 1990).

• Local evaluation is required to establish whether or not to use i.v. filters. These are claimed to remove bacterial contaminants, particulate matter and air embolus and to reduce the incidence of phlebitis (Goodinson 1990). There are those, however, who are not convinced that the cost of the filters is justified (John 1996).

• When introducing the administration set into an infusion bottle, use an air inlet filter needle to prevent contamination of i.v. fluids by the influx of air.

• Rotate peripheral devices every 48 hours, or immediately if contamination is suspected (Intravenous Nurses Association 1998). Henderson (1995) reviewed the literature and suggested that any catheter left in place for longer than 72 hours significantly increases the risk of infection.

It is essential for the patient to be instructed as to the importance of good hygiene. Patients should shower or bathe at least daily, and more often in hot weather. Studies have shown that there is no delay in healing if sutures become wet with soap and water during washing (Noe & Keller 1988). The use of an occlusive dressing eliminates the potential problem of the suture line becoming damaged during washing. Showers are preferable to a bath, as the bath and bath hoists may easily become contaminated with bacteria (Wilson 1995); during showering there is a reduced possibility of cross-infection from a previous user (Briggs & Wilson 1996). Disinfecting bath additives are not recommended for routine use as they can be easily inactivated by soap, hard water and inorganic matter (Philpott-Howard & Casewell 1994).

Greaves (1985) reported that 'a bed bath can often leave a patient dirtier after the bath than before', as organisms can survive and multiply on items such as the wash bowl and wash clothes. If the only method of washing the patient is by a bed bath, she should be supplied with her own wash bowl and disposable wash clothes. On discharge of the patient, the bowl should be terminally disinfected before being put back into general use.

The risk of extrinsic contamination is reduced by strict adherence to aseptic technique, optimum patient hygiene and maintenance of a clean environment. An increasing number of patients are being discharged home with skin-tunnelled central venous catheters or implantable ports in place and these same principles and practices of infection control in i.v. care must be maintained in the home or alternative care setting (Terry et al 1995).

PREVENTION OF CATHETER-RELATED SEPSIS

Prevention of infection involves the adoption of techniques which incorporate the principles of asepsis and hygiene. The fundamental principles of infection control must be integrated into the design of the environment and influence the choice of all equipment used by patients and staff.

The principles of infection control are to protect the patient by a system of methods which remove the potential source of infection, block the route of transfer of bacteria to susceptible patients and enhance the patient's resistance to i.v. device infection. Such methods must be research-based and take into consideration the

■ BOX 4.5

Factors which influence acquisition of infection

- Type of catheter
- Insertion of device or catheter
- Prophylactic antibiotic at catheter insertion
- Purpose of catheter
- Duration of catheter
- Intravenous therapy teams
- Care of insertion site
- Dressing
- Catheter care

available information related to bacteria pathogenicity. These practices must be regularly evaluated and updated to take into account new research findings, as well as the more adventurous surgery and high-dose chemotherapy which is resulting in an ever increasing number of patients being highly susceptible to infection.

The general measures designed to protect patients from infection include meticulous attention to all aspects of i.v. therapy. Box 4.5 highlights factors that particularly influence the acquisition of i.v. catheter-related infection.

Aseptic technique

Aseptic technique is a method which has been evolved to prevent contamination of wounds and other vulnerable sites by ensuring that only sterile items come into contact with the site and that the environment in which the procedure is being carried out is as clean and safe as possible (Mallett & Bailey 1996).

Hampton & Sheretz (1988) suggested that violation of aseptic technique increases the risk of nosocomial infection. Krakowska's (1986) study observed standards of aseptic techniques during the setting up of i.v. infusions and found that, often, only lip service is paid to written hospital procedures by some nurses and a larger number of doctors. These authors reiterated that the ward sister has a vital role to play and must be convinced that strict asepsis during i.v. work is important and that doctors and nurses must adhere to the hospital's aseptic technique policies.

Teare & Peacock (1996) found that the introduction of an infection control link nurse system raised the profile of infection control by disseminating knowledge and changing behaviour and attitudes. Haddock et al (1985) supported this view, suggesting that an enthusiastic, trained nurse is an essential component of the ward's capability to provide safe and effective i.v. therapy.

Whilst an aseptic technique can be undertaken in a variety of ways, there are basic principles that must be adhered to (Box 4.6).

Hand washing

Hand washing is the single most important procedure for preventing nosocomial infections (Philpott-Howard & Casewell 1994). Many outbreaks of nosocomial infection have been originated from the hands of health care workers (Casewell & Philip 1977). Hand washing must be convenient and acceptable and its essential importance must be recognized. Hands must be washed when going on and off duty, before and after direct patient contact, and prior to and during aseptic techniques.

The choice of hand washing technique depends on the purpose of the hand wash-

■ BOX 4.6

Principles of aseptic techniques

- Hand washing
- Sterile equipment
- Clean equipment
- Clean environment

ing and is generally based on the infection risks of the patient being cared for. Social hand washing involves washing hands with a non-medicated soap or detergent and will remove many transient microbial flora; it is suitable for when going on and off duty, and before and after brief patient care activities. Since soap can become contaminated it is important that this is supplied in a disposable dispenser which is replaced when empty (Blackmore 1987).

Hand washing with an antimicrobial hand washing product is required before all aseptic techniques and before contact with immunocompromised patients. Preparations containing chlorhexidine have been very effective in removing bacteria without causing skin damage (Kobayashi 1991).

When hands are clean, a bactericidal alcoholic handrub can be used before and during patient contact, especially when undertaking aseptic techniques. Such preparations have the added advantage over soap and antimicrobial detergents of having virucidal activity (Bellamy et al 1993), as well as being quick and easy to use. A dispenser of the bactericidal alcoholic handrub should be on the bottom shelf of all trolleys used for aseptic techniques, so that immediately prior to and during the procedure, hands can be disinfected without leaving the patient's bedside.

Correct and thorough drying of hands following hand washing is equally important, as damp hands transfer bacteria much more readily than dry ones (Gould 1995). Similarly, hands that have not been dried properly are more likely to become cracked and sore, which will increase the risk of colonization by potentially pathogenic hospital-acquired organisms and could increase the risk of cross-infection during direct patient care (Larson et al 1986).

Hot air electric hand dryers are being increasingly used in public areas and have proved useful as, unlike paper towels, they do not 'run out' and they do not have to be collected and disposed of. Nevertheless, in the clinical setting, a good quality paper towel remains the product of choice (Blackmore 1987), because the hand dryer can be slow and noisy, and warms the environment, and studies have shown that busy staff may wipe their damp hands on their clothes rather than wait for the hand dryer to dry their wet hands completely (Matthews & Newson 1987).

The bacterial counts on hands will increase with cracked nail varnish and with the wearing of rings, especially those containing stones, but these increased risks are removed by thoroughly washing hands (Jacobson et al 1985). Caution is required with the use of hand cream as an outbreak of *Klebsiella* septicaemia has been attributed to contaminated hand cream shared by nurses after washing their hands (Morse et al 1968).

Patients' hand washing is equally important. Ill patients do not always wash their hands after using the toilet, urinal or commode, and could contribute to the transfer of organisms to other body sites (Prichard & Hathaway 1988). Nurses should stress the importance of good hygiene to their patients and offer help and support to allow patients to wash their hands, as studies have shown that debilitated patients are often not offered the opportunity to wash their hands (Laurence 1983).

Sterile equipment

All surgical instruments, dressings, lotions, solutions and drugs used for or introduced by injection must be provided sterile. This equipment must also have been protected against contamination during transit, storage and use.

Regardless of how sterilization has been achieved, all items must be inspected before use to ensure that sterilization has taken place, that the packaging is intact and that the shelf life has not expired.

Clean equipment

Equipment that is not introduced into the i.v. system and does not come into contact with the i.v. site, but which is used during i.v. therapy, must be clean, including small items such as a splint and tape, and larger items such as pumps and drip poles. The items that are initially supplied clean and packaged must be stored in a dust-free, clean way. Multi-use items emphasize the importance of good hand washing to prevent cross-infection from one patient to another. Similarly, when a patient is being barrier-nursed, the minimum amount of equipment and medical and surgical supplies should be stored in the room, to eliminate the risk of unused items being used on subsequent patients. Larger items must be washed with detergent and wiped dry between patients and when spillage occurs, unless used for a known infected patient when a chemical disinfectant must be used (Ayliffe et al 1984).

Clean environment

The environment of a hospital plays an important part in the spread of hospital infection, e.g. MRSA spread during bed-making can be redispersed into the air when the bedside curtains are handled; similarly, *Pseudomonas* in sinks and bath plugs could contaminate an i.v. device during washing (Philpott-Howard & Casewell 1994). Properly trained and supervised domestic staff should clean the ward area thoroughly every day and dampen dust areas such as bed frames and curtain rails weekly to ensure that microorganisms and the material on which they thrive will be removed.

Shelves and cupboards where surgical and medical supplies are stored must be dust-free, with a stock control system operating. It is essential that stock is not stored on the floor where it may become contaminated and, equally importantly, prevent thorough cleaning of the floor.

Type of catheter

Catheter design and composition contribute to the risk of infection. Catheters need to be made of materials which do not irritate the vascular intima. Similarly, catheters which inhibit the adherence of microorganisms probably reduce the risk of infection. The larger the catheter, the greater the entry site, which increases the risk of extraluminal contamination. There is no clear evidence that multi-lumen catheters present an increased risk of infection (Lee et al 1988). However, as multi-lumen catheters are generally inserted into critically ill patients or those who are expected to receive a large number of infusions, there is an increase in catheter manipulation, which increases the risk of infection (Peruccar 1995). Similarly, if infection starts at the hub and progresses intraluminally, increasing the number of hubs will increase the risk of infection (Harrison 1997).

Several totally implantable vascular port systems are available and they are reported to be more convenient and safer i.v. devices than peripheral or central venous catheters (CVCs) (Lilienberg et al 1994). Hagle (1987) reported that implanted devices have a decreased risk of infection. However, the research studies sample groups were not matched and so caution should be adopted when comparison is made between CVCs and implanted venous access ports (Speechley & Davidson 1989). Christianson (1994) stated that as long as these ports are well managed and carefully assessed, they provide a safe venous access.

Beam et al (1990) suggested that the i.v. catheters with the highest risk of infectious complications are central catheters inserted percutaneously, usually into a subclavian or external jugular vein, as they allow easy access for the skin organisms to the transcutaneous tract and are also difficult to secure and dress.

The use of a skin-tunnelled CVC reduces the risks associated with the percutaneous CVCs. With these catheters, the tip is placed in the superior vena cava or right atrium and enters the vascular system through the subclavian vein, via a subcutaneous tunnel. There is the added advantage of a Dacron cuff situated in the subcutaneous tunnel which stimulates growth of fibrous tissue to provide stability for the catheter and a barrier to ascending organisms (Harrison 1997). Studies, in particular those where catheters were being handled by untrained staff, suggest that the incidence of catheter-related infection is reduced when skin-tunnelled catheters are used (Johnson & Oppenheim 1992).

It has been suggested that binding a non-toxic antiseptic to catheter surfaces or incorporating such substances into the catheter itself will reduce infection rates. Bach et al's (1993) animal studies demonstrated a significant protective effect against device-related colonization and infection when using these catheters. In view of the increasing use of long-term i.v. therapy, the reduction of the risk of infection by the use of a better material for catheters remains a desirable goal, and further research is required.

Insertion of intravenous devices

Placement of a device must be carried out by an experienced practitioner, as complication rates tend to be higher with inexperienced practitioners (Hrske & Tonozar 1990). Infection is more likely to occur following a difficult insertion, possibly due to a deteriorating technique, tissue trauma or disruption of skin flora (Conly et al 1989). In some hospitals, nurses have extended their role in the placement of tunnelled CVCs (Hamilton 1995).

The site of insertion is significant, with catheters placed in the lower extremities, particularly the femoral vein, having an increased risk of infection (Henderson 1995).

Tunnelled catheters must be inserted in a controlled clean environment, ideally in the operating theatre or anaesthetic room. Midline and peripherally inserted catheters and non-skin-tunnelled catheters must be inserted in a clean environment using theatre standards of aseptic technique. Peripheral devices are inserted in a wide range of environments, and aseptic techniques must be used (see Ch. 9).

Sitges-Serra et al (1995) and Elliott et al (1994) agree that the placement of all CVCs should be considered a minor operation, and therefore the skin and insertion field must be prepared for a surgical intervention, with the person undertaking the insertion wearing sterile gloves and gown. Goldmann et al (1973) recognized that some percutaneous CVCs have to be inserted in emergency conditions, but these should be replaced at the earliest opportunity.

Disinfection of the insertion site with an antiseptic solution prior to catheter insertion and during subsequent manipulation of the device is essential to prevent local catheter-associated infection. De Vries et al (1997) undertook a randomized trial of skin disinfection prior to insertion of peripheral infusion catheters using 70% alcohol and 2% alcoholic iodine. No statistical difference was seen. Maki et al's (1991) randomized study assessed the efficiency of povidone-iodine, alcohol and chlorhexidine for the prevention of infection associated with central venous and arterial catheters. This study indicated statistically that the use of 2% chorhexidine reduced the incidence of device-related infections. Chlorhexidine has the added advantage that toxicity and sensitization are uncommon, and colonization by resistant bacteria and yeast has not been seen.

Johnson & Oppenheim (1992) reviewed the literature relating to the administration of prophylactic antibiotics at the time of central venous catheter insertion and found studies which demonstrated that these antibiotics had no effect on CVC infection. Other studies which have shown reduced infection rates or increased periods of catheter use were criticized for not being blind, randomized or concurrent (MacKinnon et al 1987). These authors were unable to recommend the use of prophylactic antibiotics as a routine approach to the prevention of CVC sepsis. This opinion is supported by other authors who have reviewed similar data (Elliott 1993).

Patients' skin flora

The skin is the main source of bacteria responsible for i.v.-associated infection (Weinstein 1993). Studies have shown a direct relationship between skin colonization and positive tip culture (Balakrishnan et al 1991).

Different regions of the skin support different numbers and types of flora, which are largely determined by the degree of available humidity. Exposed dry areas have relatively low numbers of resident flora, whilst more moist areas, e.g. the axilla and groin, or as a result of sweating or fever, show larger numbers of resident flora (Wilson 1995).

It is essential to encourage the patient to shower daily and to wear clothing that is loose and light, which will keep her dry and cool. Clothing and bed linen must be changed regularly. All of these factors will help to keep the numbers of resident flora to a manageable level and so discourage endogenous infection. Loach (1997) provided a patient's view that, while cleanliness was a simple way of improving well-being, the task of washing used up so much energy that there seemed little point in making the effort. These comments reiterate the importance of nurses providing help and encouragement to the weak and vulnerable patients in their care.

Skin preparation is important in reducing the risk of site infections, and for CVCs the patient should undergo routine pre-operative care, which includes a shower or bath. Studies evaluating the effects of pre-operative bathing with detergent or a disinfectant agent have been variable. Hayek & Emerson (1988) found 3% fewer infections in the group using a detergent as compared with the group using a disinfectant. These results and others showing a reduction in the total bacterial count suggest that pre-operative bathing with chlorhexidine may be beneficial (Paulson 1993).

Purpose of the catheter

The composition of the i.v. fluid influences the risk of acquiring an i.v. device-related infection. Different infusion fluids support the growth of differing pathogens. No infusate is free of risk, and even distilled water can support the growth of *Pseudomonas* species. Koerner et al (1997) discussed an outbreak of Gram-negative septicaemia associated with contamination of infusions in a non-clinical area, and emphasized the importance of continuous staff training in infection control and the need to involve the infection control team in all structural planning for patient care areas.

Parenteral nutrition (PN) solutions are particularly good media for the growth of microorganisms. Prevention of infusion-related infection in PN can be achieved by having a PN team who make decisions on protocols for insertion, maintenance and delivery of the solutions. All PN solutions must be prepared in a laminar air flow hood using sterile techniques. Once prepared, the solution should be used immediately or stored at 4°C (see Ch. 14).

The risk of bacterial proliferation during infusion of blood and blood products is particularly high as organisms will thrive in the ambient temperature of hospital wards. Infusion must be started within 30 minutes of removing blood from the refrigerator and must be completed within 5 hours of commencement. Blood should be infused through a blood-administration set which must be changed at least 12-hourly (Blood Transfusion Service of the United Kingdom 1996).

The controversy concerning the virological safety of blood and blood products continues. Whilst all donations of blood are tested to exclude hepatitis B, hepatitis C and antibody to HIV 1 and 2, blood and blood components are not subject to further procedures to reduce the risk of virus transmission (McClelland 1996). If the blood is donated during the HIV window, the antibody test will be negative although the blood will contain the virus. Between 1985 and 1996, two cases were recorded in the UK of HIV-infected blood being transfused to patients. A total of five patients received the blood: two died and the other three became HIV antibody-positive (Mortimer & Spooner 1997). Prevention of such instances relies on donors understanding that they should not donate blood if they know they are, or suspect that they may be, HIV antibody-positive. Alternatively, the use of autologous transfusions is an option for planned surgical procedures.

Duration of the catheter

The longer the device is in situ, the more likely it is that a patient will develop a catheter-related infection (Clarke & Raffin 1990). Peripheral catheters should be removed and re-sited every 48–72 hours. Weinstein (1993) explained how, within 24–48 hours following insertion, a loosely formed fibrin sheath develops around a plastic cannula and how this forms a nidus within which organisms can multiply shielded from the host defences and antibiotics. Percutaneous CVCs can be used for longer periods. Elliott et al (1994) suggested that they should be changed after 7 days, but others have reported that, in some areas, they are left in place as long as they are needed unless CVC-related sepsis is evident (Eyer et al 1990). A skin-tunnelled central catheter is the catheter of choice for planned long-term i.v. therapy as the tunnel separates the catheter entry site into the vein from the exit site on the skin, so providing a barrier to infection by inhibiting the extraluminal spread of organisms along the outside of the catheter (Threlkeld & Cobbs 1995).

Intravenous teams

Studies have shown that an i.v. therapy team is effective in decreasing morbidity and mortality associated with i.v.-related bacteraemias (Miller et al 1996). Weinstein (1993) reported that the quality of patient care improves, as nurses are able to focus their attention on developing high standards of practice; the knowledge, skill and ability of these nurses ensure patient safety. Dougherty (1996) outlined the benefits of i.v. teams who, as well as developing the service, provide education, enhance patient care and reduce non-compliance with i.v. policies and infection rates. Scalley et al's (1992) 30-month study of i.v. cannulation, as performed by i.v. teams and non-i.v. team personnel, showed a significant cost saving in the case of the former, related to a reduction in the incidence of phlebitis; and Tomford et al's (1984) prospective controlled study found that the overall incidence of phlebitis for ward-managed i.v. catheters was 32%, compared with 15% for those cared for by an i.v. team, with the incidence of cellulitis and suppurative phlebitis reducing 10-fold under i.v. team management.

Care of insertion site

Prior to insertion, any excess hair should be removed by clipping. Shaving is not recommended as it increases the risk of skin abrasions which can harbour bacteria (Cruse & Ford 1980). Skin must be cleaned prior to cannulation. Skin preparations are applied with friction, working outwards from the insertion site in a circular pattern on an area equal to the size of dressing. For the antimicrobial solution to be effective, it should be allowed to dry for a minimum of 30 seconds (Wilson 1995). Fanning, blowing or blotting of the prepared area to speed up drying is contraindicated (Terry et al 1995). Maki et al's (1991) study of three antiseptics for skin site disinfection found that 2% chlorhexidine substantially reduced the incidence of i.v. infections. Chlorhexidine has the added advantage of continuing antibacterial activity for up to 6 hours after application to skin (Pereira et al 1997). The addition of isopropyl alcohol 70%, which kills instantly by denaturing protein, enhances chlorhexidine's action (Ayliffe et al 1992).

The insertion site must be kept clean and dry and inspected daily. Elliott et al (1994) discussed how the application of antibiotic ointment to the insertion site has been proposed as a method of reducing contamination and subsequent colonization, but others have found no benefit from applying this type of ointment. Johnson & Oppenheim (1992) suggested that its use can alter the resident skin flora and lead to superinfection with organisms not affected by the ointment.

If an occlusive dressing is to be used, it should be changed weekly unless there is evidence of infection or it becomes soiled. If a gauze dressing is being used to allow daily inspection of the site (Elliott et al 1994), it will need to be changed daily, or more often if it becomes wet or soiled. During dressing changes an aseptic technique must be maintained.

Two to three weeks following insertion of a skin-tunnelled catheter, the sutures may be removed. It is then only necessary to use a clean technique in the care of the catheter site. Dressings and applications of topical antiseptic are unnecessary, unless the patient prefers to have the site covered. Dressings do offer protection against friction from clothes and may make the patient feel more secure.

It is essential to continue to use a full aseptic technique when opening the closed central venous catheter system since, as already mentioned, the longer the catheter remains in situ, the greater is the risk of infection.

Dressings

Catheter dressings must:

- be sterile
- secure the device to prevent dislodgement and trauma
- protect the wound from external contamination
- allow easy inspection of the site
- be comfortable and cost-effective
- not cause skin excoriation or irritation.

The choice of catheter dressing remains a controversial issue, with numerous studies yielding contradictory results (Lau 1996).

The type of catheter dressing applied does appear to influence the incidence of infection (Lau 1996). Hoffman et al (1992) reviewed the literature in this area and indicated that transparent dressings may significantly increase the risk of catheter tip infection compared with gauze dressings. They suggested that this may be due to the inadequate moisture vapour permeability of such dressings, as the collection of moisture under a dressing promotes the growth of bacteria (Callahan & Wesorick 1987). Treston-Aurand et al's (1997) review of the literature supported Hoffman et al's speculation, but they argued that prospective randomized trials have not confirmed this suggestion.

Since these studies, new dressings have been developed with increased moisture permeability, which appears to prevent the accumulation of moisture on the skin surface (Keenlyside 1993). Treston-Aurand et al's (1997) study of transparent non-permeable standard polyurethane dressings, tape and gauze and transparent high-ly permeable polyurethane dressings resulted in the hospital converting to the highly permeable dressing for use with central venous catheters, which eventually led to a 25% decrease in infection rates. These authors suggested that additional definitive randomized prospective investigations are needed to clarify the complex question of which dressing is the most suitable for i.v. use.

Transparent dressings have the added advantage of only needing to be changed every 5–7 days, if the daily inspection through the dressing (which can be done without removing it) indicates that the site is satisfactory. Treston-Aurand et al's (1997) study highlighted the time spent changing tape and gauze dressings follow-ing observation of the insertion site or in re-securing the dressing – when using a transparent dressing, this time is significantly reduced.

Transparent dressings also allow the patient to shower/bath normally. They pro-vide a superior catheter fixation, thereby reducing the risk of catheter displacement as these flexible lightweight films allow freedom of movement.

All unused dressing material must be disposed of after completion of the dress-ing procedure (Roberts 1987).

Catheter care

Thrombolytic complications of catheters are often associated with catheter sepsis (Harrison 1997). It is unclear whether this is due to the occlusion requiring an increase in manipulations to unblock it, which allows the entry of microorganisms, or to the presence of the blood clot, which provides nutrients for pathogens to proliferate, lead-ing to infection. Preventing the blood from clotting in the catheter is achieved by cor-rect flushing between drugs and blood products, when the catheter is not in use, and by restricting the times when the administration set is inadvertently turned off.

DIAGNOSIS OF INTRAVENOUS-ASSOCIATED INFECTION

Intravenous catheter infection can be categorized as localized or systemic. Localized infection refers to the catheter site or catheter tunnel. The patient may complain of pain, tenderness, fever with erythema, oedema and cellulitis at the site or along the subcutaneous tunnel. Systemic infections are those which affect the body as a whole, and is not limited to a particular area. Bacteraemia and septi-caemia are examples of i.v. related systemic infections.

Intravenous-associated sepsis is not always accompanied by phlebitis and the patient may complain of chills, fever, headaches, tremors, nausea, vomiting, abdominal pain, hyperventilation and shock (Maki et al 1973).

Catheter site infection should not be confused with catheter-related sepsis. The presence of erythema or exudate at the site may indicate a localized infection and may not necessarily be a sign of catheter infection. Conversely, patients may be sep-tic with no evidence at the catheter site. Fever in a person with a central venous catheter should be attributed to the catheter until proven otherwise. Cultures from blood, catheter site, urine, wound and sputum, plus an X-ray, should be obtained in order to diagnose unexplained pyrexia in immunocompromised patients.

Peripheral devices should always be removed when device infection is sus-pected. Similarly, skin-tunnelled CVCs with obvious tunnel infection should be removed as these are very difficult to treat without removal of the catheter. CVCs are not generally removed automatically as it can make management of sepsis more difficult by removing i.v. access for antibiotics. A number of febrile patients who are diagnosed as having a catheter-related infection may be septic with bacteraemia from other sources.

Clemence et al (1995) suggested that removal of short-term CVCs where there is the suspicion of i.v. sepsis allows the catheter tip to be sent for microbiological culture, which can be helpful in diagnosing infection. Healing of the insertion site can occur once the catheter has been removed and thereby prevent re-occurrence of bacteraemia once the antibiotic therapy is completed.

Tunnelled catheters are generally left in place in an attempt to treat the bacteraemia with antibiotics. Similarly, a substantial number of patients can be cured if empirical antimicrobials are commenced. These will be chosen to include the possibility of a catheter-related infection based on the clinician's assessment of the patient, the likely bacteria responsible for the infection and the hospital's antibiotic policy. Microbiological results may take days to become available and a delay in treating an infection may be disastrous. As long as the clinician has prescribed treatment based on the best available information, adjustments to therapy can be made when laboratory results are available.

Patients with long-term CVCs who have a bacteraemia with no identified source and who fail to respond to appropriate antibiotic therapy should have the catheter removed. The 5 cm distal tip should be cut off with sterile scissors, placed in a sterile universal container and sent for culture. The problem with tip cultures is that the results are difficult to interpret; it is difficult to discriminate between catheter contamination during removal, true catheter infection or contaminated i.v. fluids.

Quantitative microbiological studies of catheter tips can increase the reliability of distinguishing between catheter-related infection and bacteraemia from another source (Maki 1977).

Blood cultures taken from a separate peripheral vein and from the catheter can be compared in the process of diagnosing catheter sepsis. If blood cultures from the catheter are positive and the peripheral vein cultures are negative, this provides a reliable diagnosis of a catheter-associated infection. If the catheter blood cultures have a significant increase in bacteria colonies compared with the peripheral blood cultures, this also suggests a catheter sepsis (Elliott et al 1994). Positive blood cultures with identical organisms can confirm a catheter as a source of infection. Rigors following the use of the catheter is generally considered highly suggestive of a catheter-related infection, although allergic reaction to the infusants has to be ruled out.

Ryan et al (1974) estimated that 75–85 % of all catheters are removed unnecessarily. Studies have been carried out on culturing catheters while they remain in position. This is achieved by passing a small sampling brush through the catheter and then culturing the brush. The aim is for the brush to pick up organisms from the tip of the catheter. Valves to prevent blood loss and air embolism are integral to the design of this sampling equipment (Markus & Budley 1989). A great deal of skill and an aseptic technique are required to use such a system.

Surveillance cultures

The value of surveillance cultures of catheter hubs and exit sites is difficult to judge. It is accepted that patients generally acquire infections endogenously, which means that surveillance cultures are occasionally useful in identifying bacteria that may need additional or different antibiotic coverage from that recommended by the antibiotic policy. This is particularly important with regard to MRSA which can easily colonize catheter sites. However, the significance of cultures from healed normal sites is difficult to interpret and can lead to a false diagnosis of a catheter site infection. Fan et al (1989) obtained cultures from hubs and sites over an 18-month period and found them to be of little value unless both cultures were positive for the same organism, which would then mean catheter removal should be considered.

Johnson & Oppenheim (1992) suggested that surveillance swabs are only of value if the clinician is prepared to remove the catheter when positive swabs are obtained. Generally reliable, problem-free catheters are retained until there is clinical evidence of infection.

TREATMENT OF INFECTION

If a patient is known or suspected to have an infection, the clinician must decide which organism is likely to be responsible and to which antibiotics it will or will not be sensitive.

There are now many different antibacterial drugs, which are classified by their chemical structure and their site of action on the bacterial cell. There are fewer antifungal and antiviral agents. Antimicrobial drugs are valuable in the treatment and, in some well researched circumstances, the prevention of infection (Wilson 1995). Unfortunately, their inappropriate use has the potential risk of toxicity and superinfection in a patient, as well as the problem of selection of resistant organisms. In view of the large number of antibiotics available, the clinician should refer to the hospital's antibiotic policy for guidance on treatment, and for complex treatment should consult the consultant microbiologist who will have a special interest and knowledge of antibiotics.

EDUCATION

Veitch et al (1997) suggested that the health service reforms have produced positive effects, by allowing many outdated and entrenched practices related to delivery of care to be discarded, enabling diversity and creative thinking. This permits nurses to be innovative and dynamic. Regrettably, negative outcomes of these changes are the lack of time a lecturer/practitioner has for a clinical commitment (Carlisle et al 1997) and the theory–practice gap between what research and theory say should happen and what actually happens in the clinical setting (Rolfe 1993).

Nurses are confronted with the tutor's requirement to implement the theory taught in the classroom and the pressures caused by constraints in the clinical setting. Similarly, students could qualify without being competent in essential nursing skills (Bradley 1998).

Dunn & Hansford (1997) emphasized the importance of new graduates being able to develop application skills and suggested a closer collaboration between educational institutions and the clinical setting. In order to meet this challenge, nurses who need further preparation in the skills with which they are unfamiliar would receive a thorough orientation when faced with new tasks. This would include education, a chance to handle the equipment, practical demonstration, supervision and support. As already mentioned, an i.v. team could play an important part in improving nurses' i.v. skills. Infection control nurses also have a responsibility to provide information and education to raise the awareness of all staff of infection prevention and control (Hospital Infection Working Group 1995).

Wilkinson's (1996) survey highlighted nurses' knowledge of i.v. therapy and found widespread dissatisfaction with the level of education provided. Larson & Hargiss (1984) conducted a prospective experiment and found that when a core of specially trained nurses is involved in the maintenance of i.v. therapy, improvements in patient comfort and decreased rates of phlebitis are seen. This author cautions that such an approach can only succeed if there is a commitment of time and money.

Dougherty (1996) outlined the importance of training, continued support and skill maintenance for staff involved in i.v. work. Tomford et al's (1984) prospective controlled trial indicated that trained i.v. therapy teams substantially reduce the risk of infection, and these data are supported by Hampton & Sheretz (1988). Clarke (1994) described the value of an i.v. special interest group – including senior nursing, pharmacy, infection control, anaesthetic and dietetic staff – whose task is to devise specific protocols and guidelines.

It is essential that patients receiving i.v. therapy are instructed about the risk (and preventive measures required to reduce this risk) of acquiring an infection. Macleod Clark (1988) reported that lack of time and manpower are the most important inhibiting factors for patients receiving adequate instruction. Twinn & Lee (1997) suggested that health education improves the quality of care and patients' satisfaction, and empowers patients to participate in care and activities to improve their own health. Audette (1994) suggested that the use of humour in i.v. care breaks the ice and helps the patient to learn faster.

OCCUPATIONAL RISK TO HEALTH CARE WORKERS

Nurses are at risk of acquiring infection in the workplace. Transmission of infection can occur through:

- skin puncture by blood-contaminated sharp objects such as needles, scalpels or scissors
- contamination of open wounds and skin lesions
- splashing of mucous membranes of the eye, nose or mouth
- human bites when blood is drawn.

It is not possible to calculate the risk to nurses, as it is not known how many people are infected with blood-borne infections in the UK. The UK Blood Transfusion Service screens all regular and new donors, but these results only provide information on a small section of the population (see Box 4.7).

It is this type of data, highlighting the number of undiagnosed carriers of infection, which gave rise to the suggestion that there is no safe patient, only safe technique; it reiterates the importance of treating all patients in the same way. This will result in staff becoming expert in undertaking procedures using a safe technique and will mean that when they are caring for a known infected patient, changes in practice will not be necessary, thereby avoiding the accidents that such changes provoke. The other advantage of using a safe technique for all patients is that when a known positive patient is treated, her confidentiality is maintained because there is no obvious change in practice between different patients on the ward.

The degree of risk is directly related to the type of incident (Table 4.2).

The number of health care workers known to have become infected as a result of occupational exposure is small, considering the frequency of exposure to blood and

---

■ BOX 4.7

Prevalence of blood-borne infection (Advisory Committee on Dangerous Pathogens 1995)

- 1 in 30 400 new blood donors found to be HIV+
- 1 in 287 000 regular blood donors found to be HIV+
- 1 in 1500 new blood donors HBsAg-positive
- 1 in 2000 new blood donors found to be hepatitis C antibody-positive

Table 4.2 Factors involved in assessing the risk of a sharps injury

High risk	Low risk
Hollow needle	Solid needle (suture)
Large needle	Small needle
Needle used to obtain blood	Flush needle
Deep penetrating	Wound scratch
Known infected patient	Non-infected patient
Advanced disease	Fit, well patient

body fluids in the clinical area (Hanrahan & Reutter 1997). Infection with hepatitis B and C has been seen, but fortunately the number of occupationally acquired acute hepatitis B infections has declined in recent years. Worldwide occupationally acquired infection of HIV has risen, with 214 cases reported before May 1995, 73 of which followed a documented occupational exposure: 65 of these were percutaneous exposure, and four occurred in the UK (Royal College of Pathologists 1995).

It must be remembered that the risk of seroconverting for HIV following an inoculation accident is low, estimated to be 1 in 320 or 0.32%; and following a mucocutaneous exposure the risk is even lower – 1 in 1000 or 0.1% (Royal College of Pathologists 1995).

While seroconversion to hepatitis B and C is higher, two studies in Japan estimated the transmission of hepatitis C following a single incident involving a known hepatitis C-positive patient to be 2.7 and 10%, respectively (Advisory Committee on Dangerous Pathogens 1995). Therefore, the post-inoculation accident management must consider all blood-borne viruses.

All health care workers are subject to regulations under the Health and Safety at Work etc. Act 1974, where employers and employees have a duty to protect, as far as is reasonably possible, those at work. The Control of Substances Hazardous to Health Regulations (COSHH) 1994 provide a framework of action designed to reduce the risk from hazardous substances, including blood-borne viruses. The Management of Health and Safety at Work Regulations (1992) cover an even broader range, involving assessment of risk, provision of health surveillance, information, instruction and training of employees. Reporting of exposure to, and incidents involving, pathogens that might jeopardize the health and safety of workers, including hepatitis B, falls within the Diseases and Dangerous Occurrence Regulations (Health and Safety Executive 1985). Similarly, the Industrial Injury Benefit Social Security Act 1975 has viral hepatitis as one of a number of prescribed industrial diseases where those affected may qualify for compensation.

Universal precautions

Universal precautions involve the appropriate use of barrier methods to prevent contamination by blood and body fluids of mucous membranes and non-intact skin, and the adoption of techniques to prevent inoculation accidents. Under these precautions, blood and body fluids of all patients are considered potentially infectious for blood-borne pathogens. Universal precautions are intended to supplement routine infection control policies such as hand washing. (Centres for Disease Control 1988; see Box 4.8).

Gloves

The use of gloves reduces the incidence of blood contamination of hands, but can-

■ **BOX 4.8**

Universal precautions

- Use of gloves
- Use of aprons
- Use of masks
- Use of eye protection
- Safe disposal of sharps
- Avoid needlestick injury
- Cover breaks in skin with a waterproof dressing

not prevent sharps injuries. Clean gloves are adequate for most nursing tasks (Rossoff et al 1993).

The likelihood of contamination depends on the following factors:

- skill and technique of the health care worker
- frequency with which the health care worker performs the procedure
- whether it is a routine or emergency procedure
- prevalence of blood-borne infections in the patient population
- terminal illness in the source patient
- the frequency and extent of blood and body fluid contact
- the number and extent of exposures
- inoculation accidents of increased risk
- skin integrity, i.e. whether it is visibly compromised
- the quality of infection control policies and procedures.

In 1991, the Medical Devices Directorate produced specifications for non-sterile, natural rubber latex examination gloves, requiring that gloves should be of a suitable strength and thickness to maximize protection whilst maintaining manual dexterity, be without perforations and be manufactured and lubricated with materials which will not harm the wearer. The use of poor-quality, low-cost gloves is neither safe nor cost-effective because glove changes during procedures would be required to ensure integrity. Gloves should be changed between patient contact, and hands and wrists should be washed thoroughly after glove removal.

Gloves should always be available for health care workers who wish to use them. Some institutions relaxed recommendations for the use of gloves by skilled phlebotomists where the prevalence of blood-borne pathogens is low; this is mainly to aid manual dexterity and sensitivity, which can be reduced by wearing gloves (BMA 1990). It can also be argued that the loss of dexterity caused by wearing gloves could make needlestick injury more likely.

The Department of Health (1990) recommended that gloves should be worn for all phlebotomy procedures when the phlebotomist is inexperienced, when the patient is restless or known to be infected with HIV or hepatitis B, or when cuts and abrasions are present on the hands of the phlebotomist.

Problems associated with the wearing of gloves do occur. Surveys have shown a high perforation rate for all gloves (Brough 1988), but this may be due to wear and tear in use or complacency and consequent carelessness when wearing gloves. For these reasons, it is essential that breaks in the skin that are likely to be contaminated with blood and body fluids are covered with a waterproof dressing.

Prevention of needlestick injuries

Preventing sharps injuries is crucial and yet poor in practice, as nurses' inability to recognize the potential of needlestick injuries persists (Gould 1994a). Jagger et al (1988) reported that 17% of all needlestick injuries occurred before or during use of a sharp, 70% during disposal and 13% after disposal.

The following list outlines good practice which should be adopted at all times:

- All employers must provide effective education and training on the safe use and disposal of sharps.
- All employees must work in accordance with health and safety procedures.
- Report any accidents, incidents or near misses immediately.
- Staff should ask for assistance when taking blood or giving injections to unco-operative patients.
- Wherever possible, replace sharps with other instruments or procedures.
- Never leave sharps lying around.
- Do not resheath used needles, unless there is a safe means of recapping (Department of Health 1990).
- Do not remove used needles from the syringe, but dispose of needles and syringes as a single unit.
- Do not bend, break or otherwise manipulate used needles by hand prior to disposal.
- Sharps should not be passed from hand to hand.
- The person using the sharp should dispose of the used sharp.
- Dispose of sharps immediately after use into a sharps container in accordance with British Standard 7320.
- Follow the manufacturer's instruction when assembling, using and sealing sharps containers.
- Place the sharps container where sharps are being used.
- Do not overfill the sharps container or attempt to press down upon sharps to make more room in the sharps container.
- Filled sharps containers must be transported in a safe manner to an incinerator to be incinerated.

Other factors that contribute to poor practice and which will increase the risk of sharps injuries include fatigue, stress, poor lighting, crowded working conditions, unsuitable furniture, and working alone with a patient who may be agitated, abusive or confused.

Hanrahan & Reutter (1997) reported that modifying behaviour had failed to reduce sharps injuries and therefore it was necessary to seek other means of prevention, e.g. safer devices. Needleless administration and phlebotomy systems which eliminate the risk of a sharps injury are now available. Bohony's (1993) study of such a system found a 68.6% reduction in needlestick injuries, whilst Prince et al's (1994) comparison of three needleless systems indicated how systems can be safe, require minimal in-servicing and yield significant cost saving.

Whitby et al's (1991) study did not fully support the safety records of these products, and they reported that sharps injuries doubled following implementation of a recapping device coupled to an education campaign. These researchers concluded that the increase in reported accidents was not caused by the device but was due to improved reporting by staff who had previously been unaware of the correct accident reporting policy to be followed.

One of the frequently stated problems with inoculation accidents is under-reporting. Murdock & Cowell (1993) undertook a survey of sharps injuries over 1 year and found that although 363 accidents were reported to the researcher, only 47 accident forms had been completed and only 27 accidents were reported to occupational health.

Houang & Hurley (1997) emphasized that knowledge of the risk alone is not sufficient to motivate correct behaviour, while Davis-Beattie & DeWit (1996) recommended a creative infection control programme based on psychological principles to improve compliance with infection control policies and procedures.

Clinical waste

All waste arising from medical and nursing care which may cause infection to those exposed to it is classified as clinical waste (Health and Safety Commission 1992). The bagging, transporting and disposal of clinical waste must comply with the Health Services Advisory Committee Guidelines (Health and Safety Commission 1992). The regulations on the safe disposal of clinical waste state that it must be disposed of in a heavy duty leak-proof yellow container and transported directly to the incinerator. Sharps must be disposed of in sharps containers which comply with the British Standards Institutions BS 7320 standards (1990).

Since 1996, a new government regulation, 'Special Waste Regulation 1996', has been adopted. Special waste involves any substances which are harmful. This Act refers to disposing, carrying or receiving special waste. Unused drugs are classified as special waste and this means that unused ampoules, infusion containers containing drugs and filled syringes all need to be disposed of in a designated special waste bin which is easily recognizable and readily available. Once these bins are full and correctly sealed, they can only be disposed of if a consignment note has been completed. These regulations also include restrictions on the mixing, storage, treatment, recycling and disposal of special waste.

It is essential that sharps are only placed in a designated sharps container. If they are inadvertently mixed with the general clinical waste, the many persons handling this waste during removal and eventual disposal could receive an inoculation injury (Burns 1988). Post-exposure care is much more complicated when the sharps source is unknown. Whilst all bags and containers must be labelled with the place of origin, it is still very difficult to accurately identify who the sharp was used on. It must be remembered that HIV and hepatitis B protected by organic matter will survive in the environment for some time (Gould 1994b).

Accident policy

When an inoculation accident or contamination of damaged skin occurs, action must be taken by:

- the injured person
- microbiology department
- occupational health.

Injured person

1. Encourage bleeding.
2. Wash area under running water.
3. Dry carefully and apply waterproof dressing.
4. Seek medical help for large wounds.
5. Obtain blood from patient on whom the needle had been used.
6. Arrange to give blood.
7. Fill in accident form.
8. Report incident to manager and occupational health.
9. Take bloods and accident form to microbiology department.

When contamination of skin occurs, the area must be washed under hot soapy water without the use of a nailbrush which could damage the skin and allow the entry of microorganisms. If contamination of eyes, nose or mouth occurs the area must be washed thoroughly with copious amounts of water and tasks 5–9 above must be undertaken.

Microbiology department

1. Test the patient's blood for hepatitis B and, if appropriate, hepatitis C and HIV. Store the remainder of blood in freezer.
2. Store the injured person's blood in freezer.

Occupational health

The patient's virology results coupled with the injured person's vaccination record will be used to decide the appropriate post-exposure prophylaxis.

Hepatitis

Hepatitis B

Following all injuries, occupational health should evaluate whether the injured person needs vaccinations, booster vaccinations or a discussion on why the accident happened and how a similar incident could be avoided in future.

Persons who have received a needlestick injury or had contaminated eyes, mouth, fresh cuts or abrasions with blood from a known hepatitis B surface antigen (HBsAg) positive patient will be offered the accelerated course of hepatitis B vaccine and hepatitis B immunoglobulin if the person has not been vaccinated. Previously vaccinated persons will receive a booster, while non-responders to hepatitis B vaccine will receive hepatitis B immunoglobulin and be considered for a booster dose of hepatitis B vaccine (Department of Health 1996).

Hepatitis C

Occupational infection with hepatitis C has become a major problem for health care workers, as there is no available hepatitis C vaccine and infection can lead to chronic carrier state and, in some cases, hepatocellular carcinoma (Mizuno & Suzuki 1997). Patients can be tested for hepatitis C and the member of staff can be tested at 3 and 6 months.

Human immunodeficiency virus (HIV)

In 1990, the Chief Medical Officer's Expert Advisory Group on AIDS considered the use of zidovudine (AZT) after exposure to HIV-positive blood and body fluids. At that time it was suggested that AZT was not a necessary component of post-exposure management (Advisory Committee on Dangerous Pathogens 1995). In 1996, the Centres for Disease Control updated the recommendations for chemoprophylaxis after HIV occupational exposure, stating that although AZT had failed in some cases to prevent seroconversion to HIV following an inoculation injury, generally a 79% decrease in the risk of seroconversion had been seen (Centres for Disease Control 1996).

In 1997, the Chief Medical Officer's Expert Advisory Group on AIDS considered the evidence for the efficacy of post-exposure prophylaxis with antiretroviral drugs for health care workers occupationally exposed to HIV and recommended that their use should be considered if a health care worker has been exposed to blood or other high-risk body fluids or tissue known to be, or strongly suspected to be, infected with HIV (UK Health Department 1997).

These latest recommendations suggest that the three drugs AZT, lamivudine and indinavir should be given for 4 weeks. Easterbrook & Ippolito (1997) stated that AZT monotherapy is obsolete, not just because combination therapy and new protease inhibitors are superior, but because of the reports of resistance to AZT, which may be the reason why there are at least 10 reports of post-exposure AZT failure

(Jochimsen 1997). Day (1996) reported that this approach was recommended by Dr Gazzard, Clinical Director of the AIDS unit at the Chelsea and Westminster NHS Trust, London, who emphasizes that these drugs should be taken immediately, which means that they should be available in accident and emergency departments across the country.

The risk of seroconversion to HIV must be balanced against the use of drugs whose efficacy and toxicity is not fully known. Easterbrook & Ippolito (1997) discussed how little is known about the long-term safety of antiretroviral drugs in uninfected individuals, outlining that one-third of patients discontinue prophylaxis because of intolerance to AZT.

A worker with occupational exposure to HIV should receive follow-up psychological support and medical care, which should include HIV testing immediately post-exposure and then at 6 and 12 weeks and 6 months following the accident. During the time that an injured person is waiting for the reassurance of a negative HIV antibody test, they must refrain from donating blood or other tissue and from breast feeding, and should limit the spread of their blood and body fluids, e.g. by adopting safer sex precautions (McKee 1996).

However reluctant a health care worker is to follow the correct post-exposure procedure, it must be emphasized that if the worse scenario occurs and a person does become infected, it is preferable to be aware of this diagnosis so that appropriate treatment and care can be provided. This could include treatment with α-interferon for hepatitis B or hepatitis C infection (Snashall 1996).

Post-exposure care is essential for the well-being of the exposed person and indirectly for future patients in their care. A surgeon thought to be infected through an occupational exposure in 1983 transmitted the virus to a patient in 1995 (Communicable Disease Report 1997). This is the second reported incident of transmission of HIV to patients during exposure prone procedures (Ciesielski et al 1992).

Education and strict adherence to correct techniques and practices and infection control guidelines are essential to protect the patient from infection and to safeguard health care workers against exposure to blood-borne diseases.

AUDIT

Audit plays an important role in monitoring quality of care based on outcomes, e.g. infection rates, by the provision of useful information. Corrective action can be taken, followed by re-evaluation and, hopefully, resolution of problems.

The Hospital Infection Working Group of the Department of Health and Public Health Laboratory Service (1995) discussed the importance of audit of infection control policies in wards and departments. They mentioned the inclusion of i.v. catheterization as a topic for audit, suggesting that the results of such audits should be fed back to each ward, with educational programmes introduced as necessary to correct deficiencies.

Elliott et al (1995) described an audit programme which assessed all areas of i.v. practice and which, by identifying areas where improvement could be made, could reduce the significant morbidity and mortality associated with i.v. therapy.

RESEARCH

The scope of i.v. therapy continues to become more complex and specialized. Nurses must be well versed in all aspects of care. Policies and procedures must be detailed and follow international guidelines and must be kept abreast of new research. All nurses involved in i.v. care are required to know all of these policies and procedures, which are reviewed regularly.

Clinical research provides a basis for the practice of i.v. therapy by validating standards of practice and by highlighting the practices which provide quality patient care (Lonsway 1987). There are many issues related to i.v. practice which could be a focus for nursing research, including:

- evaluation of skill mix and staffing levels on
  - — infection rates
  - — occlusion of catheters
  - — sharps injuries
- evaluation of educational events on
  - — infection rates
  - — occlusion of catheters
  - — sharps injuries
- product evaluation research
  - — i.v. safety devices, e.g. needleless systems
  - — improved occlusive transparent dressings
  - — catheter hubs which prevent endoluminal contamination.

CONCLUSION

Remarkable clinical success has been achieved in the treatment of many diseases. It is inevitable that even greater changes will come in the future, with new developments in medical and nursing practice. Unfortunately, modern medical, surgical and immunosuppressive treatments have increased these patients' susceptibility to infection. The provision of expert nursing care is the primary consideration, as vulnerable in-patients may have to be nursed in wards alongside patients with existing infections and be cared for by nursing and medical staff who care for both infected and vulnerable patients.

Intravenous catheter infection continues to be an important cause of mortality and morbidity for immunocompromised patients. One of the biggest challenges is the prevention of infection or, if this fails, the prompt diagnosis and treatment of the infection. It will never be possible to prevent all hospital-acquired infections, as the hospital environment, other patients and health care workers will expose the patients to exogenous infections during their stay in hospital. Similarly, many infections will be acquired endogenously. Nevertheless, every effort must be made to reduce the incidence of hospital-acquired infection.

Many issues related to the prevention of infection remain unresolved. This chapter has reviewed strategies in an attempt to help reduce the incidence of i.v.-related infection.

REFERENCES

Advisory Committee on Dangerous Pathogens 1995 Protection against blood borne infections in the workplace. HMSO, London

Audette I M 1994 The use of humor in intravenous nursing. Journal of Intravenous Nursing 17(1): 25–27

Ayliffe G A J, Coates D, Hoffman P N 1984 Chemical disinfection in hospitals. Public Health Laboratory Service, London

Ayliffe G A J, Lowberry E J L, Geddes A M, Williams J D 1992 Control of hospital infection. A practical handbook, 3rd edn. Chapman & Hall Medical, London

Bach A, Bohrer H, Motsch J, Martin E, Geiss H K, Sonntag H G 1993 Prevention of catheter related infection by antiseptic bonding. Journal of Surgical Research 55: 640–646

Balakrishnan G, Simpkins C, Grieg M, Hallworth D 1991 Catheter related sepsis. British Journal of Intensive Care 1(1): 17–22

Bauer E, Denson R 1979 Infection from contaminated elastoplast. New England Journal of Medicine 300(7): 370

Beam T R, Goodman E L, Farr B M, Maki D G, Mayhall C G 1990 Preventing central venous catheter related complications. Infection in Surgery October: 1–13

Bellamy K, Alcock R Jr, Babb J, Davies J G, Ayliffe G A J 1993 A test for the assessment of 'hygienic' hand disinfection using rotavirus. Journal of Hospital Infection 24: 201–210

Blackmore M 1987 Hand drying methods. Nursing Times 83(37): 71–74

Blank I, Oawes R K 1958 The water content of stratum corneum. The importance of water in promoting bacterial multiplication on cornified epithelium. Journal of Investigative Dermatology 31: 141–145

Blood Transfusion Service of the United Kingdom (McClelland B, ed) 1996 Handbook of transfusion medicine, 2nd edn. HMSO, London

Bohony J 1993 Fighting the needlestick battle without needles. Needleless intravenous piggy back. Medical Surgical Nursing 2(6): 469–476

Bradley S 1998 Prepared for practice? Exploring the experiences of newly qualified Project 2000 Child Branch staff nurses. Nursing Times Research 3(4): 292–302

Briggs M, Wilson S 1996 The principles of aseptic techniques in wound care. Professional Nurse 11(12): 805–810

British Medical Association 1990 The safe use and disposal of sharps. British Medical Association, London

British Standards Institution 1990 Specifications for sharps containers. BS 7320. BSI, Milton Keynes

Brough S J 1988 Surgical glove perforation. British Journal of Surgery 75: 317

Bryan C S 1987 'CDC says…': the case of i.v. tubing replacement. Infection Control 8(6): 255–256

Burns J 1988 At the sharps end. Nursing Times 84(36): 75–78

Callahan J K, Wesorick B 1987 Bacterial growth under a transparent dressing. American Journal Infection Control 15: 231–237

Carlisle C, Kirk S, Luker K A, 1997 The clinical role of nurse teachers within project 2000 course framework. Journal of Advanced Nursing 25: 386–395

Carter L W 1994 Bacterial translocation: nursing implications in the care of patients with neutropenia. Oncology Nurses Forum 21(5): 857–865

Casewell M, Phillips I 1977 Hands as a route of transmission for Klebsiella species. British Medical Journal 2: 1315–1517

Centres for Disease Control 1988 Update: universal precautions for prevention of transmission of HIV, hep B virus and other blood borne pathogens in health care settings. Morbidity and Mortality Weekly Report 30(24): 377–388

Centres for Disease Control 1996 Update: provisional public health service recommendations for chemoprophylaxis after occupational exposure to HIV. Morbidity and Mortality Weekly Report 45(22): 468–472

Chodoff A, Pettis A M, Schoonmaker D, Shelly M A 1995 Polymicrobial gram negative associated with saline solution flush used with a needleless intravenous system. American Journal of Infection Control 23(6): 357–363

Christianson D 1994 Caring for a patient who has an implanted port. American Journal of Nursing 94(11): 40–44

Cicco M, Panarello G, Chiaradia V 1989 Sources and route of microbial colonization of parenteral nutrition catheters. Lancet 1: 1258–1260

Ciesielski C, Marianos D, Ou C Y, Dumbaugh R, Witte J, Berkelman R 1992 Transmission of human immunodeficiency virus in a dental practice. Annals of Internal Medicine 116: 798–805

Clarke D E, Raffin T A 1990 Infectious complications of indwelling long term central venous catheters. Chest 97: 966–972

Clarke L 1994 Safety first. The Journal of Infection Control Nursing 21(1): 2–6 [in Nursing Times 90: 5]

Clemence M A, Walker D N, Farr B M 1995 Central venous catheter practice results of a survey. American Journal Infection Control 23(1): 5–12

Communicable Disease Report 1997 Transmission of HIV from an infected surgeon to a patient in France. Public Health Laboratory Service 7(4): 17

Conly J M, Grieves K, Peter B 1989 A prospective randomized study comparing transparent and dry gauze dressings for central venous catheters. The Journal of Infectious Diseases 159(2): 310–318

Crossley K B, Peterson A B 1995 Infections in the elderly. In: Mandell G L, Bennett J E, Dolin R (eds). Principles and practice of infectious diseases, 4th edn. Churchill Livingstone, New York, p 2737–2742

Cruse P J E, Ford R 1980 The epidemiology of wound infection – a 10 year prospective study of 62,939 wounds. Surgical Clinics of North America 60(1): 27–40

Davis-Beattie M, De Wit D 1996 Creative infection control. Journal of Hospital Infection 32: 85–98

Day M 1996 AIDS drugs limit damage done by dirty needles. New Scientist July 6: 7

De Jongh C A, Joshi J H, Newman K A 1986 Antibiotic synergism and response in gram negative bacteremia in granulocytopenic cancer patients. American Journal Medicine 80: 96–100

De Vries J H, Van Dorp W T, Van Barneveld P W C 1997 A randomized trial of alcohol 70% versus alcoholic iodine 2% in skin disinfection before insertion of peripheral infusion catheters. Journal of Hospital Infection 36: 317–320

Department of Health 1990 Guidance for clinical health care workers' protection against infection with HIV and hepatitis viruses. Recommendation of the expert advisory group on AIDS. HMSO, London

Department of Health 1996 Immunisation against infectious diseases. HMSO, London

Department of Health and Social Security 1973 Medicines Commission report on prevention of microbial contamination of medical products. HMSO, London

Dougherty L 1996 The benefits of an IV team in hospital practice. Professional Nurse 11(11): 761–763

Dunn S V, Hansford B 1997 Undergraduate nursing students' perceptions of their clinical learning environment. Journal of Advanced Nursing 25: 1299–1306

Easterbrook P, Ippolito G 1997 Prophylaxis after occupational exposure to HIV. British Medical Journal 315: 557–558

Elliott T S J 1993 Line associated bacteraemias. Public Health Laboratories Service Communicable Disease Report Review 3(7): R91–R96

Elliott T S J, Faroqui M H, Armstrong R F, Hanson G C 1994 Guidelines for good practice in central venous catheterization. Journal of Hospital Infection 28: 163–176

Elliott T S J, Faroqui M H, Tebbs S E, Armstrong R F, Hanson G C 1995 An audit program for central venous catheters associated infections. Journal of Hospital Infection 30: 181–191

Eyer S, Brummitt C, Crossley K, Siegal R, Cerra F 1990 Catheter related sepsis prospective randomized study of 3 methods of long term catheter maintenance. Critical Care Medicine 18: 1073–1079

Fan S T, Teoh-Chan C H, Lau K F 1989 Evaluation of central venous catheter sepsis by differential quantitative blood cultures. European Journal Clinical Microbiological Infectious Disease 8: 142–144

Goldmann D A, Maki D G, Rhame F S, Kaiser A B, Tenney J H, Beneath J V 1973 Guidelines for infection control in intravenous therapy. Annals of Internal Medicine 79: 848–850

Goodinson S M 1990 Good practice ensures minimum risk factors. Professional Nurse 6(3): 175–177

Gould D 1994a Sharp handling and disposal: a study. Nursing Standard 8(40): 25–28

Gould D 1994b Infection control in low risk environments. Nursing Standard 8(29): 30–32

Gould D 1995 Hand decontamination nurses opinions and practices. Nursing Times 91(17): 42–45

Greaves A 1985 We'll just freshen you up, dear. Nursing Times Supplement March 6: 3–8

Haddock G, Barr J, Burns H J G, Garden O J 1985 Reduction of central venous catheter complications. British Journal of Parenteral Therapy September: 124–128

Hagle M E 1987 Implantable devices for chemotherapy: access and delivery. Seminars in Oncology Nursing 3(2): 96–105

Hamilton H 1995 Central lines inserted by clinical nurse specialists. Nursing Times 91(17): 38–39

Hampton A A, Sheretz R J 1988 Vascular access infection in hospitalized patient. Surgical Clinics of North America 68(1): 57–71

Hanrahan A, Reutter L 1997 A critical review of the literature on sharps injuries: epidemiology, management of exposure and prevention. Journal of Advanced Nursing 25: 144–154

Harrison M 1997 Central venous catheter: a review of the literature. Nursing Standard 11(27): 43–45

Hayek L J, Emerson J M 1988 Preoperative whole body disinfectant– a controlled clinical study. Journal Hospital Infection (Supplement B): 15–19

Health and Safety Commission 1992 Safe disposal of clinical waste. Health Service Advisory Committee. HMSO, London

Health and Safety Executive 1985 The reporting of injuries, disease and dangerous occurrences regulations (RIDDOR). HS[R] 23. HMSO, London

Henderson D K 1995 Bacteremia due to percutaneous intravenous devices. In: Mandell G L, Bennett J E, Dolin R, eds. Principles and practices of infectious diseases, 4th edn. Churchill Livingstone, New York, p 2587–2598

Hoffmann K K, Weber D J, Samsa G P, William A R 1992 Transparent polyurethane film as an intravenous catheter dressing. Journal American Medical Association 267(15): 2072–2076

Hospital Infection Working Group of the Department of Health and Public Health Laboratory Service 1995 Hospital infection control guidance on the control of infection in hospitals. Department of Health, London

Houang E T S, Hurley R 1997 Anonymous questionnaire survey on the knowledge and practices of hospital staff in infection control. Journal of Hospital Infection 35: 301–306

Hrske F, Tonozar L 1990 Indications for the insertion of a central venous catheter in emergency situations. Anesthetics 39(1): 60–61

Intravenous Nurses Society 1998 Revised intravenous nursing standards of practice. Journal of Intravenous Nursing 21: S63

Jacobson G, Thiele J E, McCune J H, Farrell L D 1985 Handwashing: ring wearing and number of organisms. Nursing Research 34(3): 186–188

Jagger J, Hunt E H, Brand Elnagger J, Pearson R D 1988 Rates of needlestick injury caused by various devices in a university hospital. New England Journal of Medicine 319: 284–288

Jochimsen E M 1997 Failure of zidovudine postexposure prophylaxis in human immunodeficiency virus post-exposure management of health care workers. American Journal of Medicine 1(2): 52–55

John T 1996 Intravenous filters: panacea or placebo. Journal of Clinical Nursing 5(1): 3–6

Johnson A, Oppenheim B A 1992 Vascular catheter related sepsis: diagnosis and prevention. Journal of Hospital Infection 20: 67–78

Keenlyside D 1993 Avoiding an unnecessary outcome. Professional Nurse 2: 288–291

Kobayashi H 1991 Evaluation of surgical scrubbing. Journal of Hospital Infection 18(Supplement B): 29–34

Koerner R J, Morgan S, Ford M, Orr K E, McComb JM, Gould F K 1997 Outbreak of Gram-negative septicaemia caused by contaminated continuous infusions prepared in a non-clinical area. Journal of Hospital Infection 36: 285–289

Krakowska G 1986 Practice versus procedure. Journal of Infection Control Nursing (Nursing Times) 82(34): 64–69

Larson E, Leyden J J, McGinley K J, Grove G L, Talbot G H 1986 Physiologic and microbiologic changes in skin related to frequent handwashing. Infection Control 7(2): 59–63

Larson E, Hargiss C 1984 A decentralized approach to maintenance of intravenous therapy. American Journal of Infection Control 12(3): 177–186

Lau C E 1996 Transparent and gauze dressings and their effect on infection rates of central venous catheters: a review of past and current literature. Journal of Intravenous Nursing 19(5): 240–245

Laurence M 1983 Patients hand hygiene a clinical inquiry. Nursing Times 79(21): 24–25

Lee R B, Buckner M, Sharp K W 1988 Do multi lumen catheters increase central venous catheter sepsis compared to single lumen catheters. Journal of Trauma 28(10): 1472–1475

Lilienberg A, Bengtsson M, Starkhammar H 1994 Implantable devices for venous access: nurses' and patients' evaluation of three different port systems. Journal of Advanced Nursing 19: 21–28

Loach L 1997 Blue days. Nursing Times 93(32): 30–31

Lonsway R A 1987 Research standards and infection control the impact on IV nursing. Journal of the National Intravenous Therapy Association 10(2): 106–109

Lundgren A, Ek A 1996 Factors influencing nurses' handling and control of peripheral intravenous lines. An interview study. International Journal of Nursing Studies 33(2): 131–142

McClelland B 1996 Handbook of transfusion services of the United Kingdom, 2nd edn. HMSO, London

McKee J M 1996 Human immunodeficiency virus healthcare worker safety issues. Journal of Intravenous Nursing 19(3): 132–140

MacKinnon S, Garden O J, Gribben J C, Burns H J G, Baird D, Burnett A K 1987 The use of Hickman catheters in marrow transplant recipients. Intensive Therapy and Clinical Monitoring 8: 122–126

Macleod Clark J 1988 Communication: the continuing challenge. Nursing Times 84(23): 24–27

Maki D G 1977 A semi quantitative culture method for identifying intravenous catheter related sepsis. New England Journal of Medicine 296: 1305–1309

Maki D G, Goldman D A, Rhame F S 1973 Infection control in intravenous therapy. Annals of Internal Medicine 79: 867–887

Maki D G, Ringer M, Alvarado C J 1991 Prospective randomized trial of povidone-iodine, alcohol, and chlorhexidine for prevention of infection associated with central venous and arterial catheters. Lancet 338: 339–342

Mallett J, Bailey C 1996 The Royal Marsden NHS Trust manual of clinical nursing procedures, 4th edn. Blackwell Science, London

Markus S, Budley S 1989 Culturing indwelling central venous catheters in situ. Infections in Surgery 5: 157–161

Matthews J A, Newson S W B 1987 Hot air electric hand dryers compared with paper towels for potential spread of airborne bacteria. Journal of Hospital Infection 9: 85–88

Medical Devices Directorate 1991 Specification for non sterile, natural latex examination gloves. Department of Health, doc. no. TSS/3000.010/1

Mehtar S, Taylor P 1981 A review of bacteriological observation in the care of IV cannulae. British Journal of Intravenous Therapy June: 16–22

Miller J M, Goetz A M, Squier C, Muder R R 1996 Reduction in nosocomial intravenous device-related bacteraemia after institution of an intravenous therapy team. Journal of Intravenous Nursing 19(2): 103–106

Mizuno Y, Suzuki K 1997 Study of needlestick accidents and hepatitis C virus infection in health care workers by molecular evolutionary analysis. Journal of Hospital Infection 35: 149–154

Morse L T, William H L, Green F P 1968 Septicemia due to *Klebsiella pneumoniae* originating from a hand cream dispenser. New England Journal of Medicine 277: 472–473

Mortimer J Y, Spooner R J D 1997 HIV infection transmitted through blood product treatment, blood transfusion, and tissue transplantation. Communicable Disease Report Review 7(9): R130–132

Murdock S, Cowell F 1993 Sharp shocks. Nursing Times 89(2): 64–68

Noe J J, Keller M 1988 Can stitches get wet? Plastics and Reconstruction Surgery 28: 205

Nystrom B, Olesen-Larson S, Dankert J, Daschner F, Greco D, Gronroos P 1983 Bacteraemia in surgical patients with IV devices. A European multicentre incidence study. Journal of Hospital Infection 4: 338–349

Paulson D S 1993 Efficacy evaluation of a 4% chlorhexidine gluconate as a full body shower wash. American Journal of Infection Control 21(4): 205–209

Perceval A 1981 Microbiological hazards of parenteral nutrition therapy. Australian Journal Hospital Pharmacology 11(3): S17–S22

Pereira L J, Lea G M, Wade K I 1997 An evaluation of five protocols for surgical handwashing in relation to skin condition and microbial counts. Journal of Hospital Infection 36: 49–65

Perucca R 1995 In: Terry J, Baranowski L, Lonsway R A, Hedrick C (eds) Intravenous therapy: clinical principles and practices. WB Saunders, Philadelphia, ch 8, p 140–150

Peters G, Locci R, Pulverer G 1982 Adherence and growth of coagulase negative staphylococci on surfaces of intravenous catheters. Journal of Infectious Diseases 146: 479–482

Pettersson E 1986 A cut above the rest. Nursing Times 31(5): 68–70

Philpott-Howard J, Casewell M 1994 Hospital infection control. Policies & practical procedures. WB Saunders, London

Prichard V, Hathaway C 1988 Patients' handwashing practice. Nursing Times 84(36): 68–72

Prince K, Summers L, Knight M A 1994 Needleless IV therapy comparing 3 systems for safety. Nursing Management 25(3): 80–86

Roberts J 1987 Pennywise pound foolish. Nursing Times 83(37): 68–70

Rolfe G 1993 Closing the theory-practice gap: a model of nursing practice. Journal of Clinical Nursing 2: 173–177

Rossoff L J, Lam S, Hilton E, Borenstein M, Isenberg H D 1993 Is the use of boxed gloves in an intensive care unit safe? American Journal of Medicine 94: 602–607

Royal College of Pathologists 1995 HIV and the practice of pathology. Marks and Spencer Publication Unit of the Royal College of Pathologists, London

Ryan J A, Abel R M, Abbott W M 1974 Catheter complications in total parenteral nutrition. A prospective study of 200 consecutive patients. New England Journal of Medicine 290: 757–761

Sanderson I, Deital M 1973 Intravenous hyperalimentation without sepsis. Surgery, Gynecology and Obstetrics 136: 577–583

Scalley R D, Vans C S, Cochran R S 1992 The impact of an IV team on the occurrence of intravenous-related phlebitis. Journal of Intravenous Nursing 15(2): 100–109

Sitges-Serra A, Pi-Suner T, Garces J M, Segura M 1995 Pathogenesis and prevention of catheter related septicemia. American Journal of Infectious Diseases 23: 310–316

Snashall D 1996 Occupational factors. British Medical Journal 313: 551–554

Speechley V, Davidson T 1989 Managing an implantable drug delivery system. Professional Nurse 4(6): 284–288

Teare E L, Peacock A 1996 The development of an infection control link nurse program in a district general hospital. Journal of Hospital Infection 34: 267–278

Terry J, Baranowski L, Lonsway R A, Hedrick C 1995 Intravenous therapy. Clinical principles and practice. WB Saunders, Philadelphia

Threlkeld M G, Cobbs C G 1995 Infectious disorders of prosthetic valves and intravenous devices. In: Mandell G L, Bennett J E, Dolin R (eds) Principles and practices of infectious diseases, 4th edn. Churchill Livingstone, New York, p 783–793

Tomford J W, Hershy C O, McLaren C E, Porter D K, Cohen D I 1984 Intravenous therapy teams and peripheral venous catheters associated complications. A prospective controlled study. Archives of Internal Medicine 144(6): 1191–1194

Tramont E C, Hoover D L 1995 General or non specific host defense mechanisms. In: Mandell G L, Bennett J E, Dolin R (eds) Principles and practices of infectious disease, 4th edn. Churchill Livingstone, New York, p 30–35

Treston-Aurand J, Olmsted R N, Allen-Bridson K, Craig C P 1997 Impact of dressing materials on central venous catheter infection rates. Journal of Intravenous Nursing 20(4): 201–206

Tristram D A, Pearay L O 1992 Onlogeny of the immune system. In: Patrick C C. Infections in the immunocompromised infants and children. Churchill Livingstone, New York

Twinn S F, Lee D T F 1997 The practice of health education in acute care settings in Hong Kong: an exploratory study of the contribution of registered nurses. Journal of Advanced Nursing 25: 178–185

UK Health Department 1997 Guidelines on post exposure prophylaxis for health care workers occupationally exposed to HIV. Department of Health. PL/CO(97):1

Van Der Meer J W M 1994 Defects in host defense mechanisms. In: Rubin R H, Young L S, Russell P S (eds) Clinical approach to infection in compromised host, 3rd edn. Plenum Medical Book Company, New York, p 33–66

Veitch L, May N, McIntosh J 1997 The practice based context of education innovations, nurse and midwife preparation in Scotland. Journal of Advanced Nursing 25(1): 191–198

Wade J C 1994 Epidemiology and prevention of infection in the compromised host. In: Rubin R H, Young L S (eds) Clinical approach to infection in the compromised host, 3rd edn. Plenum Medical Book Company, New York, p 5–25

Weinstein S M 1993 Plumer's principles and practices of intravenous therapy, 5th edn. JB Lippincott, Philadelphia, p 94–111

Whitby M, Stead P, Nayman J M 1991 Needlestick injury: impact of a recapping device and an association education program. Infection Control and Hospital Epidemiology 13: 535–539

Wilkinson R 1996 Nurses' concerns about IV therapy and devices. Nursing Standard 10(3): 35–37

Williams D, Bergan T, Moosdeen F 1997 Arrival of vancomycin resistance in *Staphylococcus aureus*. Antibiotics Chemotherapy 1(2): 1

Wilson J, Richardson J 1996 Keeping MRSA in perspective. Nursing Times 92(19): 2–4

Wilson J 1995 Infection control in clinical practice. Baillière Tindall, London

Pharmacological aspects of intravenous drug therapy

Mojgan H. Sani

CHAPTER 5

INTRODUCTION

Intravenous drug infusions today are made to an extremely high standard. They must be sterile, non-pyrogenic, particle-free and usually isotonic with body plasma.

Solutions are administered intravenously in the following situations:

- to maintain fluid balance in patients who cannot take fluids by mouth
- to achieve high and predictable drug levels in acute situations, e.g. aminophylline in severe asthmatic attacks; antibiotics in life-threatening infections
- to patients in whom the gut has to be rested, e.g. Crohn's disease, following gastrointestinal surgery
- to patients who cannot tolerate drugs by mouth, e.g. if vomiting or unconscious
- when the drug is broken down in, or not absorbed from, the gastrointestinal tract, e.g. benzylpenicillin, gentamicin
- when an injection is required but injecting into skin or muscle would cause pain or trauma.

Intravenous medications are available as:

- aqueous solutions ready to administer, e.g. atropine, heparin
- powder requiring reconstitution with water or sodium chloride 0.9%, e.g. flucloxacillin, ampicillin, cefuroxime and ceftazidime
- powder supplied with special diluent, e.g. sodium fusidate
- non-aqueous solutions ready to administer, e.g. Diazemuls® and propofol.

Great care is needed when using the i.v. route, as drugs reach high concentrations in the blood and adverse reactions can be immediate and severe. Some drugs have to be given slowly in infusion fluids because the undiluted drug is an irritant to the vein, or because the serum level achieved would be dangerous after direct injection.

CHOICE OF THE ROUTE OF DRUG ADMINISTRATION

Factors which should be considered when choosing the i.v. drug administration route are detailed in Box 5.1.

Sometimes an initial period (e.g. 24 hours) of i.v. drugs such as antibiotics may be given, to ensure high plasma levels, followed by oral medication as the patient's condition improves. Clinical pharmacokinetics of drugs, therefore, play a significant role in safety and efficacy. Absorption and distribution of drugs are important factors regarding the choice of the route. Therefore, these areas will be discussed in more detail later in the chapter.

■ **BOX 5.1 Considerations for the intravenous route of drug administration**

- Risk of infection due to vascular access devices
- Increased risk of toxicity due to direct drug delivery into the circulation
- Oral bioavailability of drugs
- Clinical state of the patient (e.g. critically ill)
- Speed of response required
- Drug ineffective by the oral route
- Patient unable to take oral medication
- Cost of i.v. vs. oral administration
- Time needed for i.v. vs. oral administration
- Other routes not appropriate (e.g. erratic absorption when given intramuscularly)

BODY FLUID DISTRIBUTION BY COMPARTMENTS

The total body water (TBW) ranges from 45 to 65% of the total body weight of the human adult. Body water is distributed into two main compartments: the intracellular fluid (ICF) space and the extracellular fluid (ECF) space. Two-thirds (approximately 32 L) of the total body water is situated in the ICF space and one-third (16 L) in the ECF space. Normally about one-quarter of the ECF (4 L) is in the intravascular compartment and three-quarters (12 L) in the interstitial compartment. The membranes separating these compartments are freely permeable to water, which moves under the force of the osmotic drive until the osmolality in each compartment is equivalent.

Normal plasma osmolality is 280–290 mOsm/kg and is determined by the number of particles, not size or valence. Plasma osmolality reflects the osmolality of total body water. An isotonic solution has the same osmotic pressure as the plasma, e.g. sodium chloride 0.9%. In contrast, a hypotonic solution will have a lower osmotic pressure than plasma, e.g. sodium chloride 0.45%, and a hypertonic solution will have a higher osmotic pressure than plasma, e.g. sodium chloride 1.8%.

When 'free water' (dextrose or glucose 5%) is added into one compartment, it distributes evenly throughout the total body water, and the amount of volume added to any given compartment is proportional to its fractional representation of the total body water. For example, if 3 L of fluid is administered to the intravascular space, the above-mentioned compartment volumes will change from 16 to 17 L in the extracellular space and from 32 to 34 L in the intracellular space. Of the 3 L volume administered, only 250 ml will therefore be delivered to the intravascular volume after equilibration takes place. If the 3 L of solution are isotonic with plasma (sodium chloride 0.9% or Ringer's solution), a different fluid distribution occurs. Since there is no difference in osmolality between the infused fluid and the body fluids, there is no driving force to cause water to diffuse into the intracellular fluid space. The membrane between the interstitial fluid and the intravascular space is permeable to ions and small particles, whereas the membrane surrounding the intracellular fluid is not. Therefore, the extracellular space is the distribution compartment for the isotonic solutions such as sodium chloride 0.9%. All solutions are a combination of isotonic fluid and free water. For example, sodium chloride 0.45% can be considered as 500 ml of sodium chloride 0.9% plus 500 ml of free water. The proportion that is isotonic is distributed in the extracellular space and the other half (water) is distributed in the total body water. Therefore, isotonic solutions are distributed evenly in the extracellular space.

CLINICAL PHARMACOKINETICS

Pharmacokinetics relates to the movement of drugs within the body, and this can be subdivided into four main categories: absorption, distribution, metabolism and excretion.

Absorption

Absorption is the process by which the drug is taken into the body and is dependent on both the agent's properties and the route of administration. Bioavailability is defined as the rate and extent of absorption into the systemic circulation. In other words, absorption or bioavailability of a drug is the fraction of a dose available to the site of action following oral administration. This can be estimated by comparing the amounts of the drug excreted in the urine following oral and i.v. administration (i.e. by comparing the area under the plasma concentration against time curves (AUC) for the two routes):

Amount of drug absorbed = bioavailability × dose

The bioavailability of an i.v. drug is assumed to be 100%, as the drug is injected directly into the circulation. However, different drugs have different oral bioavailabilities (e.g. oral amoxycillin is better absorbed than oral ampicillin, as the latter has a lower bioavailability, particularly in the presence of food). Therefore, in high-risk patients, i.v. ampicillin offers a significant advantage compared with the oral formulation.

Absorption of oral drugs may be influenced by a number of factors, including gastric emptying time, intestinal transit time, acidic pH of the gastric contents, condition of the intestinal epithelium, chemistry of drugs (active or pro-drugs) and the first-pass hepatic metabolism. Each of these factors is briefly discussed in order to provide some background information regarding influences on the choice of the route, as well as to indicate when the i.v. route may be more appropriate.

Gastric emptying time If the gastric emptying time is increased, the rate of absorption is increased for the drugs absorbed in the intestine. Some drugs, such as cisapride, increase the gastric emptying time, thereby allowing more time for absorption to take place in the intestine.

Intestinal transit time Absorption of specially formulated drugs, e.g. enteric-coated (EC) or slow-release (SR), can be reduced if the intestinal transit time is increased.

Acidic pH of the gastric contents This can often influence the absorption rate; for example, most oral forms of penicillin antibiotics are much better absorbed in acidic conditions and therefore doses are taken on an empty stomach 30 minutes to 1 hour before food.

Condition of the intestinal epithelium Cardiac failure can lead to oedema of the gastrointestinal tract and this can reduce absorption of oral drugs significantly. In severe cases, antibiotic doses may have to be administered by the i.v. route to ensure that effective systemic concentrations are achieved.

Pro-drugs Some agents are formulated as pro-drugs, which are activated in the body after administration (e.g. chloramphenicol succinate). These agents (pro-drugs) need to undergo a chemical reaction within the body, e.g. hepatic metabolism, in order to become converted to active drugs.

First-pass hepatic metabolism Many drugs are absorbed in the stomach or intestine. When a drug is administered by the oral route, blood carrying the absorbed dose flows from the stomach or intestine to the liver before reaching the general cir-

Fig. 5.1 First-pass metabolism. Drugs absorbed into the bloodstream from the gastrointestinal tract undergo some metabolism in the liver before reaching the general circulation.

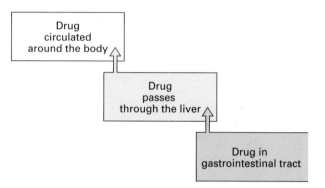

culation. The metabolism of a drug on its first journey through the liver is known as first-pass metabolism (Fig. 5.1) and this can significantly reduce the drug's bioavailability.

Distribution

Drug distribution describes the movement of drugs within the body following absorption and is influenced primarily by the molecular size, degree of ionization, tissue perfusion, and plasma and tissue drug–protein binding. It is a significant factor in deciding on an intravenous route of administration.

The term 'apparent volume of distribution' (Vd) defines the relationship between blood or plasma concentration (C) and the total amount of drug in the body (A). This relationship is expressed as:

$A = C/Vd$

Alternatively

$$apparent\ volume\ of\ distribution\ (Vd) = \frac{dose}{serum\ concentration}$$

Drugs with a small Vd (0.6 L/kg) are distributed primarily into the body water. Distribution occurs after the drug has appeared in the systemic circulation. This phase continues until equilibrium is reached. At this equilibrium, the most useful measurement would be the concentration of the drug at the site of action. A blood level measurement demonstrates a relationship between the drug concentration at the site of action and its pharmacological action. Drugs such as penicillins, cephalosporins and aminoglycosides tend to be distributed in 20–25% of body volume, which corresponds to the extracellular fluid space. More lipid-soluble compounds, such as metronidazole, rifampicin, trimethoprim, doxycycline and chloramphenicol, show a more extensive distribution due to the higher tissue penetration.

The distribution phase can be divided into the central and peripheral compartments. The central compartment consists of blood vessels and tissues which are highly perfused by blood, such as brain, heart, kidneys and liver. The peripheral compartment includes other tissues which do not receive the drug instantaneously, i.e. some time is needed for the drug to be distributed into these areas (Fig. 5.2). Among antibiotics, this particularly applies to vancomycin and teicoplanin, making the drug pharmacokinetics more complex.

Metabolism

Drug elimination from the body may occur by metabolism, excretion or both. Hepatic biotransformation, the major route of drug metabolism, is primarily depen-

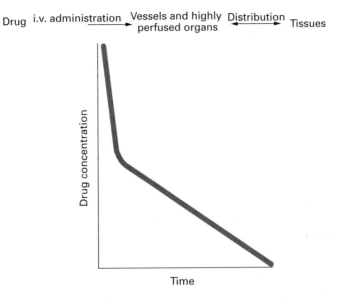

Drug $\xrightarrow{\text{i.v. administration}}$ Vessels and highly perfused organs $\xleftrightarrow{\text{Distribution}}$ Tissues

Fig. 5.2 After intravenous administration, a drug reaches the blood vessels, and thus the most highly perfused organs in the central compartment, before affecting the peripheral tissues.

dent on hepatic blood flow, drug plasma protein binding, and the hepatocytes' ability to clear drugs, i.e. the intrinsic clearance. Therefore, there is a need for dosage adjustment in patients with liver damage if the drug is dependent on hepatic metabolism.

Excretion

The kidney represents the major route of excretion of drugs and drug metabolites. A number of drugs undergo metabolism by the lungs or plasma enzymes. Some drugs undergo biliary elimination to be excreted in the faeces or to be reabsorbed at a later stage into the small intestine. This is known as enterohepatic circulation or recycling. Drug clearance is defined in terms of the rate of the blood or plasma volume that can be cleared of a drug per unit time. The elimination rate constant (k) describes the rate of disappearance of a drug from the blood and is dependent on the total body clearance (Cl) and the volume of distribution (Vd). This relationship can be described as:

$k = Cl/Vd$

The drug's half-life describes the time taken for a drug's plasma concentration to fall by 50%. The pharmacokinetic parameters such as the clearance, half-life and the volume of distribution are very useful in therapeutic drug monitoring.

THERAPEUTIC DRUG MONITORING

The therapeutic index is the ratio between the median toxic dose and the median effective dose. The therapeutic range is defined as the lowest effective serum concentration to the maximum tolerable effective serum concentration. Often there is not a clear distinction between the maximum efficacy and the risk of toxicity. Drugs with a wide therapeutic range include penicillins and cephalosporin antibiotics, and those with a narrow range include aminoglycosides, digoxin and theophylline.

Optimization of drug therapy often involves serum drug concentration measurements and monitoring in order to maintain the drug level within the therapeutic range. The therapeutic range is the range of drug concentrations with a high probability of desired clinical response and a relatively low probability of unacceptable drug toxicity. Therapeutic drug monitoring commonly includes patient-specific factors (age, weight, height, sex, history of drug exposure, concurrent disease states), along with the drug pharmacology, dose, pharmacokinetic model, route of administration, potential drug interactions, sample processing and analysis. Whilst serum concentration monitoring provides very useful information, frequent sampling may be detrimental to the patient's condition. The usefulness should always be assessed prior to sampling and should generally be restricted to therapy initiation, dosage alterations and prevention of drug toxicity.

The proper timing for taking samples is a very significant factor and it varies for different agents and routes of administration. The blood sample should ideally not be taken from the same device through which the drug has been infused. However, if it is necessary to use the device, then it should obviously be thoroughly flushed with sodium chloride 0.9% (normal saline) after drug infusion and prior to sampling.

ADVANTAGES AND DISADVANTAGES OF THE INTRAVENOUS ROUTE OF ADMINISTRATION

Advantages of the intravenous route of administration may include the following:

- The drug reaches the circulation with a minimum delay; this is important when speed is essential.
- Large quantities of fluid can be introduced over a long period of time by means of a constant infusion.
- It is suitable for substances which are not absorbed from tissue depots or the GI tract, or which would be destroyed before reaching the circulation.

Disadvantages of the intravenous route of administration may include the following:

- Once injected there is no recall, i.e. reversal is difficult and often impossible.
- Too rapid an injection may cause adverse effects on the circulation or respiration, e.g. a high blood concentration reaching the heart over a short period causing 'speedshock'. Safety demands that a slow i.v. injection be administered over a period required for the complete circulation of the blood (i.e. time taken for the blood ejected per heartbeat to go around the body and back to the heart), e.g. 1–3 minutes.
- Anaphylactic reactions may be severe in a sensitized individual, i.e. sudden massive antigen–antibody reaction.
- There is a danger of embolism (blocking of small blood vessels), e.g. if particulate matter is introduced.
- Haemolysis or agglutination may be caused by hypotonic or hypertonic solutions.
- Infection by contaminants, e.g. bacteria or pyrogens, is one of the main hazards if strict aseptic techniques are not adopted.
- Use of the wrong diluent can lead to complications, including reduced drug efficacy, damage to red blood cells, injection of particles or excess sodium load.
- Thrombophlebitis may be caused by hypertonic solutions.
- It can lead to extravasation, when the tissue is damaged by the drug, e.g. vesicant cytotoxic agents and highly alkaline drugs such as sodium bicarbonate 8.4%.
- There may be overloading due to insufficient control. This may occur if the correct equipment for drug delivery is not used, e.g. pumps, burettes.

HAZARDS OF INTRAVENOUS THERAPY

Intravenous drug therapy administration is associated with a number of hazards. These include drug incompatibilities, particulate contamination, microbial contamination, air embolism, phlebitis, infiltration and extravasation, and the risk of fluid overload.

Drug incompatibilities

A full explanation of physical and chemical drug incompatibility is given in the next section (p. 125). A summary of drug incompatibility classified into three main problems – drug/diluent incompatibility, drug/drug interaction and drug/giving set interaction – is given below.

Drug/diluent incompatibility

The choice of diluent for reconstitution and/or further dilution of the drug is an important consideration. Some specific examples are discussed below.

Frusemide is a highly alkaline drug and is therefore not compatible with dextrose (glucose) 5% infusion fluid. This is because dextrose is more acidic than sodium chloride 0.9%. However, as most patients requiring frusemide are fluid- and sodium-restricted, this presents the practitioner with a dilemma regarding the choice of the diluent and the volume used.

Amphotericin, the antifungal agent, needs to de diluted in dextrose (glucose) 5%. However, the infusion fluid has to be buffered with a phosphate buffer in order to adjust its acidity and prevent precipitation in dextrose (glucose) 5%.

Erythromycin is an irritant drug which has to be diluted well with sodium chloride 0.9%. However, this diluent cannot be used for the initial reconstitution of the powdered drug because an insoluble solid gel will be formed. Water for injections is used for the reconstitution stage and then sodium chloride 0.9% is used for further dilution.

Ampicillin has a higher stability in sodium chloride 0.9% but not in the slightly acidic glucose solutions. There is no precipitation or visible change, but polymers are formed that may play a part in allergic reactions. Ampicillin is also incompatible with drugs which themselves make infusion fluids more acidic.

Aminophylline precipitates in acidic solutions, but not in dilute solutions found in i.v. infusions. It can therefore be added to a large-volume infusion of glucose, but will precipitate if mixed with a small volume of glucose in a syringe. Aminophylline makes the solution alkaline, and therefore drugs which are unstable in alkali cannot be added as well, e.g. benzylpenicillin.

Drug/drug interaction

In an ideal situation, all drugs administered should be given into separate devices to minimize the risk of incompatibility. However, this is not always possible, particularly with critically ill patients on multiple intravenous drug therapy and with limited vascular access devices. In these situations, drugs may be given through the same device as long as they are known to be compatible. There are a number of factors that may lead to incompatibilities, but the three commonest causes are pH differences, salt factor of the agent and size of the molecules. This can be best illustrated by the following clinical examples.

pH differences All inotropes marketed in the UK are compatible with each other (all acidic pH) except for enoximone which is highly alkaline. Enoximone forms a precipitate if given through the same device as the other inotropes, such as adrenaline (epinephrine), noradrenaline, dobutamine or dopexamine. This highlights the fact that practitioners must never assume that drugs can be given through the same device even if the clinical indication (pharmacology) of the agents is similar. Compatibility is dependent on the chemistry of the drugs and not the pharmacology.

Salt factors Calcium-containing drugs must not be administered through the same administration set as an infusion containing phosphates. This is due to the cation (positively charged ions of calcium) forming a complex with the anion (negatively charged ions of phosphate). The end product will be calcium phosphate salt as a precipitate. This is why the order in which electrolytes are added when preparing parenteral nutrition (PN) is so significant, and why further additions of other drugs to the bags on the ward must be avoided (Eggert et al 1982, Henry et al 1980).

Size of the molecule Gentamicin antibiotic, given through the same device or administration set as heparinized saline, will form a complex with the heparin, leading to the inactivation of the gentamicin and/or heparin. This is due to the sizes of the two molecules interacting with each other. Gentamicin inactivation can obviously have significant implications for the septic patient. This is why the practice of flushing with sodium chloride 0.9% after the injection is recommended, rather than flushing with heparinized saline which generally offers no additional advantage for maintaining patency in the i.v. device.

Drug/administration set interaction

There are a number of drugs which are incompatible with polyvinylchloride (PVC) giving sets, e.g. glyceryl trinitrate (GTN) and nimodipine (Moorhatch & Chiou 1974). These agents are absorbed onto the PVC set and will therefore not reach the circulation until a saturation point is reached. Dose titration will be difficult if new giving sets are used each time the drug is prepared and so non-PVC sets, made of polyethylene, should be used. Drugs which are incompatible with the PVC bags are presented in glass bottles by the manufacturer, e.g. chlormethiazole, GTN, nimodipine.

Other hazards

Particulate contamination

Intravenous infusions must be free of visible particles to prevent particulate embolism. Infusions are tested by the manufacturer to ensure that non-visible particles satisfy agreed standards set in the *British Pharmacopoeia*. If a drug is added to an infusion fluid which is incompatible, particles may form. These solutions must always be discarded.

Microbial contamination

Most i.v. solutions are sterilized during manufacture by heating in an autoclave. Some solutions are unstable when heated and are sterilized by filtration. Microorganisms are filtered out by using membranes with a very small pore size. Care is needed in setting up an i.v. infusion and in giving drugs intravenously in order to maintain sterility.

Air embolism

Air embolism can occur if solution containers are allowed to empty or if they are incorrectly set up. Poor connections on the administration set also increase the chance of air embolism. They are more likely when rigid containers requiring an air inlet are used, particularly if the infusion is not stopped before the container empties.

Phlebitis

Inflammation of the vein can be caused by:

- the introduction of particulate matter
- poor venepuncture technique
- movement of the cannula within the vein
- acidic or alkaline solutions
- prolonged infusion at the same site
- cytotoxic/irritant drugs
- incorrect dilution and administration of drugs.

Infiltration and extravasation

Infiltration is the leakage of fluid into the tissues surrounding the intravenous site. This may lead to swelling. Extravasation is leakage of vesicant drugs and can result in the necrosis or sloughing of the local tissue.

Fluid overload

This is caused by excessive or overly rapid infusion of i.v. fluids. It is especially hazardous in the elderly, the very young and those with impaired renal or cardiac function.

CHEMICAL AND PHYSICAL DRUG INCOMPATIBILITY

The term incompatibility generally refers to physicochemical reactions such as precipitation or physical change in the molecule. The incompatibility may be visible as haziness or change of colour or viscosity, or it may not be visible at all. The majority of incompatibilities are classified into physical or chemical ones.

A chemical incompatibility may be related to an oxidation–reduction reaction, hydrolysis or a combination. Oxidation–reduction is defined as the gain or loss of hydrogen ions, i.e. oxidation results from the loss of electrons and reduction from gain of electrons. Oxidation and reduction may occur together and this is demonstrated by compounds normally considered to be readily oxidized, e.g. phenothiazine tranquillizers.

Incompatibilities due to acid–base reactions are manifested as precipitation, gas formation or a change in colour. Correction of acid–base reactions may be achieved by the addition of a buffer or a change of the vehicle used to prevent formation of the free acid or free base from the salt.

Hydrolysis reactions may be divided into ionic and molecular hydrolysis. Ionic hydrolysis involves the reaction with either a hydrogen (H) or a hydroxyl group (OH) of water to form an un-ionized insoluble product. For example, aluminium salts hydrolyse, resulting in insoluble basic salts and the hydroxide. Molecular hydrolysis involves the reaction of water and organic compounds such as esters and amides. This type of hydrolysis is a much slower process than the ionic one and, unfortunately, it reduces the therapeutic efficacy of the drug and is not always detectable by a physical change. Ionic hydrolysis can be prevented or reversed by the addition of any of the molecules formed as a result of hydrolysis. However, prevention of molecular hydrolysis is much more involved and requires a knowledge of molecular stability (Trissel 1997).

Physical incompatibilities are related to solubility changes or container interactions rather than a molecular change in the drug itself. For drugs that are weak acids or bases, solubility is a direct function of the pH. A drug that is a weak acid may be formulated in a specific pH to result in the desired solubility. For example, drugs such as phenytoin and methotrexate are formulated in high pH values in order to achieve desired and adequate solubility. These drugs will therefore precipitate if mixed with acidic agents due to the formation of salts. A similar rationale is applied to the salts of weak bases in alkaline solutions.

The sorption phenomenon is another form of physical incompatibility (Moorhatch & Chiou 1974). The intact drug is lost from the solution and is adsorbed onto the container material, e.g. insulins, GTN, diazepam. Glass surfaces can be modified to prevent this phenomenon, but PVC containers are more prone to the interaction. The PVC containers are made with large amounts of phthalate plasticizers to make them flexible. The lipid-soluble drugs may therefore diffuse from the solution into the plasticizer in the plastic matrix. The opposite effect of leaching of the plasticizer into the solution may also occur. Solvents may be added to prevent this leaching-out effect (Moorhatch & Chiou 1974).

Other physical incompatibilities include the salting-out reaction in which organic ions may be affected in the presence of high concentrations of electrolytes such as sodium, potassium, iron, magnesium and others. Drugs may form an insoluble complex with other solvents. For example, erythromycin or amphotericin B may form chelates (insoluble complexes) with the antibacterial preservatives in the diluents. Colour changes and gas formation are also examples of physical incompatibilities, and the latter may occur with the addition of acidic drugs to bicarbonate solutions. Some cephalosporins may contain carbon dioxide or bicarbonates in the formulation, which may result in minor explosive-like reactions in the syringe.

FACTORS AFFECTING STABILITY OF DRUG PREPARATIONS

The term instability is used to define irreversible chemical reactions rendering the drug inactive or toxic (Trissel 1997). There are a number of factors affecting the stability of drugs, including pH, light, temperature, time, and diluent for reconstitution and further dilution. These factors may render a drug unstable or inactive. This will have obvious clinical implications for the patient in terms of lack of efficacy, increased toxicity and side-effects, or both.

pH

Drug preparations, when reconstituted with the appropriate diluent, usually have the pH of maximum stability. Some are buffered or adjusted so that the pH of the resultant solution gives minimal drug degradation. Phenytoin, for example, is a highly alkaline agent which precipitates in the acidic infusion fluid dextrose (glucose) 5%. Due to its susceptibility to pH changes and thus precipitation, it should not be diluted more than 10 mg/ml.

Light

Many drugs are susceptible to light and may decompose to breakdown products which are toxic. Photodegradation may also result in a loss of therapeutic effect. For example, photodegradation of amphotericin leads to the generation of toxic by-products, with the resultant loss of potency of the drug preparation and reduced therapeutic effect.

Degradation of solutions of sodium nitroprusside is accelerated in the presence of light with the formation of cyanogen and toxic cyanide derivatives.

In order to reduce the photodegradation of solutions, such as those described above, the bulk container should be protected from light with either aluminium foil or coloured plastic. Administration sets should also be protected from light or made from coloured plastic.

Temperature

It is essential that drugs should be stored at the temperature recommended by the manufacturer to ensure their stability. Drugs which should be stored in the refrigerator include dinoprostone, disopyramide, epoprostenol and atracurium.

Time

The shelf-life of a drug is the period of time tested and approved by the manufacturer before the agent expires. Therefore, the stability time and conditions for storage, such as the temperature, recommended by the company must be adhered to. It is important to note, however, that the 'shelf-life' on the pack relates to the undiluted product. Once a drug has been reconstituted or diluted, this is reduced drastically. This information varies with each drug and can be obtained from the agent's data sheet (package insert).

Diluent

It is essential to use the correct specified diluent for the drug in order to prevent incompatibilities and loss of efficacy. This is specified in the product's data sheet produced by the manufacturer.

METHODS OF INTRAVENOUS DRUG ADMINISTRATION

Intravenous drugs can be administered by three methods:

- continuous i.v. infusion
- intermittent i.v. infusion
- bolus i.v. injection.

The choice of the method is generally based on two main factors:

- achieving sufficient concentrations in the circulation to ensure efficacy
- safety and minimization of adverse reactions and toxicity.

Antibiotics are usually administered as a bolus injection in order to achieve high peaks, so as to ensure effective antimicrobial activity. However, some antibiotics, such as vancomycin and the antifungal agent amphotericin, are administered as intermittent infusions over a few hours. This is carried out with the aim of achieving effective concentrations without unnecessary exposure to side-effects such as speed shock, e.g. 'red man syndrome' associated with the rapid administration of vancomycin.

Other drugs may need to be administered on a titrational basis via a continuous i.v. infusion. Therefore, the choice of the method of drug administration is governed by the clinical indication and licensed recommendation in order to maximize efficacy and minimize toxicity related to the drugs.

Continuous intravenous infusions

Continuous infusion of a drug may be defined as:

- Addition of a drug to a large-volume infusion bag for slow infusion.
- Addition of a drug to a small volume in a syringe for slow infusion using a

Fig. 5.3 The steadiy drug plasma concentration achieved by continuous intravenous infusion.

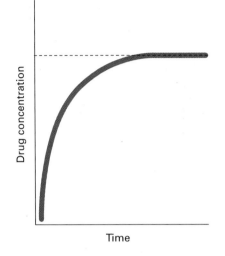

syringe pump (driver) or an ambulatory pump. The i.v. infusion is administered continuously at a specified rate in relation to the dose.

Continuous infusions are indicated when a constant therapeutic drug concentration is required, and when a drug has a rapid elimination rate or a very short half-life and can have an effect only if given continuously. The steady drug plasma concentration achieved by continuous i.v. infusion is illustrated in Figure 5.3.

Disadvantages and hazards of intermittent and continuous infusions may include:

- inappropriate dilution in the infusion fluid
- incompatibility problems with the diluent
- incomplete mixing
- miscalculation of the rate of administration required for different types of equipment, e.g. solution sets and burettes, to avoid overloading and speed shock
- increased risk of microbial contamination and particulate contamination during the preparation
- requirement for flushing the administration set and device post-infusion in order to ensure complete dose delivery
- risk of phlebitis and extravasation
- need for regular monitoring during infusion.

Intermittent intravenous infusion

Intermittent i.v. infusion may be defined as:

- Addition of a drug usually to a small-volume infusion bag connected to the primary administration set, or to a secondary administration set connected to a junction along the primary set.
- Addition of a drug to a measured volume of fluid in an in-line burette.

The i.v. infusion is administered over a set period of time at the specified rate and dose of administration.

Intermittent infusions are indicated in the following circumstances:

- when a drug must be diluted in a volume of fluid larger than is practical for a bolus injection
- when the plasma concentrations required are higher than those achievable by continuous infusion

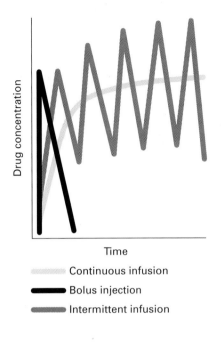

Fig. 5.4 Serum drug levels of bolus injection, intermittent infusion and continuous infusion.

Drug concentration

Time

Continuous infusion

Bolus injection

Intermittent infusion

- when a faster response is required than that achieved by a continuous infusion
- when the drug is unstable or incompatible with fluids used for continuous infusion.

Many antibiotics are administered via this method as it is a compromise between a bolus injection and continuous infusion. It achieves high plasma concentrations rapidly, ensuring clinical efficacy, and yet reduces the risks of adverse reactions associated with rapid or inappropriate administration of an antibiotic, as illustrated in Figure 5.4.

Bolus intravenous injection

This involves injection of the drug solution from a syringe into the injection port in the administration set or directly into a vascular access device. This resembles an injection directly into the vein. If the injection is to be administered over 3–10 minutes, this is referred to as a slow i.v. injection. If it is to be administered more quickly into the vein, it is called a rapid i.v. injection (sometimes referred to as an intravenous push).

Drugs given by bolus i.v. injections achieve immediate and high drug concentrations. Figure 5.5 shows how the drug plasma concentration varies over time following multidose bolus injections. It may be appropriate when time is limited or in emergencies.

Disadvantages and hazards include:

- a tendency to administer the dose too rapidly, resulting in speedshock
- damage to the veins (e.g. phlebitis or extravasation in cases of antibiotics such as erythromycin, sodium fusidate, vancomycin and acyclovir)
- volume of the diluent recommended may not be practical for the time of administration
- sudden anaphylactic reaction
- increased adverse reactions for some antibiotics (e.g. 'red man syndrome',

Fig. 5.5 Variation of drug plasma concentration over time following multidose bolus injections.

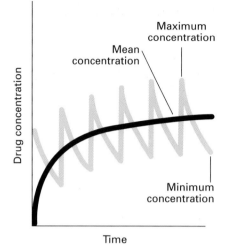

anaphylaxis and cardiac arrest with vancomycin, risk of jaundice with rapid administration of sodium fusidate).

The majority of drugs injected as a bolus should be administered as a slow i.v. injection in order to prevent speed shock and phlebitis. However, a few drugs need to be injected rapidly in order to ensure efficacy, e.g. i.v. adenosine must be administered as a rapid bolus over 2–3 seconds for the management of supraventricular tachycardia.

The choice of i.v. infusion (continuous or intermittent) versus bolus injection is dependent on the circumstances. Sometimes an i.v. infusion is necessary because a direct injection would cause a toxic level of the drug (e.g. potassium chloride is always infused as direct injection could cause cardiac arrest) or because a direct injection would cause venous irritation (e.g. high-dose benzylpenicillin, certain cytotoxics). Also if a drug is quickly metabolized or excreted, direct injections would need to be given very frequently (e.g. heparin, dopamine or dobutamine) and therefore i.v. infusion is more practical.

The decision on whether to use intermittent or continuous infusion depends on the pharmacokinetics of the drug and the clinical indication. For example, inotropes are required to be administered as a continuous infusion at titrational doses in order to achieve a targeted cardiac output and blood pressure. Patients will also need to be weaned off these infusions slowly rather than a sudden discontinuation, in order to maintain haemodynamic stability. Agents may also have a short half-life (time taken for the concentration to be reduced by 50% in the circulation), in which case, in order to maintain the clinical effect, they are required to be administered continuously.

Intermittent infusions, on the other hand, may be applicable to drugs with a longer half-life or if there is a need to achieve a high concentration in the circulation (peaks) and allow a decrease (troughs) before a subsequent dose is administered. This may well be the case for most antibacterial agents. Sometimes a drug's side-effect profile may restrict its method of administration to an intermittent infusion, because bolus injections or continuous infusions lead to high toxic concentrations or drug accumulation in the body.

Circumstances in which injection is preferred to infusion include those in which optimum blood levels are required rapidly, such as during aminoglycoside therapy or if the drug is degraded by light or is incompatible with, or unstable in, infusion fluids.

CALCULATIONS FOR INTRAVENOUS DRUG ADMINISTRATION

The basic information relating to drug calculations is given in this section. It is essential for health care professionals involved in drug prescribing, monitoring and administration to be familiar with the basic principles.

Basic information

1 g (gram) = 1000 mg (milligrams)

1 mg (milligram) = 1000 mcg (micrograms)

1 L (litre) = 1000 ml (millilitres)

Note: microgram units must always be written in full to avoid confusion with milligrams.

Percentage (%) solution = grams in 100 ml

e.g. 1% w/v lignocaine = 1 g in 100 ml

A 1% w/v lignocaine solution means that there is 1 g of lignocaine in 100 ml of solution. Therefore, an ampoule of 10 ml lignocaine 1% contains 0.1 g or 100 mg of the active drug.

1 in 1000 = 1 gram in 1000 ml (1 mg in 1 ml)

1 in 10 000 = 1 gram in 10 000 ml (0.1 mg in 1 ml)

e.g. adrenaline 1 in 10 000 = 1 gram in 10 000 ml (0.1 mg in 1 ml)

An ampoule of adrenaline 1 in 10 000 contains 1 gram or 1000 milligrams of drug in 10 000 ml. This is equivalent to 1 mg in 10 ml or 0.1 mg/ml

Calculation of flow rates

Flow rates are expressed as volumes of fluid delivered per unit time, usually as millilitres per hour (ml/h) or drops per minute (drops/min).

Calculation of flow rate in millilitres per hour (ml/h)

$$\text{Flow rate (ml/h)} = \frac{\text{volume of fluid (ml)}}{\text{time to infuse (h)}}$$

Hence, to administer 500 ml of glucose 5% over 8 hours:

Flow rate $= \frac{500}{8} = 62.5$ *ml/h*

Calculation of flow rate in drops per minute (drops/min)

It is necessary to know:

- volume of fluid to be infused
- total infusion time
- calibration of the administration set used, i.e. number of drops/ml it delivers (this information is found on the administration set package), e.g.
  — 15 drops/ml for blood sets
  — 20 drops/ml for solution sets
  — 60 drops/ml for burettes.

$$\text{Flow rate (drops/min)} = \frac{\text{volume of fluid (ml)}}{\text{total infusion time (min)}} \times \text{calibration (drops/ml)}$$

To administer 1 L of fluid over 12 hours, using a burette:

$$Flow\ rate = \frac{1000\ (ml)}{12 \times 60\ (min)} \times 60\ (drops/ml) = 83\ drops/min$$

Alternatively, use the following equations:

- For a *solution-giving set*:
  drops/min = ml/h 4 3 (i.e. calibration of 20 drops/ml)

- For a *blood-giving set*:
  drops/min = ml/h 4 4 (i.e. calibration of 15 drops/ml)

- For a *burette, microdrop set*:
  drops/min = ml/h (i.e. calibration of 60 drops/ml).

Examples

The following examples are included to demonstrate the use of differents methods or equations for i.v. drug administrations. The calculation methods are dependent on the presentation of the drug (i.e. presented as percentage weight in volume, or mg/ml and so on) and on the dosing schedule on the prescription (i.e. prescribed as mg/min or mg/h, micrograms/kg patient weight per minute or per hour, units per day and so on).

Example 1 Dopamine continuous infusion at 2.5 microgram/kilogram patient weight per minute. The patient is fluid-restricted and has a central venous catheter. The drug is diluted as 200 mg (1 ampoule) in 50 ml sodium chloride 0.9% or dextrose (glucose) 5%. The following equation may be used for administration using a syringe pump:

$$Administration\ rate\ (ml/h) = \frac{dose\ (micrograms/kg\ per\ min) \times total\ volume\ in\ syringe\ (ml) \times 60}{drug\ concentration \times 1000\ (to\ convert\ to\ mg\ in\ ampoules)}$$

$Rate = (2.5 \times 50 \times 60)/(200 \times 1000) = 0.0375\ ml/h$

Example 2 50 000 units of drug X in 50 ml of infusion fluid are to be administered at 600 units/h via a syringe pump. A quantity of 50 000 units in 50 ml solution means that 600 units is equivalent to:

$(600 \times 50)/50\ 000 = 0.6\ ml/h$

Therefore, the syringe pump is set at 0.6 ml/h.

Example 3 A lignocaine infusion 0.4% w/v in dextrose 5% polyfusor needs to be given at 1 mg/min in a volumetric pump calibrated in ml/h.

$0.4\%\ w/v\ solution = 0.4\ g\ in\ 100\ ml$
$\qquad\qquad\qquad\quad = 400\ mg\ in\ 100\ ml$
$\qquad\qquad\qquad\quad = 4\ mg/ml$

Therefore 1 mg/min = 0.25 ml/min, which is equivalent to $0.25 \times 60 = 15$ ml/h.

Example 4: Magnesium sulphate 40 mmol is to be administered over 2 hours. Magnesium sulphate is available as 10 ml of 50% w/v concentration, equivalent to 2 mmol/ml. Therefore, 40 mmol requires dilution of two ampoules of 10 ml each in a 50 ml syringe driver set at 25 ml/h for 2 hours.

ANAPHYLAXIS GUIDELINES

Anaphylaxis is an acute generalized allergic reaction and is most commonly precipitated by the injection of foreign substances, e.g. drugs, vaccines, insect stings. However, severe and even fatal reactions can also occur after food or orally administered drugs. After injections, the reaction may start within seconds or minutes. Onset may be delayed by some hours in the case of oral administration. Rarely, a similar condition can occur without obvious cause or following exercise.

A summary of signs, symptoms and management of anaphylaxis is given in Figure 5.6.

When treatment of anaphylaxis has been delayed, and shock or severe dyspnoea is present, adrenaline should be given via the intravenous route at a dose of 3–5 ml of 1 in 10 000, i.e. 0.3–0.5 mg by a very slow injection over 5 minutes. Occasionally it may be necessary to set up a continuous i.v. infusion of adrenaline. Heart rate and rhythm should be carefully monitored during i.v. administration of adrenaline, because adverse effects such as cardiac arrhythmia, myocardial ischaemia or infarction are more likely when the drug is given via this route. Adrenaline acts on the alpha-receptors, thereby reversing the vasodilation and reducing oedema and urticaria. The stimulation of the beta-receptors leads to the dilatation of the airways, increasing the force of contraction of the heart and suppressing further histamine and leukotriene release.

Volume expansion with colloids (gelatin plasma expanders such as Gelofusine or Haemaccel) and crystalloids (sodium chloride 0.9% or glucose 5%) may be required in order to restore the arterial blood pressure. Chlorpheniramine (Piriton®) may be necessary to counteract the excessive histamine release. It may be administered at a dose of 10 mg i.m. or as 10 mg in 10 ml of sodium chloride 0.9% as a very slow i.v. injection over 3–5 minutes. The i.v. route of administration may cause excessive hypotension. Hydrocortisone may be used to suppress any further allergic reactions. It is administered as a 100 mg dose by slow i.v. injection over 3–5 minutes. Secondary therapy such as aminophylline infusion, salbutamol (i.v. infusion or nebulizer), inotropes and intubation may be necessary once the patient has been transferred to the intensive care unit.

THE ROLE AND RESPONSIBILITY OF EACH PROFESSION IN INTRAVENOUS THERAPY

The following section aims to give a brief overview of the roles and responsibilities of the health care professionals involved in the practice of intravenous drug therapy. It is not intended to give a comprehensive review of the accountabilities, but to help introduce guidelines and raise awareness of the issues surrounding good clinical practice. It is recognized that with the new evolving roles of the health care professionals of all disciplines, there is scope for developing partnership in caring for the patient in an integrated multidisciplinary fashion.

Responsibilities of clinicians

Doctors are urged to restrict the use of the i.v. route to situations where there is no clinical alternative method of administration, and to keep the period of i.v. administration to a minimum. This is to minimize the problems (clinical and practical) associated with i.v. drug therapy.

Prescribing information should include the following points and be clearly written on the prescription chart:

- **approved name** of the drug to be administered intravenously
- **dose** of the drug

Fig. 5.6 Summary of signs, symptoms and management of anaphylaxis.

	Signs and symptoms	Management
Mild ↓	Urticarial rash Pruritus Rhinitus Nausea and vomiting	Antihistamines and observe
	Tachycardia Dyspnoea and cough Wheezing Malaise Angioedema	Serial vital signs (blood pressure, pulse rate) Antihistamines i.m. or i.v. and a bronchodilator, particularly in asthmatics
	Laryngeal oedema (feeling of lump in the throat, hoarseness or stridor) Hypotension Cold and clammy Sub-sternal or abdominal pain Collapse	Adrenaline

Severe anaphylactic shock

Management
↓

Discontinue administration of the suspect drug

Call medical staff

Maintain airways with 100% oxygen (intubation may be necessary)
↓

Adrenaline i.m.

Adult dose: 0.3-1 mg   i.e. [0.3-1 ml of 1 in 1000 (1 mg/ml) ampoule]
or   [3-10 ml of 1 in 10 000 (1 mg/10 ml ampoule]
or   [3-10 ml of 1 in 10 000 minijets]

Subsequent doses: Repeat the dose at 10-15 minute intervals

- **method of administration**, i.e. bolus into an administration set / cannula, intermittent infusion or continuous infusion (unless already written on the chart by the clinical pharmacist)
- **infusion fluid** in which the drug is to be diluted (unless already written on the chart by the clinical pharmacist)
- **volume** of infusion fluid (unless already written on the chart by the clinical pharmacist)

- **final concentration** of the drug infusion (unless already written on the chart by the clinical pharmacist)
- **calculated rate** at which the infusion is to be administered, e.g. 'mg per minute', 'drops per minute', 'ml per minute', or 'ml per hour', etc.
- device to be used for administration of drugs where more than one device is in use, e.g. peripheral or central venous catheter.

Responsibilities of clinical pharmacists

Pharmaceutical care can be described as monitoring and advising on the quality of prescribing and administration, as well as the drug availability, and dispensing in the correct presentation at the right time (Box 5.2).

Pharmacists are responsible for monitoring prescriptions and administration of drug therapies and alerting prescribers, nursing staff and other health care professionals to potential problems. This responsibility includes:

- Checking for the appropriate selection of specific drugs and drug regimens (dose, route, frequency, administration method, duration of therapy).
- Endorsing the prescription chart with relevant and necessary information such as drug preparation method, dilution details of infusions.
- Responding to specific enquiries raised by health care professionals regarding all aspects of drug therapies, including methods of administration, diluents and infusion fluids, drug stability, delivery systems (e.g. pumps, burettes), drug compatibility information, rate of administration, contraindication and side-effects, interactions, unlicensed drugs and their use, anaphylaxis guidelines and drug administration guidelines.
- Signing and dating the drug charts to inform health care professionals that a pharmacist has reviewed the specific prescription.
- Ensuring that the risks of drug errors are minimized throughout the process, from prescribing and dispensing to administration.
- Contribution towards training of the members of the health care team.
- Preparation of CIVAS (centralized intravenous additive service) for hazardous drugs, agents requiring specialist processes and clinical trials. In certain situations, the pharmacy department may be able to supply ready-made preparations.
- Advising on appropriate treatment for the management of extravasation and preparation of anaphylaxis boxes.

Responsibilities of nurses

The United Kingdom Central Council's *Code of Professional Conduct* (UKCC 1992a)

■ **BOX 5.2 Summary of the pharmaceutical care checklist in relation to intravenous drug therapy**

- The process of drug utilization
- Need for drugs
- Selection of specific drugs
- Selection of specific regimens
- Provision of drugs
- Correct method of administration of drugs
- Drug efficacy and toxicity
- Education and counselling
- Evaluation of effectiveness and outcome of drug therapy

for nurses states that: '*As a registered nurse, midwife or health visitor, you are personally accountable for your practice and in the exercise of your professional accountability*'. The emphasis is on acting in a manner to promote and safeguard the interests and well-being of patients, maintaining and improving one's professional knowledge and competence, acknowledging one's limitations in knowledge and expertise, and working towards achieving expertise in extended roles.

In addition to the *Code of Professional Conduct*, the UKCC's *Standards for the Administration of Medicines* document (UKCC 1992b) focuses on the fact that the nurse practitioner must be satisfied with her or his competence and mindful of her or his personal accountability with respect to the administration of intravenous drugs (section 15).

It is essential that a nurse understands when not to administer a prescribed drug. This would include circumstances when the drug chart is unclear with respect to the dose, frequency, dilution details or incompatibility problems.

Drugs may be administered by a single nurse who has demonstrated the necessary knowledge and competence. Drugs will need to be double-checked by a second nurse (or a doctor or pharmacist) if administering controlled drugs, unlicensed agents or clinical trial products, or when there are local restrictions, e.g. specialist units such as paediatrics and intensive care units where drug infusions would require specific drug calculations. The single nurse administration applies to first dose intravenous therapies as well as subsequent doses. However, if a nurse wishes to have her drug preparation checked (in any circumstances), then she is free to do so.

GOOD PRACTICE POLICY ON THE ADMINISTRATION OF INTRAVENOUS DRUG THERAPY

It is recommended that each hospital or community trust should have a local policy for i.v. drug therapy. These documents are often compiled by a multidisciplinary team of all health care professionals involved in the practice of i.v. drug administration. The group formulates the guidelines and reports back to the organization's Drugs and Therapeutics Committee which is ultimately responsible for policies and risk management related to the use of drugs. Such a document may focus on the importance of the recommendations of the independent professional bodies, as well as the principles stated within the specific local policy of a hospital/community trust.

The following steps should be taken before a nurse is authorized to administer i.v. drugs:

- *Training*. Nursing staff must be satisfied that they are competent in i.v. drug administration. Alternatively, training needs should be met by specific educational modules.
- *Policy*. Nursing staff must be aware of the local policy produced by the Drugs and Therapeutics Committee and adhere to it.
- *Prescription chart*. The instructions given on the chart must be clear and concise in order to minimize any drug errors. Nursing staff must be satisfied with the dose, frequency, dilution methods, rate and method of administration, and the equipment necessary for use.

Guide to stages of administration

- be able to read and understand the prescription without any doubts
- be aware of the drug's side-effects, contraindications and any special precautions necessary by referring to the information sources

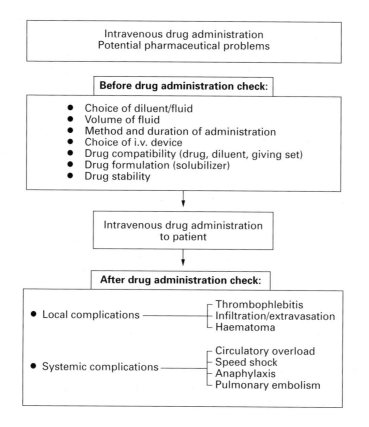

Intravenous drug administration
Potential pharmaceutical problems

Before drug administration check:

- Choice of diluent/fluid
- Volume of fluid
- Method and duration of administration
- Choice of i.v. device
- Drug compatibility (drug, diluent, giving set)
- Drug formulation (solubilizer)
- Drug stability

Intravenous drug administration
to patient

After drug administration check:

- Local complications ——— Thrombophlebitis
  Infiltration/extravasation
  Haematoma

- Systemic complications ——— Circulatory overload
  Speed shock
  Anaphylaxis
  Pulmonary embolism

Fig. 5.7 Pharmaceutical issues to be considered before, during and after intravenous drug administration.

- be certain that the dosage and method of administration are correct
- check the expiry dates of the drug, diluent and infusion fluid
- check for faults in vials, ampoules, syringes, needles and infusion containers
- prepare the drug using aseptic technique.

CONCLUSION

Figure 5.7 gives a summary of the pharmaceutical or drug-related issues that need to be considered before, during and after intravenous drug administration.

REFERENCES

Eggert L D, Ruska W J, MacKay M W 1982 Calcium and phosphate compatibility in parenteral nutrition solutions in neonates. American Journal of Hospital Pharmacy 39: 49–53

Henry R S Jurgens R W, Sturgeon R et al 1980 Compatibility of calcium chloride and calcium gluconate with sodium phosphate in a mixed TPN solution. American Journal of Hospital Pharmacy 37: 673–674

Moorhatch P, Chiou W L 1974 Interactions between drugs and plastic intravenous fluid bags: I. Sorption studies in 17 drugs. American Journal of Hospital Pharmacy 31: 72–78

Trissel L A 1997 Handbook on injectable drugs, 8th edn. American Society of Hospital Pharmacists, Bethesda, MD

United Kingdom Central Council for Nursing, Midwifery and Health Visiting 1992a Code of professional conduct. UKCC, London

United Kingdom Central Council for Nursing, Midwifery and Health Visiting 1992b Standards for administration of medicines. UKCC, London

ACKNOWLEDGEMENT

My sincere thanks to the multidisciplinary staff at Guy's & St Thomas' Hospital Trust involved in assisting me with the preparation of the *Guide to Intravenous Drug Therapy Administration 1990*. This compilation has been used for the publication of this chapter.

FURTHER READING

Trissel L A, Davignon J P, Kleinman L M et al 1988 NCI investigational drugs – pharmaceutical data. National Cancer Institute, Bethesda, MD
United Kingdom Central Council for Nursing, Midwifery and Health Visiting 1992c The scope of professional practice. UKCC, London
United Kingdom Central Council for Nursing, Midwifery and Health Visiting 1993 Midwives rules. UKCC, London

Practice

Safe administration and management of peripheral intravenous therapy

Maggie Nicol

INTRODUCTION

The nurse has a crucial role in the management of intravenous (i.v.) therapy and the prevention or early detection of complications. Many of the complications associated with peripheral i.v. therapy can be minimized or avoided by careful management. This chapter will address the following areas:

- the nurse's role in peripheral i.v. therapy
- advantages and disadvantages of the i.v. route
- care of the peripheral i.v. site
- preparation and management of i.v. infusions
- maintaining patency in indwelling i.v. cannulae
- the use of extension sets, three-way taps and other i.v. equipment
- drug calculations and checking procedures
- i.v. drug administration
- removal of peripheral i.v. cannulae.

THE ROLE OF THE NURSE IN PERIPHERAL INTRAVENOUS THERAPY

The care of the peripheral i.v. site and administration of i.v. infusions have long been the responsibility of the nurse. However, until relatively recently, i.v. cannulation and the administration of i.v. drugs were the responsibility of the doctor. Intravenous cannulation is now increasingly being undertaken by nurses, and theoretical preparation for i.v. drug administration is now included in most pre-registration nursing programmes. Newly qualified nurses require only a period of supervised practice before being able to administer i.v. drugs. The legal and professional aspects of the nurse's role in i.v. drug administration are addressed in Chapter 1. This chapter deals with the practical aspects of drug administration and the management of peripheral i.v. cannulae.

ADVANTAGES AND DISADVANTAGES OF THE INTRAVENOUS ROUTE

Advantages

The intravenous route for the administration of drugs and fluids has a number of advantages. Some drugs are painful or cause damage to the tissues and so cannot be given by intramuscular (i.m.) or subcutaneous injection. Intravenous drug administration enables a more rapid onset of action and the achievement of constant plasma concentrations. It overcomes many pharmacological variables, such as absorption of the drug and drug metabolism, and enables drugs to be accurately titrated according to the desired effect. Unlike the i.m. route, i.v. therapy is relatively painless once i.v. access has been established. The i.v. route also allows fluid and electrolyte imbalances to be promptly corrected, and nutritional needs to be met when the gastrointestinal route is not available.

Disadvantages

There are also a number of disadvantages associated with the i.v. route. Drugs given intravenously have a rapid onset of action and once given cannot be removed from the circulation. This means that any adverse reaction may be severe and rapid. Also, if the drug is administered too quickly, toxic levels of plasma concentration may quickly be reached, resulting in 'speed shock'. This may lead to collapse, shock and cardiac arrest (Weinstein 1997).

If a number of different drugs are being administered simultaneously, there is a risk of interaction or incompatibility, and when drugs are added to an i.v. solution, precipitation may occur, leading to particulate matter and the risk of embolism. Some drugs may degrade or become unstable in solution, resulting in a less than therapeutic, or even adverse, effect.

All i.v. therapy requires venous access, which breaches body defences and creates a portal for the entry of microorganisms, increasing the risk of infection (Clarke 1997). In addition, most drugs and solutions are irritant to the vein, causing phlebitis and/or thrombophlebitis. There is also a risk of a number of other complications (see Ch. 7).

CARE OF THE PERIPHERAL INTRAVENOUS SITE

Prevention of contamination

Hands must be washed and dried thoroughly before any manipulation of the cannula, i.v. fluid, administration set or i.v. site. This has consistently been shown to be one of the most important factors in the prevention of cross-infection (Crow 1996). When changing the dressing, there is a risk of contact with blood and so gloves should be worn. If a non-touch technique is used, the gloves do not need to be sterile, unless otherwise indicated by the patient's condition (e.g. immunosuppressed). They should be well-fitting gloves, to allow dexterity and careful manipulation of the dressing and cannula. Unless otherwise indicated by the patient's condition (e.g. MRSA), an apron is not necessary provided the uniform or clothing is clean.

Observation of the site

The cannula site should be inspected at least once a day and every time that i.v. drugs are administered, and this may necessitate removal of bandages and even the dressing itself, depending on the type used (see below). Observe the site for redness (phlebitis, thrombophlebitis), heat (infection) and swelling (extravasation or infiltration) (see Ch. 7). The cannula site should not be painful. There is likely to be some degree of discomfort associated with the cannula and the patient may feel a 'coolness' in the limb during bolus drug administration, but it should not be painful between drug administrations or while an infusion is running. Some drugs may cause venous pain during administration but this should be minimized by slow administration. If the patient is complaining of continuous pain, the cannula needs to be re-sited.

Types of dressing

The peripheral i.v. site should be covered with a dressing that is sterile and easy to

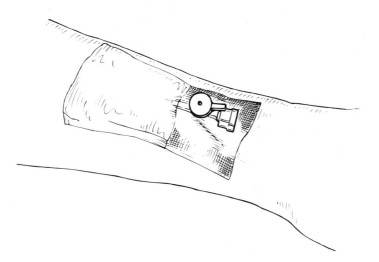

Fig. 6.1 Transparent dressing.

apply and remove, keeps the site free from exogenous infection, secures the cannula in place and allows easy visual inspection of the site (RCN 1994, Wilson 1994). Many manufacturers now produce dressings specifically for i.v. cannulae which are designed to meet the above criteria. Sterile gauze and unsterile tape have been shown to be cheap and effective (Maki & Ringer 1987), but do not allow visualization of the site. Also, the cannula has to be held in place by unsterile tape, which has been shown to increase the risk of infection (Oldman 1991).

Transparent dressings (Fig. 6.1) have the advantage that the whole site is visible and so any complications are immediately apparent, allowing swift intervention. However, some research (Hoffman et al 1992, Elliott 1993) suggests that there is a build-up of moisture under the dressing which leads to increased bacterial growth. The conditions required for optimum wound healing, i.e. warm, moist environment, are also those in which bacteria thrive and multiply and so all dressings are likely to create the same conditions to some extent. However, randomized studies of transparent dressings have shown differences in pooling of moisture and newer dressings have been shown to offer improved moisture vapour transmission (Maki & Ringer 1991, Kiernan 1997).

Sterile, self-adhesive gauze dressings (Fig. 6.2) provide secure fixing of the cannula but do not allow easy visual inspection of the site. Some manufacturers have addressed this problem by combining gauze and a transparent dressing to allow visualization of the vein. One manufacturer has designed a dressing such as this which also incorporates a small gauze pad to sit under the wings of the cannula to increase patient comfort. The puncture site is also covered by a small aluminium pad which has bacteriostatic properties and encourages moisture to move to the surface, leaving the surface in contact with the skin dry, and thus further discouraging bacterial growth.

The choice of dressing is usually dictated by local infection control policy, availability and cost. Whichever dressing is chosen, it must be sterile, keep the area covered, hold the cannula firmly in place to prevent irritation of the lining of the vein wall, and preferably allow visualization of the site. It must also be applied correctly. Nelson et al (1996) reported an increase in the incidence of inflammation around the site when dressings were not applied in accordance with the manufacturer's instructions.

Fig. 6.2 Sterile, self-adhesive gauze dressing.

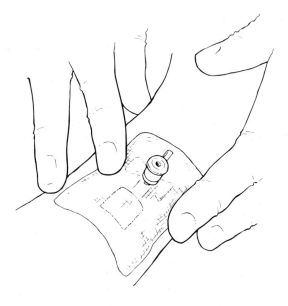

Frequency of dressing change

An i.v. site should be treated as a surgical wound. If the dressing is clean and secure, it is neither necessary nor cost-effective to change it until the cannula is removed or re-sited (Maki & Ringer 1987). However, unless the dressing allows visualization of the insertion site, it may be necessary to remove it in order to inspect the cannula site. As with any wound, there is a risk of introducing infection during dressing change and there is an additional risk of movement or even displacement of the cannula during the process (Vost & Longstaff 1997). However, if the dressing is wet or bloodstained or, in the case of the transparent type, there is haemoserous fluid collecting around the site, the dressing must be changed.

Thorough hand washing and strict asepsis are vital to prevent cross-infection (Crow 1996) and if there is likely to be contact with blood, gloves should be worn. These should be sterile and close-fitting to permit dexterity. A small dressing pack containing sterile gloves is ideal for this, although the gloves are usually fairly large as they have to accommodate a range of hand sizes.

If the site requires cleaning, normal sodium chloride 0.9% will normally be sufficient (Elliott et al 1994), although other solutions such as chlorhexidine or povidone-iodine may be used according to local policies and procedures. Whichever cleansing agent is used, the site should always be allowed to dry before applying the dressing (Kiernan 1997). Great care is required during removal of the old dressing to avoid displacement of the cannula. If the patient is confused or unable to cooperate by keeping still, help should be sought. Scissors should never be used to remove old tape or dressings because of the risk of accidentally cutting the cannula.

Bandaging

Bandaging of the peripheral i.v. site is often avoided because it means that the dressing and vein are no longer visible, increasing the risk that complications may go undetected. It is also likely to inhibit the moisture permeability of transparent dressings and so defeat the purpose of using such a dressing. Bandaging may also increase the temperature of the area, providing extra warmth which may encourage bacterial growth. However, many patients prefer to have their i.v. site bandaged as it feels more secure, does not catch on clothing and cannot accidentally become dislodged. One study (Stonehouse 1996) found that 60% of patients complained that the port of the cannula frequently caught on bed linen and nightwear, making it painful. Also, some patients prefer not to be able to see the cannula. If the patient is confused, bandaging is often necessary to secure the cannula.

If bandaging is deemed necessary, a light 'cling'-type bandage should be used, and not a crepe bandage as this is designed to apply pressure which may interfere with the infusion. The limb should be bandaged lightly to prevent pressure on the vein, and the bandage must be removed every time a drug is administered or at least once a day to allow inspection of the site. The site should be inspected more frequently if the patient complains of pain or discomfort.

Use of splints

Great care must be taken if using a splint as nerve damage may result from pressure of the splint during prolonged use. If the cannula is sited in the forearm, the bones provide a natural splint and additional support is not usually necessary. However, if the cannula is in the hand where the wrist flexes, or in the antecubital fossa, a splint may be necessary to ensure consistent functioning of the infusion.

A splint should be padded to promote comfort and be lightly bandaged into place. It should be removed and reapplied at least once a day and the area inspected for redness or sores developing. Any complaints of pain or discomfort from the patient should be investigated without delay. Splints should be disposable or covered in a non-porous material that can be cleaned easily and effectively to prevent cross-infection between patients.

PREPARATION OF THE INTRAVENOUS INFUSION

Inspection of infusion fluid

Most i.v. infusion fluids are manufactured in plastic infusion bags, although some (e.g. Intralipid) are in a glass bottle. The bag of prescribed infusion fluid should be removed from its outer packaging and checked for leakage. If the bag is wet, this may mean that it has leaked and, however minimal, the contents cannot be assumed to be sterile and so should not be used. The infusion fluid should be checked to ensure that the expiry date for use has not passed, the solution is clear and there are no particles present. Particles may indicate contamination of the fluid during the manufacturing process, although this is extremely rare, or precipitation of some component of the solution through improper storage. Either way, the solution must not be used and should be returned to the pharmacy so that the manufacturers can be alerted. If a solution containing particles is infused, it may cause particulate irritation of the venous endothelium (Falchuck et al 1985). It may even cause blockage of lung vasculature due to a build-up of layers of phagocytic cells around the particle, creating a granuloma (Walpot 1989).

Adding drugs to infusions

Many i.v. drugs are administered by continuous or intermittent infusion. Strict aseptic technique must be used when adding drugs to an infusion bag or burette. The injection port should be disinfected according to local policy, and the drug injected using a 25G needle. The injection membrane is designed to close completely after puncture and prevent the entry of microorganisms provided a 25G needle is used. The solution must then be mixed thoroughly to ensure even distribution. A label should be affixed to the container to indicate the date and time that the drug was added and should include the signature of the nurse(s) involved.

Choosing the administration or 'giving' set

The nurse must choose an appropriate administration set, commonly referred to as a 'giving set'. A standard administration set, which does not have a filter chamber, is suitable for most i.v. infusions, with the exception of the following:

- *Blood and blood products.* A blood administration set, which has an integral filter chamber, must be used (see Ch. 13).
- *Platelets.* A special administration set is usually supplied with the platelets.
- *Neonates and paediatrics.* A burette should be used. This has a chamber into which a small amount of fluid from the bag is run before infusion to the patient. This prevents accidental overinfusion of large volumes of fluid and so may also be used with elderly patients with heart failure to prevent accidental overload. It may also be used for drug administration as the chamber allows mixing and dilution of the drug before slow administration. Care is required to ensure thorough mixing of the drug with the infusion fluid. Failure to mix thoroughly may result in a high concentration of the drug being administered over a short period of time.

The various administration sets will deliver different numbers of drops per millilitre (ml). This will have to be taken into consideration when calculating the drip rate of the infusion (see calculations later in this chapter). The different rates are:

- standard administration set – 20 drops/ml
- blood administration set – 15 drops/ml
- burette – 60 drops/ml.

Priming and connecting the administration set (Box 6.1)

Most administration sets have a date of sterilization on the packaging but may not have an expiry date by which they must be used. If the outer packaging is intact, has never been allowed to get wet and does not appear damaged in any way, the contents may be assumed to be sterile. On opening the outer packaging, both ends of

---

■ BOX 6.1

Priming the administration set

- Close the flow control clamp before inserting the spike of the administration set into the fluid bag, as this prevents fluid running into the set before you are ready.
- Rest the bag of fluid on a flat surface to prevent accidental puncturing of the side of the bag when the spike is inserted.
- Remove the protective cover from the inlet port on the bag, and the protective cap from the spike of the administration set and push this firmly into the inlet port using a twisting movement to ensure it is fully inserted.
- Hang the bag on the infusion stand and squeeze the drip chamber several times until half full of fluid. Do not overfill it or you will be unable to see the drops forming.
- Expel all remaining air from the set by gradually opening the flow control clamp and allowing the fluid to flow slowly through the set.
- The protective cap on the end of the administration set should remain in place throughout to keep it sterile until use.
- If the infusion is in a glass bottle, an air inlet will be needed (Fig. 6.3).

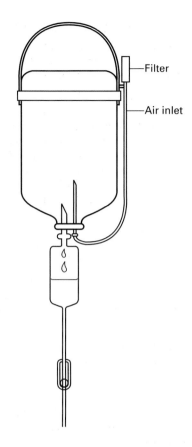

Fig. 6.3 Glass bottle with air inlet.

—Filter

—Air inlet

■ **BOX 6.2**

Connecting the administration set to the cannula

- The hands must be clean and gloves should be worn.
- If necessary, remove any bandaging and check the site for redness, swelling, heat or pain (see Ch. 7).
- Place a sterile gauze square under the end of the cannula when connecting the administration set to absorb any blood that leaks back from the cannula during connection (it must be sterile as it will come into contact with the exposed end of the cannula).
- With the exposed end of the administration set in your non-dominant hand and the sterile gauze in position underneath the end of the cannula, remove the cap or injectable bung on the end of the cannula.
- Swiftly insert the end of the administration set and luer-lock into position.
- To reduce the flow of blood through the cannula as you connect the administration set, apply pressure to the vein just beyond the tip of the cannula (see Fig. 6.4).
- Discard the gauze in the clinical waste system.

---

the giving set are covered by protective caps to allow handling of the set without desterilization of the part that will be inserted into the fluid bag or the end that will be connected to the cannula.

Box 6.2 describes how to connect the administration set to the cannula, and Box 6.3 describes how to change an existing infusion.

Fig. 6.4 Occlusion of vein.

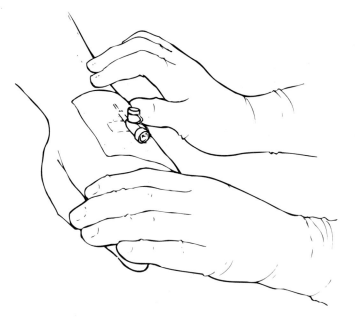

■ **BOX 6.3**

Changing an existing infusion

If connecting a new bag to an existing infusion, inspect the infusion fluid as described in the text (p. 145). At the bedside:

- Close the roller clamp on the administration set. Alternatively, bend the administration set back on itself and place the tubing in the clamp grippers at the back of the roller clamp. This will cease the flow of the infusion fluid; when the new infusion container has been connected, release the tubing from the clamp grippers and the infusion will continue at its preset rate.
- Remove the old infusion from the stand and pull out the administration set, taking care not to contaminate the spike.
- Remove the protective cover from the inlet port of the new infusion bag and insert the spike of the administration set, twisting until fully inserted.
- Replace the bag on the infusion stand and adjust the roller clamp to the prescribed flow rate.

Securing the administration set

It is necessary to support the tubing of the administration set to prevent it pulling and causing trauma to the vein wall or dislodgement of the cannula. This may be achieved by using a piece of hypoallergenic tape approximately 4 inches long. Position the tubing so that it is not pulling the cannula then stick the tape onto the tubing first before applying it to the skin. Pinch it over the tubing to promote maximum adhesion. This will prevent the tubing from sliding through the tape. Now apply the tape to the skin (see Fig. 6.5).

Avoid applying the tape over the dressing at the puncture site as this may prevent moisture loss through the dressing and increase the temperature at the site,

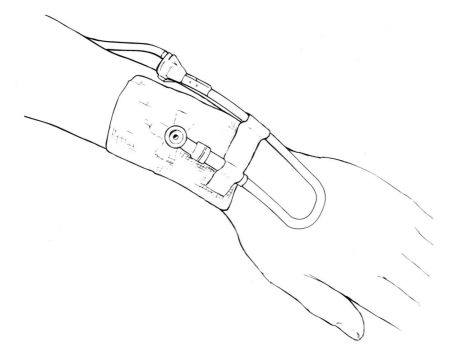

Fig. 6.5 Fixing of tubing with tape.

thus encouraging bacterial growth. The creation of a loop of tubing before fixation to the skin will prevent traction on the cannula. However, the loop should not be too large, as it may become kinked, and should lie flat against the skin to minimize the risk of it getting caught and causing dislodgement of the cannula.

Documentation/record-keeping

All aspects of i.v. therapy should be documented according to local policy. This will usually include the following:

- The time the infusion started.
- The batch number of the fluid. This is recorded on the i.v. prescription chart so that in the event of an adverse reaction, the manufacturers will be able to trace the fluid back to the production stage.
- Most patients with an i.v. infusion will require a fluid balance chart. The new infusion and completion of the old should be recorded.
- There is usually space on the i.v. prescription chart for the signature of the nurse(s) who administered the infusion. The number of nurses (one or two) required to check i.v. infusions will vary according to local policy (see 'Checking procedures', p. 154).

Changing administration sets

Although the Department of Health guidelines (DHSS 1973) and manufacturers' instructions advise that all administration sets should be changed every 24 hours, recent research has shown that this is not necessary except in the following situations:

- parenteral nutrition (Snydman et al 1987)
- blood and blood products (these are usually changed more frequently than every 24 hours)
- infusions to which drugs have been added (Wilson 1994).

A number of studies have shown that during infusions of clear fluids, such as sodium chloride 0.9% and dextrose 5%, there was no increase in infection rates if administration sets were left unchanged for 48–72 hours (e.g. Buxton et al 1979, Maki et al 1984, Maki & Ringer 1991). Snydman et al (1987) found that burettes could also be safely changed every 72 hours. This clearly represents huge cost savings, but it is important that patient care is not compromised. Any cost savings will quickly be lost and greater costs incurred if the patient should develop a systemic infection from a contaminated administration set (Vost & Longstaff 1997).

Contamination of infusion fluid during manufacture is now extremely rare. However, infusion fluid is easily contaminated when drugs are added or administered via the cannula and so the administration set should be changed every 24 hours.

Accurate documentation is necessary to ensure that all involved know when the set is due to be changed. Documentation will vary according to local policies but will usually involve the use of an adhesive label on the set to indicate the date when changing is due and a record in the nursing notes. Thorough hand washing and strict asepsis are important with any manipulation of the administration set. The use of connections, extension sets and three-way taps should be kept to a minimum as each connection increases the risk of infection entering the system (Lamb 1995).

EXTENSION SETS, THREE-WAY TAPS AND OTHER EQUIPMENT

Extension sets and three-way taps

Advantages

The use of extension tubing and three-way taps increases the convenience of use of the peripheral cannula. Two infusions may be administered at the same time, or a second infusion may be given intermittently without having to remove the administration set between infusions, thus reducing the risk of contamination. Use of an extension set means that manipulations of the administration are further away from the cannula, thus reducing the risk of movement of the cannula itself which may cause trauma to the vein wall. They also have the advantage that if needles are being used for bolus doses through an injectable bung, they are kept well away from the patient. This is particularly useful in children and those with needle phobias.

Disadvantages

Any extra connection within the administration system increases the risk of infection, and three-way taps have been shown to encourage the growth of microorganisms. They are difficult to clean due to their design, as microorganisms can become lodged and are then able to multiply in the warm, moist environment. When the three-way tap becomes colonized, the microorganisms are carried in the i.v. solution to the cannula, which then becomes colonized (Moro et al 1994). Three-way taps should be changed every time the administration set is changed, which is costly, and their benefits must be weighed against the increased risks. The addition of in-line filters greatly reduces the risk of infection, but they are relatively expensive and their use is contraindicated with some drugs and solutions (see page 152).

Injectable caps or bungs

For intermittent bolus drug administration, an injectable bung (Fig. 6.6) has several advantages. The injectable membrane is made of latex rubber that closes completely despite numerous punctures with a small needle (25G is recommended), thus preventing the entry of microorganisms. The surface of the bung can be disinfected

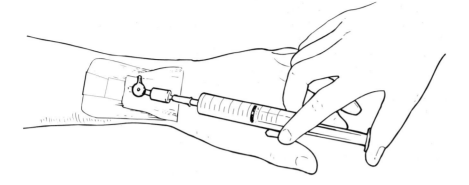

Fig. 6.6 Ported cannula with injectable bung attached.

easily and effectively prior to each drug administration (Speechley 1984). The use of a needle with a small lumen also means that the drug is injected in a slow, controlled fashion. This allows the drug to be diluted by the blood flow in the vein, thus reducing chemical irritation to the vein wall. However, because a needle is used, there is a risk of needlestick injury.

Some cannulae are equipped with an integral injection port covered by a coloured protective cap. These are designed for drug administration by attaching the syringe directly onto the injection port, and as no needle is required, the risk of needlestick injury is reduced. However, as with three-way taps or stopcocks, there is a danger that the injection port will become contaminated, particularly as the protective cap frequently becomes loose, and the area is difficult to clean effectively (Clarke 1997). When the drug is administered, any microorganisms present are then flushed into the circulation. The fact that no needle is used may also inadvertently result in a faster rate of administration.

Needleless systems

The risks attached to needlestick injuries have prompted the development of needleless systems. These appear to have all the advantages of the injectable bung without the disadvantage of using a needle. Their design involves a rubber membrane and valve mechanism which opens to admit a syringe tip but closes after removal of the syringe to provide a secure barrier against the entry of microorganisms. Needleless systems also permit the attachment of an administration set and so intermittent infusions may be attached without removing the cap and opening the system, which should also reduce the risk of infection. However, there are as yet few reports into the use of needleless systems and so the potential for contamination of these devices is not yet clear (Brown et al 1997).

When selecting a needleless system, the following should be considered: ease of use, versatility, cost and perceived benefits to patients and staff (Dougherty 1997). The cost is significantly higher than an ordinary injectable bung and this is likely to influence their use in general clinical areas. However, their use should be considered with patients who are particularly vulnerable to infection and in areas where a needlestick injury would carry a high risk, such as patients with hepatitis or HIV.

In-line filters

The role of in-line filters is still a matter for debate. In-line filters (0.2 μm) prevent particulate matter, fungi, bacteria and endotoxins from entering the system

(Weinstein 1997) and thus will reduce the frequency with which administration sets need to be changed. This has been shown to produce savings in terms of equipment and nurses' time (Cousins 1988). Particulate matter has been implicated as a major cause of infusion phlebitis, and in-line filters have been shown to significantly reduce the incidence of infusion phlebitis (Allcutt et al 1983, Francombe 1988). However, they have been reported to be incompatible with a number of drugs such as insulin (Butler 1980) because the drug adheres to the filter. Also, due to the presence of cellular components, blood, blood products and fat emulsions cannot be administered via a 0.2 μm filter (Cousins 1988).

In a review of the available evidence regarding the use of in-line filters, Johns (1996) concluded that if cost was not an issue, their use to reduce the incidence of complications such as phlebitis would seem prudent. However, as cost is inevitably an issue and as phlebitis, although painful, is usually transient and rarely life-threatening, the use of in-line filters is likely to be restricted to those who are immunodeficient or immunocompromised and those receiving multiple infusions with many additives, such as patients in intensive care and high-dependency units (Adams et al 1986).

MAINTAINING PATENCY OF INDWELLING CANNULAE

Many i.v. cannulae are left in place without an infusion attached. These are often used for the administration of intermittent bolus doses of drugs such as antibiotics or to provide access for the administration of emergency drugs should the patient's condition suddenly deteriorate. In order to maintain patency of these cannulae, regular flushing is necessary. Until relatively recently, heparin diluted in sodium chloride 0.9% was used for this purpose; however, heparin is no longer routinely used.

Flushing solution

Goode et al (1991), in a meta-analysis of the effects of heparin and sodium chloride 0.9% flushes in adult patients, concluded that sodium chloride 0.9% was as effective as heparin in maintaining patency. Early studies demonstrated that the addition of heparin to i.v. solutions reduced the incidence of phlebitis. However, Goode et al (1991) found no statistical basis to conclude that heparin was more effective than sodium chloride 0.9% in increasing duration of the cannula. In fact, one study (Barrett & Lester 1990) found that cannulae flushed with heparin had a statistically higher incidence of phlebitis than those flushed with sodium chloride 0.9%.

The use of sodium chloride 0.9% avoids the risk of side-effects of heparin, such as thrombocytopenia or iatrogenic haemorrhage, which may occur even with very small amounts (Passonnate & Macik 1988). It also eliminates the risk of heparin incompatibility with drugs such as gentamicin and other antibiotics (Goode et al 1991). In addition, there are cost savings in terms of drugs and staff time. In many NHS Trusts, sodium chloride 0.9% flushes do not require a doctor's prescription but are a standing order as part of the i.v. drug administration policy.

Amount

In most instances, 5 ml of sodium chloride 0.9% is sufficient – 2 ml before and 3 ml after administering the drug. If more than one drug is being administered, more will be needed so that the cannula can be flushed after each drug to prevent mixing in the cannula. If an infusion is in progress and the injection port of the administration set is being used, a larger volume of solution will also be needed to ensure adequate flushing.

Frequency of flushing

The frequency of flushing in order to maintain patency varies widely between and even within institutions. Goode et al (1991) found that some studies recommended flushing every 8 hours, whilst others recommended every 12 hours. A study by Dunn & Lenihan (1987) compared the two frequencies and found no difference in device duration, incidence of phlebitis, infiltration, patency or clotting. The current literature supports flushing before and after every drug administration to check patency and to ensure there is no mixing of drugs in the cannula with possible adverse reactions.

Flushing technique

The technique used to flush i.v. cannulae may also be important in maintaining patency. Some studies (Dunn & Lenihan 1987, Nicoll 1990) suggest that patency is enhanced by the positive pressure that is maintained by using a closed system with a resealable injection cap, preventing the backflow of blood into the cannula and clotting. Shearer (1987) suggested that this can be achieved by withdrawing the flush syringe while exerting pressure on the plunger of the syringe and injecting the last 0.5 ml of solution.

REMOVAL OF PERIPHERAL INTRAVENOUS CANNULAE

Hands must be washed and dried thoroughly, and as there may be contact with blood, gloves should be worn. A sterile gauze square should be used to apply pressure to the puncture site immediately after (not during) removal of the cannula. Firm pressure should be applied (the patient may be able to do this) until the bleeding stops and a small self-adhesive dressing applied. Relying on gauze and tape to provide sufficient pressure to stop the bleeding should be avoided, as it is rarely successful and often results in extensive bruising (Godwin et al 1992).

After removal, the cannula should be inspected to check that it is intact. If the i.v. site is inflamed and painful, and infection of the cannula is suspected, the tip of the cannula may be sent to the pathology laboratory for microculture. If there is pus or exudate present around the cannula, the site should be cleaned with sodium chloride 0.9% prior to removal of the cannula to prevent contamination of the tip during withdrawal. If a plastic cannula has been used, this may be disposed of in the normal clinical waste bags. If it is a steel 'butterfly' winged infusion device it must be discarded into a sharps container.

PREPARATION FOR INTRAVENOUS DRUG ADMINISTRATION

Intravenous training programmes

Until recently, i.v. drug administration was viewed as part of the extended role of the nurse, an additional role that was adopted only after considerable experience as a qualified nurse. However, now that i.v. drug administration is firmly established as part of the nurse's role, theoretical preparation for i.v. drug administration is now included in most pre-registration nursing programmes. Although there are presently no national guidelines and no nationally recognized system of certification, most courses address the following aspects:

- anatomy and physiology
- fluid and electrolyte balance
- infection control
- prevention and management of complications of i.v. therapy
- drip rate and drug calculations
- care of the i.v. site
- i.v. drug administration technique
- use of infusion devices
- legal/professional issues.

Approved drug lists

In many NHS Trusts there is one or a number of 'approved lists' of drugs that may be administered by nurses who have undergone appropriate training. Many also have additional lists of 'specialist' drugs which may be administered intravenously by nurses working within certain specialist practice areas, e.g. coronary care units. Any drugs not included on the approved drugs list (or appropriate specialist list) should not be administered by nurses but by the prescribing doctor. The drugs on the approved list are those whose action, method of administration and side-effects are well known and many hospitals supply additional information about these drugs in the i.v. drug administration policy.

Any nurse administering a drug which is not included in the approved or (if appropriate) specialist list, may find the Trust refuses to accept vicarious liability in the event of an incident (see Ch. 1). Thus it is important to decline to administer drugs that are not on the list. Doctors should be advised that the approved list is constantly being updated as new drugs become available and others are no longer used. The procedure for including new drugs on the approved and specialist lists will vary from institution to institution but is usually relatively simple. When the drug has been approved, nurses may administer it intravenously and the Trust will be vicariously liable as long as Trust policies and procedures were followed.

Checking procedures

Drug checking procedures in the UK have changed over the past decade. In 1986, the UKCC issued an advisory paper which stated that it was no longer necessary for two nurses to check all drugs prior to administration (UKCC 1986). The Royal College of Nursing (RCN) supported this view but felt that the practice should continue in the case of i.v. drugs because 'mistakes cannot be easily rectified' (RCN 1987). In 1995, a survey of acute NHS Trusts in the Thames regions (Nicol 1995) revealed that although most drug administration policies (46 of the 48 Trusts that responded) permitted single-person administration for oral, intramuscular and subcutaneous drugs, over half (28 of the 46) still required i.v. drugs to be checked by two people, one of whom must be a registered nurse.

There is no research evidence available to support either method, and the literature on drug errors suggests that neither method is sufficiently foolproof to prevent errors occurring. A review of the psychological literature (Nicol 1997) suggested that an increase in the number of people involved in a task often resulted in a decrease in individual effort. However, these experimental studies invariably involved some simple and often pointless task such as rope pulling or hand clapping. Thus, any comparison with an important activity such as drug administration is at best speculative (Nicol 1997). However, the literature on drug errors is full of evidence that simply having two people involved in drug administration does not eliminate errors.

It is vital that the nurse administering the drug is completely satisfied that he is giving the correct drug and does not rely on another person to confirm this even if two-person checking is required by the policy. The five 'rights' identified by Clayton (1987) – the *right patient*, gets the *right drug*, in the *right dose*, by the *right route*, at the *right time* – provide a simple but comprehensive framework for checking.

The 'right patient'

A study by Gladstone (1995) found that, of the 79 drug incidents examined, 10 (12.7%) involved the incorrect patient. In addition, anecdotal evidence suggests that patients sometimes answer to the wrong name, perhaps because they assume that the nurse knows who they really are and that it was just a slip of the tongue; or perhaps they did not actually hear what was said.

Checking the name band, if the patient is wearing one, is probably the safest method, or asking the patient to state her name and/or date of birth. In the Gladstone (1995) study, nurses were asked to rank statements in order of perceived frequency as being the cause of drug errors. The statements 'drug errors occur when the nurse fails to check the patient's name band with the prescription chart' and 'drug errors occur when nurses are distracted by other patients/events on the ward' received high rankings. These findings were supported in a small observational study of drug administration in hospital wards (Nicol 1995). The high level of distractions in the ward environment was evident, as were the number of interruptions during drug administration. The feelings of personal guilt and loss of clinical confidence reported by nurses who have made drug errors, even when no harm has come to the patient (Wolf 1994), should convince nurses of the need to check and double-check that it is the right patient.

Having ascertained that it is the right patient, it is important to check that the drug has not already been given and that the patient does not have any known allergies to the drugs prescribed. With a new patient, this should be checked verbally if there is no mention in the records.

The 'right drug'

The drug must be correctly prescribed using generic (not trade) names and abbreviations should be avoided. The prescription must be clearly written, signed and dated by the prescribing doctor. It must include the patient's name, hospital number, name of the drug, strength, dose, route, frequency and timing of administration (Scales 1996). It is the nurse's responsibility to know the normal dose of the drug so that prescription errors can be detected. A source of reference such as the *British National Formulary* (BMA/RPSGB 1998) should be readily available to allow speedy checking if unsure.

It is also necessary to check compatibility of the drug with any diluent used, with other drugs being given and with any infusions that are running. Most i.v. drugs will be diluted with sterile water for injections to a volume of at least 10 ml (except in paediatrics). This is to reduce the chemical irritation of the lining of the vein (see Ch. 7) and also facilitates slow administration of the drug. Although there are some exceptions, most drugs should not be mixed with others before administration as this may cause chemical degradation of one or both agents, precipitation or unknown chemical reactions.

If a number of drugs are being given by bolus doses, the cannula must be flushed between each drug to prevent mixing, leading to precipitation or chemical reactions in the cannula. Sodium chloride 0.9% is normally appropriate for this but a few drugs (e.g. amphotericin) are incompatible with sodium chloride 0.9%, in which case dextrose 5% should be used instead. The BNF provides comprehensive infor-

■ **BOX 6.4**

Knowledge a nurse must possess before administering intravenous drugs

- The action of the drug including any patient assessment necessary prior to administration, e.g. checking blood pressure prior to administering a hypotensive agent
- The recommended dosage range
- Possible side-effects
- Any special precautions during and after administration, e.g. protection from light
- The type of diluent to be used
- The method of administration, e.g. by slow i.v. bolus, intermittent infusion, etc.
- Compatibility with other drug therapy and infusions
- Any patient monitoring required following/during administration

mation regarding the compatibility of various drugs with common infusion fluids. If in doubt, flush the cannula well before and after administration of the drug.

The knowledge required when administering i.v. drugs, or indeed drugs by any route is summarized in Box 6.4.

The 'right dose'

As discussed previously, it is the nurse's responsibility to ensure that the dose that has been prescribed is appropriate and so nurses must know the recommended dosage range. The dose should be clearly written using recognized abbreviations only. The abbreviations for milligrams (mg) and micrograms (µg) look very similar when handwritten and so micrograms should be written in full or the abbreviation 'mcg' should be used to avoid confusion. Administration of the correct dose may involve calculations and it is vital that nurses are competent to perform the type of calculations required in their clinical area.

The 'right time'

Timing of i.v. drug therapy is important as correct intervals are necessary to ensure that therapeutic levels are maintained.

The 'right route'

Drugs suitable for i.v. administration should be labelled accordingly and the data sheet should include specific instructions for administration by this route (Scales 1996). Some intramuscular preparations may not be suitable for i.v. use and the appropriate dose may well vary. However, because the use of i.v. drugs is expanding so rapidly, some drugs are being given intravenously before the manufacturer has obtained a product licence for that route. If a drug is prescribed for i.v. administration but the ampoule and data sheet state that it is for i.m. or subcutaneous use only, the nurse should check with the pharmacy before administration.

Drug errors, and even fatalities, have occurred when drugs have been given by the wrong route, often because the i.v. dose is much smaller than that given intramuscularly. For example, pethidine 100 mg is a common dose when prescribed intramuscularly, but only 10–12 mg would be given intravenously. Oral preparations (or doses) must never be given by any other route and it may not even be appropriate to crush tablets for administration via a nasogastric tube. This should be checked with the pharmacy.

UKCC guidelines

The UKCC guidelines for the administration of medicines (UKCC 1992) advise against administering drugs that the practitioner has not prepared himself. The only exception to this is when taking over the care of a patient who is already receiving i.v. drugs by continuous infusion. In order to be fully accountable, the nurse must take full responsibility for the drugs given and that includes ensuring that the correct drug and diluent are prepared. Intravenous drugs for individual patients should be prepared and then administered immediately. Mistakes can easily occur if a number of drugs for different patients are prepared together.

DRUG CALCULATIONS

It is vital that the nurse is competent to perform the mathematical calculations required to administer the correct dose of the drug. Unlike oral tablets, the patient has no means of knowing whether the drug in the syringe is in fact correct: a syringe containing 250 mg of an antibiotic will look exactly the same as one containing 750 mg. Even totally different drugs may look exactly the same in the syringe.

There are three types of i.v. drug calculation that all nurses are likely to need to be able to perform competently: (1) calculation of the volume of injection for an i.v. bolus (see below); (2) calculation of the number of drops per minute (drops/min) for gravity infusions and drip-regulating infusion devices; and (3) calculation of the number of millilitres per hour (ml/h) for volumetric infusion devices (see Ch. 5).

Calculation of volume of injection

$$Volume\ to\ be\ given = \frac{what\ you\ want \times what\ it's\ in\ (vol.)}{what\ you've\ got}$$

Example Flucloxacillin 125 mg has been prescribed. The stock ampoules are 250 mg and you have diluted it to 10 ml with water for injection. The calculation would be:

$$\frac{125 \times 10}{250} = \frac{1250}{250} = 5\ ml$$

Professional responsibility

The importance of being competent to accurately perform the mathematical calculations necessary for drug administration cannot be overstressed. Nurses may have their own methods, which may vary from the example above. It is vital that nurses seek help if they have difficulty in this area. There are several books and packages available for nurses, and most hospital pharmacists are prepared to offer help and advice. Although checking with another nurse may be advisable where calculations are involved, the administering nurse must never rely on the second person to perform the calculation. It is particularly important when working with student nurses that the qualified nurse is able to demonstrate the way in which the dose was calculated, not just the answer. Every nurse administering i.v. drugs has a professional responsibility to ensure that he has sufficient knowledge of all aspects of i.v. therapy, including calculations.

INTRAVENOUS INFUSION DEVICES

Intravenous pumps and syringe drivers are increasingly being used to control i.v.

infusions in general wards as well as specialist clinical areas. Many drug errors occur as a result of failure to set or operate the pump correctly (Cousins 1995). In a study of drug errors in a district general hospital (Gladstone 1995), 50% of the errors involving the i.v. route were found to involve the use of an infusion device. Nurses must take individual responsibility to ensure that they are fully conversant with any device being used.

Training is sometimes provided by the company representatives, particularly when new equipment has been purchased, but probably the most common method is 'on-the-job' learning. McConnell (1995) found that the most frequently identified methods of initial learning were 'trial and error' and reading the instruction manual. All devices will vary slightly in design, but there are a number of common features and nurses should ensure that they are familiar with the following aspects of any device being used.

Power supply

The device may operate on mains electricity, battery or both. There may be an alarm to warn the user of a low battery or power failure. If not, the user will have to check the pump at least every hour. If the pump runs on rechargeable batteries, it is important to keep them fully charged during and between uses by keeping the pump plugged into the mains. The batteries are usually only designed for short-term use such as transfer to another hospital or theatre. If the pump runs on disposable batteries, it is important to know what size and type are required and where spares are obtained.

Administration set/cassette/syringe

Most devices require a specific administration set, cassette or syringe, and the use of any other type may result in over- or under-infusion. If the pump is designed to use a variety of administration sets or syringes, it normally needs to be programmed with information regarding the type and size being used.

Setting up the device

All administration sets, cassettes and syringes are designed to be easily inserted and so, if force is required, an incorrect procedure is being followed. When using syringe drivers, it is important that the barrel of the syringe and plunger are correctly positioned to prevent inaccurate infusion and/or siphonage. Many Trusts have a policy regarding the documentation and frequency of checking of i.v. devices during infusion.

Alarm systems

Most modern devices have a number of alarms designed to alert the user to a variety of potentially dangerous situations (e.g. 'air in line' or 'occlusion'). If the device has no alarm system, frequent checking to ensure accurate administration is vital. Most devices have a mute facility which will silence the alarm whilst the problem is being dealt with and then automatically reset itself. However irritating, the alarm system should never be disabled as it is very easy to forget to switch it on again.

Maintenance

All i.v. devices require regular maintenance and must not be used if the 'expiry date' for the next routine service has passed. The outer casing should be kept clean and dust-free using a cloth and hot, soapy water. They must not be immersed. Pumps with mains and battery facilities should be plugged into the mains when stored to ensure that the battery remains fully charged.

BOLUS DRUG ADMINISTRATION (INTRAVENOUS PUSH)

The hands must be clean and gloves may be necessary to protect the nurse when administering drugs such as cytotoxic therapy or antibiotics, or if the patient's condition requires it, e.g. MRSA.

The prescribed drug and any diluent should be checked carefully, including expiry date, and the drug prepared according to the manufacturer's instructions. Supplementary instructions may be included in the prescription, e.g. 'to be diluted in 100 ml of sodium chloride 0.9%', and other information, such as the optimum rate of administration, is often included in the i.v. drug administration policy. Drugs for i.v. administration should be prepared in a clean part of the ward where there is minimal distraction, to permit full concentration, particularly if calculations are involved.

Drugs for one patient should be prepared and then administered immediately. This reduces the risk of the drug(s) being given to the wrong patient. Also, some drugs may be stable for a short period only when reconstituted and so should be administered immediately. A flush of sodium chloride 0.9% should also be prepared (a small number of drugs are not compatible with sodium chloride 0.9%, e.g. amphotericin B, in which case dextrose 5% should be used instead). The amount required will depend on the number of drugs being given as the cannula will need to be flushed after each drug and at the end. If only one drug is being administered, 5 ml of sodium chloride 0.9% is sufficient. If a continuous i.v. infusion is in progress, and the solution is not compatible with the drug being given, the tubing will need to be flushed and so a larger volume will be required.

If a drug requires a very precise rate of infusion (e.g. mcg/kg per min), it will need to be administered via an infusion pump or syringe driver. Drugs given by intermittent bolus dose or 'i.v. push' should be given slowly to prevent speed shock. Slow i.v. administration is also necessary to minimize trauma to the intima of the vein as a result of chemical irritation by the drug.

Explain the procedure to the patient. This is important to gain cooperation and consent, but also if for some reason the patient has already received the drug, she will alert you to this. Adopt a comfortable posture (sitting is probably best) in a position that allows easy access to the cannula. Face the patient so that any adverse reaction may be observed, and if the patient is undergoing cardiac monitoring, this should also be in view. It is important to be in a comfortable position to avoid rushing the administration. Anecdotal evidence suggests that you are also less likely to be interrupted when sitting down with a patient, and interruptions increase the likelihood of errors occurring.

Check the patient's identity against the prescription again. This may involve checking the name band or asking the patient her name or date of birth (see 'Checking procedures', p. 154).

Check the i.v. site for signs of infection, phlebitis or discomfort/pain. If the site is bandaged, this must be removed to allow inspection of the site. If there is an infusion running, the i.v. bolus may be administered via the small injection port which is situated approximately 4 inches from the end of the administration set. Although some cannulae have an integral injection port, this should not be used for drug administration as it is difficult to keep the port clean (see 'Injectable caps and bungs', p. 150). Thoroughly disinfect the rubber membrane of the injection port or injectable cap/bung according to local policy and allow to dry.

Administer a small amount of the sodium chloride 0.9% flush before administering the drug itself to confirm the patency of the cannula. If the patient complains of pain at the site, this may be due to infiltration. By administering a small amount of flush solution first, it will only be sodium chloride 0.9% rather than some potentially more damaging substance that has been administered into the surrounding tissues. If the injection port on the administration set is being used, unless the infusion is sodium chloride 0.9%, it will be necessary to flush the tubing before and after administration.

The drug should be administered according to the manufacturer's instructions, the prescription and/or local policies and procedures, using a small (25G) needle through the injectable rubber cap or port. The use of a 25G needle encourages slow administration and also minimizes the risk of injecting foreign particles, such as rubber or glass, which may be drawn into the syringe during preparation of the drug (Clarke 1997).

Administer the remaining flush or, if a number of drugs are being given, flush between each one to prevent mixing in the cannula (see 'Flushing technique', p. 153). After administration, dispose of needles, glass ampoules, etc. immediately into a sharps disposal container. Ensure that the patient is comfortable and advise her to report any side-effects. Document the drug administration according to local policies and procedures.

CONCLUSION

Intravenous therapy has become a routine part of the nursing care of patients in hospital, and increasingly those in community settings as well. The i.v. route clearly has several advantages, but there are risks. The nurse's role in the safe management of i.v. therapy is crucial. Through good practice, strict asepsis and thorough checking, many of the risks of i.v. therapy may be minimized, if not avoided altogether. The principles of asepsis are vital to the prevention of infection and must be rigorously applied when caring for the site, manipulating the apparatus and preparing and administrating i.v. drugs and infusions. Hand washing continues to be shown to be the most important factor in the prevention of cross-infection (Crow 1996). Minimizing the use of three-way taps, cannula hubs and connections will also reduce opportunities for microbial contamination.

Drug errors are potentially more serious when using the i.v. route. Any drug administered in error cannot be recalled and the effect is likely to be rapid. Many i.v. preparations require dilution prior to administration and often involve mathematical calculations, which increase the risk of error when nurses are busy. Furthermore, patients are not able to detect potential errors in the same way as they are with oral drugs when they are familiar with the tablets they normally receive. Intravenous therapy, like all aspects of nursing care, requires careful management, but good standards of nursing practice will ensure that the risks involved are minimized.

REFERENCES

Adams S D, Killien M, Larson E 1986 In-line filtration and infusion phlebitis. Heart & Lung 15(2): 134–140

Allcutt D, Lort D, McCullum C 1983 Final in line filtration for intravenous: a prospective hospital study. British Journal of Surgery 70: 111–113

Band J D, Maki D G 1979 Safety of changing intravenous delivery systems at longer than 24 hour intervals. Annals of Internal Medicine 91: 173–178

Barrett P J, Lester R L 1990 Heparin versus saline flush solutions in a small community hospital. Nursing Research 40(6): 325

British Medical Association/Royal Pharmaceutical Society of Great Britain (BMA/RPSGB) 1998 British national formulary, no. 36. The Pharmaceutical Press, London

Brown J D, Moss H A, Elliott T S J 1997 The potential for catheter microbial contamination from a needleless connector. Journal of Hospital Infection 36: 181–189

Butler L D 1980 Effect of in-line filters on the potency of low dose drugs. American Journal of Hospital Pharmacy 37: 935–938

Buxton A, Highsmith S, Garner J et al 1979 Contamination of intravenous infusion fluid: effects of changing administration sets. Annals of Internal Medicine 90: 764–768

Clarke A 1997 The nursing management of intravenous drug therapy. British Journal of Nursing 6(4): 201–206

Clayton M 1987 The right way to prevent medicine errors. RN June: 30–31

Cousins D 1988 Cost savings in IV therapy. Care of the Critically Ill 4(1): 30–35

Cousins D H 1995 Medication errors: make infusion pumps safer to use. Pharmacy in Practice October: 401–406

Crow S 1996 Prevention of intravascular infections: ways and means. Journal of Intravenous Nursing 19(4): 175–181

Department of Health and Social Security 1973 Addition of drugs to intravenous fluids. HMSO, London

Dougherty L 1997 Needleless injection systems. RCN IV Special Interest Group Newsletter, July

Dunn D L, Lenihan S F 1987 The case for the saline flush. American Journal of Nursing 6: 689–699

Elliott T 1993 Line associated bacteraemias. Communicable Disease Report Review 3: 91–95

Elliott T, Faroqui M, Armstrong R 1994 Guidelines for good practice in central venous catheterization. Journal of Hospital Infection 28(3): 163–176

Falchuck K, Peterson L, McNeil B 1985 Microparticulate induced phlebitis: its prevention in in-line filtration. New England Journal of Medicine 312: 78–82

Francombe P 1988 Intravenous filters and phlebitis. Nursing Times 84(26): 34–35

Gladstone J 1995 Drug administration errors: a study into the factors underlying the occurrence and reporting of drug errors in a district general hospital. Journal of Advanced Nursing 22: 628–637

Godwin P G, Cuthbert A C, Choyce A 1992 Reducing bruising after venepuncture. Quality in Health Care 1: 245–246

Goode C J, Titler M, Rakel B et al 1991 A meta-analysis of effects of heparin flush and saline flush: quality and cost implications. Nursing Research 40(6): 324–330

Hoffman K, Weber D, Samsa G, Rutala W 1992 Transparent polyurethane film as an intravenous catheter dressing: a meta-analysis of the infection risks. Journal of the American Medical Association 267: 2072–2076

Johns T 1996 Intravenous filters, panacea or placebo. Journal of Clinical Nursing 5: 3–6

Kiernan M 1997 Know how: IV insertion sites. Nursing Times 93(37): 72–73

Lamb J 1995 Guidelines on intravenous therapy. Nursing Standard 9(30): 32–35

McConnell E 1995 How and what staff nurses learn about the medical devices they use in direct patient care. Research in Nursing and Health 18: 165–172

Maki D G, Ringer M 1987 Evaluation of dressing regimens for prevention of infection with peripheral intravenous catheters. Journal of the American Medical Association 258: 2369–2403

Maki D G, Ringer M 1991 Risk factor for infusion-related phlebitis with small peripheral venous catheters. Annals of Internal Medicine 114: 845–854

Moro J L, Vigano E F, Lepri A C 1994 Risk factors for central venous catheters-related infections in surgical and intensive care units. Infection Control and Hospital Epidemiology 15: 253–264

Nelson R S, Tebbs S E, Richards N, Elliott T S J 1996 An audit of peripheral catheter care in a teaching hospital. Journal of Hospital Infection 32(1): 65–69

Nicoll L 1990 Heparin versus saline as a flush solution for intermittent intravenous devices. Research Review 6: 3–4

Nicol M J 1995 Drug administration: checking the facts. Unpublished MSc thesis, RCN, London

Nicol M J 1997 Drug administration: is checking necessary? Managing Clinical Nursing 1(3): 82–86

Oldman P 1991 A sticky situation: a microbiological study of adhesive tape used to secure IV cannulae. Professional Nurse Feb: 265–269

Passonnate A, Macik D G 1988 Case report: the heparin flush syndrome – a cause of iatrogenic haemorrhage. Nursing Research 40(6): 326

Royal College of Nursing 1987 Drug administration: a nursing responsibility. RCN, London

Royal College of Nursing 1994 Intravenous line dressings: principles of infection control. RCN, London

Scales K 1996 Legal and professional aspects of intravenous therapy. Nursing Standard 11(3): 41–46

Shearer J 1987 Normal saline flush versus dilute heparin flush. National Intravenous Therapy Association 10: 425–427

Snydman D R, Donnelly-Reidy M, Perry L K, Martin W J 1987 Intravenous tubing containing burettes can be safely changed at 72 hour intervals. Infection Control 8: 113–116

Speechley V 1984 The nurse's role in intravenous management. Nursing Times 80(18): 31–32

Stonehouse J 1996 Phlebitis associated with peripheral cannulae. Professional Nurse 12(1): 51–53

United Kingdom Central Council for Nursing, Midwifery and Health Visiting 1986 Administration of medicines: an advisory paper. UKCC, London

United Kingdom Central Council for Nursing, Midwifery and Health Visiting 1992 Standards for the administration of medicines. UKCC, London

Vost J, Longstaff V 1997 Infection control and related issues in intravascular therapy. British Journal of Nursing 6(15): 846–857

Walpot H 1989 Particulate contamination of IV solutions and drug additives during long-term intensive care (parts 1 & 2). Anaesthetist 38: 544–548, 617–621

Weinstein S M (ed) 1997 Plumer's principles & practice of intravenous therapy, 6th edn. JB Lippincott, Philadelphia

Wilson J 1994 Preventing infection during IV therapy. Professional Nurse 9(6): 388–392

Wolf Z R 1994 Medication errors: the nursing experience. Delmar Publishers, New York

Local and systemic complications of intravenous therapy

Julie Lamb

CHAPTER 7

INTRODUCTION

In the course of a year, over 500 million peripheral cannulae are sited on patients throughout the world to enable the delivery of effective treatments. A decade ago more than 13 million were used in the UK for the administration of drugs (Baxter Healthcare 1988). In the United States it is estimated that as many as 80–90% of patients, from a total of approximately 27 million, require placement of a vascular access device (Perdue 1995).

Like most clinical procedures, intravenous (i.v.) therapy involves significant risks of damaging side-effects. It is recognized that in i.v. therapy there are risks that are iatrogenic, with problems not necessarily arising from the patient's treatment, but from device-related complications, the clinical status of the patient or the administering practitioner.

Patients who require i.v. therapy are likely to be those who, because of illness, are susceptible to infection. The insertion of a cannula that penetrates the body's skin defence mechanism will result in an additional potential hazard for these patients. If we accept that many patients are going to receive i.v. therapy then we also need to accept that a high percentage of them will be exposed to the possible risks and problems associated with that therapy (Jacques 1992).

The potential for complications is always present in the patient receiving i.v. therapy. Complications increase hospital stays, duration of therapy and nursing and medical responsibilities and can put the patient at risk of other medical problems. In addition, the patient experiences further discomfort and the hospital's overall expenses are increased.

This chapter will review the most common local and systemic complications of i.v. therapy, identifying the procedural and clinical management measures.

SOURCES AND MECHANISMS OF INTRAVENOUS DEVICE INFECTIONS (Fig. 7.1)

Cannula colonization

Microorganisms adhere to the surface of the cannula and can be detected by culturing the tip of the device when it is removed. Cannula colonization is frequently used as a measure of i.v. device infection and is strongly associated with bacteraemia (Graham et al 1991, Mermel et al 1991).

Cause

Following the insertion of a plastic cannula into a vein, a loosely formed fibrin sheath collects around the intravascular portion of the device within 24–48 hours,

Fig. 7.1 Sources of intravenous device-related infections.

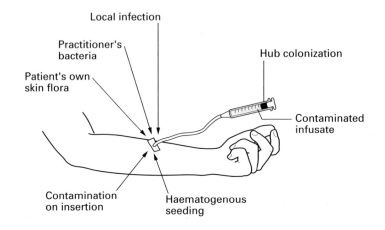

Local infection

Practitioner's bacteria

Hub colonization

Patient's own skin flora

Contaminated infusate

Contamination on insertion

Haematogenous seeding

forming a nidus (Weinstein 1997). This helps the bacteria adhere to the cannula and resist microbial agents circulating in the blood, which means it can be difficult to treat cannula-related infections without removing the device.

Three main sources yield the bacteria responsible for i.v.-associated infection:

- the air
- the skin
- the blood.

Clinical features

Clinical symptoms of a local infection are purulent drainage at the i.v. insertion site which may be accompanied by tenderness, erythema, warmth or induration of the vein.

Prevention

The cannulation procedure may introduce bacteria from the skin into the vein, so insertion should be considered as a minor surgical procedure and carried out with a high standard of asepsis (Wilson 1994).

Where possible, the skin should not be shaved, as the microscopic damage caused increases microbial colonization and therefore the risk of infection (Maki 1976, Wilson 1994, Perdue 1995, Weinstein 1997). Cannulae should be firmly secured to prevent movement which may transfer skin microorganisms from the skin and increase the risk of mechanical phlebitis.

Tape has been implicated as a source of infection, and therefore tape in direct contact with the insertion site should be sterile (Sheldon & Johnson 1979).

The principles of good i.v. practice include the use of sterile dressings to secure peripheral cannulae; despite this, however, the use of non-sterile tapes to secure peripheral i.v. cannulae was identified in a 'point of prevalence single day' study as a widespread practice in adult hospitals in the UK (Goodinson et al 1988).

There is conflicting evidence related to the type of dressing used and the incidence of infection. Transparent film dressings have some advantages over gauze as they allow easy visibility of the insertion site to detect for early signs of infection or phlebitis. Their principal disadvantage is the build-up of skin flora that occurs beneath the dressing. Some studies have demonstrated that the incidence of cannula-related infections increases by 50% if the film dressing is left on for 7 days (Maki & Will 1984). Others have shown no difference between films left on for 7 days and gauze changed every 2–3 days (Ricard et al 1985), or between gauze replaced every other day and films left on for the lifetime of the cannula (Maki & Ringer 1987). New transparent films with a high moisture permeability may be associated with reduced skin colonization (Maki et al 1991).

Action

Treat as directed by a clinician.

Airborne contamination

The number of microbes per cubic foot of air will vary according to the particular area involved.

Cause

Where infection exists, bacteria will escape in body fluids, contaminating clothing, bedding and dressings. Activity such as bed-making sends bacteria flying into the air on particles of lint, pus and dried epithelium (Weinstein 1997).

Prevention

Increased activity causes a rise in the amount of airborne particles, providing an environment that interferes with aseptic technique and potentially contributes to contamination (Weinstein 1997). These contaminants can easily pervade unprotected i.v. solutions.

Activity should be kept to a minimum, particularly when dressing wounds and open lesions or when performing an i.v. procedure.

Action

Treat as directed by a clinician.

Skin contamination

Skin flora has been implicated as a major source of microorganisms in i.v.-related sepsis (Elliot 1988).

Cause

Numerous epidemics of device-related bacteraemias have been linked to the carrying of the epidemic strains of bacteria on the hands of hospital personnel (Henderson 1990).

Because not all bacteria are removed by scrubbing, meticulous care must be observed to avoid contaminating sterile equipment. Touch contamination is a potential hazard of infection because hospital personnel move about frequently, touching both patients and objects (Weinstein 1997). Frequent and proper hand washing is vital.

Action

Treat as directed by a clinician.

Blood contamination

The blood may harbour potentially dangerous microorganisms.

Cause

Care must be taken to prevent bacterial contamination from blood spills when obtaining blood samples and performing cannulation.

It is more likely, however, that the problem in the blood will be viral in origin, e.g. hepatitis virus and acquired immunodeficiency syndrome (AIDS) retrovirus. The hepatitis virus is transmitted easily and is destroyed only by heat or gas sterilization.

Prevention

Correct care of all i.v. equipment is essential.

Action

Proper labelling of blood samples that may be contaminated is necessary to prevent the spread of any infection amongst health care staff.

Contamination of infusion system

Extrinsic contamination may occur via the administration set, the drug delivery sites and additional equipment such as extension sets, fluid containers and cannulae (Fig. 7.2). Each time the i.v. apparatus is manipulated, the likelihood for contamination increases. Careless management of i.v. systems will increase the potential for contamination.

Some bacteria, such as *Klebsiella*, grow rapidly in i.v. solutions, particularly dextrose 5%. Dextrose, as well as being a source of carbon and energy, includes the extra nutrients needed to support the growth of 10 million organisms per millilitre (Weinstein 1997).

Prevention

Prior to use, containers of fluid should be examined, preferably against a light and dark background, for cracks, defects, turbidity and particulate matter; plastic containers should be squeezed to detect any punctures (Goodinson 1990a). Accidental puncture may occur without being evident and thereby provide a point of entry for microorganisms (Maki et al 1973). Any container with a crack or defect must be considered as faulty and disregarded; glass containers lacking a vacuum when opened should not be used.

Infusion fluid can be easily contaminated when drugs are added or given into the cannula, when fluids or administration sets are changed and when blood and blood products are given (Wilson 1994); an aseptic technique is therefore essential.

Close observation of the fluid is required prior to administration; if discoloration is overlooked, the subsequent infusion of a few hundred millilitres of contaminated fluid will result in shock or possibly even death (Weinstein 1997).

Action

Treat as directed by a clinician.

Intravenous fluids/solutions

Cause

Studies have identified that i.v. fluids and sets can become contaminated while in use (Weinstein 1997). The larger the container, the greater the proliferation of bacteria.

Prevention

Intravenous fluids may be inadvertently contaminated by complacent techniques in the manipulation of equipment. Studies have demonstrated that, although the infu-

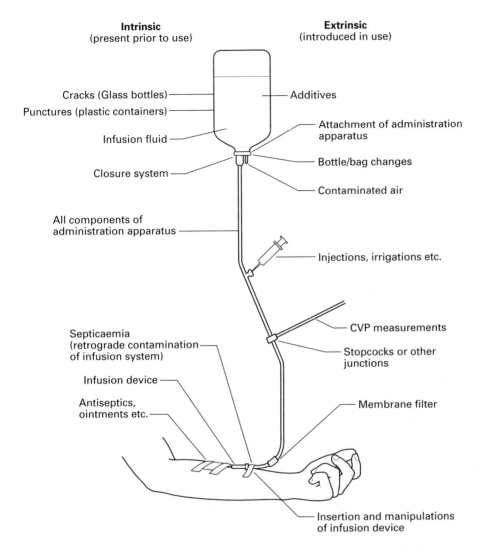

Fig. 7.2 Potential mechanisms for contamination of intravenous infusion systems.

sion fluid is more likely to be contaminated after 72 hours than after 48 hours, the difference is not statistically significant (Maki et al 1987).

Contamination is more likely to occur in high-dependency settings where i.v. catheters are used for central access or haemodynamic monitoring.

Proper hand washing and aseptic technique are essential to minimize contamination. Regular changing of administration sets has also been recommended to prevent contamination (DHSS 1972).

Action

Treat as directed by a clinician.

Injection ports

Cause

As the injection port site is at the distal end of the tubing, it has the potential to be exposed to patient excreta and drainage, resulting in possible contamination.

Prevention

The injection port should be swabbed for a minimum of 1 minute with an appropriate antiseptic such as isopropyl alcohol 70%. Alternatively, swabbing the injection cap for 30 seconds with an antimicrobial (povidone-iodine) provides acceptable disinfection (Weinstein 1997).

Meticulous aseptic technique must be observed when using injection ports.

Action

Remove and replace injection port if contaminated.

Three-way taps/stopcocks

Cause

Three-way taps are vulnerable to the transfer of bacteria to the host as their ports are open to moisture and contamination.

Prevention

A sterile catheter plug attached at the time the tap is added and then changed following each use will minimize the risks of contamination.

If fluid leakage is found at injection sites, connections or vents, the i.v. administration set or offending tap should be replaced. Adherence to aseptic technique is essential.

Action

Replace three-way tap or stopcock if contaminated.

Skin preparation

Microorganisms found on the hands of health care staff contribute to hospital-associated infections. Commonly this results in the contamination of some part of the i.v. system due to poor compliance with aseptic technique and, in particular, hand washing.

The importance of hand hygiene in the control of infection is not in doubt, but persuading clinicians to comply with advice appears to be a problem (Keenlyside 1992). Krakowskas' (1986) study found that out of 18 medical personnel questioned, only 11% always washed their hands before peripheral cannulation, and 5% admitted to never washing their hands. Maki (1989) believes that nurses are, in general, far better informed and a more effective force for ensuring compliance with infection control procedures than other medical personnel.

The number of resident bacteria on the hands may be greatly reduced by washing with soap and water (Elliott 1988) and this method of hand washing is adequate prior to placing peripheral cannulae (Simmonds 1983). Gloves should be worn if contamination with blood is anticipated.

Adequate preparation of the patient's skin and adherence to asepsis are vital for the cannulation procedure, during which the skin, the body's first defence barrier, is breached, providing a vulnerable port for the migration of bacteria.

Alcohol is frequently used to cleanse the skin prior to venepuncture and, when applied with friction for 1 minute, is as effective as 12 minutes of scrubbing and reduces the bacterial count by 75%. Too frequently the use of alcohol consists of a quick wipe, which fails to reduce the bacterial count significantly (Weinstein 1997).

Iodine preparations remain one of the most reliable agents for skin cleansing, providing bactericidal, fungicidal and sporicidal activity; however, 70% alcohol solutions are an acceptable alternative if used vigorously and for at least 1 minute after washing the site (Maki 1976). Patient allergy should be established prior to use. The solution should be applied liberally, allowed to dry for at least 30 seconds and wiped off with 70% alcohol (Maki 1976, Weinstein 1997). More recently chlorhexadrine in 70% alcohol has proved to be an effective skin-cleansing agent.

Infusion particulate matter

Studies have identified that particulate contamination is present in all i.v. fluids and administration sets (Weinstein 1993). Enormous efforts are being made by manufacturers to provide high-quality i.v. infusions, but their efforts can be negated by the numerous manipulations prior to infusion.

The administration of drugs is a significant cause of contamination. An improper technique in the preparation and reconstitution of drugs can result in the formation of insoluble particles. The risks are minimized when drugs are prepared in laminar flow cabinets by trained pharmacy staff.

Particulate matter infused via i.v. fluids may produce pathological changes that can have a detrimental effect on critically ill patients.

Particles although minute may cause considerable harm. They travel through the venous system, ending in the capillary bed of the lung. Particles larger than the capillary diameter (7–12 µm) will become lodged in the lung, leading to cellular damage or tissue death (Weinstein 1997).

Glass ampoules

Glass ampoules may be responsible for the injection of thousands of glass particles into the circulation. Turco & Davis (1972), in a study prompted by the frequency of high-dose administration of frusemide, showed that a dose of 400 mg, which at that time required the breaking of 20 ampoules, could add 1085 glass particles larger than 5 µm to the injection (Weinstein 1997).

Manufacturers are leaning towards the use of plastic ampoules in an effort to reduce this risk.

Antibiotic injectables

Studies have been performed in relation to particulate matter in commercial antibiotic injectable products (Weinstein 1993). They showed particulate contamination levels of bulk-filled antibiotics to be 2–10 times greater than those of stable antibiotic solutions and lyophilized antibiotics.

Particulate matter in i.v. injections may be responsible for much of the phlebitis that frequently occurs with the administration of these drugs.

Reducing the level of contaminants

Filters are available to prevent unwanted material from entering an infusion or vein or to extend the duration of use of the administration set. Their inception was based upon the need to reduce the risks of contamination and there are arguments both for and against their use. A knowledge of specific filter characteristics, use and correct handling is important for patient safety. Inappropriate or faulty handling can cause plugging of the filter, resulting in the patient not receiving the prescribed fluid. A ruptured filter may go undetected and introduce filter fragments, bacteria and air into the i.v. system.

Research has shown that the use of in-line filters reduces the incidence of phlebitis by removing particulate contaminants from the infusion (Francombe 1988, Johnson 1994).

Up to 70% of particles present in an i.v. system are contributed by the addition of drugs to the system. Filters have the potential to eliminate entrained air and remove

■ BOX 7. 1

Phlebitis grading – Dinley grading scale

1+ Pain at site, no erythema, no swelling, no induration, no palpable venous cord

2+ Pain at site with erythema, some degree of swelling, or both, no induration, no palpable cord

3+ Pain at site with erythema and swelling and with induration or a palpable venous cord less than 3 inches above the i.v. site

4+ Pain at site, erythema, swelling, induration and a palpable venous cord greater than 3 inches above the i.v. site

5+ Vein thrombosis along with all the signs of 4+

particles present in fluids and drugs. They can also retain microbes inadvertently introduced into the i.v. system and some may even retain endotoxins released by many bacteria (Horibe et al 1990, Richards & Thomas 1990).

There are few situations in i.v. therapy delivery in which the use of filters is essential.

CLINICAL FEATURES OF LOCAL COMPLICATIONS OF INTRAVENOUS THERAPY

Phlebitis

Phlebitis is a complication frequently associated with i.v. therapy. Various investigators have reported that infusion-related phlebitis affects 25–70% of all hospitalized patients (Perucca & Micek 1993). Approximately 60% develop clinical phlebitis indicators between 8 and 16 hours following insertion (Perucca & Micek 1993).

Phlebitis is defined as the acute inflammation of the intima of the vein. It is characterized by pain and tenderness along the course of the vein, erythema and inflammatory swelling with a feeling of warmth at the site (Scalley et al 1992, Bohony 1993, Perucca & Micek 1993, Perdue 1995) (Box 7.1).

Experimental studies have ruled out infection as being the major source of phlebitis (Maki 1976).

Cause

Factors which substantially increase the risk for infusion phlebitis include:

- improper cannula material, length and gauge
- lack of skill of the individual inserting the cannula
- incorrect anatomical site for cannulation
- prolonged duration of cannulation
- infrequent dressing changes
- properties and character of the infusion fluid
- host factors, such as age and clinical status.

The three most common causes of irritation are:

- mechanical, such as rubbing of the cannula against the vessel wall
- contamination by microscopic particles that may be transferred to (and by) infusion fluids and drugs
- chemical reasons related to the nature of fluid being administered.

■ BOX 7.2

Prevention of phlebitis

- Refrain from using veins in the lower extremities
- Select veins with ample blood volume when infusing irritant substances
- Avoid veins in areas over joint flexion
- Anchor cannulae securely to prevent movement
- Frequently inspect the i.v. site
- Remove the cannula at the first sign of discomfort and inflammation

Prevention and action

Phlebitis is often associated with the length of time the cannula has been in place. Changing the cannula every 72 hours regardless of whether tenderness or erythema have developed will reduce the risks of phlebitis, and diluting drugs and slowing the infusion rate will eliminate some of the causes (Millam 1988, Perucca & Micek 1993, Perdue 1995) (Box 7.2).

Pathophysiology

When the vein wall is punctured by an i.v. cannula, an injury to the skin occurs as well as trauma to the vessel wall. Patients receiving i.v. therapy may experience temporary discomfort from the venepuncture. Usually the initial discomfort associated with the venepuncture resolves. However, occasionally trauma and injury to the vessel wall can precipitate the development of phlebitis (Perucca & Micek 1993).

The phlebitic process involves a series of physical and chemical reactions that occur in response to the tissue injury. Soon after venepuncture, the damaged tissue releases large quantities of histamine, bradykinin and serotonin. Histamine stimulates dilation of the vessel. The blood flow to the area is increased, which results in redness and increased warmth at the insertion site. Increased permeability allows fluid and protein to shift from the interstitial space. The collection of fluid and protein results in oedema and pain at the venepuncture site. If the cannula is left in situ, the clinical indicators of phlebitis continue to increase in severity. The immune system causes leucocytes to concentrate at the inflamed insertion site, resulting in further oedema and pus formation in the inflamed tissue. The leucocytes release endogenous pyrogens into the bloodstream, stimulating the hypothalamus to increase body temperature. As the leucocytes circulate to the bone marrow, more leucocytes are released into the bloodstream, elevating the white blood cell count (Perucca & Micek 1993).

Chemical phlebitis

Cause

Chemical phlebitis is associated with a response of the vein intima to certain chemicals infused into the vascular system. An inflammatory response can follow the administration of solutions and/or medications or can be a result of the cannula material used for venous access.

Solutions or drugs with a high pH or osmolality predispose the vein intima to irritation. The more acidic the solution, the greater the potential for phlebitis.

The rate of infusion can be a significant component in the onset of phlebitis.

Prevention and action

The slower the rate of infusion, the less the propensity for venous irritation. Rapid infusion rates irritate the vessel walls by providing a larger concentration of medications and solutions. Slower rates provide longer absorption times, with haemodilution of smaller amounts of solutions and medications (Perdue 1995).

Clinical trials have shown that the prophylactic use of transdermal glyceryl trinitrate will reduce the incidence of phlebitis and infusion failure (Khawaja et al 1989). A study by Wright et al (1985) showed that the frequency of infusion failure was three times lower with glyceryl trinitrate than with placebo patches. The decrease was of similar magnitude whether the failure was due to extravasation or phlebitis. Headaches, however, were more common but were relieved by simple analgesics.

Mechanical phlebitis

Cause

Mechanical phlebitis is associated with the placement of the cannula. Cannulae placed in areas of flexion can result in the onset of mechanical phlebitis; as the limb is moved, the cannula irritates the intima of the vein, causing friction. A large cannula placed in a small vein which rubs against the wall of the tunica intima will also cause friction.

Various investigators have related the incidence of phlebitis to the design of the infusion device (Kerrison & Woodhill 1994). Gaukroger et al (1988) looked at the incidence of phlebitis in 700 surgical patients randomized to receive either Teflon or Vialon cannulae and the results showed a 46% reduction in thrombophlebitis when Vialon was used. McKee et al (1989) examined the incidence of thrombophlebitis in patients with 'difficult' veins, such as oncology patients requiring repeated cannulation; Teflon and Vialon were again compared and 191 cannulae evaluated. The results showed a 36% decrease in thrombophlebitis when Vialon was used.

However, a study by Payne James et al (1991) showed that despite the theoretical superiority of Vialon as a cannula material, under controlled conditions there appeared to be little difference in its inherent capacity to cause thrombophlebitis.

Prevention

A large cannula placed within a small vein will irritate the intima causing inflammation and phlebitis. Therefore, the smallest gauge cannula appropriate to delivery of the prescribed therapy should be used, and, additionally, siting the cannula away from joints and bony prominences will be beneficial.

Cannulae must be anchored securely, otherwise they have the potential to slide in and out of the vein, resulting in phlebitis.

Action

Remove and replace the cannula if phlebitis is present.

Bacterial phlebitis

Bacterial phlebitis is an inflammation of the intima of the vein associated with a bacterial infection and is the rarest type of phlebitis (Perdue 1995). It has the potential to predispose the patient to the systemic complication of septicaemia.

Hand washing is the principal method of preventing nosocomial infections.

Post-infusion phlebitis

Post-infusion phlebitis is associated with inflammation of the vein that usually becomes evident within 48–96 hours of cannula removal (Perdue 1995). The vein is reddened and inflamed, symptoms are often accompanied by pain, and is estimated to affect up to 70% of all infusions (Francombe 1988).

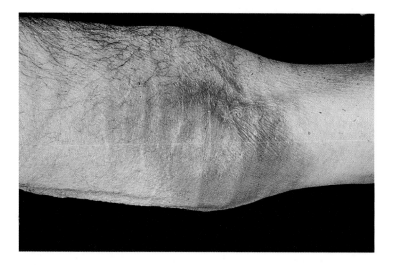

Fig. 7.3 Phlebitis at the cannula site.

Following removal, the venepuncture site should be observed for erythema, oedema and drainage; the site should be palpated for warmth and vein induration (Perdue 1995). Measures for its prevention are identical to those used in phlebitis (Fig. 7.3).

Thrombophlebitis

Thrombophlebitis is the inflammation of a vein associated with thrombus formation. It is characterized by varying degrees of histopathological change, including infiltration, oedema and, in extreme cases, haemorrhage and necrosis of the vein wall. Local redness, pain, warmth, stiffness and a palpable cord are usually present (Goodinson 1990b).

Clinical features

Diagnostic features of thrombophlebitis include fever, tachycardia, leucocytosis, lymphadenopathy and positive blood cultures. Symptoms and signs usually last days or weeks, although Hästbacka et al (1965) reported that symptoms may persist for months. It is possible for suppuration (Ross 1972, Curry & Zallen 1973, Arnold et al 1977), septicaemia (Arnold et al 1977), pulmonary embolism (rarely) (Swanson & Aldrete 1969) and even death (Frazer et al 1977) to result (Lewis & Hecker 1985).

Pathophysiology

It has been suggested that thrombus formation results from:

- changes in the blood
- changes in the characteristics of the flow of blood
- changes in the vessel wall (Lewis & Hecker 1985).

It is thought that chemical irritation causes much of the inflammation in thrombophlebitis. Prostaglandins may be released or stimulated by histamine, adenosine-5-triphosphate (ATP) and prostaglandin E_1 during the inflammatory response.

Prostaglandins $PGE_1 + PGE_2$ increase local vascular permeability. Early histological changes such as swelling of the endothelial cells and leucocyte infiltration to the tunica media are then initiated.

When the vein wall is traumatized, platelet phospholipase A_2 is stimulated to form biologically active compounds which increase vascular permeability. In addi-

■ BOX 7.3

Factors which contribute to the formation of a thrombosis

- Placement by an unskilled professional
- Multiple cannulation attempts
- Use of a cannula that is larger than the vein lumen
- Poor circulation with venous stasis
- Administration of medicines incompatible with solutions
- Administration of solutions or drugs with a high pH or tonicity
- Ineffective filtration
- Use of cannula materials that are thrombogenic

tion, other platelet-produced metabolites, PGG_2, PGH_2 and thromboxane A_2, become activated as platelet-releasing agents, which may also be involved at the endothelial surface. Humoral agents released in response to venous irritation may provoke venoconstriction. If the flow of blood in the vein is diminished, irritant infusates are not rapidly diluted with blood and this together with stasis would predispose to thrombophlebitis (Lewis & Hecker 1985).

Prevention

Preventative measures include avoiding the placement of cannulae in the lower extremities where the veins are small, which allows pooling of blood with resultant damage to the vein intima and subsequent clot formation. The selection of an appropriate venous device, i.e. the smallest and shortest device possible to deliver the prescribed therapy, minimizes the potential for injury to the endothelial lining of the vessel wall (Elliot 1991, Perdue 1995). Veins over flexion areas should be avoided and cannulae should be anchored securely to prevent movement. Too much movement of the cannula at the entry site can drag organisms from the skin into the bloodstream (Millam 1988).

Factors which contribute to the formation of a thrombosis are presented in Box 7.3.

If thrombophlebitis goes untreated, the vein becomes sclerosed and is unavailable for future therapy. Although the inherent danger of an embolism always exists when a thrombus forms, these thrombi are generally well attached to the vein wall and do not migrate. The risk of septicaemia or bacterial endocarditis is greater, particularly if the inflammation is the result of sepsis (Perdue 1995).

Action

The infusion should be discontinued immediately and the cannula removed. Cold compresses should be applied to the site initially to decrease the flow of blood and increase platelet adherence to the clot already formed. A warm compress should then be applied and the limb elevated.

Infiltration

Infiltration is the inadvertent administration of a non-vesicant solution or drug into surrounding tissues as a result of dislodgement of a cannula (Perdue 1995). It is one of the most common complications of i.v. therapy.

Cause

Complete infiltration occurs when the cannula slips out of the vein or is forced completely through the vessel wall on insertion (Fig. 7.4A). Partial infiltration occurs when only the tip of the cannula remains in the vein or the vessel wall does not seal around the cannula, allowing some but not all of the fluid to infiltrate (Fig. 7.4B).

Rigid steel needles substantially increase the risk of infiltration, which can occur any time following placement. With plastic cannulae, it usually becomes apparent after the first day as it commonly results from poor initial placement (Bohony 1993).

A misconception surrounding infiltration is that the infusion rate will always slow or stop if the cannula becomes dislodged from the vein. In fact the fluid will continue to flow into the surrounding tissues until the interstitial pressure overcomes the gravity pressure of the infusion (Millam 1988).

Clinical features

The clinical symptoms of infiltration are coolness, leakage at the site, and swelling

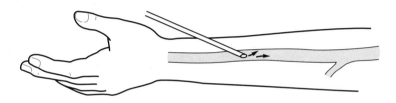

Fig. 7.4 A. Complete infiltration.

i   The cannula is infusing solution into a patent vein.

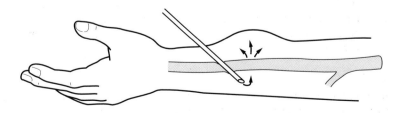

ii   The cannula tip has pulled out of the vein and is infusing into the surrounding subcutaneous tissue.

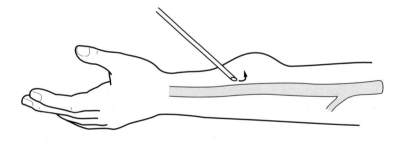

iii The cannula tip has passed through the vein wall and is infusing into surrounding subcutaneous tissue (occurs more commonly with steel needle winged devices).

Fig. 7.4 B Partial infiltration.

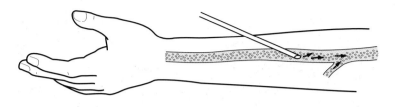

i   The cannula is infusing into a patent vein with blood freely flowing through a side branch.

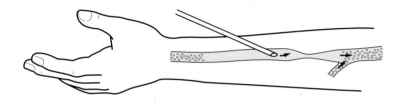

ii Constriction has occured around cannula. Pressure has increased and resistance is apparent. The valve closes and dilution of the infusate with blood before the side branch ceases.

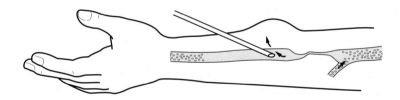

iii Complete occlusion. Due to the pressure around cannula, its tip may increase the hole made on insertion, which will increase the liklihood of the infusate leaking into the surrounding tissues.

and tenderness around the site (Bohony 1993). If a large amount of fluid is trapped in the subcutaneous tissue, the skin may appear taut or stretched with the patient complaining of tightness and discomfort around the site (Fig. 7.5). The amount of discomfort experienced by the patient will be determined by the type of solution or drug being infused (Perdue 1995).

Prevention and action

To prevent infiltration it is essential that the infusion is monitored regularly and the cannula removed once infiltration has been identified. If the solution being infused is isotonic, the patient will experience minimal suffering; however, a warm compress may help to alleviate discomfort and assist in absorbing the infiltrated fluid by increasing circulation to the area (Perdue 1995).

Not all infiltrations can be avoided, but adhering to certain measures can aid in their prevention and minimize their severity. Flexion areas should be avoided, the cannula anchored securely and the site protected from excessive and unnecessary movement.

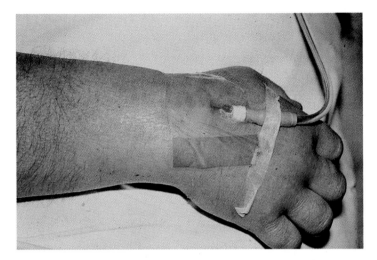

Fig. 7.5 Infiltration of fluid into subcutaneous tissue around the cannula site.

Health care staff should be aware of infusion failures, and attempts to restart or encourage sluggish infusions by winding tubing around scissors or pens or by nipping the tubing should be discouraged as they increase the pressure within the vein, which damages it. The risk of solutions or drugs leaking into the surrounding tissues is therefore increased (Dougherty 1992).

Patient education plays a key role in the prevention of infiltration, along with early recognition and treatment of the clinical features.

Extravasation

An estimated 80% of hospitalized patients have i.v. cannulae inserted to deliver fluids and/or drugs. Approximately 50% of these cannulae fail (Yucha et al 1993).

Extravasation is the inadvertent administration of a vesicant or irritant solution into the surrounding tissues. A vesicant solution is one that causes the formation of blisters with subsequent sloughing of tissues due to tissue necrosis (Perdue 1995). Drugs that contribute to extravasation necrosis are most often osmotically active or ischaemia-inducing, or cause direct cellular toxicity (Weinstein 1997) (Box 7.4).

Cause

Solutions which differ in osmolality and pH behave differently on extravasation; they will produce varying amounts of pain and will be reabsorbed at different rates. Hypertonic infiltrates will enlarge in size, while hypotonic solutions will reabsorb into surrounding tissues quite quickly. This is associated with the osmosis of fluid from the plasma and surrounding tissues into the infiltrated region driven by the concentration gradient that speeds movement of water from the infiltrate into the surrounding tissue cells and capillaries (Yucha et al 1993). Vasoconstrictive drugs such as noradrenaline and dopamine act by causing local vasoconstriction, resulting in tissue ischaemia (Flemmer & Chan 1993).

Clinical features

The patient may complain of pain or burning at the site of extravasation, which will progress to signs of erythema and oedema. The infusion will slow in rate and, if a bolus is being administered, pressure will be felt on the syringe.

Tissue sloughing is usually apparent within 1–4 weeks due to tissue necrosis (Perdue 1995). Necrosis can involve a small superficial area of tissue loss which, fol-

■ **BOX 7.4**

Drugs capable of causing severe tissue damage (non-cytotoxic)

- Amphotericin
- Acyclovir
- Ganciclovir
- Phenytoin
- Potassium chloride (if greater than 40 mmol/L)
- Hypertonic solutions of sodium bicarbonate (greater than 5%)
- Vancomycin

lowing debridement (and if infection-free), will granulate. It may also involve large areas and take in deep structures, including underlying connective tissues, muscles, tendons and bone, which may result in the need for surgical wide excision, debridement, grafting or even amputation to restore tissue integrity (Weinstein 1993). Percutaneous extravasation in neonates with circulatory compromise or nutritional defects has been found to be associated with significant morbidity (Flemmer & Chan 1993). Quick and appropriate therapy becomes critical when the probability of morbidity may include partial- or full-thickness skin loss, infection, deep tissue necrosis with nerve or tendon damage, loss of limb function or loss of the limb itself (Flemmer & Chan 1993).

Prevention (Box 7.5)

It is essential that an extravasation be identified early before a large volume of fluid infiltrates the interstitial tissues. The intravenous site should be examined at frequent and regular intervals. As time progresses after extravasation, it becomes increasingly difficult to accurately palpate and measure the borders of induration, suggesting that surface assessments are most accurate when performed within a short period of extravasation (Yucha et al 1993).

When an extravasation is suspected, the infusion must be discontinued immediately. The flow rate should never be increased to determine the infiltration of a vesicant solution nor should a blood return be considered as a reliable method to ascertain the presence of an extravasation (Perdue 1995).

The i.v. site should always be checked for patency prior to, during and following administration. It is advisable to administer such drugs through a fast running infusion via a side port, as a free-flowing infusion will indicate a patent cannula and, should extravasation occur, the tissue damage will be reduced due to the concentration of the vesicant drug being diluted (Perdue 1995). Vesicant/irritant agents should not be administered in areas of flexion and the hands should be avoided due to the close network of tendons and nerves that would be destroyed if extravasation were to occur (Perdue 1995).

Most establishments have written protocols and procedures related to the management of such an event. Only trained staff knowledgeable in the administration of vesicant drugs should administer these agents.

If a cannula has been in situ for longer than 24 hours, it is prudent to consider replacing it, preferably on the opposite limb, prior to administration.

Knowledge of vesicant potential of solutions and drugs and the recognition of the clinical features and preventative measures are imperative for the safe administration of these drugs.

■ **BOX 7.5**

Prevention or minimization of the risks of extravasation

- Correct positioning of the cannula using the smallest gauge possible
- Correct site placement – use the forearm; avoid sites near joints
- Administer through a recently sited cannula
- Consider a central venous catheter for slow infusions of high-risk drugs
- Verify correct placement prior to vesicant administration
- Administer by slow i.v. push into side arm port of a fast-running i.v. infusion of compatible solution
- Administer vesicant drugs first
- Observe the site continuously
- If in doubt, stop and resite cannula
- Ask the patient to report any sensation of pain, burning or stinging

In the event of an extravasation, treat promptly and document all the details in the patient's notes.

A major part of the prevention of such problems is the education of patients. Asking them to promptly report any sensation of pain and burning will assist in minimizing tissue damage.

Action

Regardless of the mechanism causing injury, the treatment goals are to promote rapid absorption of the irritant and to decrease vascular constriction. Extravasated antibiotics and electrolytes in hypertonic solutions or with non-physiological pH may cause direct cellular injury. The primary goal in such cases is to increase absorption. Extravasated vasopressors causing vasoconstriction and ischaemia may lead to tissue necrosis, making the primary objective the rapid reversal of the vaso-constriction (Flemmer & Chan 1993).

Cold or warm compresses are applied to the site – a cold compress for alkylating and antibiotic vesicants and irritant solutions, and a warm compress for the vinca alkaloid compounds (Perdue 1995). The limb should be elevated and observed reg-ularly.

Detailed guidelines on the management of extravasation are given in Chapter 16.

Risk factors

The patient Extravasation injuries commonly occur in seriously ill patients and appear to be more prevalent in children, elderly people and patients who require frequent venepunctures, such as those receiving chemotherapy. Patients who are unable to communicate pain produced by extravasated fluid are more likely to develop tissue injury. These include neonates, young children, and anaesthetized and comatose patients (Root & Stanley 1993).

The status of the patient's venous access is an important contributory factor. Fragile veins will increase the potential for extravasation. Elderly and debilitated patients are more likely to have poor venous access. Patients with generalized vas-cular disease are more likely to extravasate, as are those with elevated venous pres-sure and those with obstructed venous drainage, perhaps following axillary surgery or radical mastectomy (Root & Stanley 1993).

Critically ill patients often have reduced clotting factors and can be thrombocytopenic, which will inhibit the formation of a firm homeostatic plug at the cannula site and increase the risk of leakage.

Venous spasm as a result of changes in body temperature, raised blood pressure or psychological factors may lead to extravasation.

Cannulation and administration technique Many extravasation injuries occur as a result of inexperienced staff establishing venous access and administering drugs. If a vein is punctured repeatedly before a successful device is secured, drugs are more likely to leak into the surrounding tissues.

The type of cannula used can also affect the incidence of extravasation. It has been shown that correctly positioned steel needles extravasated drugs twice as often as those with plastic cannulae (Root & Stanley 1993).

Patients receiving drugs via infusion pumps should be closely monitored, as continued pumping of fluid after displacement of the cannula leads to mechanical compression of the tissues, resulting in severe tissue damage (Fig. 7.6).

The drug The factors which increase the prevalence of extravasation are:

- the drug's ability to bind to DNA, i.e. doxorubicin
- the drug's ability to cause direct cellular toxicity, i.e. vinca alkaloids
- the drug's ability to cause local tissue ischaemia, i.e. vasopressors
- formulations with high osmolality, i.e. glucose 20%
- formulation pH outside the range 5–9, i.e. phenytoin
- formulations likely to precipitate, i.e. diazepam.

Cannula occlusion

Cause

Cannulae can become occluded with blood when infusion containers run dry and when flush solutions are not administered appropriately (Perdue 1995).

If incompatible-solutions are administered, this may also result in precipitate formation within the cannula, with subsequent occlusion.

Fig. 7.6 Extravasation of sodium bicarbonate.

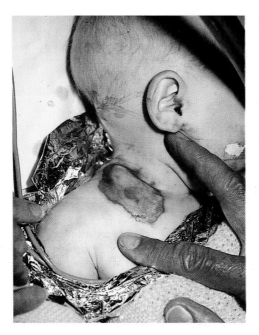

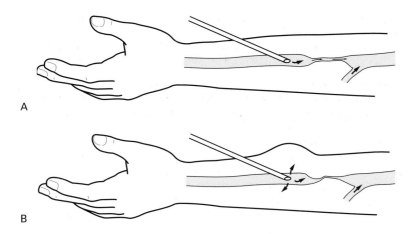

Fig. 7.7 A. Vein constriction. **B.** Vein occlusion.

A

B

Prevention

The prevention of cannula occlusion requires proper care and maintenance. When a cannula occludes, the infusion will slow and eventually stop.

Flushing the peripheral cannula prior to and following each drug administration will assist in reducing the potential for occlusion. For most central venous catheters, it is recommended to use heparinized sodium chloride 0.9% to prevent formation of a fibrin sheath at the end of the catheter which may occlude the end of the catheter lumen(s).

Action

Cannulae should not be flushed to forcefully dislodge an occlusion as this will release the offending particle into the venous circulation, creating the potential for embolus (Perdue 1995). If undue resistance is felt against the syringe plunger, then the cannula should be removed.

Venous spasm

A spasm is a sudden, involuntary contraction of a vein resulting in temporary cessation of blood flow through a vessel (Fig. 7.7).

Cause

Stimulation by cold infusates or by mechanical or chemical irritation may produce spasms (Perdue 1995).

Clinical features

The patient may experience cramping or pain above the venepuncture site.

Action

The infusion should be discontinued, the administration rate decreased or the drug diluted further. If the spasm is the result of a cold solution, warm compresses, which will cause venous dilation and increase blood supply, should be applied above the venepuncture site to relieve the spasm and the pain (Perdue 1995).

Infection at the venepuncture site

Cause

Infections occurring at the venepuncture site are usually local in the absence of any phlebitis grading found at the cannula entry site (Perdue 1995).

Prevention

The cannula should be observed for signs of clinical complications at least daily or whenever the i.v. system is manipulated.

Action

Once identified, the cannula should be removed and cultured along with any drainage from the site. An appropriate dressing should be applied and antibiotics prescribed if necessary. The site should be monitored until the infection has resolved (Perdue 1995).

Mechanical problems which may affect the intravenous system

Regular observation of the patient receiving i.v. therapy is required to maintain an accurate flow rate and complication-free therapy.

The practitioner needs to determine whether there are any mechanical factors which could interfere with fluid delivery.

Cause

The following could interfere with the flow rate:

- Positioning the infusion container less than 36 inches above the i.v. insertion site prevents gravity from overcoming vascular pressure and will stop the infusion.
- Kinks in the i.v. administration set tubing or the cannula will prevent flow.
- Taping at the cannula site can obstruct the cannula lumen, particularly if tape is placed directly over the bevel of the cannula.
- Small gauge cannulae can slow fluid delivery.
- Cannulae sited near joints may occlude when the patient moves.

Other factors such as the presence of tortuous veins, venous spasm, infiltration, phlebitis and loss of patency may all affect accurate fluid delivery (LaRocca & Otto 1993).

Prevention and action

Careful and accurate patient assessment and appreciation of the risk factors will reduce the amount of problems encountered. A working knowledge and understanding of good clinical practice in i.v. therapy will assist in the prevention of a majority of complications.

Ecchymosis and haematoma

Ecchymosis is a term used to denote the infiltration of blood into the tissues, whereas haematoma usually refers to uncontrolled bleeding at a venepuncture site, usually creating a hard and painful lump (Perdue 1995).

Prevention and action

Their occurrence is often the result of a poor venepuncture technique which has caused trauma to the vein wall or they may occur in patients who have a tendency to bruise easily. Staff should be trained to an acceptable standard of competency and should take time to consider which patients are vulnerable to bruising prior to venepuncture.

Ecchymosis can also develop if a tourniquet is put on too tightly or left on for too long (Millam 1988).

The presence of both ecchymosis and haematoma limits the capability of veins for future use and produces damage to tissues. If a haematoma is severe, it may limit the use of a limb (Perdue 1995).

CLINICAL FEATURES OF SYSTEMIC COMPLICATIONS OF INTRAVENOUS THERAPY

Septicaemia

Any local i.v. site infection carries the risk of becoming a systemic infection. If the patient's health is already compromised, this complication can progress quickly and may prove fatal. Infection of the i.v. site can be caused by poor adherence to aseptic technique during procedures and manipulations; failure to maintain a clean site or closed delivery system; and failure to change administration sets and cannulae at regular intervals. Aseptic technique is the key preventative measure in reducing the likelihood of infection associated with i.v. therapy. Hand washing is the most basic, but often the most ignored, of all the techniques to minimize infection (Elliott 1991).

Patients are more at risk if they are malnourished, immunocompromised, less than 1 or greater than 60 years of age, or if they already have an infection at another site (Weinstein 1997).

Each time the delivery system is opened for direct access, the risk of contamination increases. An i.v. system provides the opportunity for bacteria to enter the bloodstream and cause serious infectious complications. To all intents and purposes, the patient receiving i.v. therapy has a hollow conduit directly connecting his bloodstream to the outside world and its abundant microflora. One of the patient's most important host defences is totally abrogated – the intact skin (Maki 1976).

Septicaemia is a pathological state or pyrogenic reaction that is usually accompanied by systemic illness. It occurs when pathogenic bacteria invade the bloodstream. The presence of bacteria in blood is described as bacteraemia, and where bacteraemia is associated with symptoms of infection (e.g. rigors, fevers), this is termed septicaemia (Wilson 1994). Infection will depend upon the ability of the bacteria to survive and proliferate. The factors which influence their survival are:

- the specific organisms present
- the number of such organisms
- the resistance of the host
- environmental conditions.

Contributing factors

These can be divided into two primary categories: those that make the patient susceptible to infections, i.e. the patient's disease state or their treatment; and those that allow microorganisms to enter the bloodstream (Perdue 1995), as described below.

Solution container The solution container can be a focal point not only for contamination but also for microbial growth. *Klebsiella, Enterobacter, Serratia* and *P. cepacia* show rapid growth within 24 hours in dextrose 5% in water solutions. Blood products also provide a rich source for *Klebsiella* microorganisms to grow and parenteral nutrition solutions support the growth of *Candida* species (Perdue 1995).

Solution containers that are allowed to hang for longer than 24 hours may also cause septicaemia, as bacteria proliferates in solutions with greater than 24 hours of use (Bennet & Brachman et al 1986, Hampton & Sheretz 1988).

Stopcocks Studies have demonstrated that three-way taps when used have been the cause of microorganisms entering the i.v. system (Perdue 1995).

Microorganisms can enter the system from the hands of health care staff during manipulations, from syringes used to flush or draw blood samples, from residual blood that remains in the port following use and from a failure to keep a sterile cap on the tap when not in use (Perdue 1995).

Cannula material and structure Larger cannulae, such as central venous catheters, come into contact with a greater area of skin, produce a larger hole in the skin, are generally more difficult to secure and are more often used for purposes that require more frequent entries into the i.v. system. Although there is no conclusive evidence, some studies have identified that the use of multi-lumen catheters increases the risk of infections up to as much as 12.8% due to the increased number of entry sites into the vascular system (Perdue 1995).

Catheters constructed from more rigid materials can also increase the potential for infection by encouraging thrombogenesis and an inflammatory response that may facilitate colonization.

Microorganisms are able to adhere to some cannula materials more readily than to others. The *Candida* species have been shown to attach to polyvinylchloride catheters much better than to polytetrafluoroethylene catheters. Differential adherence of microorganisms to catheters of various compositions may influence the microbiology of infection (Perdue 1995).

Cannula insertion site Skin organisms can enter into the transcutaneous tract (the space between the cannula and the subcutaneous tissue) when the cannula is inserted (Perdue 1995). Studies have identified that microbial growth occurs when i.v. entry sites are not cleaned properly and when dressings are not changed. These microorganisms migrate along the tract and enter the bloodstream producing bacteraemia and fungiaemia (Maki & Ringer 1991).

Haematogenous seeding Microbes can be transmitted from a remote site or other source of infection, i.e. surgical wound, and seed on the i.v. cannula. Factors that affect cannula seeding include the causative pathogen, degree and duration of bacteraemia, the patient's clinical status and the length of time that the cannula has been in situ (Perdue 1995).

Skill of the practitioner Studies have demonstrated that a good insertion technique will reduce the potential for infection (Henderson 1988, Hampton & Sheretz 1988).

Cannula-related infections can be greatly reduced by the insertion of peripheral cannulae and by a skilled team approach to the administration of care of both peripheral and central catheters. In their studies of patients receiving parenteral nutrition, Hampton & Sheretz (1988) found that infection rates were reduced from 25–30% to 3–5% by such an approach. In comparative trials, Maki & Ringer (1991) concluded that the availability of a team of nurses who are highly experienced in i.v. therapy and who place cannulae, providing close surveillance of infusions, resulted in a twofold lower rate of infusion phlebitis and an even greater reduction in catheter-related sepsis (Perdue 1995).

Clinical presentation

The patient with septicaemia will usually present with chills, fever, malaise and headache, which occur when the pathogenic organisms first invade the circulation. As the fever increases, pulse rate increases and weakness occurs with accompanying symptoms of flushed face, backache, nausea, vomiting and hypotension. If the infection goes undetected or untreated, symptoms become more severe, and cyanosis, tachypnoea and hyperventilation can occur. As the offending organisms overcome the system, vascular collapse, shock and death can occur (Perdue 1995).

Prevention

Prevention strategies support the use of air-eliminating, bacterial retentive filters. Intravenous delivery systems should be considered as potential ports for infection.

Effective hand washing techniques, cannula/catheter management protocols, adherence to accepted standards of practice, administration set changes and proper cannula care will all assist in the prevention of septicaemia in the patient receiving i.v. therapy (Weinstein 1997).

Action

Treat the patient as clinical symptoms dictate.

Pulmonary embolism

Cause

Pulmonary embolism occurs when a mass, usually a blood clot, becomes free floating and is carried by the venous circulation to the right side of the heart and into the pulmonary artery or the artery to the lobes, occluding arterial apertures at major bifurcations. If the pulmonary artery is obstructed, the patient will experience cardiac disturbances. If multiple emboli are passed into the pulmonary circulation, the patient will experience pulmonary hypertension and right-sided heart failure (Perdue 1995).

Clinical features

Clinical manifestations include dyspnoea, pleuritic pain or discomfort, apprehension, cough, unexplained haemoptysis, sweats, tachypnoea, cyanosis and low-grade fever.

Prevention

Preventative measures include:

- use of a filter to remove particulates from solutions and drugs
- administration of blood through a micro-aggregate filter
- avoiding the use of lower extremities for cannulation in adult patients
- prevention of trauma to the vein intima, by ensuring that practitioners are skilled, by using the smallest and shortest cannulae appropriate for the prescribed therapy, by the use of large veins when irritating solutions are being administered, and by the use of correct fixation and securing techniques to prevent cannula movement
- use of good judgement when i.v. systems are being flushed – if, for example, there is any resistance within the device, undue force should not be employed as a blood clot may be released into the vascular system
- examining solution containers for particulates prior to use
- clipping of excessive hair and the proper cleansing of the i.v. site to remove the potential for hair to be severed and carried into the circulation when the skin is breached (Perdue 1995).

Action

Medical and nursing intervention will include administration of oxygen to maintain correct blood gas levels, a lung scan and a prothrombin time prior to initiating anticoagulant therapy.

Air embolism

Cause

Air embolism occurs when air enters a systemic vein and travels to the right ventricle via the vena cava. The bubble of air in the ventricle impedes its pumping ability, thus reducing the blood to the pulmonary vasculature. The pulmonary arterioles then become occluded by tiny air bubbles pumped into them. As a result of the reduced output from the right ventricle, the venous pressure rises considerably. Further, the flow of blood from the left ventricle into the systemic circulation decreases and cyanosis occurs. Reduced blood flow to the brain causes syncope and the arterial blood pressure falls as a result of reduced cardiac output. A loud continuous churning sound is often heard over the precordit. It is known as a Mill House murmur and is produced by the presence of air and blood in the right ventricle. This classic murmur confirms the diagnosis, but it is not always present (Stanton Ostrow 1981).

Although air embolism is a significant possible complication with air-dependent containers, it is much more frequently associated with central venous catheters. Fatal embolism may occur when small bubbles accumulate dangerously and form tenacious bubbles that block the pulmonary capillaries (Weinstein 1997).

If a vented container is allowed to run dry, air enters the tubing and the fluid level drops to the proximity of the patient's chest. The pressure exerted by the blood on the walls of the veins controls the level to which the air drops in the tubing. A negative pressure occurs when the extremity receiving the infusion is elevated above the heart (Weinstein 1997).

With a central venous catheter, the greatest danger of air embolism occurs during insertion. This is because once the large-bore needle is in the vein, it must be disconnected at the hub while the catheter is threaded into the vein (Stanton Ostrow 1981).

Clinical features

When an air embolism occurs, the clinical symptoms demonstrated can be chest pain, shortness of breath and shoulder or back pain, depending upon the location of the embolus. The patient will appear cyanotic, hypotensive with a weak and rapid pulse, and may faint or lose consciousness. If left untreated, shock or cardiac arrest may follow (Weinstein 1997).

Prevention

Placing the patient in the Trendelenburg position during the insertion reduces the risk and is essential as this position increases the intrathoracic pressure, reducing the chance of air being sucked into the vein during the negative phase of inspiration. During inspiration, the intrathoracic pressure is below that of the atmosphere, and therefore negative. It is therefore during the inspiratory phase of respiration that the possibility exists for air to enter the vein.

A further preventative measure is to ensure that the patient is not hypovolaemic, as hypovolaemia can generate an increased 'sucking' force (Stanton Ostrow 1981).

Infusion via central venous catheter poses a greater risk of air embolism when the solution container empties than an infusion via a peripheral vein. This is because the central venous pressure is lower than the peripheral venous pressure, and consequently there is a greater propensity towards negative pressure which could suck air into the circulation (Weinstein 1997).

All connections of an administration set must be tight. Any faulty openings or defects within the set allow air to be emitted into the flowing infusion. If a stopcock is used, the outlets not in use must be completely shut off. The regulating clamp on the administration set should be located no higher than the chest level of the patient. The lower the clamp, the greater is the chance of any defects occurring above it, where positive pressure can force the solution to leak out (Weinstein 1997).

Preventative measures include:

- lying the patient flat and performing the Valsalva manoeuvre whenever central catheters are being inserted or discontinued or the tubing is being changed
- the use of air-eliminating filters
- changing solution containers before they empty completely
- use of luer-lock connections on all parts of the i.v. delivery system
- purging all i.v. administration sets prior to use.

Action

In the event that air does enter the venous system, the patient should be turned onto the left side in a modified Trendelenburg position. This will decrease the flow of air into the vein during inspiration by decreasing intrathoracic pressure. The left lateral position allows the pulmonary artery to become inferior to the body of the right ventricle. The air bubble therefore rises into the right ventricle, relieving the obstruction to the pulmonary vasculature bed. Trendelenburg's position will then help to stop the flow of air into the vein and the left lateral position will improve the pumping ability of the right ventricle.

In addition to correct positioning, the patient will require oxygen by mask rather than cannula to achieve as high an oxygen concentration as possible, monitoring of vital signs and reassurance (Stanton Ostrow 1981).

Cannula embolism

Cause

Cannula embolism may occur when a piece of cannula shears within the vein and enters the systemic circulation. This can occur with the placement of a through-the-needle cannula if the cannula is pulled back and then threaded forward, resulting in the needle piercing or severing the cannula. Cannula embolism may also occur during the insertion of an over-the-needle cannula if the needle is either partially or totally withdrawn and then re-inserted.

Prevention and action

If it is suspected that a cannula embolism has occurred, the patient must be observed for signs of cyanosis, hypotension, increased central venous pressure, tachycardia, fainting and loss of consciousness. The severity of the symptoms and the treatment plan depend on the location of the embolism (Perdue 1995).

Circulatory overload

Cause

Circulatory overload will occur when an infusion is given too rapidly, which increases venous pressure and creates the potential for cardiac dilation and pulmonary oedema. If undetected, congestive cardiac failure, shock and cardiac arrest may result.

Clinical indications will be venous dilation with engorged neck veins, increased blood pressure, rapid respiration and shortness of breath (Weinstein 1997).

Prevention

Although this problem is less common today due to the increasing use of electronically controlled infusion devices, it may still occur for one or more of the following reasons:

- too rapid an i.v. rate, either wrongly prescribed or incorrectly set
- 'positional' i.v. cannulae
- manipulation of the clasp control by the patient
- impaired renal or cardiopulmonary status of the patient (Millam 1988).

Action

When suspected, the infusion should be discontinued or slowed to a minimal rate, and administration of diuretics and chest physiotherapy ordered for the patient.

Speed shock

Cause

Speed shock can occur when large volumes of fluid are given over a short period of time. It can also occur when an i.v. drug is given too quickly. A rapid injection permits the concentration of a drug in the plasma to reach toxic proportions, flooding the organs rich in blood, such as the heart and the brain. As a result syncope, shock and cardiac arrest may follow (Weinstein 1997).

Prevention

When administering drugs, patients should be observed for dizziness, facial flushing and headache, as these symptoms can quickly progress to chest tightness, hypotension, irregular pulse and anaphylactic shock. In such situations the infusion or injection should be immediately discontinued and the patient treated as the clinical symptoms dictate (Perdue 1995).

Prevention measures will include a sound knowledge of the drug and its recommended rate of administration by the practitioner. Electronic flow control devices are endorsed for use with critical medications.

Action

Administer i.v. solutions and medications at the recommended rate.

Allergic reactions

Cause

An allergic reaction is a response to a drug or solution to which the patient is sensitive. Reactions may be immediate or delayed; the most common reactions are those that occur as a result of the administration of antibiotics and blood products (Perdue 1995).

Clinical features

If experienced, the patient may complain of chills, fever, either with or without urticaria, erythema and itching. Depending upon the internal response to the allergen, shortness of breath with or without wheezing and angioneurotic oedema could manifest (Perdue 1995).

Prevention

All patients receiving i.v. therapy should be monitored continuously at the commencement of therapy for the possible onset of an allergic reaction.

To reduce the likelihood of reactions occurring, the patient's previous and known drug allergies or sensitivities should be established, assessed and recorded prior to any drug administration. Proper screening and filtration of blood products can assist in the prevention of blood product reactions (Perdue 1995).

Action

If such symptoms occur, the infusion must be discontinued immediately and antihistamines and/or steroids administered. Any adverse drug reaction must be reported to the pharmacist.

INTRAVENOUS THERAPY TEAMS

The general nurse who expands her role to develop cannulation and i.v. skills within other clinical responsibilities will improve upon current standards of practice. However, it is well recognized that the use of a skilled and dedicated i.v. team will significantly improve the quality of i.v. care provided. This issue is particularly relevant to the common complication of phlebitis. Studies have shown that, on average, a reduction of as much as 80% in a hospital's phlebitis rate can be achieved through the use of an i.v. team. A hospital with an i.v. team can have a phlebitis rate of 5% compared with 25% in hospitals without (Mendez-Lang 1987).

The concept of i.v. therapy teams has become widely accepted in the USA and hospitals there have recognized and embraced the merits of such teams. In the 1970s, individual nurses in the UK began to practise cannulation and direct injection of drugs into the vein. Initially these nurses all held senior status, but as demand increased, the i.v. team concept developed. However, there are still only a few hospitals which provide a full hospital-wide service (Dougherty 1994).

It is well established that an i.v. team enhances the level of care provided by an institution, the quality of patient care being improved because specialist nurses, relieved from other responsibilities, are able to focus their attention on developing high standards of performance.

It has been demonstrated that i.v. teams decrease the incidence of phlebitis, in part by controlling factors related to its development (i.e. cannula size, type, cannula siting and dwell time; Scalley et al 1992). The severity of the phlebitis occurring in hospitals serviced by such teams is also reduced. As it is the more severe levels of phlebitis that cause most of the increases in length of hospital stay (Mendez-Lang 1987), it can be seen that the skill level of an i.v. team contributes directly to a reduction in both the cost of treating phlebitis and the cost of hospital stay. Looking at the actual figures, Mendez-Lang (1987) estimated that, in a 500 bed hospital, an i.v. team saved approximately US$408 034 per year in the costs associated with phlebitis.

There are other cost-generating complications of i.v. therapy on which i.v. teams have had an impact. Miller et al's (1996) study documented a threefold decrease in catheter-related bacteraemia after the institution of an i.v. therapy team. This translated into 29 fewer cases of i.v.-related bacteraemia in the first year of the i.v. therapy team's operations. Bearing in mind that, in 1991, the estimated saving in one hospital on the reduction of bacteraemias was US$124 096 (Miller et al 1996), through the implementation of an i.v. team, it is clearly evident that the costs associated with i.v. complications are considerable, and consequently the savings that can be made are also significant.

Maki et al (1973) advocated the implementation of the team approach in an attempt to control infusion-related septicaemia, and Speechley (1984) found a reduction in phlebitis and infiltration due to early detection and prompt action provided by an i.v. team.

An i.v. team can increase the quality of patient care in other areas. For example, patients experience less pain during cannulation because of the expertise of i.v. therapy teams, who are more adept at placing cannulae. A consequence of this is that fewer supplies are used (Miller et al 1996). Few procedures are so easily affected by stress as the execution of a difficult venepuncture (Dougherty 1996).

The aim of an i.v. team is to administer safe and successful i.v. therapy in the best interests of the patients, the hospital and the nursing profession. This is achieved by:

- developing skills and imparting knowledge
- encouraging further education and knowledge in i.v. therapy
- collaborating in the development and implementation of continuing nurse education
- developing nursing practice in i.v. therapy
- keeping abreast of the latest scientific, medical and nursing advances and their implications (Dougherty 1996).

A decentralized approach to i.v. therapy with the integration of i.v. skills into the general nursing staff may help to improve current standards and assist in reducing levels of complications, but if ward nurses are expected to assume these skills among a multiplicity of other tasks and duties, the procedure cannot be given their full attention and would therefore be relegated to a suboptimal service provision.

Appropriate training, continuous support and the maintenance of i.v. skills are vital. Practitioners who are expert in their skills, who know what to look for, who are aware of and understand the associated risks, and who are able to deal with them properly will significantly reduce i.v.-related problems and, as a consequence, improve patient care.

CONCLUSION

To optimize the potential for a patient receiving i.v. therapy to have a complication-free outcome, the provision of i.v. care must be considered within a multiprofessional framework. All parties need to be working in partnership towards the common goal of a successful conclusion to patient therapy.

The nurse must consider her position from a legal and professional outlook. In relation to the UKCC's *Scope of Professional Practice* (UKCC 1992), nurses should embrace the expansion of their roles in the delivery of i.v. therapy only when they have the accompanying knowledge base and competence to ensure that they can deliver a service of excellence to their patients, of whom an estimated 80–90% will require i.v. therapy during their hospital stay (Massoorli 1995).

There are certain hazards associated with i.v. therapy, and it is important to address indifferent attitudes concerning i.v. care and management practices.

Various investigators suggest that there is a degree of complacency surrounding the importance of asepsis, yet it is conclusively demonstrated that poor attention to asepsis in i.v. therapy is the cause of much morbidity and even mortality, particularly in the vulnerable patient groups (Maki 1976, Elliot 1991, Keenlyside 1992, Lamb 1995).

It is evident that the longer i.v. therapy continues, the greater is the risk of complications. A working knowledge and appreciation of correct standards of practice, knowing what to look for, being aware of the risks and dangers involved in therapy and being able to manage them effectively will help to reduce i.v.-related complications.

REFERENCES

Arnold R E, Elliott E K, Holmes B H 1977 The importance of frequent examination of infusion sites in preventing post-infusion phlebitis. Surgery, Gynaecology and Obstetrics 145: 19

Baxter Healthcare Ltd 1988 Principles and practice of intravenous therapy. Baxter Healthcare, Compton

Bennet J V, Brachman P S et al 1986 Hospital infections, 2nd edn. Little, Brown, Boston, p 561–574

Bohoney J 1993 Nine common IV complications and what to do about them. American Journal of Nursing October: 45–49

Curry J T, Zallen R D 1973 Reduction of thrombophlebitis associated with indwelling catheters. Journal of Oral and Maxillofacial Surgery 31: 636

Department of Health and Social Security 1972 Guidelines on the administration of parenteral infusion fluids. HMSO, London

Dougherty L 1992 Intravenous therapy. Surgical Nurse 5(2): 10–13

Dougherty L 1996 The benefits of an IV team in hospital practice. Professional Nurse 11(11): 761–763

Elliot T S J 1988 Plastic devices: new fields for old microbes. Lancet 1: 30–31

Elliot T S (ed) 1991 Successful IV therapy. Viggo-Spectramed, Sweden

Flemmer L, Chan J S L 1993 A paediatric protocol for management of extravasation injuries. Paediatric Nursing 19(4): 355–358

Francombe P 1988 Intravenous filters and phlebitis. Nursing Times 84(26): 34–35

Frazer I H, Eke N, Laing M S 1977 Is infusion phlebitis preventable? British Medical Journal 2: 232

Gaukroger P B, Rogers J G, Manners T A 1988 Infusion thrombophlebitis: a prospective comparison of 645 Vialon and Teflon cannulae in anaesthetic and post-operative use. Anaesthetic & Intensive Care 16(3): 265–271

Goodinson S M 1990a Good practice ensures minimum risk factors. Complications of peripheral venous cannulation and infusion therapy. Professional Nurse 6(3): 175–177

Goodinson S M 1990b The risks of IV therapy. Professional Nurse 5(5): 235–238

Goodinson S M et al 1988 A survey of I.V. catheters and other inserts. Paper presented at the Second International Conference on Infection Control

Graham D R, Keldermans M M, Klemm L W, Semenza N J, Shafer M L 1991 Infectious complications among patients receiving home intravenous therapy with peripheral, central or peripherally placed central venous catheters. American Journal of Medicine 91(suppl. B): 95S–101S

Hampton A A, Sheretz R J 1988 Vascular access infections in hospitalised patients. Surgical Clinics of North America 68(1): 57–66

Henderson D K 1988 Intravascular device-associated infection: current concepts and controversies. Infect Surg 365–371, 398–399

Henderson D K 1990 Bacteraemia due to percutaneous intravascular devices. In: Mandell G L et al (eds) Principle and practice of infectious disease, 3rd edn. Churchill Livingstone, London

Horibe K et al 1990 Evaluation of the endotoxin retention capabilities of in-line filters. Journal of Parenteral Enteral Nutrition 14: 56–59

Hästbacka J, Tammisto T, Elfving G, Tiitinen P 1965 Infusion thrombophlebitis: a clinical study based on 1048 cases. Acta Anaesthesiologica Scandinavica 10: 9

Jacques S 1992 Managing IV therapy in immunocompromised patients: a nursing viewpoint. In: Lee H A, Barnett M I (eds) Proceedings of the Symposium on Managing the Complications of Intravenous Therapy. Pall Biomedical Ltd, Portsmouth, p 47–51

Johnson S 1994 A time and money saver? Cost comparison of IV therapy with and without Pall 96 filters. Professional Nurse November: 94–96

Keenlyside D 1992 Every little detail counts: infection control in IV therapy. Professional Nurse January: 226–232

Kerrison T, Woodhill J 1994 Reducing the risk of thrombophlebitis. Professional Nurse July: 662–666

Khawaja H T, O'Brien B J, Buxton M J, Weaver P C 1989 Cost minimization study of transdermal glyceral trinitrate in reducing failures of peripheral intravenous infusions. British Medical Journal July: 97

Krakowska G 1986 Practice versus procedure. Nursing Times (Journal of Infection Control Nursing) 34(63): 64–69

Lamb J 1995 Peripheral IV therapy. Nursing Standard 9(30): 32–35

LaRocca J C, Otto S E 1993 Pocket guide: IV therapy, 2nd edn. Mosby, St Louis

Lewis G B H, Hecker J F 1985 Infusion thrombophlebitis. British Journal of Anaesthetics 57: 220–233

McKee J M, Shell J A, Warren T A, Campbell V P 1989 Complications of intravenous therapy: a randomised prospective study – Vialon vs Teflon. Journal of Intravenous Nursing 12(5): 288–295

Maki D G 1976 Preventing infection in intravenous therapy. Hospital Practice April: 95–104

Maki D G 1989 Risk factors for nosocomial infection in intensive care. Archives of Internal Medicine 149: 30–35

Maki D G, Botecelli M S, LeRoy M, Thielke T 1987 Prospective study of replacing administration sets for intravenous therapy at 48 v 72 hour intervals. Journal of the American Medical Association 258(13): 1777–1781

Maki D G, Goldmnan D, Rhame F 1973 Infection control in intravenous therapy. Annals of Internal Medicine 73: 867–887

Maki D G, Ringer M 1987 Evaluation of dressing regimens for prevention of infection with peripheral intravenous catheters, gauze, a transparent polyurethane dressing and an idaphor transparent dressing. Journal of the American Medical Association 258: 2396–2403

Maki D G, Ringer M 1991 Risk factor for infusion-related phlebitis with small peripheral venous catheters. Annals of College of Physicians 114(10): 845–854

Maki D G, Ringer M, Alvarado C J 1991 Prospective randomized trial of povidone-iodine, alcohol, and chlorhexidine for prevention of infection associated with central venous and arterial catheters. Lancet 338: 339–343

Maki D G, Will L 1984 Colonisation and infection associated with transparent dressings for central venous, arterial and Hickman catheters: a comparative trial. In: Twenty-fourth Interscience Conference on antimicrobial agents and chemotherapy. American Society for Microbiology

Masoorli S 1995 When IV practice spells malpractice. RN August: 53–55

Mendez-Lang M 1987 Cost savings approach for justification of an IV team. National Intravenous Therapy Association September/October: 348–356

Mermel L A, McCormick R D, Springman S R, Maki D G 1991 Epidemiology and pathogenesis or infection with Swann Ganz catheters: a prospective study using molecular epidemiology. American Journal of Medicine 91(3b): 97

Millam D 1988 Managing complications of IV therapy. Nursing 18(3): 34–42

Miller J, Goetz A, Squier C, Muder R 1996 Reduction in nosocomial IV device related bacteraemias after institution of an iv therapy team. Journal of Intravenous Nursing 19(2): 103–106

Payne James J J, Rogers J, Bray M J, Rana S K, McSwiggan D, Silk D B A 1991 Development of thrombophlebitis in peripheral veins with Vialon and PTFE-Teflon cannulas: a double blind randomized, controlled trial. Annals of the Royal College of Surgeons at England 73: 322–325

Perdue M 1995 Intravenous complications. In: Terry J, Baranowski L, Lonsway R A, Hedrick (eds) Intravenous therapy: clinical principles and practice. WB Saunders, Philadelphia

Perucca R, Micek J 1993 Treatment of infusion related phlebitis. Journal of Intravenous Nursing 16(5): 282–286

Ricard P, Martin P, Marcoux J A 1985 Protection of indwelling vascular catheters: incidence of bacterial contamination and catheter-related sepsis. Critical Care Medicine 13: 541–543

Richards C, Thomas P 1990 Use of endotoxin retentive IV filters with paediatric total parenteral nutrition solutions. Journal of Clinical Pharmacy and Therapeutics 15: 53–58

Root T R, Stanley A P 1993 Extravasation. In: The cytotoxics handbook, 2nd edn. Radcliffe Medical Press, Oxford, ch 9, p 77–91

Ross S A 1972 Infusion phlebitis. Nursing Research 21: 313

Scalley R, Van C, Cochran R 1992 The impact of an IV team on the related occurrence of intravenous related phlebitis. Journal of Intravenous Nursing 5(2): 100–109

Sheldon D L, Johnson W C 1979 Cutaneous mucomycosis: two documented cases of suspected nosocomial infection. Journal of the American Medical Association 241: 1032–1033

Simmonds B P 1983 Guidelines for prevention of intravascular infection. American Journal of Infection Control 11(5): 183–199

Stanton Ostrow L 1981 Air embolism and central venous lines. American Journal of Nursing November: 2036–2038

Swanson J T, Aldrete J A 1969 Thrombophlebitis after intravenous infusion – factors affecting its incidence. Rocky Mountain Medical Journal 66: 48

Turco S, Davies N M 1972 Glass particles in intravenous injections. New England Journal of Medicine 287: 1264–1265

United Kingdom Central Council for Nursing, Midwifery and Health Visiting 1992 Scope of professional practice. UKCC, London

Weinstein S M (ed) 1993 Plumer's principles and practice of intravenous therapy, 5th edn. JB Lippincott, Philadelphia
Weinstein S M (ed) 1997 Plumer's principles and practice of intravenous therapy, 6th edn. JB Lippincott, Philadelphia
Wilson J 1994 Preventing infection during IV therapy. Professional Nurse March: 388–392
Wright A, Hecker J F, Lewis G B H 1985 Use of transdermal glyceryl trinitrate to reduce failure of intravenous infusions due to phlebitis and extravasation. Lancet 299: 1148–1150
Yucha C, Hastings-Tolsma M, Szeverenyi N 1993 Differences among IV extravasation using four common solutions. Journal of Intravenous Nursing 16(5): 277–281

FURTHER READING

Allwood M, Wright P 1993 The cytotoxic handbook, 2nd edn. Radcliffe Medical Press, Oxford
Davis N M 1995 Potassium perils. American Journal of Nursing March: 14
Department of Health and Social Security 1976 Addition of drugs to intravenous fluids. DHSS, London
Elliott T S (ed) 1990 A guide to peripheral IV cannulation for medical and nursing staff. Viggo-Spectramed, Sweden
Feldstein A 1986 Detect phlebitis and infiltration before they harm your patient. Nursing 16(1): 44–47
Haley R W 1996 Managing hospital infection control for effectiveness. American Hospital Publishing, Chicago
Haynes S 1989 Infusion phlebitis and extravasation. Professional Nurse 5(3): 160–161
Hecker J F 1989 Failure of intravenous infusions from extravasation and phlebitis. Anaesthesia and Intensive Care 17(4): 433–439
Hill G 1995 The KCl killer. Journal of the Medical Defense Union Spring: 10–11
Hunter E S, Bell E, Staub M A, Coyle G 1995 Relationship of local IV complications and the method of intermittent IV access. Journal of Intravenous Nursing July / Aug 18(4): 202–206
IVAC UK Ltd 1990 History of IV therapy. IVAC, UK
Jones A M, Stanley A 1997 Probe high extravasation rates. Pharmacy in Practice June: 292–296
Livesey J, Richardson S 1993 Securing methods for peripheral cannulae. Nursing Standard 7(31): 31–34
Maki D G 1987 Prospective study of replacing administration sets for intravenous therapy at 48- vs 72-hour intervals. Journal of the American Medical Association 258(13): 1777–1781
Mallet J, Bailey C (eds) 1996 The Royal Marsden NHS Trust manual of clinical nursing procedures, 4th edn. Blackwell Science, Oxford
Millam D 1987 IV therapy 30 years ago. National Intravenous Therapy Association 10: 118–121
Terry J, Baranowski L, Lonsway RA, Hedrick C (eds) 1995 Intravenous therapy. Clinical principles and practice. WB Saunders, Philadelphia
Wilkinson R 1996 Nurses' concerns about IV therapy and devices. Nursing Standard 10(35): 35–37
Wright A 1996 Reducing infusion failure: a pharmacologic approach: a review. Journal of Intravenous Nursing 19(2): 89–97

Intravenous flow control and infusion devices

Shelley Dolan

CHAPTER 8

INTRODUCTION

'Man is only man at the surface. Remove his skin, dissect, and immediately you come to machinery.' (Auden 1938)

During the 1990s in the UK and some parts of Europe, there has been a move towards primary health care, and in particular the provision of intravenous (i.v.) therapy, in the community. This trend has provided some of the impetus for the recent advances in infusion device technology. Reliability and safety issues have become paramount now that patients are receiving their therapy in a non-monitored environment.

Flow control can be defined as the delivery of i.v. fluids and medications at an appropriate rate and in a constant, accurate manner in order to achieve a therapeutic response and prevent complications such as over- or under-infusion (Dougherty 1996a) (Box 8.1).

This chapter outlines when to use an infusion device, how to select the device in order to meet the needs of the patient, and the nurse's responsibilities with regard to the purchasing and maintenance of i.v. equipment.

GRAVITY FLOW

In spite of the age of technology, it is important to recognize that there are still many clinical situations where patients in the hospital or home care setting will require

---

■ BOX 8.1

Complications of inadequate flow control

Over-infusion

- Fluid overload with accompanying electrolyte imbalance
- Metabolic disturbances during parenteral nutrition
- Toxic concentration of medication which may result in 'speed shock'
- An increase in venous complications caused by reduced dilution of irritant substances
- Air embolism if containers run dry earlier than anticipated

Under-infusion

- Dehydration
- Metabolic disturbances
- A delayed response to medications or below therapeutic dose
- Occlusion of i.v. device due to slow cessation of flow

■ BOX 8.2

Advantages and disadvantages of gravity flow

Advantages
- Low cost
- Familiar to all staff
- Easy to set up
- Infusion of air is less likely
- Minimizes risk of extravascular infusion

Disadvantages
- Cannot be used for arterial infusions
- Variability of drop size
- Infusion rates limited
- Risk of free flow
- Requires frequent observation and adjustment

minimal i.v. input and where their therapy can be delivered with a simple administration set utilizing gravity flow. Indeed, in some areas the cost of electronic devices will be prohibitive or demand will overwhelm the hospital's supply, and it is therefore important that safe therapy can still be provided without these devices (Box 8.2).

Indications for use
Indications for use of a gravity flow administration set are as follows:

- delivery of fluids without additives
- administration of drugs or fluids where adverse effects are not anticipated if the infusion rate varies slightly
- where the patient's condition does not give any cause for concern and no complication is predicted (Dougherty 1996a).

When an infusion depends on gravity for its flow there will be a limitation to its rate and accuracy of delivery, and therefore for intensive or multimodality therapy, a flow control device should be used (Hunt & Rapp 1996). It also requires a nurse to calculate the rate of administration, using the following formula:

$$\frac{Quantity\ to\ be\ infused\ (ml) \times no.\ of\ drops/ml}{No.\ of\ hours\ over\ which\ infusion\ to\ be\ delivered \times 60\ min}$$

$$= no.\ of\ drops/min \hspace{3cm} \text{(Gatford 1990)}$$

It should be noted that the number of drops per millilitre (drops/ml) is dependent on the administration set and the viscosity of the fluid. An increased viscosity will cause a larger drop size. Crystalloid fluid being administered by gravity flow is delivered at the rate of 20 drops/ml, whereas red blood cells given via a blood set are delivered at 15 drops/ml (Dougherty 1996a). If greater safety is required, a burette administration set can be utilized, particularly if large bolus volumes could be harmful, e.g. in children or in those patients with cardiac failure. The burette set has a discreet 150–200 ml chamber which can be filled from the infusion bag each hour. This allows the nurse to ensure that the patient receives no more than the pre-

---

■ **BOX 8.3**

Factors which affect rate of gravity flow infusions

- Condition and size of vein
- Gauge size and length of device
- Type and location of device
- Partial or total occlusion of device
- Administration set
- In-line devices
- Type and viscosity of fluid
- Temperature of fluid
- Height of container
- Roller clamp control
- The patient

---

scribed hourly rate. This does, however, require a greater degree of nurse–carer intervention, but can help to avoid the danger of free flow.

There are many factors which will affect the rate of flow of gravity flow infusions (Box 8.3).

Venous access device and administration set

When an infusion is running via a peripheral venous access device, the flow may be influenced by the following factors:

- The gauge size and length of the device.
- The location of the device, e.g. over a joint.
- The position of the device within the vein, e.g. if the bevel of the device is against the inner wall of the vein, flow will be slow (Weinstein 1997).
- The condition and size of the vein, e.g. small or thrombosed veins.
- Kinking or pinching of the device or administration set.
- Occlusion of the device caused by clot formation or fibrin sheath. This can occur as a result of restricted venous circulation, e.g. blood pressure cuff on the infusion arm, restraints on or above device, the patient lying on the arm receiving the infusion, blood backtracking down the device due to an empty infusion bag, or container lowered preventing gravity flow.
- Other in-line devices, e.g. filters.

Fluid and container

The type and viscosity of the infusion fluid, as well as the temperature at which it is delivered, may influence flow rates (Sagar & Bomar 1980), as cold or irritating solutions may cause venous spasm, impeding the rate of flow (Weinstein 1997). A warm pack placed on the vein proximal to the device will offset this reaction.

For gravity flow to be effective, the infusion will need to be suspended at an adequate height above the patient. The amount of fluid within the container exerts a pressure and any change in gravity by raising or lowering the container will affect the flow rate (Weinstein 1997). Generally, the greater the infusion rate required, the higher the infusion will need to be placed; thus, increasing the distance between the bag/bottle and the patient will increase the rate (MDA 1995a). The optimum height of the container above the patient is 0.9 m and changes in the patient's position may require further adjustment, e.g. ambulant patients or during transportation.

Roller clamp control

The roller clamp used to control flow may become loose and slip or even distort the administration set tubing, and this results in a phenomenon known as 'cold flow' (Dougherty 1996a). Any marked stretching or tension on the tubing can also render the clamp ineffective (Sagar & Bomar 1980).

The patient

Patients may occasionally tamper with the roller clamp control or inadvertently adjust the height of the infusion container without realizing the effect it will have on flow rate. Flexing of the arms may also influence flow if the device is sited near a joint.

FLOW CONTROL DEVICES

Certain groups are more at risk of complications associated with flow control (Box 8.4) and it is in these circumstances that a flow control device must be utilized. There are also a number of other factors to consider when selecting the appropriate infusion system for a particular situation, e.g. risks to the patient, delivery parameters and environmental features (Box 8.5).

MDA classification

In order to aid the selection, the Medical Devices Agency (MDA) of the Department of Health, in collaboration with users, manufacturers and technical and clinical specialists, has developed a classification of pumps according to the perceived risk and suitability of a device for a specific clinical purpose, as follows:

- *neonatal* – the highest risk category
- *high-risk infusions* – these are typically the infusion of fluids in children where fluid balance is critical or the infusion of drugs, e.g. cardiac inotropes or cytotoxic drugs, where consistency of flow and accuracy are important
- *lower risk infusions* – these would include the delivery of simple electrolytes, parenteral nutrition (PN) and infusional antibiotics (MDA 1995a).

There are now a vast range of infusion devices and these have been grouped into four main types (see Box 8.6):

- those using a syringe
- gravity controllers
- infusion pumps
- ambulatory pumps.

■ **BOX 8.4**

Groups at risk of complications associated with flow control (adapted from Dougherty 1996a)

- Age – infants, young children and the elderly
- Patients with compromised cardiovascular status, impairment/failure of organs or major sepsis
- Postoperative or post-trauma patients
- Patients suffering from shock
- Stressed patients
- Patients receiving multiple medications, whose clinical status may be changing rapidly

■ **BOX 8.5**

Factors to consider when selecting an appropriate infusion system

Risk to patient of:
- Over- or under-infusion
- Uneven flow
- Inadvertent bolus
- High delivery pressure
- Extravascular infusion

Delivery parameters
- Infusion rates and volume required
- Degree of short- and long-term accuracy required
- Alarms required
- Ability to infuse into chosen site (venous, arterial, subcutaneous)
- Suitability of infusing the type of drug (half-life, viscosity)

Environmental features
- Ease of operation
- Frequency of observation and adjustment
- Type of patient (child, very sick)
- Mobility of patient

■ **BOX 8.6**

Types of equipment available

Using a syringe
- Syringe infusion pumps
- Syringe drivers
- Anaesthetic pumps
- Patient-controlled analgesia (PCA) pumps

Gravity controllers
- Drip rate controllers
- Volumetric controllers

Infusion pumps
- Drip rate pumps
- Volumetric pumps
- Patient-controlled analgesia (PCA) pumps

Ambulatory pumps
- Continuous infusion
- Multimodality pumps
- Patient-controlled analgesia pumps

All infusion devices have advantages and disadvantages (Table 8.1) as well as a range of features (Table 8.2).

PUMPS USING A SYRINGE

Syringe infusion pumps

These are devices in which a syringe containing fluid or a drug in solution is fitted into the pump and the plunger of the syringe is driven forwards at a predetermined rate. These pumps are usually set to run at millilitres per hour (ml/h) (MDA 1995a).

Application

Syringe infusion pumps are designed for the accurate delivery of fluids at low flow rates (MDA 1996). Syringe pumps are therefore ideally selected for the safe infusion of fluids and drugs to neonates or children and drugs to adults. Most pumps will accept different brands and sizes of syringes; some will automatically read the brand and size whilst others must be manually programmed (MDA 1995a).

Features

When using syringe infusion pumps in the neonatal and high-risk settings, it is essential that the devices have the following:

- Internal rechargeable battery that will provide power (if the mains power fails) without interruption and without losing memory of set parameters or patient data.
- The syringe barrel and plunger must be located securely in order to ensure accurate function. If the syringe is incorrectly inserted, there should be activation of an alarm and automatic disablement of the pump so that the infusion cannot continue.

Although not essential, it is recommended that the pump has the ability to record and recall its service or technical history (MDA 1996). Comprehensive alarm and tamper prevention features are also important considerations.

Neonatal In addition to the above, the syringe pumps which fulfil this category must have the following features (MDA 1996):

- high accuracy – both in the short and long term
- consistency of flow delivery with very low flow rates
- flow rate increments in ml/h
- very short occlusion and low pressure alarm times
- very low bolus volume on release of occlusion.

High-risk infusion pumps These pumps will typically be used with children or adults but *not* neonates, and will be used to deliver fluid where fluid balance is critical, e.g. in the critically ill child, or to deliver drugs where an accurate titration is essential, e.g. cardiac inotropes such as adrenaline or dobutamine (Oh 1995).
The pumps which fulfil this category have the following features:

- high accuracy – both in the long and short term
- consistency of flow delivery
- short occlusion and low pressure alarm times
- low bolus volume on release of occlusion (MDA 1996).

Table 8.1 Advantages and disadvantages of intravenous equipment

Type of device	Advantages	Disadvantages
Syringe driver	• Small and lightweight enough to fit into a pocket or waist belt • Size limitations mean minimum of functions • Capital and resource expenditures are low • Universal syringes and extension sets can be used • Easy to use	• Battery-driven but electrical capacity is low and continuous pumping is not possible – most give a small bolus every few minutes • Very few alarms are provided. Warning indicators are generally limited to an alarm to indicate occlusion or the end of the infusion; they may also have a flashing light to indicate that the pump is running (MDA 1995a) • Small battery size means ensuring a spare battery is available at all times • Volumetric accuracy is variable; depends on the disposables, e.g. size of syringe; type of tubing used • At very low infusion rates, there is a danger that the drug solution can migrate into the plastic of the tubing thus reducing the amount delivered to the patient (MDA 1995a)
Syringe pump	• Usually calibrated in ml/h • Precise delivery at low flow rates • Easy to use	• Free flow possible with older models (without plunger clamps) • Problems with mechanical backlash • Occlusion pressures on older models tend to be rather high
Gravity controller Drip rate controller	• Fairly inexpensive • Used with standard gravity administration sets • Simple to use • Quick alarms, no bolus • Very low infusion pressure • Counts drops accurately • Infusion of air unlikely	• Cannot be used for arterial infusions • Infusion rates limited • Not accurate volumetrically
Volumetric controller	• Calibrated in ml/h • Easy to use • Quick alarms, no bolus • Very low infusion pressure • Infusion of air unlikely • Minimizes risk of extravascular infusion	• More expensive than drip rate controllers • Usually require a dedicated set • Cannot be used for arterial infusions • Infusion rate limits variable volumetric accuracy

(cont'd)

Table 8.1 (cont'd)

Type of device	Advantages	Disadvantages
Infusion pumps Drip rate pumps	• None	• Very high occlusion alarm pressures • Very high alarm delays and high bolus on release of occlusion • High delivery pressure • Very few alarms • Not accurate volumetrically
Volumetric pumps	• Calibrated in ml/h • Wide flow rate range • Comprehensive alarm systems • Air-in-line detection • Good volumetric accuracy • Low occlusion alarm pressure settings • Secondary infusion facility • Can be used on venous and arterial infusions • KVO facility	• More expensive that other pumps • Requires dedicated sets • Can be more complicated to use • Problems if incorrect set loaded
Ambulatory infusion pumps	• Small, lightweight • Usually calibrated in ml/h • Varying sizes of reservoirs – up to 250 ml • Comprehensive alarm systems	• Older models have few alarms • Requires dedicated sets • Disposables can be more expensive

Lower risk infusion pumps The pumps which fulfil this category have the following features (MDA 1996):

• lower accuracy over the long and short term
• less consistent flow
• rudimentary alarm and safety features
• higher occlusion alarm pressure
• poorer overall occlusion alarm response.

Safety issues

• Use the smallest syringe that the device will accept and that which is able to hold the required volume of drug. A smaller syringe ensures improved consistency of flow and occlusion response times are decreased (MDA 1995a).
• If using several pumps simultaneously with one patient in a high-dependency or critical care setting, ensure that the pumps can be mounted horizontally as this makes checking of the rate easier and thus minimizes the potential for errors. It also enables more pumps to be attached to one intravenous stand.

Cost implications

Syringe pumps represent a high capital outlay per pump. Some syringe pumps only utilize a dedicated administration set, but the majority are designed to use standard non-dedicated syringes and extension sets. It is important to recognize that the

Table 8.2 Equipment features

Type of feature	Description of function
Air-in-line detector	Detects air bubbles in the tubing. The sensitivity is usually adjustable via the device configuration
Occlusion response alarm	This is the time taken for the device to alarm with the onset of occlusion and is inversely proportional to the occlusion alarm pressure setting at any given flow rate. It is an advantage to have as low an occlusion alarm pressure setting as possible
Occlusion sensors	These detect a complete tubing restriction upstream or downstream of the device. The downstream occlusion alarm response can usually be set for different occlusion pressures. The sensitivity level can be adjusted to suit the needs of the hospital. However, it is important to distinguish between total occlusions resulting from kinked sets or blocked catheters and partial occlusions caused by phlebitis or extravasation. Most infusion devices are not designed or intended to detect extravasation and are unlikely to alarm under clinical care
Occlusion alarm pressure	The pressure in the infusion set at which the pump alarms when occluded
Occlusion alarm time	The time taken from the moment of the occlusion occurring to the alarm sounding, e.g. time to alarm following infusion at 1 ml/h = 30 min
Bolus release facility	When an occlusion occurs, pumps continue pumping until the pressure reaches a level required to trigger the alarm. During this time, a bolus of infusate is building up and stored mainly by expansion of the infusion set. If time before the alarm is more than a few minutes, this bolus can be shot into the vein if the occlusion is released (unless deliberately removed), e.g. bolus following release of occlusion at all flow rates – neonatal, 0.3 ml; high-risk, 0.6 ml
VTBI/KVO settings	VTBI = volume to be infused KVO = keep vein open; this setting varies depending on the device, e.g. 5 ml/h or programmed rate, whichever is less
Safety clamp	This prevents accidental fluid flow by automatically occluding the tubing whenever the pump door is opened
Delivery accuracy	Long-term accuracy should not deviate by more than 5%. Short-term accuracy determines the delivery accuracy of device over minute-by-minute intervals

other resource implication will be the maintenance and service costs once the pump is out of warranty.

Anaesthesia pumps

These are syringe pumps which use 20, 30 or 50 ml syringes. They are different from all other syringe pumps in that they are designed to allow changes in flow rate and bolus to be made while the pump is infusing.

All other pumps require the user to stop the pump first.

Application

These pumps are only to be used in operating departments, high-dependency and critical care areas. They are designed to provide induction of anaesthesia or sedation and therefore have to be able to provide much greater flow rates and larger boluses than other devices, e.g. several hundred ml/h.

Special features

These pumps often have a number of special features:

- built-in drug information system
- software enabling for a 'smart-card' system which can automatically calibrate the pump for the drug being delivered
- programming for the individual patient's body weight and the drug concentration being used
- computer interface for control and for connection to the patient monitoring system; some pumps have the ability to change drug rates depending on changes in the patient's haemodynamic status (Schumaker et al 1995).

Safety issues

Due to the ability of the pump to give large boluses and to run at high rates, it is essential that they are only used in high-dependency areas. Senior management must ensure that these pumps *never* follow the patient out of these areas to a general ward (MDA 1995a).

Cost implications

These pumps are relatively expensive in terms of the initial outlay, although most will utilize non-dedicated syringes and infusion sets. The additional cost will be maintenance and servicing.

Patient-controlled analgesia pumps

Background

The literature demonstrates that in the late 20th century, patients who have undergone surgery report that they experience severe unrelieved pain (Kuhn et al 1990). Kuhn et al's work showed that 40% of postoperative patients ($n = 33$) reported that the 'postoperative period had been very painful'. The authors postulated several reasons for the inadequacy of analgesia, the most likely being that clinicians are still concerned about the possibility of opiate dependency and therefore choose minimal dosages. This research and several other studies led to a report being produced by the Royal College of Anaesthetists and the Royal College of Surgeons (RCS & RCA 1990). This report recommended that patients should have access to pain teams and that one of the pain control methods which should be available for patients was patient-controlled analgesia (PCA).

Although often regarded as a recent advance, the concept of patient-managed or-controlled analgesia has its roots in the 1960s both in the USA and in the UK. In the USA in the late 1960s, Dr Sechzer devised an experimental approach to measuring pain experienced by postoperative patients. He taught patients to press a button when they felt pain and a nurse observer would then administer a bolus of i.v. analgesia. Meanwhile in the UK, in the late 1960s, Scott was experimenting with a hand-held spring-loaded clamp which controlled an i.v. bottle containing a solution of glucose 5% with 300 mg pethidine. His patients were taught to grip the clamp each time they experienced pain – the clamp would then close automatically and prevent further analgesia doses if the patient fell asleep (Levy & Williams 1992).

These two early devices were superseded in the 1970s by technological advances that harnessed a syringe to a clockwork driver such as the 'Cardiff Palliator' which was a syringe driver originally used on women in labour (Levy & Williams 1992).

PCA allows the patient to self-medicate small doses of opiates which should be sufficient to maintain fairly constant plasma concentrations (Tammisto & Tigerstedt 1982). After the delivery of a small bolus, a lock-out is activated which ensures that the patient cannot receive an inappropriate dose.

One of the advantages of the PCA system is that the patient can deliver the dose when they choose. For this reason it is sometimes known as 'demand analgesia'. It is recognized that there are many factors that influence the intensity of the pain experience and it therefore seems wise to individualize the approach to a patient's pain relief (Watt-Watson & Donovan 1992).

It is important to recognise that PCA is not a universal panacea for all postoperative pain and is not successful in some patients. Indeed, recent research has indicated that there may be no significant advantages of PCA over intramuscular opiate injections (Snell et al 1997).

An important factor in the success of PCA is patient education and compliance, both of which will be influenced positively by a well-designed device (MDA 1995a).

There are now several varieties of PCA pump, which deliver the analgesia via a syringe, a reservoir bag or from a disposable elastane balloon (the reservoir and disposable devices will be discussed later in this chapter).

Application

PCA is most commonly used in the postoperative setting, but it has proved useful in other areas of acute and chronic pain, such as the acute pain resulting from severe mucositis caused by anti-cancer chemotherapy (Bakitas-Whedon 1991) or the chronic pain caused by the bony metastases of cancer or 'benign' back pain.

More recently, PCA has also been employed in the paediatric setting. Although most centres showed that it was used mainly with the older child and adolescent (Rodgers et al 1988), some have used it with children as young as 6 years old (Berde 1989).

Features

These devices are similar to the syringe infusion pumps described previously, but they have the following special features (MDA 1995a):

- a hand-held button or switch which allows the patient to deliver a pre-set bolus
- a preset lock-out time between boluses
- the ability (some models) to deliver a continuous background or basal infusion, providing a continuous low rate of analgesia
- a loading dose to be delivered on setting up the pump
- a memory log which can be accessed by the clinician to ascertain the number and frequency of boluses used, and the total volume of opiate used in a given time.

Safety issues

The general safety issues as described previously for syringe infusion pumps apply, but the following apply particularly to the PCA pump.

The whole idea of PCA is that the patient takes an active role in their therapy. In order to do this, the patient must firstly receive an explanation of PCA and then, if they consent to this type of therapy, they should be trained in its use. It is therefore essential that the pump is 'user-friendly'. The following safety design features are therefore recommended:

- simple to follow steps for accessing a bolus
- an easily depressed or gripped device (some patients may have peripheral sensory problems).

All PCA pumps must have the facility to lock out the programming device from the patient. If there is any concern that the patient's respiratory function or conscious level could be altered then it may be safer to select a bolus-only setting. This means that there will be *no* background infusion of opiate and the patient can only receive a bolus dose when they push the button.

It is imperative that the nursing and junior medical staff have received training and understand the particular settings of the PCA pump.

Cost implications

Depending on the number of functions available, these pumps can be expensive. Some pumps use a dedicated administration set, while others accept a standard syringe and administration set.

Syringe drivers

Syringe drivers are sometimes known as miniature syringe pumps.

Applications

Syringe drivers are used in the following situations:

- when the patient is mobile in hospital or receiving treatment at home and in the community for delivering cytotoxic chemotherapy where a small volume is delivered over several days or weeks
- when the ambulant patient requires continuous pain relief via the subcutaneous, i.v. or epidural route.

Safety issues

Syringe drivers are designed to be set over hours or a day (24 h). When using the hourly driver, the rate is set in 'mm/h'; the 24-h driver, however, should be set to 'mm/24 h'. Manufacturers have endeavoured to clearly label the devices but care should still be taken when setting up the driver (MDA 1995b).

Syringe drivers are not suitable for neonatal infusions because of their limited alarm function. They should not be used for other high-risk infusions such as catecholamine infusions.

Cost implications

These devices represent a relatively small capital and resource expenditure, and most utilize standard syringes and administration sets. Other costs include maintenance, servicing and replacement batteries.

GRAVITY CONTROLLERS

These are electronic devices which achieve the prescribed rate of an infusion by constricting an administration set. These controllers rely solely on the height of the fluid bag above the patient as the device has no pumping action.

The rate of the infusion is monitored by a sensor which is attached to the drip chamber of the administration set. The sensor ensures that there is no over-infusion of fluid, but if there is any resistance to flow, i.e. occlusion in access device or administration set, there may be under-infusion of fluid. If the device has not delivered the prescribed volume of fluid the controller will alarm. Some models of controller have a 'flow status' system which then allows the clinician to view whether there is any resistance to flow (MDA 1995a).

Gravity controllers can be further subdivided into two types: the drip rate controller and the volumetric controller.

Drip rate controller

These controllers have no pumping action, as described above, and are powered by mains or battery. They tend to have few controls and are therefore very easy to operate.

Application

These controllers are suitable for most of the lower risk infusions such as simple fluid infusions, e.g. sodium chloride 0.9% or dextrose 5%. Drip rate controllers are not recommended for the infusion of PN because of the likelihood that the small drop size will result in inaccuracies of flow rate.

Safety issues

The accuracy of a drip rate controller is dependent upon the sensor counting drops. However, several factors can influence the volume of fluid in each drop (MDA 1995a):

- the shape, condition and size of the hole in the administration set from which the drop falls
- the drip rate that has been set
- the type of fluid, its osmolality, temperature and surface tension.

Therefore, if volumetric accuracy is important, another device should be selected.

Cost implications

Although these devices are only suitable for lower risk infusions, they are considerably cheaper than the more sophisticated devices. Therefore, it is always advisable to plan carefully the functions that are required from a device. Most drip rate controllers utilize standard administration sets.

Volumetric controller

These devices are set in 'mm/h'. They have a drop sensor and may need a dedicated administration set or a disposable 'add-on' rate clip. Volumetric controllers usually have more settings and alarms than the drip rate controllers, but although they can compensate for the drop size, their accuracy is still only ± 10% and therefore they are still only suitable for lower risk infusions.

Cost implications

Generally the volumetric controller is more expensive than the drip rate controller, but it is still cheaper than a volumetric pump. However, in resource terms these controllers can be quite expensive as most will only utilize a dedicated administration set.

INFUSION PUMPS

These devices pump fluid from an infusion bag, bottle or infusor via an administration set.

Drip rate pumps

When setting up these pumps, the user selects a rate by choosing the number of drops/minute. There is a drop sensor attached to the drip chamber of the infusion set. The device pumps the fluid by the peristaltic action of rollers (rotary peristaltic) or by mechanical 'fingers' that 'pinch off' the tubing.

Features

These pumps have very few alarms and few indications to alert the clinician to any malfunction.

Safety issues

Drip rate pumps have the following major problems:

- no air-in-line detection
- poor occlusion response coupled with resulting high pressures
- poor alarm response, particularly with regard to occlusion or extravasation.

For the above reasons, these pumps are *not recommended* and are not currently sold in the UK (MDA 1995a).

Volumetric pumps

These are the preferred option for larger flow rates and the wide range of devices available ensures that there is a volumetric pump available for all patient sizes, including neonates.

They usually weigh between 3 and 5 kg, and are designed to be 'stationary', i.e. attached to an i.v. pole or a bed rail (Sheldon & Bender 1994).

All volumetric pumps have the facility to work on mains or battery, with most batteries needing to be recharged by plugging in the pump even when it is not in use. Most of these pumps have lead cadmium batteries which will last for approximately 2–3 hours when fully charged.

The infusion rate is set using ml/h and most devices can be programmed to between 1 and 1000 ml/h, although when used at rates below 5 ml/h, accuracy may decrease. Most pumps use a linear peristaltic pumping action, although there are other mechanisms with devices using a cassette or other dedicated administration set (MDA 1995a).

Application

Volumetric pumps have a comprehensive range of safety and alarm features and can therefore be recommended for use in neonatal and higher risk infusions (MDA 1995a), as well as a variety of care settings (Box 8.7).

Features

General Some pumps have a drop sensor which they use for safety monitoring and alarms, e.g. 'empty infusion bag', but unlike the drip rate pumps this sensor is not integral to the rate mechanism.

In most volumetric pumps the infusion pressure is limited so that above a certain level the pump will alarm (MDA 1995a).

■ BOX 8.7

Care settings for use of volumetric pumps

Acute care settings

- Fluids – both crystalloid and colloid
- Antimicrobials
- Blood and blood products
- Cardiac drugs – inotropes and anti-arrhythmics
- PN, electrolyte infusions such as magnesium, calcium, phosphate
- Dialysate used in haemodialysis or more commonly in the continuous filtration methods, such as continuous veo-venus haemodiafiltration (CVVHD)
- Rapid fluid resuscitation (Tinker & Zapol 1991)
- Forced diuresis regimens
- Fluid management of cardiac bypass and other invasive critical care procedures
- Experimental therapies used in critical care, such as surfactant for acute respiratory distress syndrome (ARDS) and the antimediator therapy for severe sepsis (Lamy et al 1996)

General wards

- Fluid management
- Blood transfusions – particularly in the elderly or those with a degree of cardiac failure
- Pre-hydration regimens prior to nephrotoxic drugs such as anti-cancer chemotherapy (Holmes 1990)
- PN and electrolyte infusions (as 'acute care')
- Infusional antimicrobials – particularly in the care of patients who are immunocompromised either through their disease, as in cancer, or as the result of suppressant therapy after an organ transplant

All of the above may be used in neonatal and paediatric care, but with particular emphasis on the management of critical fluid balancing. It should be noted that in the neonate or small child, it is more accurate (and therefore safer) to use syringe pumps, if the aim is to deliver infusions at rates of less than 5 ml/h (MDA 1995a).

Home-care setting

- Fluids
- Antimicrobials
- Anti-cancer chemotherapy
- Pain control
- Peritoneal dialysis fluid
- PN, electrolyte infusions
- Recently, studies in the USA have demonstrated that the infusion of cardiac inotropes may be safely accomplished (Mayes et al 1995)
- There has also been some work in the USA looking at long-distance control of devices via the telephone system. Utilizing this system a patient's haemodynamic parameters are constantly monitored and relayed back to a central control via the telephone cables. A clinician can alter the programming of the pump and thus change the rate of an infusion using remote control. However, authors working with this system are anxious to assert that this kind of long-range therapy requires careful patient selection and does not obviate the need for good home care peripatetic nursing (Sheldon & Bender 1994).

It should be noted that for some applications patients at home may prefer a portable pump (Boutin & Hagan 1992).

Special Most volumetric pumps have the following special features (MDA 1995a):

- air-in-line detector
- automatic alarm and cessation of the pump if air enters the infusion system
- comprehensive alarm systems
- volume to be infused (VTBI) setting – preset by clinician, after which the pump displays a digital read-out of the cumulative total infused
- when the infusion is completed, automatic switching to a keep vein open (KVO) setting
- computer interface
- technical memory log
- drug library
- simple anti-tamper devices
- primary and secondary infusion settings
- technical incident log.

Safety issues

These pumps have an excellent safety record (MDA 1995a); however, because of their increased sophistication, it is essential that the correct administration set is used. Some devices may allow the use of a non-dedicated PVC set, but many require a dedicated set.

As these pumps can deliver rates of up to a 1000 ml/h, care must be taken to ensure that the pump rate is set correctly, e.g. taking particular care to set 10 ml/h rather than 100 ml/h. This is especially important in the paediatric setting and for this reason some centres prefer to incorporate a burette administration set (Thompson 1990).

In the acute care setting, care must also be taken to ensure that pumps that are not currently in use are left plugged into the electrical supply. This can become extremely important if a critically ill patient needs to be moved and cannot manage without supportive drug therapy. The pumps need to be fully charged so that they can be powered by their battery (Oh 1990).

Cost implications

The capital outlay on a volumetric infusion pump will depend on its technical sophistication and the number of functions it performs, but generally these pumps represent the top of the market and consequently carry a high price. However, most manufacturers will consider discounts, rental facilities and purchasing the pumps through a contract, e.g. by purchasing the same company's disposable administration sets.

AMBULATORY PUMPS

These pumps are small portable devices that will fit easily into a pocket, a handbag or a waist belt. They can utilize a small syringe but most use a reservoir bag of 100–250 ml that can be housed in a plastic 'wallet' that clips onto the pump. Most of these pumps are pre-programmable and they are therefore an ideal choice for the patient who can be taught a few basic care rules whilst in hospital and can then receive a preset dose of drug over several days or weeks. These pumps are powered by a small battery and so patients are advised to have a spare battery available.

Application

Like ambulatory syringe pumps, these devices are best suited to small volumes of solution. Depending on the reservoir size, a dose regimen can be set up for weeks or months.

Ambulatory pumps are therefore well suited for anti-cancer chemotherapy, long-term antibiotic therapy, anticoagulant therapy and pain control (Sheldon & Bender 1994).

Increasingly manufacturers are providing a variety of ambulatory pumps which include a PCA function.

Features

These pumps have the same safety features as listed in the section on PCA syringe pumps (p. 205).

As it may be necessary for patients and/or their carers to access any of the controls, e.g. to change a dose, the settings should be 'user-friendly' with buttons or a soft pad large enough to be visualized and activated easily.

Safety issues

As these pumps are predominantly used in the home and community setting, it is essential that they are reliable and require the minimum maintenance. In the last 5 years, manufacturers have greatly improved the reliability and durability of their designs (Sheldon & Bender 1994).

Cost implications

The ambulatory pump market is growing steadily with new more sophisticated models constantly being introduced. There is, therefore, a wide range of pricing between the older less advanced models and the more sophisticated ones, with, for example, those with PCA function retailing at £2000–3000.

IMPLANTED PUMPS

In recent years, as biotechnology has advanced, so has the manufacture of dedicated devices. Implanted pumps have been developed for those ambulatory patients who need long-term low-volume therapy. These pumps are small and are implanted subcutaneously, often in the area just below the umbilicus. The drug is then infused through an internal catheter into a vein, an artery or an area of dedicated tissue (Sheldon & Bender 1994).

Application

These pumps were designed to target chemotherapy or biological behaviour modifiers directly to a site of cancer (Holmes 1990). Regional anti-cancer chemotherapy is used at the following sites (Otto 1995):

- intra-arterial chemotherapy – hepatoma, metastatic colorectal cancer, osteosarcoma, glioblastoma, astrocytoma and tumours of the head and neck
- intraperitoneal chemotherapy – localized ovarian cancer (although more recently, combination systemic regimens have become more popular)
- intrathecal or intraventricular chemotherapy – acute lymphocytic leukaemia, brain tumours and palliation for metastatic disease in the brain.

More recently, implanted pumps have been successfully developed to be used in long-term anticoagulant and pain management therapy (Sheldon & Bender 1994).

Features

There are several devices available, all working on the principle of a periodically 'topped up' port. In some pumps, the device is powered by the vaporization of a 'charging' fluid in a reservoir adjacent to the drug reservoir. The pressure of this vapour exerts a pressure on some bellows which, in turn, force the drug out through a filter and flow restrictor to the dedicated implanted catheter. In another device, a septum port is periodically filled and then programmed telemetrically (Otto 1995).

Safety issues

In dealing with implanted devices, access to the device will be solely through repeated filling of reservoirs. Therefore, although there is less for the patient and carer to learn about the device, education concerning the aseptic technique is essential (Otto 1995).

Patients must also be trained to recognize any alteration in the appearance of the site of the implanted pump, e.g. signs of infection or any signs that the pump has become dislodged or that it is no longer working, and the necessity for quick reporting to their relevant referral team.

DISPOSABLE PUMPS

For the last 10 years the market in disposable devices has been steadily growing. These non-electronic devices have several advantages for the patient in that they are generally very lightweight and small so that they can be easily worn even whilst performing physical exercise. They are usually very 'user-friendly', requiring the minimum of input from the patient. They do not require a battery and are therefore less expensive and the patient does not have to remember to carry a spare battery. Finally they can be purchased pre-filled, thus minimizing patients' and carers' exposure to needles and ampoules.

Application

These lightweight infusors have been used predominantly in the ambulatory and home-care setting, but because of their predictable small-volume, low-rate capacity, they have also been used in acute care settings. The following are the most common uses:

- anti-cancer chemotherapy
- anticoagulant therapy
- pain control – particularly coupled with a disposable PCA device such as the 'wrist watch' attachment (Levy & Williams 1992).

Due to their low cost, there are reports of these infusors being used in the ITU setting when all the available electronic pumps are being used (Davidson et al 1993).

One advantage that these infusors may have in an acute setting is that they look very different from all the other pumps used, which may help to minimize errors when many pumps per patient are being set.

Features

The disposable pumps work on the principle of an elastomeric balloon which is situated inside a plastic cylinder. When the balloon is filled, the resulting hydrostatic pressure inside the balloon is enough to power the infusion. The drug is then infused through a small-bore administration set which usually has a rate restrictor at the patient end (Davidson et al 1993).

Cost implications

The disposable infusor pumps are intended to be filled only once, the usual reservoir size being 50–70 ml; the infusor is then discarded. The infusors can also be purchased prefilled by private pharmaceutical companies or hospital pharmacies. Another cost advantage of the disposable non-electronic pump is that there are no maintenance or servicing costs.

MANAGEMENT OF FLOW CONTROL DEVICES

Any technical equipment will only function optimally if it is cared for in an appropriate manner and all such devices are supplied with recommendations from the manufacturer as to servicing and maintenance. Whichever department is concerned with the technical management of these devices, it is imperative that clinicians have a direct input into this area.

Indeed, clinical practitioners are bound by their professional codes to recognize their individual responsibility and accountability for practice. For nurses in the UK, the United Kingdom Central Council (UKCC) for Nursing, Midwifery and Health Visiting states in the *Code for Professional Conduct* that (UKCC 1992):

'As a registered nurse, midwife or health visitor you are personally accountable for your practice and, in the exercise of your professional accountability must ... act always in such a manner as to promote and safeguard the interests and well-being of patients and clients.'

A nurse, whether he is working clinically with patients or as a manager responsible for a care environment, must recognize that it is unacceptable to use any device that is:

- not suitable
- has not been maintained
- is partly broken
- is unknown to the user (Cuthrell 1996).

Every year government agencies, such as the Medical Devices Agency, receive many reports of patient untoward incidents or errors involving flow control devices.

It is the recognition of the need for clinical staff to be closely involved with the monitoring of device management that has led to increasing nurse involvement in 'focus' groups concerned with product design (Hasler 1996).

Selection and procurement

It is during the initial planning and selection stage that care should be taken to ensure that all relevant personnel are involved in the process. It is recommended that this group consists of the following personnel:

- Clinical representatives – it is essential that there is some representation from those directly involved with patient care and using the device. A member of the i.v. team may also be invited.
- Supplies or administrative personnel who are familiar with the process of ordering, supply and delivery.

- Accountant or financial adviser.
- Biomedical engineer or personnel who are involved with the maintenance and servicing of equipment.
- Directorate manager or personnel with a link to the manager with responsibility for the relevant budget.

Clinical representative

It is essential that there is involvement from personnel who have been working in the environment that requires new equipment. This representative should have experience in the specific needs of the area but also the relevant literature on devices; in some areas a nurse with this degree of experience may be the clinical nurse specialist or the senior sister.

Medical staff, particularly anaesthetists or intensivists, may also wish to be involved. However, it is the nurses who are at the bedside frequently setting up and changing rates on devices, as well as discovering faults and sending the devices for repair, and therefore it is recommended that a nurse be present. An important addition to this group would be a member of the i.v. team whose experience will be a valuable resource in the selection and the management of devices (Dougherty 1996b).

Prior to a meeting of the above personnel, the clinical staff should discuss the clinical needs for a device and devise a written specification which should include the following:

- the reason for choosing the equipment and the benefits to be gained from a particular device
- the problems that might occur
- whether it is user-friendly
- type of patient – neonate, child, adult
- type of infusion category – neonatal, high-risk, low-risk
- environment – home-care, ambulatory, general ward use, theatres and anaesthetics, acute care
- portability
- budget limit for capital purchase and ongoing expenditure on disposables
- devices already used in the same environment – standardizing of devices (where possible) to facilitate training and minimize the risk of user error (Leggett 1990, Dougherty 1996b).

Supplies or administrative personnel

It is important to include personnel who have experience in liaison with manufacturers and in the arrangement of purchasing deals that may include standing orders for disposables. Such staff will also have experience and knowledge of the reliability of different manufacturers concerning delivery of disposables, and also customer care and after-care.

Accountant or financial adviser

It is imperative that an accountant or financial adviser is involved in the initial stages when contracts are being discussed. They may also be very helpful in the negotiation of any trial periods or discounts on bulk purchasing.

Biomedical engineer

Although clinical staff will be aware of clinical needs, it is important that any device should also be considered from a mechanical and scientific viewpoint. Technical reports such as those produced by the MDA can be helpful, but expert technical help and experience are vital. Most large biomedical engineering departments build up a library of devices which have been evaluated and they can therefore offer valuable advice on how a device will perform over time.

Directorate manager

It is advisable that any purchasing of equipment be standardized, where possible, throughout directorates and even throughout a Trust. Devices are often moved with patients through various wards, and departments' standardization of equipment may help to minimize user error and ensure ease of training of personnel (MDA 1995a).

A directorate manager may be able to influence or liaise with other directorates to ensure that there is a more streamlined approach to the selection and purchasing of devices. In some areas in the UK, several hospital Trusts have joined together to form groups with greater purchasing power for device selection and purchasing, e.g. North London Group.

Staff development and training

The strategic development of training programmes is recommended by the MDA (MDA 1995a). The MDA further recommend that the need for such ongoing staff development and training should be recognized and operationalized at a senior level. The aim of such training programmes should be:

- to optimize patient safety and minimize the probability of incident or error
- familiarity with all the functions and flexibility of devices
- knowledge of any technical and software developments during the life of the device.

Each establishment will need to plan the type of training programme best suited to their environment and needs. Including the clinical staff in the devising of these programmes will improve motivation and ensure appropriate strategies (Cuthrell 1996).

Although each area will undoubtedly have individual needs, the following items could be regarded as the core of any programme (MDA 1995a):

- the type of device to use for a particular clinical function
- how to load disposable administration sets into all devices used in the area
- the optimum mounting of pumps (particularly syringe pumps) for ease of viewing the digital display and to ensure that the pump is securely anchored
- prevention of air entrainment and free-flow
- pump configuration and functions
- cleaning and storage issues.

Every training programme should ideally be multidisciplinary and must be part of a continuous education programme. All new staff should be introduced to new devices as part of their orientation and all training must be carefully documented.

Care should be taken that all nurses working with devices are provided with training, including those working part-time or as locums, but nurses also have a professional responsibility and accountability to ensure that they are trained in any devices that they use in caring for patients (UKCC 1992).

It is inevitable in a busy clinical environment that there will be occasions when teaching time is difficult to find, and therefore a minimum safety requirement is the availability of written material for each device. This written material should take the carer through the basic setting up and priming of the device and then through its functions and alarm settings to enable the user to problem-solve (Table 8.3).

Table 8.3 Problem-solving (adapted from Dougherty 1996)

Problem	Cause	Prevention	Action
Alarms			
Occlusion	Occlusion in intravenous device or administration set	Ensure device is flushed and remains patent Do not allow infusion bags to run dry	Locate occlusion – if in tubing then change relevant equipment; if within the i.v. device, attempt to remove the occlusion
	Kinking of administration or extension set tubing	Ensure tubing is taped to prevent kinking Reposition tubing within pump whenever set is removed to prevent crushing	If tubing kinked, reposition and tape to prevent further kinking; change position within pump
	Phlebitis/infiltration or extravasation	Observe site regularly for signs of swelling, erythema or pain	Remove device immediately and resite
Air	Air bubbles in administration set	Ensure all air is removed from administration set prior to use Change infusion bags on time to prevent them running dry	Remove all air from administration set and restart infusion
	Set wrongly loaded	Ensure that the tubing is correctly positioned within the air-in-line detector	Check set is loaded correctly and reload if necessary
Over- or under-infusion	Incorrect rate setting	Ensure that the rate is correctly set and checked regularly within the first hour. Check rate setting at start of each shift	Check patient's condition Inform medical and nursing staff, and complete an incident form
	Technical fault with equipment	Ensure regular servicing and maintenance of the equipment	Remove equipment from use immediately and label to prevent further use Report incident to medical and nursing staff – note serial number, problem. Inform MDA
Electrical malfunction	Not charging at mains Low battery	Check that lead is pushed in adequately Ensure that the equipment is kept plugged in where necessary	Remove pump and ensure that the lead is fitted correctly and then leave on charge for 24 hours until it is fully charged
	Batteries require frequent replacement	Do not use small rechargeable batteries in drivers or ambulatory pumps	Request that works/EBME department check plug/fuse

(cont'd)

Table 8.3 (cont'd)

Problem	Cause	Prevention	Action
Mechanical malfunction	Device soiled inside mechanism	Maintain equipment and keep clean and free from contamination and dust	Remove administration set and clean pump according to manufacturer's recommendations, e.g. do not use alcohol-based solutions on inside of mechanisms
Unstable pump	Mounted on old, poorly maintained or incorrect stands	Ensure that the correct stands are used, and kept maintained. Replace old stands	Remove stand from service and send for repair. Change to correct stand
	Equipment not correctly balanced on stands	Ensure that equipment is correctly balanced on stand or use more than one stand	Balance equipment on stand or use two stands if more equipment required

These instructional cards can often be obtained from the manufacturer and affixed to the device.

Finally, it is important that any training is research-based and reflects current knowledge. It may be useful to incorporate a 'news bulletin' or 'factsheet' to provide up-to-date information about new changes or recommendations, e.g. the recent recommendations to avoid the use of mobile phones in clinical areas as they may alter the function of devices (MDA 1997).

Storage of devices and tracking strategies

Care should be taken to comply with the manufacturer's instructions regarding storage of their equipment. The following general rules apply:

- Any device that has a battery back-up facility needs to be plugged in continuously even when not in use – it is therefore necessary for storage areas to have enough electrical sockets.
- Pumps powered by small removable batteries (such as ambulatory pumps) should be stored without their batteries.
- All devices should be stored clean and ready for use.
- If possible, devices should be stored in a central collection area where they can be logged in and out – a bar code and light pen system can be utilized. This system can help to prevent devices being stored in inappropriate places such as cupboards or window sills and it also ensures that pumps are available.

All devices will at some time need repairing or updating and it is therefore essential that each department keeps a log or tracking system for its devices. If a tracking system is used, it is possible for a designated person to identify a particular device that has malfunctioned more times than expected or to be able to check that all the department's devices are returned.

Another use for a tracking or logging system is to ensure that all devices are routinely maintained and serviced at least as often as the manufacturer's recommendations.

Routine tracking of all medical devices is becoming commonplace in many areas and although it requires some resource allocation, this can be justified as part of the institution's risk management programme. As medical litigation becomes more common, patients and their families are becoming more aware of their right to be cared for in an institution that has an optimum safety network (Hayden 1992).

Maintenance and servicing

All devices need to be maintained and serviced as directed by the manufacturer. Once the devices are out of their warranty period (usually 1–3 years), they will often need an annual service. Most of these devices are easily portable and in the hospital setting they could be difficult to locate. Therefore, to enable the pumps to be easily located, a tracking system maintained by a designated person is essential.

Each institution or department should have guidelines which ensure the following:

- careful cleaning and decontamination of pumps prior to handling by service and maintenance personnel
- immediate withdrawal of a device from the clinical area if it has been dropped or subjected to other damage
- documentation of all service and maintenance checks and of any repair work carried out for each individual pump – utilizing a bar code or the manufacturer's code number can be useful.

It is important to rigorously discourage any mending of devices by clinical staff or carers in the hospital or community setting. Devices today are complex machines and should only be attended to by designated biomedical engineers or the manufacturer. It should be noted that if a device malfunctions and causes a patient incident, its service history will be checked and if a non-designated person has carried out any work on the device, the manufacturer may have a case in law to place the responsibility onto the institution (Weinstein 1997).

Most countries have a system of reporting whether a device has been involved in a patient incident. In the UK, if a device is involved in an incident it is recommended that it is reported to the MDA. There are strict guidelines for reporting such an incident, including the retention for examination of any related disposable such as the syringe/reservoir or administration set that was used (MDA 1995a).

It is vitally important that such patient incidents are reported to a central body, because it is this reporting that can provide the necessary large data base to recall a device from general sale and thus help to protect future patients.

Reporting errors with devices

The continuous infusion of i.v. drugs is increasing in popularity as technological advances in equipment and pharmacological improvements in drugs are introduced into clinical practice. Such technology, however, also introduces potential new complications (Kelly & Brull 1995). Every year the MDA receives many reports of adverse patient incidents where a device has been used. Some of these incidents are due to the malfunctioning of equipment, but many reflect user error.

During the last 15 years, there have been 21 device-related deaths and at least as many near deaths requiring intervention in the form of resuscitation or antidotes reported to the Department of Health (Box 8.8). A further 280 incidents of overinfusion which may have caused severe patient distress have also been reported. This probably only represents a fifth of the number of actual incidents, due to massive underreporting (Richardson 1995).

A large proportion of reports have been identified as being due to user error and not to failure of infusion pumps. In all cases of unidentified incidents, the pumps have been serviced and returned to use with no further failure. This indicates that some form of user error was also involved in these incidents (Richardson 1995).

Anecdotal evidence suggests that the majority of clinicians, nursing staff and

■ **BOX 8.8**

Device-related deaths (*Richardson 1995*)

- A patient died when diamorphine was infused via a clockwork pump which was not accurate enough for the purpose
- A patient died when a drug was infused at nearly 50 times the required rate; the pump had been returned from the serving department and set at a high rate which was not reset by nursing staff prior to use
- A patient died because a pump designed for use with a dedicated administration set was used with a standard set
- A patient died when no drug was infused because an in-line tap was closed. The pump drive mechanism was badly worn and slippage meant that the alarm was not activated
- A patient died when the roller clamp on the administration set was not closed; when the pump was opened it caused a massive over-infusion of drug

pharmacists have little or no knowledge or understanding of the types and suitability of pumps for intravenous infusions (Pickstone et al 1994). Inadequate understanding of equipment makes it difficult to interpret information correctly and diagnose false alarms (McConnell 1995, Sinclair 1988). Nurses who do not understand the purpose, capabilities, limitations and functioning of a device may be unable to point out malfunctions, which will increase liability (McConnell 1995).

Fitter (1986) stated that critical care nurses in Europe reported inadequate training to be a major problem with machine use in direct patient care for a variety of reasons:

- New equipment frequently arrived on the unit for almost immediate use.
- Nurses had difficulty in getting time off to attend extracurricular training courses.
- Device use education was, in some instances, limited to on-the-job training from partially knowledgeable colleagues or learned from an equipment supplier's manual.
- There was inadequate time to learn from supplier's demonstrations which may be narrow in scope and skewed to favour the device (see McConnell 1995).

As a result the nurses judged their device education inadequate.

Nurses caring for patients with mechanical devices need to fulfil their professional responsibility to protect their charges and should therefore possess comprehensive device knowledge, which includes a conceptual understanding of the technology involved. The nurse should be aware of the underlying physical properties and principles of the device, in addition to factors such as primary functions, limitations and safety features (McConnell 1995). It will only be when the nurse is fully conversant, competent and proficient in the use of mechanical devices in direct patient care that the potential for error will be at its minimum. However, there are also some additional management tools that can be used to ensure safety:

- a network for near-miss reporting
- a compassionate and professional attitude to incident reporting – this may encourage reporting
- a computerized database of all incidents – to allow for the recognition of repeated similar errors to be collated and management action to be taken
- regular updates for clinical staff on errors reported and the management action taken
- awareness of the MDA reporting system as noted above.

As technological advances make further inroads into device development, more pumps can now incorporate a failure/error log, which may be useful for local data collection.

Following the Clothier report requested by the Department of Health in the UK (MDA 1995c), many manufacturers are now investigating tamper-proof devices. These programmes are still in their development stages, although some pumps already incorporate a 'lock-out' panel often useful when caring for small children.

Disposal of devices

It is imperative that all obsolete or failed devices are removed from the clinical area immediately. It is *not* safe to remove devices from the bedside into a ward office in order to deal with it later. Clinical staff are often busy and this kind of practice may lead to errors – it is therefore recommended that a designated person outside of the individual clinical area have the responsibility for checking that obsolete or malfunctioning pumps are removed.

The MDA has compiled a list of devices which should now be considered either for immediate replacement or for replacement over the next few years (MDA 1995a). Each institution will need written documentation for the procedure to be followed when a device is to be condemned and to document this removal from the hospital database.

The practice of sending out-of-date medical equipment to developing countries is *not* recommended as all safety issues will be further compounded in countries and regions that have no technical back-up facilities.

Audit of practice

Once an institution or community team has established management guidelines to facilitate all the areas covered in the management of devices, it is imperative that an audit process is organized.

It is recommended that the audit be performed by the Health and Safety Committee or similar body which can review documentation and practice from a global perspective.

This audit could take the following form:

- review of documentation
- review of data collection
- interviews with all levels of the multidisciplinary clinical team
- spot checks of clinical practice.

CONCLUSION

There has been an emphasis on safety and the prevention of error throughout this chapter. However, this is with due recognition to the huge contribution that flow control devices make to our clinical care. Indeed, many aspects of therapeutic care that we perform today would not be possible without the aid of these devices.

It is also known from experience and the literature that our patients are increasingly keen to learn about the devices used in their treatment, and they are sometimes now being involved in the development or selection of devices (Boutin & Hagan 1992). It should therefore be our aim to ensure continuous education for all our personnel, patients and their families in this area as in other clinical areas.

Finally, it is by becoming more knowledgeable and therefore more confident that we as health care personnel will be able to enter the debate with manufacturers and work together to ensure the highest standards of clinical excellence for our patients.

REFERENCES

Auden W H 1938 A certain world. Penguin books, UK

Bakitas-Whedon M 1991 Bone marrow transplantation: principles, practice, and nursing insights. Jones and Bartlett, Boston, MA

Berde C 1989 Paediatric post-operative pain management. Paediatric Clinics of North America 36: 921–940

Boutin J, Hagan E 1992 Patient's preference regarding portable pumps. Journal of Intravenous Nursing15(4): 230–232

Cuthrell P 1996 Managing equipment failures: nursing practice requirements for meeting the challenges of the Safe Medical Devices Act. Journal of Intravenous Nursing 19(5): 264–268

Davidson J A H, Boom S J, Dryden C M, Simon E J 1993 The use of a PCA system as an infusion pump. British Journal of Intensive Care May: 105–106

Dougherty L 1996a Intravenous management. The Royal Marsden NHS Trust manual of clinical nursing procedures, 4th edn. Blackwell Science, London, ch 23, p 310–337

Dougherty L 1996b The benefits of an IV team in hospital practice. Professional Nurse 11(11): 761–763

Fitter M 1986 The impact of new technology on workers and patients in the health services. Loughlinstown House, Dublin

Gatford G H 1990 Nursing calculations, 3rd edn. Churchill Livingstone, Edinburgh

Hasler R A 1996 Human factors design: what is it and how can it affect you? Journal of Intravenous Nursing 19(3) S5–S8

Hayden L S 1992 Risk management strategies. Journal of Intravenous Nursing 15(5): 288–290

Holmes S 1990 Cancer chemotherapy. Austen Cornish, London

Hunt M, Rapp R 1996 Intravenous medication errors. Journal of Intravenous Nursing 19(3): S9–15

Kelly D, Brull S J 1995 The cost of modern technology. Journal of Clinical Anaesthesia 7: 80–81

Kuhn S, Cooke K, Collins M, Jones J M, Mucklow J C 1990 Perceptions of pain relief after surgery. British Medical Journal 300: 1687–1689

Lamy M, Eisele B, Kernecke H et al 1996 Antithrombin III in patients with severe sepsis: a randomised placebo controlled double blind multicentre trial. 9th European Congress on Intensive Care Medicine proceedings of 24–28 September, Glasgow, pp 385–390

Leggett A 1990 Intravenous infusion pump. Nursing Standard 4(28): 24–26

Levy D M, Williams A 1992 Recent developments in the management of post-operative pain. The Pharmaceutical Journal September 12: HS12–15

McConnell E A 1995 How and what staff nurses learn about medical devices they use in direct patient care. Research in Nursing and Health 18: 165–172

Mayes J, Carter C, Adams J 1995 Inotropic therapy in the home care setting: criteria, management, and implications. Journal of Intravenous Nursing 18(6)

Medical Devices Agency (MDA) 1995a DB 9503. Device bulletin – infusion systems. Medical Devices Agency, London

Medical Devices Agency (MDA) 1995b MDA 9506. Hazard notice. Graseby Medical MS16, MS16A, & MS26 ambulatory syringe pumps. Medical Devices Agency, London

Medical Devices Agency (MDA) 1995c The report of the expert working group on alarms on clinical monitors in response to recommendation II of the Clothier Report. The Allitt Inquiry, DoH, London

Medical Devices Agency (MDA) 1996 Evaluation 283 – syringe infusion pumps. Medical Devices Agency, London

Medical Devices Agency (MDA) 1997 DB 9702. Device bulletin – electromagnetic compatibility of medical devices with mobile communications. Medical Devices Agency, London

Oh T E 1990 Intensive care manual. Butterworths, London

Otto S E 1995 Advanced concepts in chemotherapy drug delivery: regional therapy. Journal of Intravenous Nursing 18(4): 170–176

Pickstone M, Jacklin A, Langfield B, Wootton R 1994 Intravenous infusion of drugs measuring and minimising the risks. British Journal of Intensive Care 5: 338–343

Richardson N 1995 A review of drug infusion incidents: the situation from the national perspective. British Journal of Intensive Care February (Suppl): 8–9

Rodgers B, Webb C, Stergios D, Newman B 1988 Patient controlled analgesia in paediatric surgery. Journal of Paediatric Surgery 23: 259–262

Royal College of Surgeons/Royal College of Anaesthetists 1990 Working party of the commission on the provision of surgical services. Pain after surgery. RCS/RCA, London

Sagar D, Bomar S 1980 Intravenous medications. Lippincott, Philadelphia

Schumaker W, Ayers S M et al 1995 Textbook of critical care, 3rd edn. WB Saunders, Philadelphia

Sheldon P, Bender M 1994 High-technology in home care. Nursing Clinics of North America 29: 507–519

Sinclair V 1988 High technology in critical care: implications for nursing's role and practice. Focus on Critical Care 15(4): 37–41

Snell C C, Fothergill-Bourbonnais F, Durocher-Hendriks S 1997 Patient controlled analgesia and intramuscular injections: a comparison of patient pain experiences and postoperative outcomes. Journal of Advanced Nursing 25: 681-690

Tammisto T, Tigerstedt L 1982 Narcotic analgesics in postoperative pain relief in adults. Acta Anaesthesia Scandinavia 74(suppl. 1): 161–164

Thompson J 1990 The child with cancer. Scutari Press, London

Tinker J, Zapol W M 1991 Care of the critically ill patient, 2nd edn. Springer-Verlag, London

United Kingdom Central Council for Nursing, Midwifery and Health Visiting 1992 Code of professional conduct for the nurse, midwife and health visitor, 3rd edn. UKCC, London

Watt-Watson J H, Donovan M I 1992 Pain management – nursing perspective. Mosby Year Book, London

Weinstein S M 1997 (ed) Plumer's principles and practice of intravenous therapy, 6th edn. JB Lippincott, Philadelphia

Obtaining peripheral venous access

Lisa Dougherty

INTRODUCTION

Venepuncture and cannulation are the most commonly performed invasive procedures in the UK (Peters et al 1984). Neither of these procedures is based simply on technical skill, each requiring adequate knowledge of the relevant anatomy and physiology, the impact that such a procedure can have on a patient and the expected outcomes of therapy. The ability to assess the patient and make an informed choice on the selection of the vein and the device to be inserted is based on observation, nursing judgement, the use of clinical and nursing notes and the ability to problem-solve. The aim should be to provide the patient with a functional, comfortable peripheral vascular access device.

The procedures are defined as follows:

- venepuncture – the insertion of a needle into a vein usually to obtain a blood specimen
- cannulation – the process of introducing a hollow tube made of plastic into a peripheral blood vessel to enable the administration of drugs or fluids, which can remain in situ for variable periods of time

PSYCHOLOGICAL EFFECT ON PATIENT

Venepuncture and cannulation have become routine procedures for both doctors and nurses to perform, but for a patient who is unfamiliar with the procedure, it may be a frightening experience (Plumer 1987). The importance of never underestimating the effect on a patient of having a blood test or a cannula inserted is highlighted in the literature (Dougherty 1992, Hecker et al 1983, Middleton 1985, Speechley 1987).

Age certainly appears to play a role in the amount of pain and distress associated with needles. Agras et al (1969) showed that the incidence of injection fear in the general population rises sharply from 0 to 15 years and then there is a steep decline ending at 30 years of age, suggesting that the fear is short-lived. However, both Wilson Barnett (1976) and Coates et al (1983) found that hospitalized patients under 40 years of age responded more negatively to injections than those aged 40 and over. Age has also been correlated to the level of distress associated with routine venepuncture and this could account for the variability in degree of distress and pain reported (Bennett-Humphrey & Boon 1992).

Gender does not appear relevant in children and adolescents, but in adults it appears that women (particularly those under the age of 45) are more anxious about needles than men (Coates et al 1983). Van den Berg & Abeysekera (1993) found that more female patients had greater pain scores and more responses during the cannulation procedure, suggesting that female patients may need more care and attention during the procedure. However, it must be remembered that men tend to have been socialized to appear brave and not express pain (Levine & De Simone 1991).

Coates et al (1983) found that anxiety was often related more to the fear of having a needle inserted than the pain of the needle itself, and this is supported by Bennett-Humphrey & Boon (1992) and reflected in patients' own accounts of venepuncture and cannulation. Buckalew (1982) described how she became anxious before and after chemotherapy and identified one of the sources of her anxiety as the pain of having i.v. infusions started. One bad experience of an infiltrated i.v. infusion had led to feelings of extreme anxiety prior to venepuncture and cannulation. She listed fear, anticipation of pain and severe anxiety as being more painful than the pain of the procedure itself.

Fears and phobias

Agras et al (1969) performed a study on a population of a medium-sized city to discover the incidence and predict the prevalence of common fears and phobias. The results showed that the bulk of the population was affected by common fears such as visiting the dentist and the sight of blood. This is also supported by Marks (1988). Mild phobias affect a significant but lesser portion of the population and severe disabling phobias are much less common. Interestingly, Agras et al (1969) discovered that 57 out of 1000 individuals had sought advice from a physician about a severe fear or phobia related to a medical procedure, such as blood tests and injections, in order to minimize their fearful response.

Humans have a natural tendency to be squeamish at the sight of blood, and discomfort, faintness and nausea are triggered by cues involving blood such as blood sampling (Marks 1988). This natural, mild human fear usually causes no difficulty in normal life and is only termed a phobia if it becomes severe and causes a marked or even life-threatening handicap. These patients avoid blood or injury cues to avert fainting as it is the fear and anticipation of a faint that brings on the anxiety. Blood phobia is defined as a fear and avoidance of situations involving direct and indirect exposure to blood or injuries and its prevalence in the general population is 3.1–4.5 %. Those with blood phobias usually also have injection phobia (Ost 1992). Injection phobia is the fear and avoidance of receiving various types of injection and having a blood sample drawn through venepuncture (Ost 1992).

Early work in the field of injection fear was performed on dental patients, who tend to have high levels of anxiety and rank their common fears as pain, blood and needles (Berggren 1992). However, Ost (1992) discovered that it was often fear of the pain rather than the fear of the injection that led to phobic reactions, highlighting the anticipatory effect of fear and anxiety on the perception of pain. Phobias can be acquired in various ways and Ost (1991) suggested three pathways to fear acquisition:

- conditioning
- vicarious acquisition
- transmission of information and/or instruction.

Fears of blood and injection tend to start in childhood and this may be as a result of modelling. Parents who exhibit fear of a particular situation may pass these onto their children through vicarious conditioning (Marks 1988, Ost 1992). Some parents may pass fears more directly to their children by warning them against specific situations. However, these fears tend to disappear in adulthood because of repeated exposure to the feared situation (Mavissakalian & Barlow 1981). But if the exposures are traumatic, the memory of the experience may induce a conditioned response. Auerbach et al (1976) found that anxiety states in dental patients were related to previous dental contacts of an aversive nature.

In a study performed by Ost (1991) more than half the patients (53.5%) ascribed the origin of their phobia to direct experiences of the conditioning type. Condition theory seems to accommodate the way in which the majority of both injection (57%)

■ **BOX 9.1**

'Jab-fear woman is saved from herself' (Morris 1996)

'Doctors were forced to carry out a life-saving caesarean operation on a woman too terrified of needles to agree to an anaesthetic injection ... the women had agreed in principle to a caesarean but because of her needle phobia insisted on gas rather than an injection ... the judge decided that L's extreme needle phobia rendered her incapable of weighing relevant treatment information.'

'The fear that condemned a man to die in agony from rabies' (Verity 1993)

'Mark Sell enjoyed the reputation as an action man. He was fearless in his high risk job ... only one thing frightened him – needles. And when he was bitten by a friend's dog in Thailand 2 months ago, he refused to have an anti-rabies injection that might have saved his life ... 'He couldn't stand to even look at a syringe, it was that bad,' his father Terry said yesterday. 'He was a brave man ... but he was terrified of injections.'

and blood (49%) phobics acquired their phobias (Ost 1991). Steel et al (1986) also recognized that diabetic injection phobias were usually acquired as a conditioned response.

Problems can result from blood and injection phobic conditions and serious consequences can arise for the patient whose survival depends on injections and blood tests, such as diabetics (Steel et al 1986) (see Box 9.1). It has been found that phobias in adults rarely disappear spontaneously without treatment (Agras et al 1972), but once the cause of the phobia is ascertained treatment with exposure or behaviour therapy can be successful (Marks 1988, Rachman & Wilson 1980).

The skilled practitioner

'Only a skilled practitioner should perform a venepuncture on an anxious patient with limited or difficult veins.' (Weinstein 1993)

The skill of the practitioner appears to be relevant to the feelings attached to the procedure of venepuncture and cannulation and is recounted in patients' experiences. Kaplan (1983) described his major fear as having the novice intern taking bloods and being poked, prodded and probed time after time. Cohn (1982) described how staff would not listen to his warnings about his veins and what would or would not work.

Both Buckalew (1982) and Kaplan (1983) stressed that patients should not have to endure unnecessary assaults because of inexperienced practitioners. It appears that patients feel less anxious when the procedure is performed by a skilled practitioner, and also equate the skill of giving injections with caring behaviour. Larson (1984) and Mayer (1987) found that cancer patients identified 'knows how to give an i.v. and manage equipment' as the most important caring behaviour.

Vasovagal reactions

The critically ill patient is susceptible to fears, which become exaggerated, triggering an undesirable autonomic nervous system response known as a vasovagal reaction. Such a reaction may present as syncope. Sympathetic reaction may follow and result in vasoconstriction. This limits available veins, complicates the procedure and makes therapy more difficult (Weinstein 1993). It has been well established that fainting or vasovagal syncope is a common feature of venepuncture and cannulation (Kaloupek et al 1985, Pavlin et al 1993). Although typically benign and self-limited, these episodes may cause traumatic injury if unanticipated and are considered stressful and embarrassing by patients. Symptoms include feeling faint, light-headed, sweaty, hot, cold or nauseated (Pavlin et al 1993).

Pavlin et al's study investigated how to identify subjects who are at greatest risk of vasovagal reaction and provided direction for future methods of prevention or treatment. They found that patients responded to various aspects, including psychological stress, pain, anticipated pain, the sight of blood and the act of donating of blood. Only the age of the patient, the duration of cannulation and prior history of fainting were identified as independent predictors of vasovagal reaction (Kaloupek et al 1985, Pavlin et al 1993).

The number of attempts at venepuncture and the duration of cannulation had equally strong associations with developing symptoms but were not independent of each other. The incidence of reaction was 16.6% in patients aged 40 or less; those with a history of fainting (33.3%) reacted 50% of the time; and 12% of female patients reacted compared with 9% of males. Pavlin et al (1993) strongly recommended the use of a reclining chair to prevent the mechanical trauma that may occur during syncope; it also permits rapid change from the upright to the horizontal. However, the study did not show that selecting the horizontal position before venepuncture would alter the incidence of vasovagal reaction.

PAIN RELIEF

Inducing pain during a procedure can provoke feelings of incompetency and frustration in the nurse and lack of confidence, apprehension, distress and even hostility in the patient (Millam 1995). Investigations into the pain associated with venepuncture and cannulation in both adults and children have concentrated on influencing variables such as age, sex, device and vein site, as well as the relief of physical pain caused by the insertion of needles.

A study by Van den Berg & Abeysekera (1993) investigating venous cannulation in a large sample of patients (1422) considered a range of influencing factors during the insertion of a cannula. These included arm used, vein site, cannula size and pain on cannulation. Pain was assessed by a verbal analogue scale and observation of patients' responses. Use of the cephalic vein and a larger gauge (16 g) cannula produced more responses, but reported pain was reduced when lignocaine was used.

Cannula design has also been implicated in the degree of reported pain, with thin-walled cannulae appearing to cause less pain than thick-walled cannulae (Ahrens et al 1991). This evidence reinforces the necessity for careful selection of vein, device design and size. Hecker et al (1983) performed a study using glyceryl trinitrate (GTN) ointment to increase vasodilation and facilitate easier venous access. They recommended its use to reduce patient trauma and save time.

There are a number of methods for reducing pain in invasive procedures. The two most commonly used are (1) an injectable skin wheal for lignocaine or sterile sodium chloride 0.9%, and (2) the application of a topical anaesthetic. Although some of the ointments or sprays do not achieve sufficient dermal anaesthetic for the insertion of i.v. devices, a topical anaesthetic cream has been found to be useful in alleviating the pain of venepuncture. Hallen et al (1984) provided evidence of good pain relief when the cream was applied for at least 60 minutes prior to the procedure. The ease of venepuncture and reduction of experienced pain produced by using both GTN and a local anaesthetic cream can lead to a less traumatic experience. However, these ointments did not influence patients' perception of pain, but may have implications for how they go on to perceive future experiences (Gunwardene

& Davenport 1990). Vasoconstriction seen as blanching (37%) has also been noted following removal of some creams, and has necessitated the use of local heat to aid vasodilation (however, no increased absorption occurs). In 30% of patients, erythema of the skin is noticeable, and 6% experience a mild oedema. These disappear within hours. Rare minor adverse side-effects include alteration in temperature sensation, itching and rash (Millam 1995).

The issue of local anaesthetic by injection is a controversial one. Anaesthetists commonly use local anaesthetic, although in a recent study only 73% of anaesthetists were aware of the research recommending the use of injectable local anaesthetic for the siting of cannulae 18g or larger. This use has now increased from 12 to 65%. The research showed that the pain of cannulation using cannulae 22 g or larger was reduced significantly by prior subcutaneous infiltration with 1% lignocaine when compared with cannulation without infiltration. Moreover, there was no increased difficulty associated with cannulation (Dennis et al 1995, Harrison et al 1992).

Use of transcutaneous electrical nerve stimulation (TENS) for procedural pain associated with i.v. needlesticks is based upon the gate control theory (see Ch. 2, p. 42). Coyne et al (1995) investigated whether the application of TENS decreased the complaints of pain and unpleasantness with i.v. needle insertion. Their double-blind randomized study was conducted on 71 patients who were placed in one of three groups – placebo TENS, TENS or control. The use of modified brief intense TENS did not produce a reduction in pain (sensory or affective) associated with cannulation, although Lander & Fowler-Kerry (1992) (with children) and Webster et al (1992) (with adults) showed a decrease in procedural pain. The obvious benefits are the lack of long-term side-effects or complications. Continued investigation into this non-invasive method of pain relief is required.

IMPROVING VENOUS ACCESS

Difficult venepunctures are time-consuming and traumatic for the patient. Application of a tourniquet, taping and stroking of veins, vigorous swabbing, clenching the hand to pump up veins, hanging the forearm downwards and application of local warmth are all commonly used aids for cannulation (Hecker 1988).

The application of the tourniquet promotes venous distension. The tourniquet should be tight enough to impede venous return while not affecting arterial flow (Millam 1993). It should be applied around the upper forearm to promote dilation of the veins and time should be allowed for the veins to fill. A blood pressure cuff may also be used, with the cuff being inflated to a pressure just below the diastolic pressure. A tourniquet can be applied over a thin layer of clothing if there is a chance that it could cause injury or bruising of the skin. This is particularly true of elderly patients, those with extremely fragile veins and thrombocytopenic patients, making it necessary to release the tourniquet as soon as the vein is entered or not apply it at all. It should not pinch the patient's skin once it is tightened and should not be left on for long periods of time as it may have an effect on the results of certain blood tests and can even result in ecchymosis. If venous access is difficult, it may be necessary to release the tourniquet and allow refilling; then, once it is tightened, the search for the vein may continue (Perucca 1995, Whitson 1996).

Other methods used to improve venous distension include lowering the extremity below the level of the heart, and opening and closing the fist (the action of the muscles forces blood into the veins, causing them to distend). Light tapping of the vein may be useful, but it can be painful and may result in the formation of a haematoma; again, elderly patients and those with fragile veins are most at risk.

When these methods fail, applying a warm compress in the form of a heat pack or electric heating blanket or immersing the limb in a bowl of hot water for 10–15 minutes helps to increase vasodilation and promote venous filling (Dougherty 1996, Middleton 1985, Perucca 1995). GTN patches have also been successfully used to aid vasodilation (Gunwardene & Davenport 1990, Hecker et al 1983) as well as reducing the incidence of chemical phlebitis and increasing site survival time (Hecker 1988).

SITE PREPARATION

Asepsis is vital when performing venepuncture or cannulation, as the skin is breached and a foreign object is introduced into a sterile circulating system. The two main sources of microbial contamination are:

- cross-infection from practitioner to patient
- skin flora of the patient (Maki 1991).

It is therefore essential that the nurse employs good hand washing and drying techniques (Hart 1996). In order to adequately clean the skin and remove the risk presented by the skin flora, the patient's skin should be washed with soap and water if visibly dirty (Speechley 1984); then, firm and prolonged rubbing with an antiseptic solution such as chlorhexidine in 70% or 2% aqueous solution is recommended (De Vries 1997, Maki 1991).

The prepared area should be 2–3 inches in diameter and a solution applied with friction from the insertion site outward (Perucca 1995). It is imperative during the skin cleansing procedure not only to use the most effective antiseptic, but also to clean the skin for a long enough period of time – 30 seconds to a minute for peripheral cannulation (Mallett & Bailey 1996, Millam 1992, Rowland 1991, Weinstein 1993). For the antimicrobial solution to be effective and ensure coagulation of the organisms, and to prevent stinging as the needle pierces the skin, the area should be allowed to air dry for a minimum of 30 seconds. Fanning, blowing and blotting of the prepared area are contraindicated.

Skin cleansing is a controversial subject and it is acknowledged that a cursory wipe with an alcohol swab does more harm than no cleaning at all as it disturbs the skin flora (Mallett & Bailey 1996). The skin must not be touched or repalpated once it has been cleaned. If it is necessary to repalpate, then the same cleaning regimen should be repeated.

The question of whether to shave the insertion site remains controversial. Maki (1976) could not demonstrate a relationship between the presence of hair and bacterial counts, and felt the removal of hair was of doubtful value. Weinstein (1993) suggested that shaving might cause microabrasions and therefore encourage microbial growth. She also felt that antiseptics used to clean the skin would also clean the hair. Depilatories are not recommended because of allergic reactions which could cause skin eruptions (Perucca 1995). Electric razors or scissors are acceptable for clipping and removing excess hair but must be cleaned between patients to prevent cross-infection.

SELECTING AN APPROPRIATE ENVIRONMENT

It is important that the patient is provided with privacy, but it may be that the patient wishes to have a friend or relative with them during the procedure for support or distraction (Dougherty 1994). Adequate lighting of the environment is essential for performing accurate venous assessment and achieving successful venepuncture or cannulation. It may be necessary to use a bedside light or to increase the lighting if it is not sufficient.

The next step is to ensure that the patient is in a comfortable position. It is helpful to place a pillow or a rolled towel under the extended arm for support and to provide a firm, flat surface. It is also vital that the nurse is in a comfortable position and it may be necessary to adjust the height or position of the bed or chair to ensure unnecessary bending or twisting.

The temperature of the environment is also a consideration. The room should be warm enough to encourage vasodilation, but if it is too warm, the patient may feel faint. If the room is too cold then the patient's venous access will be more difficult to assess. As Sagar & Bomar (1982) stated:

'A sufficiently warm room not only provides a feeling of comfort to the patients but by promoting dilation and filling of the veins will facilitate selection and entry of the vein.'

APPROACH TO THE PATIENT

How the practitioner approaches the patient may have a direct bearing on that person's response to the venepuncture or cannulation procedure (Weinstein 1993). An efficient, unhurried approach will reinforce the nurses' competence. A nurse who feels unsure of her abilities will transmit that feeling to the patient (Sagar & Bomar 1982). The practitioner should ensure that all the equipment is prepared in advance and is on hand at the patient's bedside, as leaving the room during the procedure to get additional equipment may lead a patient to question the nurse's competence and may promote anxiety as a result.

Once the environment has been prepared, the practitioner must discover if the patient has ever undergone such a procedure before; if not, an explanation should be given and the patient encouraged to ask questions. In order to eliminate fear of the unknown, it may be useful to show the patient what the equipment looks like, as well as providing information about the general aspects of i.v. therapy, drugs, etc. and being honest about the discomfort that may be experienced.

Patients may previously have had a bad experience of venepuncture or cannulation, and as a result may feel anxious prior to insertion. The practitioner should listen to what the patient says about previous experiences and, in order to gain trust and encourage compliance, the patient should be involved in the decision-making. Being offered a choice of where the device is to be sited is important to patients (Dougherty 1994). Even being asked to point out areas to be avoided, such as previous painful sites or areas of poor venous access, represents a degree of choice and patients may feel more in control of their i.v. therapy if they are encouraged to become active participants (Hudek 1986). Mills & Krantz (1979) found that patients given a choice of arm for blood donation showed reduced self-rated discomfort and pain relative to no choice. However, some patients may feel that they are happy to make the choice of which arm to use, but that any more detail should be left to the experts (Dougherty 1994). The final step is encouraging the patients to use individual coping skills, as well as employing interventions such as distraction or relaxation techniques. Only once the patient is fully informed can consent be obtained.

CHOICE OF VEIN

'The choice of vein may be the deciding factor in the success of the infusion and the preservation of veins for future therapy. The most prominent vein is not necessarily the most suitable.' (Weinstein 1993)

It is important to make a full assessment of the patient and his veins before the vein and device are chosen. The main factors which should be considered are the clinical status of the patient, the location and condition of the vein, and the purpose and duration of the therapy.

The clinical status of the patient

Injury or disease may prevent the use of a limb for venepuncture or cannulation for a variety of reasons. There may be a reduction in the venous access due to amputation, fracture or a cerebrovascular accident. Surgery often dictates which arm can be used. Veins should be avoided in the affected arm of an axillary node dissection such as a mastectomy, as the circulation may be impaired. This can lead to impaired lymphatic drainage, which can influence venous flow regardless of whether there is any obvious lymphoedema (Rowland 1991). If it is necessary to cannulate the affected arm, permission should be sought from the doctor and the patient's arm should be closely monitored for any signs of an increase in swelling. An oedematous limb should be avoided as there is danger of stasis of lymph predisposing to complications such as phlebitis and cellulitis (Millam 1992, Rowland 1991).

Positioning of the patient may dictate the site of choice, e.g. if a patient is to be turned on one side during an operation. The upper arm is preferred for an i.v. infusion, as the increased venous pressure in the lower arm may interfere with the free flow of the solution (Weinstein 1993). The placement of a cannula into the affected limb of a patient who has had a cerebrovascular accident is contraindicated. This is due to the reduced or absent neurological sensation in the limb, which prevents the patient from detecting pain as a result of an infiltration or developing phlebitis. There is also often limited venous access because of reduced mobility (Perucca 1995).

An extremity where an arteriofistula or graft is situated should not be used for routine peripheral cannulation. It is usually inserted only for dialysis and requires special consideration when selecting the site. Patients who are in shock or dehydrated will have reduced peripheral circulation, making venous access difficult. Not only do the veins not dilate sufficiently, but they may also collapse more quickly. Patients who are obese tend to have veins located deep in the subcutaneous tissue and fat, making the veins much more difficult to palpate. A hand vein may be the only easily accessible vein (Millam 1992). Malnourished patients may have more obvious venous access; however, there is a lack of subcutaneous support, and the veins may be mobile and more friable.

In the elderly, there is a thinning of elastin fibres in the skin and a loss of subcutaneous supporting tissue. In addition, the skin undergoes a generalized loss of water and loose skin folds appear. There is also a loss of fat on the dorsal aspects of the hands and arms. Veins and bones of the hand become prominent (Whitson 1996) but tend to be tortuous and fragile, have narrow lumens and may be thrombosed.

The type of medication currently being taken by patients may influence the condition of the vein. Those taking anticoagulants or on long-term steroid therapy may present with fragile, friable veins and thin, dry parchment skin, and have the potential to bruise. Another problem may be restriction of a patient's mobility, especially if the best veins for cannulation lead to a patient being unable to use a crutch or other lifting/mobilizing aids. It may also be important to consider which is the dominant arm and if it is more appropriate to use the non-dominant arm.

Type of treatment

The purpose of the therapy and the type of solution/medications to be infused or administered dictate the rate of flow required. If large quantities are to be administered or a solution with a high viscosity, such as packed cells, then a large vein with adequate blood flow will be required. It is also useful to select a large vein when using hypertonic or irritant solutions. These types of solution cause trauma to smaller vessels, leading to phlebitis, as the supply of blood is not sufficient to dilute the drugs (Weinstein 1993). If vesicant drugs are to be administered, small veins or those over joints should be avoided due to the local damage and tissue necrosis which may occur in the event of an extravasation.

Length of therapy

The length of therapy often dictates the choice of vein. It is recommended that the most distal site should be selected for cannulation or venepuncture. If a prolonged course of therapy is required, sites can be maintained for longer by starting at the lowest point of the arm and working upwards. However, patient comfort and co-operation are required and, if infusions or therapy are to be administered over an extended period of time, areas of joint flexion and the dorsal surface of hands should be avoided.

Patient preference

Patients have reported anxiety and pain associated with the location of the cannula (Dougherty 1994). Allowing patients to choose the site may help to reduce anxiety and improve compliance (Hudek 1986). Both Middleton (1985) and Dougherty (1992) stressed the importance of positioning the cannula away from a joint and, where possible, in the non-dominant arm to allow the patient maximum use of the arm. Patients have also identified that the veins in the wrist and the back of the hand are often the most painful and awkward places to have a cannula sited, causing discomfort and restricted movement. Overall, patients prefer the veins of the forearm – they are more convenient, cannulation appears to be less painful, the cannula remains in situ for longer and allows flexion and movement, enabling the performance of normal daily activities (Dougherty 1994).

Location of the vein

The superficial veins of the upper extremities are used for venepuncture and cannulation because they are located just beneath the skin in the superficial fascia (Fig. 2.10, p. 34). Cannulation of the lower extremities is usually avoided due to the risk of complications such as thrombophlebitis and pulmonary embolism (which is caused by a thrombus extending into deep veins). Stagnant blood in varicosities and pooling of infused drugs cause untoward reactions when a toxic concentration reaches the circulating blood (Weinstein 1993). If a cannula is inserted into a lower limb, it should be changed as soon as another more appropriate site can be found. The Center for Disease Control, Atlanta, recommends the use of upper in preference to lower extremity sites in adults for cannulation. If these veins are used, the dorsum of the foot and the saphenous vein of the ankle are the sites of choice (Millam 1992).

Most superficial veins of the upper extremity are available for venepuncture and cannulation but may not be practical for a variety of reasons.

The median cubital veins

The median cubital veins (median cephalic and basilic) in the antecubital fossa are usually selected for venepuncture. Their size and superficial location makes them easy to palpate and they are well supported by muscular and connective tissue. They are chosen for venepuncture because they are capable of providing copious and repeated blood specimens without damage to the vein, providing a good technique is used (Mallett & Bailey 1996). However, for use in cannulation a number of problems are associated with these veins.

Firstly, their location over an area of joint flexion means that any motion could dislodge the cannula and cause infiltration of the infusion fluid, extravasation of the drug or result in mechanical phlebitis (Perucca 1995, Weinstein 1993). However, some authors recommend their use as they are large and will enable large volumes of fluid, viscous solutions or irritant drugs to be rapidly diluted and circulated, thus reducing the risk of chemical phlebitis (Millam 1992).

The joint is a difficult area to splint and the piston-like movement of a device over the joint could lead to the dragging of microorganisms from the skin into the circulation, leading to infection (Goodison 1990a). The general feeling is to avoid the use of the antecubital fossa for long-term cannulae and therapy, as one infusion of a long duration may traumatize the vein, limiting those vessels that most readily provide ample quantities of blood when needed (Weinstein 1993). Also, because of their close proximity to the arteries and nerves (the median cephalic vein crosses the brachial artery), special care must be taken to prevent accidental arterial cannulation.

The cephalic vein

The size and position of the cephalic vein make it an excellent vein for transfusion administration. It readily accommodates a large gauge cannula, and by virtue of its position on the forearm, a natural splint is provided for the cannula (Weinstein 1993). However, its position at a joint may increase complications such as mechanical phlebitis and even general discomfort and patient compliance. The presence of tendons controlling the thumb can lead to these obscuring the vein during insertion of a device (Hadaway 1995), and care must be taken not to hit the radial nerve.

The basilic vein

This is a large vein, which is often overlooked due to its inconspicuous position on the ulnar border of the hand and forearm. It is found on palpation when the patient's arm is placed across the chest, with the practitioner opposite the patient (Hadaway 1995). Venepuncture access can be awkward due to its position and it can be difficult to observe. There is also a tendency for this vein to have many valves, which can hinder the advancement of the cannula. It tends to roll easily and a haematoma may readily occur if the patient flexes his arm, which squeezes blood from the engorged vein into the tissues.

The median veins

The median veins in the wrist may appear to be suitable for venepuncture, but they are usually situated between two branches of the median nerve, which results in extremely painful venepuncture. The veins are thin-walled and small and are associated with bruising, phlebitis and infiltration (Millam 1992). However, the median vein tends to be easy to stabilize and accessible (Hadaway 1995) and can be used if absolutely necessary.

The dorsal venous network

The dorsal venous network of the hand allows for successive sites in proximal locations. They can usually be visualized and palpated easily. The digital veins are small and may be prominent enough to accommodate a small-gauge needle as a last resort for fluid administration, but may be of more use for venepuncture. With adequate taping, the fingers can be immobilized, thus preventing the cannula from piercing the posterior wall of the vein and leading to bruising or infiltration.

The metacarpal veins

The metacarpal veins are accessible, easily visualized and palpated and are well suited for i.v. use, as the device lies flat between the joints and metacarpal bones of the hand, thus providing a natural splint (Weinstein 1993). They tend to be smaller veins than those of the forearm and may prove difficult in infants due to excessive subcutaneous fat. These veins are contraindicated in the elderly as there is diminished skin turgor and loss of subcutaneous tissue, making the vein difficult to stabilize and often take longer to fill (venous distension takes longer due to slower venous return and reduced competence of venous valves), and they are difficult to secure (Whitson 1996). These veins are a better option for short-term or outpatient i.v. therapy.

Condition of the vein

The assessment should start with the visual inspection of both upper limbs, followed by palpation of the veins likely to be used. Visual inspection will enable the practitioner to avoid areas of phlebitis, infection or oedema, bruised or inflamed veins, or any veins which have undergone multiple punctures. If previous phlebitic or infiltrated areas are used for cannulation, accurate site assessments cannot be performed. Also if damaged veins are used, greater injury to the skin and vein will occur (Perucca 1995).

Palpation of the vein is an important assessment tool. It helps to determine if the vein is located in the superficial fascia or deep tissue. Stroking the vein downward and observing the venous refill are helpful in determining the condition of the vein. This procedure also enables the practitioner to differentiate veins from arteries and to locate valves (Weinstein 1993, Dougherty 1996). Palpation should be performed before every cannulation, even if the vein appears large and easy to cannulate. To palpate a vein, place one or two fingers over it and press lightly; then release pressure to assess the vein's elasticity and rebound filling (Millam 1992). Always use the same finger(s) to palpate veins, in order to develop sensitivity for assessing them. Usually the index finger and the third forefinger of the non-dominant hand have the most sensitivity (Perucca 1995); the thumb should not be used as it is not as sensitive and a pulse may be detected which could be confused with an aberrant artery (Weinstein 1993).

An ideal vein feels soft and bouncy as it is palpated. It should refill quickly once it has been depressed and should be straight, visible and well supported (Dougherty 1996). Using veins which are tender, schlerosed, thrombosed, fibrosed or hard is unacceptable and can result in pain and undue stress (Weinstein 1993).

A thrombosed vein may be detected by its lack of resilience and its hard cord-like feeling, and it tends to roll easily.

Arteries tend to be placed much deeper than veins and have thicker, tougher walls. Veins do not pulsate – arteries do! Aberrant arteries pulsate and are located superficially in an unusual location. It is estimated that 1:10 people have an aberrant artery in the antecubital fossa, and they can also frequently occur in the hand or wrist (more commonly on a thin emaciated person) (Perucca 1995). Aberrant arteries should not be used for peripheral cannulation, because if drugs are administered, spasm will result, followed by contraction, necrosis and gangrene. If an artery is cannulated, the patient may complain of severe pain in the hand or arm and bright red blood will be observed.

Valves are folds of epithelium present in larger vessels to prevent backflow of blood into the extremity. They can be detected by a small visible bulge in the vein and on palpation. There is little or no documentation about the specific location of valves, probably due to the great variations among individuals (Hadaway 1995). They tend to occur at points of branching and junctions. Applying a tourniquet impedes venous flow so that when suction is applied (as in blood withdrawal), the valves compress and close the lumen of the vein; this prevents the backward flow of blood and interferes with the process of venepuncture. In palpating the vein and locating the valves, the practitioner can ensure that the needle is placed above a valve to facilitate blood withdrawal. When cannulating, valves can also prevent the advancement of the cannula and, if forced, can cause pain and rupture of the vessel.

DEVICE SELECTION

The practitioner must always select the device to be used only after assessing the condition and accessibility of the individual patient's vein. The selection should be based on:

- the needs of the patient
- the number of samples required
- the use and location of the device
- the type of fluid/drug to be administered (Weinstein 1997).

In general, the smallest gauge needle or cannula possible should be used to prevent damage to the intima of the vein (Perucca 1995, Peters et al 1984, Weinstein 1997). The measurement used for needles and cannulae is standard wire gauge (swg), which measures the internal diameter – the smaller the gauge size, the larger the diameter. Standard wire gauge measurement is determined by how many cannulae fit into a tube with an inner diameter of 1" (1 inch = 25.4 mm) and uses consecutive numbers from 13 to 24 (Mallett & Bailey 1996). Needles tend to be odd-numbered, e.g. 19g, 21g, etc., whilst cannulae are even-numbered, e.g. 18g, 20g, etc. Most manufacturers simply refer to the gauge or the Charriere, commonly known as 'French', which relates directly to catheter size, i.e. 1 Ch = 0.33 mm.

Venepuncture

The device most commonly used to perform venepuncture for blood sampling is a straight steel needle or a steel winged infusion device (see Box 9.2). Either of these can then be attached to a standard syringe or a vacuum system. The optimum gauge for blood sampling is 21g which enables blood to be withdrawn at a reasonable speed without undue discomfort to the patient or possible damage to the blood cells (Mallett & Bailey 1996). However, the choice of whether to use a needle or a winged infusion device, and of which size is the most suitable, is dependent on the patient's venous access and the experience of the practitioner at handling the equipment. The advantages and disadvantages of each system are outlined in Table 9.1.

Vacuum systems

Using a syringe has many inherent problems. The correct syringe size needs to be selected according to the volume of blood required, and if a large volume is required, e.g. 40–50 ml, the syringe may become cumbersome and difficult to manipulate, especially if attached to a straight steel needle. It also leaves the practitioner with the need to decant the blood into bottles, which can increase their risk of spill and contamination by blood.

The vacuum system is a safer system and has increased the efficiency of blood sampling. It consists of a plastic holder which contains or is attached to a sterile disposable double-ended needle or an adaptor. Once the needle is in the vein, the rubber-topped tube is pushed onto the needle and the rubber sheath covering the shaft of the needle is forced back, allowing the blood to flow into the tube. The tube is vacuumed in order that the exact amount of blood required for the test is withdrawn, and the filling ceases once that occurs.

■ BOX 9.2

Procedure for venepuncture (using a winged infusion device)

- Explain the procedure to the patient and give him the opportunity to voice any concerns, express any preferences or ask any questions. Ensure the patient gives his consent; this is usually implied when the patient rolls up his sleeve and places his arm in a position ready for the procedure to be performed. However, the practitioner should also get the patient to verbally consent to the procedure.
- Check the patient's identity by asking for name and date of birth. These must be checked against the information on the request forms. It is vital that the practitioner ensures that the correct samples are taken from the correct patient.
- Gather all the equipment that will be required.
- Wash hands with an appropriate bactericidal solution.
- Position yourself and the patient, ensuring there is adequate lighting and ventilation.
- Apply the tourniquet and use methods to encourage venous access.
- Assess and select the vein, and release the tourniquet.
- Select the device based on the vein size, location, etc.
- Reapply the tourniquet.
- Apply the cleaning solution to the selected vein for a minimum of 30 seconds and allow to air dry. Do not repalpate the vein or touch the skin.
- Remove the device from the packaging and inspect it for any faults.
- Stabilize the vein by applying manual traction on the skin.
- Hold the wings firmly and insert the needle (bevel up) through the skin at the selected angle and observe for backflow of blood into the tubing.
- Level off the needle (by decreasing the angle of the needle to the skin) and advance slightly in order to stabilize the needle within the vein.
- Gently release the skin tension and, if necessary, tape one wing to stabilize the device.
- Attach syringes or vacuumed bottles and withdraw the required volume of blood.
- During filling of the last bottle/syringe, release the tourniquet to decrease the pressure within the vein.
- Place a sterile swab over the insertion site, remove the needle and apply pressure.
- Discard the needle into a designated sharps container.
- Apply firm digital pressure directly over the puncture site until bleeding has ceased.
- Cover with a clean dressing and/or an adhesive plaster to prevent leakage or introduction of bacteria, and advise the patient to keep it in place until healing is complete.
- Transfer blood into bottles where necessary and label all bottles with relevant details.

Samples may be obtained one after another by removing the filled tube and replacing it with another. As the tube is removed the rubber sheath slips back over the needle, preventing blood from leaking into the holder and contaminating the practitioner. This makes it a closed system and there is no risk to the practitioner of contamination during the venepuncture and no need to decant the blood. The exact volumes are obtained and the only items to dispose of are the needle and holder. In

Table 9.1 The choice of device for venepuncture (reproduced with kind permission from Mallett & Bailey 1996)

Device	Swg	Advantages	Disadvantages	Uses
Needle	21	Cheaper than winged infusion devices Easy to use with large veins	Rigid; difficult to manipulate with smaller veins in less conventional sites May cause more discomfort	Large, accessible veins in the antecubital fossa Used when small quantities of blood are to be drawn
Winged infusion device	21	Flexible due to small needle shaft; easy to manipulate and insert at any site Causes less discomfort	More expensive than steel needles	Veins in sites other than ante-culbital fossa Used when quantities of blood greater than 20 ml are required from any site
	23	As above Smaller swg and therefore useful with fragile veins	As above, plus there can be damage to cells which can cause inaccurate measurement, especially if measuring certain blood values, e.g. potassium	Small veins in more painful sites, e.g. inner aspect of the wrist Used especially if measurements are related to plasma and not cellular components

some hospitals, the holders are re-used if no obvious blood contamination is noted, disinfected at the end of the day or discarded after each use.

The disadvantage of this system is that it is more expensive. If the bottles are not vacuumed properly they have to be discarded and the suction in the tubes can sometimes cause collapse of smaller veins, making blood withdrawal more difficult. It is important always to remove the last tube from the holder prior to removing the needle, as it can cause backflow of blood out of the needle, leading to possible contamination of the practitioner.

Winged infusion devices

The steel winged infusion device, commonly referred to as a 'butterfly', is used for venepuncture and short-term intravenous therapy, as well as single-dose medications. The device comprises a steel needle with a pair of flexible wings and plastic tubing. The wings enable the device to be easily grasped during insertion and once placed in the vein, the wings are flattened and provide an anchor for stabilization. The device is available in a variety of gauge sizes – as small as 25swg for use in children – and the tubing is available in various lengths depending on the type of therapy. The steel needle is inflexible and so greatly increases the risk of vein damage, infiltration and extravasation. Tully et al (1981) found, when steel needles were compared with plastic cannulae, that they were significantly associated with infiltrations but that the risk of phlebitis was much lower. Therefore, this device is recommended for non-vesicant therapies only.

■ BOX 9.3

Suggested procedure for cannulation (using the one-handed technique)

- Explain the procedure to the patient and give him the opportunity to voice any concerns, express any preferences or ask any questions. Ensure the patient gives his consent.
- Gather all the equipment that will be required.
- Wash hands with an appropriate bactericidal solution.
- Position yourself and the patient, ensuring there is adequate lighting and ventilation.
- Apply the tourniquet and use methods to encourage venous access.
- Assess and select the vein, and release the tourniquet.
- Select the device based on the vein size, location, etc.
- Open a pack and place a sterile towel under the patient's arm.
- Reapply the tourniquet.
- Apply the cleaning solution to the selected vein for a minimum of 30 seconds and allow to air dry. Do not repalpate the vein or touch the skin.
- Remove the device from the packaging and inspect it for any faults.
- Stabilize the vein by applying manual traction on the skin.
- Ensure the cannula is in the bevel up position and, placing the device directly over the vein, insert the cannula through the skin at the selected angle according to the depth of the vein.
- Wait for the first flashback of blood into the flashback chamber of the stylet.
- Level the device by decreasing the angle between the cannula and the skin and advance the cannula slightly to ensure entry into the lumen of the vein.
- Withdraw the stylet slightly and a second flashback of blood will be seen along the shaft of the cannula.
- Maintaining skin traction with the non-dominant hand, slowly advance the cannula off the stylet and into the vein with the dominant hand.
- Release the tourniquet and apply pressure to the vein above the cannula tip and remove the stylet.
- Dispose of the stylet into an appropriate sharps container.
- Attach an injection cap, extension set or administration set and flush to check patency, observing the site for signs of swelling or leakage, and ask the patient if any discomfort or pain is felt.

Cannulation (Box 9.3)

A cannula is defined as a hollow plastic tube used for accessing the vascular system (Weinstein 1993). The first plastic cannula was introduced in 1945. There are two main types: over the needle and inside the needle. The inside-the-needle type of device (where the device is pushed through the needle until the desired length is within the vein) is not recommended for routine use by the Intravenous Nursing Society, due to the risk of puncture and shearing, and has been superseded by the midline and peripherally inserted central catheters.

The over-the-needle type of cannula is the most commonly used device for peripheral venous access and is available in various gauge sizes, lengths, composition and design features. The cannula is mounted on the needle and once the device is pushed off the needle into the vein, the needle is removed. Nightingale & Bradshaw (1982) listed some of the desirable properties for a peripheral venous cannula (see Box 9.4).

■ BOX 9.4

Properties of a cannula

- Sterility
- Sharp-tipped introducing needle
- Non-toxic/non-irritant material
- Thin walls
- Good flow rates
- Wide range of gauge sizes and lengths
- Easily secured
- Strong, firm components
- Comfortable grip
- Radio-opaque
- Kink recovery
- Non-tapering shaft
- Smooth insertion
- Quick and easily observable flashback

Needle and cannula design

A sharp-tipped introducer facilitates penetration into the vein and the type of graduation from the cannula to the needle can affect the degree of trauma to the vessel and the cannula tip, allowing negligible resistance to tissue penetration. A thin smooth-walled cannula tapering to a scalloped end causes less damage than one which is abruptly cut off.

If the distance from the bevel of the introducing needle to the tip of the cannula is short (less than 1.0 mm), it will minimize the risk of flashback of blood with the needle tip in the vessel lumen and the cannula tip still outside it. The cannula should have a non-tapering shaft in order to reduce the overall size. The incidence of complications such as thrombophlebitis is higher when the tapering portion is inside the lumen of the vein (Nightingale & Bradshaw 1982, Peters et al 1984). Turbulent flow is also decreased with parallel-sided cannulae, which improves flow rates.

It has been shown that the incidence of vascular complications increases as the ratio of cannula external diameter to vessel lumen increases. Therefore, most of the literature recommends the use of the smallest, shortest gauge cannula suitable for any given situation (Lewis & Hecker 1985, Millam 1992, Nightingale & Bradshaw 1982, Perucca 1995, Weinstein 1993). Flow rate through a cannula is related to its internal diameter and is inversely proportional to its length. Therefore, as the length of the cannula increases, so does the likelihood of vascular complications. A large, long device will fill the vessel, preventing good blood flow around it and causing mechanical trauma to the vessel; both factors would contribute to the development of phlebitis.

The walls of the device should therefore be thin to provide a large internal diameter, so that maximum flow rates may be achieved whilst reducing complications (see Table 9.2); note, however, that flow rates vary between different manufacturers. A short bevel reduces the risk of trauma to the endothelial wall of the vein, which could lead to infiltration from a puncture to the posterior wall. When a needle with a long bevel is inserted into the vein, blood may leak into the tissue before the entire bevel is within the lumen of the vein (Weinstein 1993), resulting in haematoma or extravasation.

Material

The ideal material is one that is non-irritant and does not predispose to thrombus

Table 9.2 Gauge sizes and average flow rates (using water)

Gauge	Flow rate (ml/min)	General uses
14g	350	Used in theatres or emergency for rapid transfusion of blood or viscous fluids
16g	215	As 14g
18g	104	Blood transfusions, PN, stem cell harvesting and cell separation, large volumes of fluids
20g	62	Blood transfusions, large volumes of fluids
22g	35	Blood transfusions, most medications and fluids
24g	24	Medications, short-term infusions, fragile veins, children

formation (Payne-James et al 1991). Ideally it should be radio-opaque or contain a stripe of radio-opaque material for radiographic visualization. Much controversy exists over the advantages and disadvantages of the available cannula material (Perucca 1995), which ranges from polyvinylchloride and Teflon to various polyurethane and elastomeric hydrogel materials. There are certain properties of materials that increase the risk of thrombogenicity and bacterial colonization.

Surface irregularities These are created during manufacturing and consist of pits, ridges and grooves. They are usually revealed by scanning with an electron microscope. These defects act as ideal sites for bacterial colonization and may cause turbulent flow. This in turn enhances platelet adhesion, platelet disintegration and thrombogenesis, leading to thrombophlebitis.

Chemical composition It appears that bacteria have affinities for certain materials, in particular certain types of synthetic polymer; this affinity is lowest in steel. This was demonstrated by Maki (1976) who found that the incidence of bacteraemia was lowest when steel needles were used (0.2%), while plastic cannula rates ranged from 0 to 8%. Crow (1987) also suggested that some plastic catheters actually appeared to promote the growth of organisms such as *Staphylococcus epidermidis*.

Flexibility There may be enhancement of the flexibility of a material in fluids at body temperature. Absorption of water by the cannula material enhances its plasticity and therefore makes it less likely to cause mechanical trauma (McKee et al 1989).

Recent studies have compared the different types of material available, such as Teflon and Vialon, with a view to finding the material with the lowest potential risk for phlebitis. Gaukroger et al (1988) carried out a randomized, controlled trial ($n = 645$) comparing Teflon and Vialon cannulae. They found an overall thrombophlebitis rate of 51.9%, with Vialon at 40.9% and Teflon at 63.5% ($P < 0.001$), using the Dinley grading scale. However, it appeared that the phlebitis scores for both types of device increased with the duration of infusion. This result was also reflected in studies by McKee et al (1989) and Kerrison & Woodhull (1994). By contrast, Payne-James et al (1991) found that, although Vialon was theoretically superior as a cannula material, under controlled conditions there appeared to be little difference in the capacity of both materials to cause thrombophlebitis. It must be noted that studies comparing catheter materials often use different phlebitis scales and calculations for creating a total score for each device. Other variables to consider are the differences in catheter size, skin preparation, the use of dressings and the type of solution being infused.

Sterility and packaging

All packaging should be inspected for integrity before use and when opened should enable the practitioner to maintain sterility prior to insertion. The device itself should also be inspected to ensure that it is complete, there are no barbs and the needle is not bent in any way. Some manufacturers suggest that the stylet is twisted to release the cannula and make advancement off the needle into the vein easier. All components and connections should be checked to ensure they are firmly fixed.

Flashback chamber

The flashback chamber is an important aspect of the cannula as it is this which allows the practitioner a visual sign of success on insertion of the device. The flashback should be quick and easily seen in the chamber, but not so rapid that it leaks from the end of the hub. Some devices have small plugs on the end of the chamber which prevent blood spills.

Grip

The practitioner should be able to perform the cannulation smoothly and comfortably, so the design of the cannula for grip is also important. Some devices have a fingerguard to help stabilize the device which also helps with the advancement of the device into the vein.

Other features

It is vital that the cannula can be easily secured to the skin to reduce piston-like movement within the vein and prevent accidental removal. Some devices have wings which can help with securing.

Other devices have ports for intermittent injections. There has always been controversy attached to ported devices and their use is favoured more in Europe than in the USA. The advantage of such a device is the ability to administer drugs without interfering with continuous infusion. However, the caps are often not replaced properly, leaving the system exposed to contamination and at risk of air entering (although this seems highly unlikely). The ports have also been found to be inadequately sterilized with a swab, as there is no flat surface. These devices may also tempt the practitioner into not removing the dressing and inspecting the site but merely administering the drug via the port. Opinion is divided as to the risk of infection associated with ported devices (Cheeseborough & Finch 1984) and it has been recommended that side ports, if used, should be equipped with a bacterial filter (Brismar et al 1984).

Midline catheters

The midline catheter is a more recent introduction to the peripheral venous access range. There are over-the-needle and through-the-needle designs. Midline catheters provide venous accessibility along with an easy and hazard-free insertion (Box 9.5). The catheter is introduced into an antecubital vein with the tip extending into the upper arm. As the catheter is in a larger vein, it is useful for patients who are requiring frequent resites of their peripheral cannula or who have exhausted their lower arm peripheral veins, or those who present with poor venous access, but who do not require a central venous catheter. The device can stay in situ for weeks or even months depending on the type of material.

Benefits to the patients include less frequent resiting of the device and a reduction in associated venous trauma (Mallet & Bailey 1996). The main problem associated with these devices is the risk of mechanical phlebitis, which usually occurs within the first week following insertion. This can be resolved by close observation, resting

■ **BOX 9.5**

Midline catheter insertion

- Explain the procedure to the patient and give him the opportunity to voice any concerns, express any preferences or ask any questions. Ensure the patient gives his consent.
- Gather all the equipment that will be required.
- Wash hands with an appropriate bactericidal solution.
- Position the patient by fully extending the arm and abducting at a 45° angle.
- Apply the tourniquet and use methods to encourage venous access.
- Assess and select the vein. The vein site should be two to three finger breadths above or one finger breadth below the bend of the elbow (antecubital fossa). The basilic is better as it tends to be straighter and larger. Release the tourniquet.
- Measure from the selected insertion site to the axilla.
- Select the gauge size based on the vein size, location, etc.
- Open a sterile pack and place a sterile towel under the patient's arm.
- Apply sterile gloves.
- Cut the catheter to the desired length.
- Apply the cleaning solution to the selected vein, working outwards to an area of 4–5" in diameter for 1 minute and allow to air dry.
- Remove and discard gloves. Do not repalpate the vein or touch the skin.
- Reapply the tourniquet.
- Don a second pair of sterile gloves.
- Drape the arm with a fenestrated drape.
- Stabilize the vein – the veins above the antecubital fossa tend to be deeper and more mobile.
- Insert introducer needle and, once flashback is observed, advance into the vein until stabilized.
- Release the tourniquet.
- Apply digital pressure on the vein above the tip of the introducer needle and remove the stylet.
- Insert the catheter and advance slowly through the introducer until it reaches the desired length.
- Do not force the catheter; if any resistance is encountered, reposition the patient's arm at a different angle, rotate the wrist or get the patient to open and close the fist. Apply a heat pack above the insertion site (Perucca 1995).
- Remove the guidewire and attach flushing solution.
- Flush the catheter with sodium chloride 0.9% and check for patency, discomfort and swelling.
- Gently retract the introducer and remove according to manufacturer's instructions.
- Secure the device and apply a dressing.
- It may be necessary to instruct the patient to keep his arm straight and rest it for about 1 hour.

the limb and the use of heat. However, if it does not resolve, it will become necessary to remove the catheter and resite it in another vein, preferably in the opposite arm if possible. It has been suggested that the more skilled the practitioner in placing these devices, the longer they remain in situ and the fewer complications they present. X-ray verification of the tip is not required and it is because of this that some institutions do not recommend that vesicant drugs are administered via this type of catheter. This is because of the risk of extravasation, which would not be easily detected.

TECHNIQUES USED DURING INSERTION

Stabilizing the vein

Skin stabilization is one of the most important elements for successful venepuncture or cannulation (Perucca 1995). Superficial veins tend to roll, and to prevent this, the vein must be anchored in a taut, distended and stable position. The wrist and hands are flexible and so hand veins are often easier to immobilize than veins in the forearm (Millam 1993).

Veins are stabilized by applying traction to the side of the insertion site or below it using the non-dominant hand. This will also provide counter-tension, which will facilitate a smoother needle entry. Where and how traction is applied will depend on the vein and the preference of the practitioner.

Various methods can be used. The thumb can be used to stretch the skin downwards or the hand of the practitioner can be placed under the patient's arm and traction applied with the thumb and forefinger on either side, creating an even traction. Also, a vein can be stretched between forefinger and thumb, but this can cause problems for the trainee. Draping the hand over a pillow will create a degree of tension in the skin and help to stabilize hand veins. Problems arise when the thumb is too close to the venepuncture site and prevents the correct angle of approach; and sometimes, once the skin has been pulled taut, the position of the vein alters slightly to the side of the vessel and necessitates relocation.

Stabilization of the vein must be maintained throughout the procedure until the needle or cannula is successfully sited. If the tension is released halfway through the procedure, it can result in the needle penetrating the opposite wall of the vein and causing a haematoma formation.

Device placement

It is important that the needle enters the skin with the bevel up. This is to aid a smooth venepuncture, as the sharpest part of the needle will penetrate the skin first and will produce less trauma to the skin and vein. It also reduces the risk of piercing the vein's posterior wall (Weinstein 1997). The method of inserting the needle bevel down to prevent extravasation in small veins is described by Weinstein (1993), but this is not a commonly used or recommended technique.

The angle of the needle varies with the type of device used and the depth of the vein in the subcutaneous tissue. The literature recommends a range of 10–45° (Millam 1992, Perucca 1995, Weinstein 1997). A vein located superficially, such as a hand vein, certainly requires a smaller angle of approach, whilst a large or deeply placed vein will require a greater angle. Once the device is in the vein, the angle will always be reduced in order to prevent puncturing the posterior wall of the vein (Perucca 1995).

The approach to the vein can be accomplished using either the direct or indirect method. The direct method is when the device enters the skin directly into the vein. The advantage is that the vein is entered immediately. However, with small, fragile veins, this method may lead to the vein bruising more easily or puncturing of the posterior wall. For these types of vein, the indirect method may be preferable. To achieve this, the device is inserted through the skin, then the vein is relocated and the device advanced into the vein. It is a form of tunnelling and may be useful in veins which are palpable and visible for only a short section. This method enables a more gentle entry and thus reduces trauma to the vein.

Flashback into the tubing of a winged infusion device or into the flashback chamber of a cannula is an indication that the initial entry into the vein has been successful. This may be accompanied by a popping or 'giving way' sensation felt by the practitioner (and sometimes the patient). This is felt when there is resistance from the vein wall as the device enters the lumen of the vein. It tends to be more obvious when inserting devices into large, strong-walled veins and more difficult to discern in thin-walled veins with a small blood volume (Millam 1992). If the device punctures the posterior wall, the flashback will stop. However, it must be remembered that with small-gauge cannula or hypotensive patients, the flashback may be slow, due in the latter case to the lower blood pressure.

Advancing the device

During venepuncture, once the needle has successfully entered the vein, it needs only to be advanced slightly in order to stabilize it and prevent dislodgement during blood sampling. The distance it should be advanced will depend on the length of the needle and the size and position of the vein.

There are several methods of advancing the cannula into the vein. It should be advanced gently and smoothly and the technique will often depend on how the practitioner was taught, although for the student, it may be necessary to try other approaches in order to find the most suitable.

- *The one-handed technique*. This is the most common method used by nurses (see Box 9.3). The same hand which performs cannulation also withdraws the stylet and advances the cannula into the vein. This allows skin traction to be maintained while the device is advanced and, if the patient is uncooperative, enables the practitioner to hold onto the patient's arm.
- *The one-step technique*. In this case, when the cannula has entered the vein, the practitioner slides it off the stylet in one movement. The disadvantage with this method is that the stylet must remain completely still in order to prevent damage to the vein. It is best accomplished on a straight vein and is more helpful if the cannula has a small fingerguard which can be used to 'push' the cannula off.
- *'Floating'*. Floating the cannula into the vein is useful if the device comes up against a valve. Once the device has entered the vein, advancement is usually prevented and then the stylet can be removed and a syringe or an infusion of sodium chloride 0.9% can be attached; as the fluid opens the valve, the device can be advanced and 'floated' into the vein.
- *The two-handed technique*. This is when the practitioner uses one hand to perform the cannulation and then releases skin traction to use the hand to hold and withdraw the stylet, while the dominant hand advances the cannula off the stylet. Millam (1992) suggested that this method prevents blood spill, but it requires the release of skin traction which can often lead to the puncturing of the posterior vein wall, particularly in mobile or fragile veins. It may be an easier technique to learn but is not recommended unless the vein is straight, large and well supported by subcutaneous tissue.

Once the cannula is advanced into the vein, the tourniquet should be released. Then, using a finger just above the location of the tip of the cannula, apply pressure (to prevent blood spillage) and remove the stylet completely. An injection cap or administration set can then be attached.

If the cannulation is unsuccessful, the stylet should never be reintroduced into the cannula. The result of this could be shearing or puncturing of the cannula wall, which could lead to pieces of cannula breaking off and causing an embolism. A new device should be used for each venepuncture or cannulation. It is bad practice to re-use equipment, for a number of reasons:

- The needle has become contaminated; although the skin has been cleaned, there is still the opportunity for any microorganisms on the skin or just below the skin to contaminate the device.

- The needle will not be sharp and cannula tip fraying may occur.
- If there is blood in the flashback chamber or tubing, it will make it difficult to assess success on the second attempt.

If bruising occurs during the procedure, the tourniquet should be released immediately and the device removed and pressure applied to prevent haematoma formation. If the tourniquet is reapplied to the same arm too soon after a venepuncture, a haematoma will form.

REMOVAL OF NEEDLE

On completion of venepuncture, pressure should not be applied until the needle has been fully removed or it will cause the needle to be dragged out of the vein, causing pain and venous damage. Once a needle or cannula has been removed, firm digital pressure should be applied over the puncture site. This is to prevent leakage and haematoma formation. In some patients, it may take longer for bleeding to cease, especially if the patient is on medication which interferes with clotting mechanisms, e.g. warfarin or heparin, or if their disease predisposes them to bleeding, e.g. thrombocytopenia or haemophilia. Weinstein (1993) instructs patients to elevate the arm which causes a negative pressure in the vein, collapsing it and facilitating clotting, although it is not recommended in cardiac patients. In the past, patients were also encouraged to apply pressure and bend the arm when the venepuncture had been performed in the antecubital veins. Dyson & Bogod (1987) found that flexing the elbow after venepuncture produced visible bruising compared with subjects who kept their arm straight. They concluded that the common practice of flexing the elbow after venepuncture was not an efficient way of preventing bruising in the antecubital fossa. It has also been suggested that the practitioner should apply the pressure, rather than the patient, as this also reduces the incidence of bruising (Godwin et al 1992). The nurse should remain with the patient until bleeding has stopped and only then should a dressing be applied.

SECURING DEVICE

It is important on completion of a successful cannulation that the device is secured to prevent mechanical phlebitis and accidental dislodgement. Clean tape may be used, providing it does not come into contact with the insertion site as this may contaminate and obscure the site, making observations for early signs of phlebitis difficult (Fig. 9.1). The cannula may then be dressed using a recognized dressing such as dry sterile gauze or a transparent dressing (Maki & Ringer 1987). Any tubing should also be taped to prevent pulling on the cannula. If the device is located over a joint, or in an uncooperative, confused patient or child, the joint should be splinted to prevent movement and possible dislodgement. The use of the correct type of splint is important. The choice will depend on the type of joint being splinted, e.g. elbow or wrist. Complications such as contracture, particularly in patients with oedema and muscle weakness, can arise if hands are not correctly immobilized on a splint in order to ensure a functional position (Weinstein 1997).

CARE OF THE DEVICE

Once sited and dressed, the cannula should be flushed with either a solution of sodium chloride 0.9% or heparinized saline. The frequency and type of solution

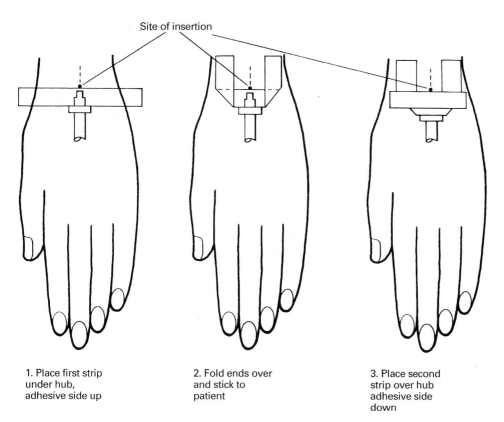

Site of insertion

1. Place first strip
under hub,
adhesive side up

2. Fold ends over
and stick to
patient

3. Place second
strip over hub
adhesive side
down

Fig. 9.1 Taping a peripheral cannula. (After Mallett & Bailey 1996.)

are still in question (Goode et al 1991), but most authors agree that it is the technique that ensures patency of the device (Baranowski 1993, INS 1998, Kamitomo & Olson 1996, Mallett & Bailey 1996, Shearer 1987). The recommended technique is to use turbulent flow (brisk flush), achieved by a push–pause method, and to complete with a positive pressure (achieved by maintaining pressure on the plunger of the syringe whilst removing the needle from the injection cap) (Perucca 1995).

RESITING/REMOVAL OF CANNULA

It has been recommended that peripheral cannulae should be resited every 48–72 hours to reduce the risk of phlebitis (Goodinson 1990b). However, this may be difficult to achieve in certain groups, such as oncology or paediatric patients. In these cases, it may be preferable to ensure careful monitoring of the site, and to remove and resite the cannula at the first indications of tenderness, infiltration or phlebitis. The device should be removed carefully, using slow, steady movement and keeping the hub parallel to the skin, in order to prevent damage to the vein. Pressure should then be applied for at least 1 minute, and the site covered with a sterile dressing. The sites should be alternated whenever possible to allow time for cannula sites to rest and recover, and for any local complications (e.g. phlebitis or infiltration) to resolve. On removal, the cannula integrity should be checked, as well as its length to ensure that the complete device has been removed.

SAFETY OF THE PRACTITIONER

While performing venepuncture or cannulation, both of which are invasive and potentially hazardous procedures, manual dexterity is required. Practitioners may feel that this, along with sensitivity, is reduced when wearing gloves (BMA 1991). The Department of Health (1990) have recommended that gloves should be worn in the following circumstances:

- when the practitioner is inexperienced in venepuncture
- when the practitioner has cuts or abrasions on the hands which cannot be covered by a dressing alone
- when the patient is restless and there is risk of a blood spill
- when the patient is known to be infected with HIV or hepatitis.

It must always be remembered that whilst the use of gloves will protect practitioners against unexpected spill or contamination, they will not prevent a needlestick injury if practice is not safe. The solution is to use a good technique at all times.

Systems are now available that reduce the risk of accidental needlestick injury, e.g. vacuum collection systems, needleless injection caps and retracting stylets on cannulae, and these should be used wherever possible.

PROBLEM-SOLVING TECHNIQUES

Anxious patient

Some patients may be anxious prior to venepuncture or cannulation because of:

- previous traumatic experiences
- fear of needles or blood
- ignorance about what the procedure involves.

Prevention

- Approach the patient in a calm and confident manner.
- Explain what the procedure involves and show them the equipment if appropriate.
- Offer the patient the opportunity to lie down or recline during the procedure.
- Use all methods of improving venous dilation to ensure success on the first attempt.
- Listen to the patient's previous experiences and involve him in site selection.

It may be necessary to refer the patient if anxiety and fear are of phobic proportions.

Difficulty in locating a suitable vein

Some patients may have limited venous access due to:

- excessive previous use
- shock or dehydration
- anxiety
- fragile, thready veins, e.g. in the elderly or in patients on anticoagulant therapy
- thrombosed veins as a result of treatments, e.g. cytotoxic therapy.

Prevention

- Alternate sites wherever possible to avoid overuse of certain veins.
- Use the methods described above to reduce anxiety.

Action

- Reassure the patient.
- Use all methods of improving venous access before attempting the procedure.
- Do not attempt the procedure unless you are experienced.

Spurt of blood on entry

When the bevel enters a large or superficial vein, before the entire bevel is under the skin it may result in a small spurt of blood on the patient's skin and cause a small blood blister.

Prevention

- Select a less superficial vein where possible.
- Enter the vein smoothly and without hesitation.

Action

Reassure the patient that there is nothing to be concerned about, and wipe away any blood after removal of the needle.

Missing the vein on insertion of the needle

The needle fails to be inserted directly into the vein due to:

- inadequate anchoring
- collapse of the vein
- incorrect position of practitioner or patient
- inadequate palpation
- poor vein choice
- lack of concentration
- failure to penetrate the vein properly due to incorrect insertion angle.

Prevention

- Ensure good position and lighting.
- Better preparation and concentration.
- Use good technique and accurate vein selection.

Action

- Withdraw the needle and manoeuvre gently to realign it and correct the angle of insertion.
- Check during manoeuvring that the patient is not feeling any pain.
- If the patient complains of pain, remove the needle.
- If unsuccessful then remove the needle.
- Where necessary, pass to a colleague with more experience.

Blood stops flowing through the device

In this case, blood flashback is seen and then the blood stops flowing due to:

- venospasm
- bevel of needle up against a valve
- penetration of the posterior vein wall by the device
- possible vein collapse.

Prevention

- Try to locate valves prior to insertion and insert the device just above the valve.
- Carefully level off once in the vein to prevent penetration.
- Use a good angle of approach to the vein.

Action

- Massage the veins above the needle tip to pull blood into the vein.
- Release and tighten the tourniquet.
- Gently stroke the vein above the needle to relieve venous spasm.
- Withdraw the needle slightly to move the bevel away from the valve.
- If the vein wall is penetrated, remove the device.

Difficulty in advancing

On advancing the needle/cannula, the practitioner may have difficulty, which could be due to:

- stopping too soon after insertion
- removing the stylet too far and being unable to advance the cannula which is now no longer rigid enough to be advanced
- encountering a valve
- not releasing the cannula from the needle prior to insertion
- poor anchoring or stretching of the skin
- releasing the tourniquet too soon, causing the vein to collapse.

Prevention

- Ensure the tourniquet remains sufficiently tight until insertion is completed.
- Ensure the cannula is released from the stylet prior to insertion, to allow for smooth advancement.
- Ensure that a sufficient length of the cannula is inserted into the vein before stylet withdrawal.
- Use good technique.
- Assess the vein accurately, observing for valves, and avoid where possible.

Action

- In the event of early stylet removal or encountering a valve, connect a syringe of sodium chloride 0.9%, flush the cannula and advance at the same time in an effort to 'float' the device into the vein.
- Tighten the tourniquet and wait for vein to refill.

Difficulty in flushing once the cannula is in situ

Sometimes, the cannula has been successfully inserted, but on checking patency by flushing, the practitioner has difficulty because:

- the cannula tip is up against the valve
- the cannula has pierced the posterior wall of the vein
- the cannula tip is resting on the wall of the vein
- there is an occlusion.

Prevention

- Avoid areas along the vein where there may be valves.
- Ensure careful insertion to prevent puncturing the posterior wall of the vein.

Action

- Withdraw the cannula slightly to move it away from the vein wall or valve and attempt to flush.
- If the vein wall is pierced, remove the cannula.
- Attempt to withdraw the clot and clear the occlusion.

COMPLICATIONS

Pain

Pain can be caused by any of the following:

- tentative stop–start insertion (often a problem with hesitant or new practitioners)
- hitting an artery, nerve or valve
- poor technique – inadequate anchoring causes skin to gather as the needle is inserted
- alcohol is not allowed to dry adequately before insertion, resulting in stinging pain
- using a frequently punctured, recently used or bruised vein
- anxious patient, may have low pain threshold
- use of large-gauge device
- use of veins in sensitive areas.

Prevention

- Use methods to relax and relieve anxiety.
- Avoid use of bruised, used or sensitive areas.
- Use local anaesthetic creams or injections.
- Ensure good technique is employed.

Action

- Reassure the patient and explain, especially in the case of nerve pain, that it may last for a few hours.
- Depending on the cause (e.g. nerve or artery), it may be necessary to remove the device immediately.
- Document the incident.

Haematoma

This is bruising which occurs during the insertion procedure or after removal. It can be caused by:

- failure to remove the tourniquet promptly or before removing needle
- penetration of the posterior vein wall
- incorrect choice of needle to vein size
- fragile veins
- patients receiving anticoagulant therapy
- spontaneous rupture of the vessel on application of the tourniquet or cleaning of the skin
- inadequate pressure on venepuncture site.

Prevention

- Remove the tourniquet before removing the needle.

- Use good vein and device selection.
- Employ careful technique.
- Be aware of patients with fragile veins or those on anticoagulant therapy.
- Apply adequate pressure on removal of the needle/device.
- Do not apply the tourniquet to a limb where recent venepuncture has occurred.
- Do not leave the tourniquet for any longer than is essential.

Action

- Remove the needle immediately.
- Apply pressure to the site for a few minutes.
- Elevate the extremity if appropriate.
- Reassure the patient and explain the reason for the bruise.
- Apply a pressure dressing if required.
- Apply an ice pack if bruising is extensive.
- Do not reapply the tourniquet to the affected limb.
- Document the incident.

Syncope/vasovagal reaction

Patients may feel faint, light-headed, sweaty, hot, cold or nauseated (Pavlin et al 1993) or go on to a vasovagal reaction which is characterized by bradycardia and hypotension (Kaloupek et al 1985). It can be caused by:

- fear of needles or blood
- a hot stuffy environment
- feeling very hungry
- being pregnant
- feeling unwell.

Prevention

- The practitioner should have a confident reassuring manner and approach.
- A facility for the patient to lie down during the procedure should be available.
- Spend time prior to the procedure discussing fears and anxieties with the patient.
- Be aware of which patients are more vulnerable.

Action

- The patient who feels faint should be encouraged to put his head between his legs; this may be difficult especially if the patient has the device in the vein.
- Try to get the patient to lie down.
- If the patient faints then the vein will collapse; therefore it may be useful to secure the device in case the patient requires any medication as a result of a reaction, so that it can be used once the patient has recovered.
- It may be necessary to remove the device and resite it once the patient has recovered.
- Document the incident.

Hitting an artery

This is characterized by pain and a spurt of bright red blood caused by accidental puncture of an artery.

Prevention

Adequate assessment and recognition of arteries prior to performing the procedure will help to prevent the occurrence.

Action

- Remove the device immediately and apply pressure to the puncture site for up to 5 minutes.
- Reassure the patient.
- Do not reapply the tourniquet to the affected limb.
- Document the incident.

Hitting a nerve

If a nerve is accidentally hit on insertion of the needle into the vein, this will result in severe shooting pain (Yuan & Cohan 1987).

Prevention

Prevention is achieved by ensuring that the location of superficial nerves is known.

Action

- The needle should be removed immediately.
- Reassure the patient and explain that the pain may last for a few hours and the area may feel numb. Explain that the pain can sometimes last for a few days and that, if it continues or gets worse, medical advice should be sought.
- Document the incident.

BLOOD TESTS

Blood tests are routinely performed to:

- indicate relatively common disorders
- enable diagnosis
- follow the course of a disease
- regulate therapy (Weinstein 1993).

Each blood test requires a different type of tube which contains a specific additive to enable the serum or plasma to be analysed or the blood to be collected in an anti-coagulated form or as a clotted sample (see glossary of terms in Box 9.6). It is important, following collection of blood, that the specimen tubes are inverted to mix the blood with the additives (Noe & Rook 1994). However, excessive agitation of the sample may alter the test results (Cella & Watson 1989).

General sources of variability

Increased capillary hydrostatic pressure can cause water to shift from the intravascular to the interstitial space. This increases the concentration of the constituents of blood, a process called haemoconcentration. It can result from a systemic increase in capillary pressure such as that seen with prolonged standing and from local effects such as prolonged application of the tourniquet during venepuncture. Therefore, the time of standing prior to venepuncture and the time of tourniquet application should both be kept to a minimum. The recommendation for tourniquet application is not more than 1 minute prior to venepuncture and not more than 2–3 minutes for the entire procedure (Cella & Watson 1989).

Rapid flow of blood through small-bore needles, especially if exposed to large negative pressures, leads to haemolysis. This can be minimized by the use, where possible, of large-bore needles, moderate flow rates and moderate negative pressures. Blood samples may become contaminated with infusion fluid and therefore blood should not be taken from a site above an infusion, but where feasible should

■ **BOX 9.6**

Glossary of terms used in blood sample analysis

- *Anticoagulated blood* – sample of blood collected in a tube containing an anticoagulant such as EDTA or lithium heparin, which prevents the blood from clotting
- *Clotted blood* – sample of blood collected in a plain glass or plastic tube and allowed to clot
- *Blood serum* – extracellular fluid of clotted blood, i.e. the fluid that remains when the cellular elements of clotted blood have been removed
- *Blood plasma* – extracellular fluid of anticoagulated blood, i.e. the fluid that remains when the cellular elements of anticoagulated blood have been removed
- *Haemolysis* – the rupture of red cell membranes causing release of haemoglobin, which can occur if blood is withdrawn through a very small-gauge needle or if withdrawal is very slow and prolonged

be obtained from a site in the opposite arm or below the infusion site (Noe & Rook 1994). Some institutions advise that the infusion should be switched off for a certain period of time prior to taking blood from the arm with an infusion. However, there appears to be no defined time and care must be taken that the cannula does not become occluded during this period.

Equipment

The vacuumed tubes often used for collecting samples of venous blood come in various sizes appropriate to the age of the patient and the type of laboratory analysis. The colour of the top or stopper usually indicates the presence and type of additive. Care must be taken to ensure that the correct tube is used for the test to be performed.

If a needle and syringe are used, when decanting the blood into the sample tube, it should be allowed to flow gently down the inside of the tube. If using vacuumed bottles, a 21g or larger needle should be used to prevent haemolysis (Cella & Watson 1989).

Haematology tests

The full blood count is the most commonly requested and performed blood test. It is not one but rather a group of tests, including the following:

- a count of the cellular elements of blood – red blood cells, white blood cells and platelets
- the measurement of haemoglobin concentration in the blood
- assessment of size and appearance of the cells.

It is generally used to investigate anaemia, but in the oncology setting is used extensively to assess leucopenia and thrombocytopenia (Higgins 1995a).

Method of collection

Blood for a full blood count is usually collected in a tube which contains K2 EDTA. Screening for haemostasis and thrombosis, as well as anticoagulant control, is carried out using a bottle containing citrate. In all of these tests, it is vital that the correct volume of blood is withdrawn into the bottle or the results can be inaccurate.

Measurement to evaluate fluid and electrolyte status

Electrolyte imbalances are serious complications in the critically ill patient and must be recognized and corrected immediately. Levels of potassium, sodium, calcium, chlorides and phosphorus are all measured and their accuracy is largely dependent on the proper collection and handling of the samples.

Method of collection

Potassium Alterations can occur due to any of the following:

- A tight tourniquet and vigorous opening and closing of the fist can elevate the potassium by 27 mEq/L (Cella & Watson 1989, Weinstein 1993).
- Haemolysis should be prevented as this releases potassium from blood cells into serum and causes elevation in serum potassium levels.
- Leucocytes and platelets are rich in potassium and, at high levels, can release potassium during the clotting process.

Calcium Variations in sample collection technique can also affect the results. Acid–base changes can occur from prolonged tourniquet application and variations in the amount of heparin in the collecting bottle/syringe can alter the measured calcium ions.

Liver function tests

These tests may be useful in diagnosing kidney and liver disease or in determining the effectiveness of treatment; they include albumin, globulin and total protein. Bilirubin tests differentiate between impairment of the liver by obstruction and haemolysis.

Kidney function tests

Creatinine and blood urea nitrogen are both used to measure kidney function.

Blood sugar tests

The test for blood sugar is used to detect any disorders of glucose metabolism; for example, raised levels may indicate diabetes or chronic liver disorder, and low levels may indicate overdose of insulin, tumours of the pancreas or insufficiency of the endocrine glands (Weinstein 1993).

Fasting blood sugar usually requires the patient to fast for 8 hours before the blood is taken. It must be remembered that results will be elevated above baseline if the patient is receiving parenteral glucose, regardless of the site from which the sample is withdrawn.

Glucose tolerance tests involve a fasting blood sugar, followed by the patient drinking a quantity of glucose; blood and urine samples are then taken at 30, 60, 90, 120 and 180 minutes after ingestion of the glucose.

Acid–base balance and enzymes

When deviations occur in the normal acid–base ratio, a change in pH results and is accompanied by a change in bicarbonate concentration.

Method of collection

Carbon dioxide measurement is performed by collecting the blood in a heparinized syringe which is put immediately on ice; a heparinized tube; or a dry tube without any anticoagulant. The containers should always be filled to the top with blood and it is important that the patient avoids clenching the fist. This is because muscular activity in the arm raises carbon dioxide levels in the blood (Weinstein 1993).

Acidity (pH) is measured once blood has been collected in a heparinized 2 ml syringe which is capped off or in a vacuumed bottle containing heparin. It should not be agitated and should be packed in ice after collection.

Enzymes Tests such as amylase, acid and alkaline phosphatase, AST, ALT and LDH will be inaccurate if the sample is haemolysed.

Blood typing

Blood typing is a common test required to be carried out on all blood donors and all patients who may require a blood transfusion. The ABO system denotes four main groups – A, B, AB, O – and the antigens such as D, E, C, etc. belong to the Rh system. Other tests include direct or indirect Coombs' tests (Weinstein 1993).

Identification of the patient and clear and correct labelling of the sample bottle and request form are essential. The patient must give his full name and date of birth, and the sample and form must be signed by the practitioner collecting the blood.

Method of collection

Venous blood is collected and allowed to clot. Usually one bottle is enough, but occasionally the laboratory may request two or three samples to be collected.

Antibiotic assays

Some antibiotics, e.g. vancomycin and aminoglycosides, are potentially nephrotoxic and ototoxic. Therefore, patients receiving these drugs should have serum sent regularly for antimicrobial assay. The purpose is to avoid toxic accumulation and to check that therapeutic levels are being achieved.

Method of collection

Levels should be sent every 2–3 days or daily in the presence of marked renal failure. Pre-dose levels are taken just before administration of the antibiotic. Post-dose levels are usually taken 1 hour after bolus injection or the end of an infusion. It is important that the samples are taken at standardized times so that the results can be interpreted accurately and the dosage adjusted accordingly.

Serum samples of blood should be collected in a plain tube, usually 10 ml directly from a vein. Neither pre- nor post-dose levels should be taken from a cannula or catheter because the device may have been contaminated by previous administration of antibiotic.

Blood cultures

This test is usually performed during febrile illnesses and when a patient is having chills with a spiking fever. The number of bacteria in the blood of an infected individual is too low for visual confirmation of bacteraemia, so a blood culture sample may be taken in order to culture the bacteria in a nutrient solution (which rapidly increases the number of any bacteria present) to enable identification of microorganisms (Higgins 1995b, Weinstein 1993).

Most laboratories provide two bottles for blood cultures. One is for culturing aerobic bacteria and has oxygen in the headspace above the liquid media. The second has a gas mixture and no oxygen, for culture of anaerobic species (Higgins 1995b).

Method of collection

Blood for cultures must be taken from a peripheral vein and not from an indwelling cannula or catheter, which might itself be contaminated. The only exception is when it is the cannula or catheter which is suspected of being the cause of infection. This would necessitate obtaining two sets of cultures: one from the catheter/cannula and one from a peripheral vein. Both sets should be clearly marked with the site from which they were taken. It is also important to sample blood before administration of antibiotics, otherwise the bacteraemia is suppressed, making isolation difficult.

It is important to collect blood samples without introducing any contaminating bacteria from the skin or the environment which would multiply and therefore confuse the true result. It has been suggested by some institutions that the practitioner should wear sterile gloves; however, it is more important that the site of the venepuncture should be cleaned thoroughly with an approved antiseptic solution. The blood should then be collected and injected via the rubber septum (cleaned with an antiseptic swab) into the blood culture bottles.

The volume of blood required varies depending on the type of bottle used, but it is between 5 and 10 ml/bottle. It is recommended that a separate syringe and needle be used to decant blood into each bottle. Some laboratories recommend taking a second sample not less than an hour later. The bottles should be clearly labelled and transported immediately to the laboratory or placed in an incubator maintained at 37°C (Higgins 1995b).

General considerations

High-risk samples

These samples should be clearly labelled and identified as high risk. They are usually double-bagged, with the request form separated from the sample to prevent accidental contamination. Staff asked to take blood from high-risk patients should be informed of the risk and ensure universal precautions are practised when sampling.

Special preparation

The practitioner must be aware of the activities or habits which may influence the results of blood tests, and ensure that the patient is aware of any activities that will need to be restricted prior to venepuncture (Box 9.7). If a patient is to have bloods taken which require a dietary restriction, e.g. a special diet, fasting or omitting medications, the practitioner must ensure that the patient understands what is required and the reasons for it. Verbal instruction should be reinforced with written information to ensure that patients' and practitioners' time is not wasted.

Sampling from a central venous catheter

Care must be taken when sampling from a central venous catheter as inaccurate laboratory values may be reported from blood specimens obtained via this route. This is because it is difficult to ensure that a drug is completely flushed from the catheter prior to taking a blood sample, and residual drug, such as an antibiotic or anticoagulant, could affect the results of the test. The proximal lumen of a multi-lumen catheter is the preferred site from which to obtain the sample. All infusions should be stopped before the catheter sample is obtained. The first sample withdrawn (usually 5–10 ml of blood) should be discarded (Cella & Watson 1989). An

■ **BOX 9.7**

Activities that may need to be restricted prior to venepuncture

- Vigorous exercise
- Ingestion of alcohol
- Intramuscular injections
- Certain surgical procedures
- Smoking
- Previous blood transfusions
- Immunizations
- Traumatic venepunctures (especially for haematology tests)
- Anxiety
- Pain
- Dehydration

alternative method is to flush the catheter with sodium chloride 0.9% and then flush back and forth several times to clear the catheter prior to removing the blood (Holmes 1998, Perucca 1995). An important aspect of care once the sample has been withdrawn is to ensure adequate flushing of the catheter to reduce the risk of clot formation and subsequent infection. Vacuum systems can be used with the aid of an adaptor.

Needlestick injury

The risk of a needlestick injury should be reduced by using safety or needleless systems whenever possible. If a needlestick injury does occur, the area should be made to bleed and washed under running water. Usual steps following such an injury include testing both patient and practitioner for hepatitis B, documentation of the accident and reporting the incident to the occupational health department.

CONCLUSION

Following the reduction in junior doctors' hours, one of the responsibilities actively taken on by nurses has been the practice of venepuncture and cannulation. The nurse is both accountable and responsible for maintaining the technical expertise and high level of skill necessary for performing these procedures (UKCC 1992). The practitioner must ensure that she has knowledge of the anatomy and physiology of the venous system, how to choose the appropriate vein and equipment, as well as the associated complications, in order to meet the physical, social and psychological needs of the patient undergoing venepuncture and cannulation.

REFERENCES

Agras S, Sylvester D, Olivean D 1969 The epidemiology of common fears and phobias. Comprehensive Psychiatry 10(2): 151–157
Agras W S, Chapkin H N, Olivean D C 1972 The natural history of phobia. Archives of General Psychiatry 26: 315–317
Ahrens T, Wiersma L, Weilitz P B 1991 Differences in pain perception associated with intravenous catheter insertion. Journal of Intravenous Nursing 14(2): 85–89
Auerbach S M, Kendall P C, Cutter H F, Levitt N R 1976 Anxiety, locus of control, type of

preparatory information and adjustment to dental surgery. Journal of Consulting and Clinical Psychology 44(5): 809–818

Baranowski L 1993 Central venous access devices – current technologies, uses and management strategies. Journal of Intravenous Nursing 16(3): 167–194

Bennett-Humprey G, Boon C M J 1992 The occurrence of high levels of acute behavioural distress in children and adolescents undergoing routine venepuncture. Paediatrics 90(1): 87–91

Berggren U 1992 General and specific fears in referred and self-referred adult patients with extreme dental anxiety. Behavioural Research Therapy 30(4): 395–401

Brismar B, Malmborg A S, Nystrom B, Strandberg A 1984 Bacterial contamination of intravenous cannula injection ports and stopcocks. Clinical Nutrition 3: 23–26

British Medical Association 1991 A code of practice for the safe use and disposal of sharps. BMA, London, p 20–21

Buckalew P G 1982 On the opposite side of the bed: a nurse clinician's experience of anxiety during chemotherapy. Cancer Nursing 5(6): 435–439

Cella J H, Watson J (eds) 1989 Obtaining peripheral blood specimens. In: Cella J H, Watson J (eds) Nurses' manual of laboratory tests. FA Davis, USA, appendix 1, p 481–486

Cheeseborough J S, Finch R 1984 Side ports – an infection hazard? British Journal of Parenteral Therapy 5(4): 155–157

Coates A, Abraham S, Kaye S B, Sowerbutts T, Frewin C, Fox R M, Tattersall M H N 1983 On the receiving end – patient perception of the side effects of cancer chemotherapy. European Journal of Cancer Clinical Oncology 19(2): 203–208

Cohn K H 1982 Chemotherapy from an insider's perspective. The Lancet 1: 1006–1009

Coyne P J, MacMurren M, Izzo T, Kramer T 1995 Transcutaneous electrical nerve stimulator for procedural pain associated with intravenous needlesticks. Journal of Intravenous Nursing 18(5): 263–267

Crow S 1987 Infection risks in intravenous therapy. National Intravenous Therapy Association 10: 101–105

Dennis A R, Leeson-Payne C G, Langham B T, Aikenhead A R 1995 Local anaesthesia for cannulation – has practice changed? Anaesthesia 50: 400–402

Department of Health 1990 Guidance for clinical health workers: protection against infection with HIV and hepatitis viruses: recommendations of the Expert Advisory Group on AIDS. HMSO, London

De Vries J H, van Dorp W T, van Barneveld P W C 1997 A randomised trial of alcohol 7% versus alcoholic iodine 2% in skin disinfection before insertion of peripheral infusion catheters. Journal of Hospital Infection 36: 317–320

Dougherty L 1992 Intravenous therapy. Surgical Nurse 5(2): 10–13

Dougherty L 1994 A study to discover how cancer patients perceive the intravenous cannulation experience. Unpublished MSc thesis, University of Surrey, Guildford

Dougherty L 1996 Intravenous cannulation. Nursing Standard 11(2): 47–51

Dyson A, Bogod D 1987 Minimising bruising in the antecubital fossa after venepuncture. British Medical Journal 294: 1659

Gaukroger P B, Roberts J G, Manners T A 1988 Infusion thrombophlebitis: a prospective comparison of 645 Vialon and Teflon cannulae in anaesthetic and postoperative use. Anaesthesia and Intensive Care 16(3): 265–271

Godwin P G R, Cuthbert A C, Choyce A 1992 Reducing bruising after venepuncture. Quality in Health Care 1: 245–246

Goode C J, Titler M, Rakel B, Ones D S, Kleiber C, Small S, Triolo P K 1991 A meta-analysis of effects of heparin flush and saline flush: quality and cost implications. Nursing Research 40(6): 324–330

Goodinson S M 1990a Keeping the flora out. Professional Nurse 5(11): 572–575

Goodinson S M 1990b The risks of IV therapy. Professional Nurse 5(5): 235–238

Gunwardene R D, Davenport HT 1990 Local application of EMLA and glyceryl trinitrate ointment before venepuncture. Anaesthesia 45: 52–54

Hadaway L 1995 Anatomy and physiology related to intravenous therapy. In: Terry J, Baranowski L, Lonsway R A, Hedrick C (eds) Intravenous therapy in intravenous therapy: clinical principles and practices. WB Saunders, Philadelphia, ch 6, p 81–110

Hallen B, Olsson G L, Uppfeldt A 1984 Pain free venepuncture. Anaesthesia 39: 969–972

Harrison N, Langham B T, Bogod DG 1992 Appropriate use of local anaesthesia for venous cannulation. Anaesthesia 47: 210–212

Hart S 1996 Aseptic technique. In: Mallett J, Bailey C (eds) The Royal Marsden NHS Trust manual of clinical nursing procedures, 4th edn. Blackwell Scientific, London, ch 1

Hecker J 1988 Improved techniques in IV therapy. Nursing Times 84(34): 28–33

Hecker J F, Lewis B H, Stanley H 1983 Nitroglycerine ointment as an aid to venepuncture. The Lancet 1: 202–206

Higgins C 1995a Haematology testing. Nursing Times 91(7): 38–40

Higgins C 1995b Measuring renal function with urea and creatinine tests. Nursing Times 90(51): 35–36

Holmes K 1998 Comparison of push pull versus discard method from central venous catheters for blood testing. Journal of Intravenous Nursing 21(5): 282–285

Hudek K 1986 Compliance in intravenous therapy. Journal of Canadian Intravenous Nursing Association 2(3): 7–8

Intravenous Nursing Society (INS) 1998 Revised intravenous nursing standards of practice. Journal of Intravenous Nursing 21(15): 1S

Kaloupek D G, Scott J R, Khatami V 1985 Assessment of coping strategies associated with syncope in blood donors. Journal of Psychosomatic Research 29(2): 207–214

Kamimoto V, Olson K 1996 Using normal saline to lock peripheral intravenous catheters in ambulatory cancer patients. Journal of Intravenous Nursing 19(2): 75–78

Kaplan M 1983 Viewpoint: the cancer patient. Cancer Nursing 6(2): 103–107

Kerrison T, Woodhull J 1994 Reducing the risk of thrombophlebitis –comparison of teflon and vialon cannulae. Professional Nurse 9(10): 662–666

Lander J, Fowler-Kerry S 1992 TENS for children's procedural pain. Pain 52: 209–216

Larson P J 1984 Important nurse caring behaviours perceived by patients with cancer. Oncology Nursing Forum 11(6): 46–50

Levine F M, De Simone L L 1991 The effects of experimenter gender on pain report in male and female subjects. Pain 44: 69–72

Lewis G B H, Hecker J F 1985 Infusion thrombophlebitis. British Journal of Anaesthetics 57: 220–233

McKee J M, Shell J A, Warren T A, Campbell V P 1989 Complications of intravenous therapy: a randomised prospective study – Vialon vs Teflon. Journal of Intravenous Nursing 12(5): 288–295

Maki D G 1976 Preventing infection in IV therapy. Hospital Practice 11(4): 95–104

Maki D G 1991 Improving catheter site care. Royal Society of Medicine Services Ltd, London, p 3–28

Maki D G, Ringer M 1987 Evaluation of dressing regimes for prevention of infection with peripheral IV catheters. Journal of American Medical Association 258(17): 2396–2403

Mallett J, Bailey C (eds) 1996 Venepuncture. In: Mallet J, Bailey C (eds) The Royal Marsden NHS Trust Manual of Clinical Nursing Procedures, 4th edn. Blackwell Scientific, London

Marks I 1988 Blood injury phobia: a review. American Journal of Psychiatry 145(10): 1207–1213

Mavissakalian M, Barlow D H 1981 Phobia, psychological and pharmacological treatment. The Guildford Press, New York, ch 1, p 4–9

Mayer D K 1987 Oncology nurses' versus cancer patients' perceptions of nurse caring behaviours: a replication study. Oncology Nursing Forum 14(3): 48–52

Middleton J 1985 Don't needle the patient. Nursing Mirror 161(4): 22–24

Millam D 1992 Starting IVs – how to develop your venipuncture skills. Nursing 92: 33–46

Millam D 1993 How to teach good venipuncture technique. American Journal of Nursing 93(7): 38–41

Millam D 1995 The use of anaesthesia in IV therapy. Journal of Vascular Access Devices 1(1): 22–29

Mills R T, Krantz D S 1979 Information, choice and reactions to stress. A field experiment in a blood bank with laboratory analogue. Journal of Personality and Social Psychology 3(4): 608–620

Morris S 1996 Jab-fear woman is saved from herself. Mail on Sunday [article]

Nightingale K W, Bradshaw E G 1982 A review of peripheral cannulae. British Journal of IV Therapy 3(4): 14–23

Noe D A, Rook R C 1994 (eds) Specimen collection procedures in laboratory medicine – the selection and interpretation of clinical lab studies. Williams and Wilkins, Baltimore, appendix 1, p 870–873

Ost L G 1991 Acquisition of blood and injection phobia and anxiety response patterns in clinical patients. Behavioural Research and Therapy 29(4): 323–332

Ost L G 1992 Blood and injection phobia: background and cognitive psychological and behavioural variables. Journal of Abnormal Psychology 101(1): 68–74

Pavlin D J, Links S, Rapp S E, Neesley M L, Keyes H J 1993 Vasovagal reactions in ambulatory surgery centre. Anaesthesia Analgesia 76: 931–935

Payne-James J J, Rogers J, Bray M J, Rana S K, McSwiggon D, Silk D B 1991 Development of thrombophlebitis in peripheral veins with Vialon and PTFE–Teflon cannulas: a double blind randomised controlled trial. Annals of the Royal College of Surgeons of England 73: 322–325

Perucca R 1995 Obtaining vascular access. In: Terry J, Baranowski L, Lonsway R A, Hedrick C (eds) Intravenous therapy: clinical principles and practices. WB Saunders, Philadelphia, ch 21, p 377–391

Peters J L, Frame J D, Dawson S M 1984 Peripheral venous cannulation: reducing the risks.
British Journal of Parenteral Therapy 5: 56–58

Plumer A 1987 Principles and practice of intravenous therapy, 4th edn. Little, Brown, Boston,
ch 12, p 172–177

Rachman S J, Wilson G T 1980 The effects of psychological therapy, 2nd edn. Pergamon Press,
Oxford

Rowland R 1991 Making sense of venepuncture. Nursing Times 87(32): 41–43

Sagar D P, Bomar S K 1982 Intravenous medications. JB Lippincott, Philadelphia, ch 2,
p 12–21

Shearer J 1987 Normal saline flush vs dilute heparin flush. A study of peripheral intermittent
IV devices. Journal of Intravenous Nursing 10: 425–427

Speechley V 1984 The nurse's role in intravenous management. Nursing Times 80(18): 31–32

Speechley V 1987 Nursing patients having chemotherapy. In: Tiffany R, Borley D (eds)
Oncology for nurses and health care professionals – cancer nursing, 2nd edn.
Harper & Row, London, vol 3, ch 3, p 74–121

Steel J, Taylor R, Lloyd G 1986 Behaviour therapy for phobia of venepuncture. Diabetic
Medicine 3: 481

Tully J L, Friedland G H, Baldrini L M, Goldmann D A 1981 Complications of intravenous
therapy with steel needles and teflon catheters: a comparative study. The American Journal
of Medicine 70: 702–706

United Kingdom Central Council for Nursing, Midwifery and Health Visiting 1992 Scope of
professional practice. UKCC, London

Van den Berg A A, Abeysekera R M 1993 Rationalising venous cannulation: patient factors
and lignocaine efficacy. Anaesthesia 48(1): 84

Verity E 1993 The fear that condemned a man to die in agony. Daily Mail, 1 July 1993 [article]

Webster D, Pellegrini L, Duffy K 1992 Use of transcutaneous electrical neural stimulation for
fingertip analgesia: a pilot study. Annals of Emergency Medicine 21: 1472–1475

Weinstein S M 1993 Plumer's principles and practice of intravenous therapy, 5th edn.
JB Lippincott, Philadelphia

Weinstein S M 1997 Plumer's principles and practice of intravenous therapy, 6th edn.
JB Lippincott, Philadelphia

Whitson M 1996 Intravenous therapy in the older adult: special need and considerations.
Journal of Intravenous Nursing 19(5): 251–255

Wilson Barnett J 1976 Patients' emotional reactions to hospitalisation: an exploratory study.
Journal of Advanced Nursing 1: 351–358

Yuan R T W, Cohan M D 1987 Lateral antebrachial cutaneous nerve injury as a complication
of phlebotomy. Journal of Canadian Intravenous Nurse Association 3(3): 16–17

Vascular access in the acute care setting

Katie Scales

CHAPTER 10

INTRODUCTION

Intravenous access is necessary for the reliable and predictable administration of drugs and fluids (Soni 1989). The nature of the access is dependent upon the severity of illness or the potential for deleterious change in the condition of the patient.

In acute care, access may also be required for haemodynamic monitoring, haemofiltration or dialysis, or to facilitate transvenous pacing or biopsy procedures. These procedures usually require central venous access. Central venous access is also the route of choice if the drugs or fluids to be administered are irritant to peripheral veins or have the potential to cause tissue necrosis should extravasation occur (Park & Manara 1994).

The local concentration of a drug often determines the degree of irritation to the vessel. High concentrations of drugs entering a small, low-flow vessel will cause a high intravascular concentration and can result in local inflammation (phlebitis). The same drug further diluted or delivered into a high-flow vessel will result in a lower intravascular concentration and less inflammation (Soni 1989). The ability to further dilute drugs will depend largely on the clinical condition of the patient, e.g. their ventricular or renal function.

Once seen as a last resort, the use of central venous access is now commonplace for an increasing number of patients in both the hospital and outpatient setting (Baranowski 1993). Despite this trend, the use of more traditional access routes should not be forgotten. The use of central venous access is not without risk and health care workers must evaluate the relative advantages and disadvantages when selecting the most appropriate route for intravenous therapy. In view of the significant morbidity and mortality associated with central venous catheters, their use should be reserved for patients who will truly benefit from them (Seneff 1987a).

PERIPHERAL VENOUS ACCESS

Peripheral access should not be excluded from the management of acute care patients. It is associated with fewer complications than central access, but there are also limitations to its use.

There are many sites of potential peripheral venous access, and some are more advantageous than others. Arm veins have the benefit of easy access but the disadvantage of flexure points and close proximity to arterial structures. Leg veins can hamper mobility and are associated with increased risk of venous thrombosis.

The choice of site and the size of cannula will be determined by the indication for its placement (Soni 1989). For example, patients who require fluid resuscitation need a large cannula in a large vein which can be accessed at the first attempt. By contrast, patients who require elective drug administration need a smaller cannula with more attention paid to patient convenience and comfort.

In acute settings such as the A&E department or the anaesthetic room, large-gauge cannula are often selected to facilitate large-volume fluid replacement in patients who are considered to be at high risk. A 14 or 16 gauge cannula is usually selected. A 2.5-inch, 16 g peripheral cannula is capable of infusing twice the amount of fluid as an 8-inch, 16 g central catheter (Seneff 1987a).

In the conscious patient, these large peripheral cannulae can be associated with significant pain. Research demonstrates that the pain associated with insertion, and the residual pain of the in situ cannula, can be reduced by the infiltration of local anaesthetic prior to cannulation (Langham & Harrison 1992). Dennis et al (1995) demonstrated that despite the publication of conclusive research, 46% of the anaesthetists surveyed were unaware of it. They also concluded that junior anaesthetists were less likely to use local anaesthesia than their more experienced colleagues.

Soni (1989) believes infection to be a grossly underestimated problem with peripheral cannulae and emphasizes the need for peripheral cannulae to be replaced every 48 hours. This view is well supported by the literature, which concludes that 72 hours is the longest time that a peripheral cannula should be allowed to remain in situ (Collin et al 1975, Maki & Ringer 1987).

In the shocked patient whose peripheral circulation is shut down, the palpation of peripheral vessels may be impossible. It is relatively commonplace to attempt central venous access in the absence of peripheral veins; however, in patients with trauma to the trunk and abdomen, central venous access may prove equally difficult and potentially hazardous.

CUT-DOWN VENOUS ACCESS

This once common technique has become largely redundant since the establishment of central venous access as a routine method of administration in the critically ill patient.

In the event that cut-down access is required, a large vein which is not prone to anatomical inconsistency is usually selected (Soni 1989). It is important to have an understanding of the related anatomy if complications are to be avoided. For example, when cutting down to a vein in the antecubital fossa, it is important to know that the area also contains the brachial artery and the median nerve. The most common sites for cut-down access are the veins of the antecubital fossa and the saphenous vein at the ankle (Soni 1989). This procedure is usually restricted to medical personnel as it requires a surgical technique to locate and access the vein.

A technique for venous cut-down of the saphenous vein at the ankle, as recommended by Soni (1989), is given in Box 10.1.

CENTRAL VENOUS ACCESS

In the past, central venous cannulation was mainly restricted to thoracic surgery. Seneff (1987a) suggested that the increase in popularity of central venous catheters (CVCs) parallels a proliferation in newer techniques for cannulation and invasive monitoring technology. In 1989, the American Food & Drug Administration (FDA) estimated that 3 million CVC procedures were performed annually in the USA (McGee et al 1993). This compares with an estimated 200 000 performed annually in the UK (Elliot 1993).

Central veins are usually considered to be veins which lie within the thorax and which are in direct continuity with the right atrium (see Fig. 10.1). Access to the central veins can be achieved from several approaches: internal or external jugular, subclavian, femoral or peripheral veins. Each site has its relative indications and most appropriate technique.

■ **BOX 10.1**

A technique for venous cut-down of the saphenous vein at the ankle

- Locate the vein – 2 cm above and anterior to the medial maleolus.
- Make a transverse incision in the skin over the vein.
- Locate the vein using blunt dissection with forceps or scissors.
- Place ties around the vein, a lower one tying off the vessel, and another one higher up.
- Incise the vein, taking care not to cut through it, and introduce the cannula into the vessel.
- Flush the cannula to check patency.
- Use the upper tie to secure the cannula.

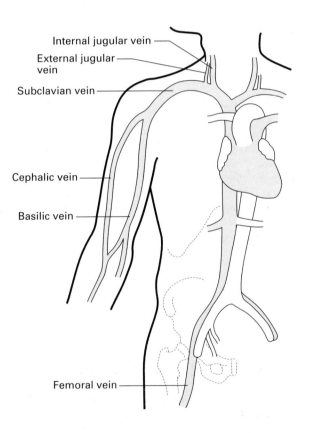

Internal jugular vein

External jugular vein

Subclavian vein

Cephalic vein

Basilic vein

Femoral vein

Fig. 10.1 The central veins.

SITE SELECTION

The antecubital fossa

This is an established route into the central venous system and has the advantage of a low incidence of thoracic complications (Seneff 1987a). It is also advantageous for the patient who cannot tolerate the supine position traditionally required for CVC insertion.

The first report of a peripherally inserted central venous catheter (PICC) was in

1929 when Forssman, a German physician, passed a 4 Fg ureteric catheter up to his heart via a wide-bore needle in his cubital fossa (Abi-Nader 1993). The use of the basilic or saphenous vein catheter was reported by Hughes & Magovern (1959) for the assessment of central venous pressure.

In these early years, the catheter materials were relatively rigid and resulted in a high incidence of thrombosis, malposition, sepsis and phlebitis (Abi-Nader 1993). In 1962, the first silicone elastomer (Silastic) catheter was introduced, but there was no method of advancing this soft, malleable catheter into the central circulation. In the 1970s a spring stylet was introduced which produced enough rigidity for the catheter to be threaded into the central circulation (Abi-Nader 1993). A range of PICC devices are now available.

The antecubital fossa permits percutaneous cannulation of the basilic and cephalic veins or cut-down cannulation of the brachial vein (Seneff 1987a).

Complications as a result of PICC insertion remain minor in comparison with other central access routes (Seneff 1987a). Deep vein thrombosis of the arm and pulmonary embolism are two significant thrombotic complications and Seneff suggested that their incidence is proportional to the length of time that the catheter remains in situ. Controversy exists about this length of time – early studies from the 1960s (utilizing older catheter materials, e.g. polyethylene) suggested that a PICC inserted via the antecubital fossa should not be left in situ in excess of 72 hours. More modern catheter materials, such as elastomeric polyurethane or silicone, which are considered to be more flexible and biocompatible, are designed for more prolonged use. A retrospective study by Lam et al (1994) demonstrated an average catheter placement in an acute care hospital of longer than 2 weeks. However, in the intensive care setting, Soni (1989) highlighted the risk of infection and compared a PICC to a peripheral cannula, recommending its replacement every 2–3 days.

Soni (1989) suggested that CVC placement via the antecubital fossa is a relatively easy technique with few insertion complications and a low incidence of pneumothorax. The main complication is the failure to thread the catheter past the axilla in a high percentage of cases. He also noted that a small number of catheters end up in neck veins rather than chest veins when inserted via this route.

The femoral vein

The femoral vein is a well established access route with relatively consistent anatomy. The femoral artery lies lateral to the femoral vein in the region of the inguinal ligament, and the femoral nerve lies lateral to the artery. This is usually a relatively easy access site for the inexperienced operator, and should the femoral artery be punctured, pressure is easy to apply.

Some medical personnel shy away from the femoral vein as a routine access route because of the potential risk of infection. Indeed, Seneff (1987a) suggested that use of the femoral vein should be restricted to 24 hours in view of the infection risks. However, in reality, intensive care units which do utilize this route find that the risks are no greater than that of the internal jugular site (Soni 1989).

There is also concern over the incidence of false aneurysm in the femoral artery. Again, in practical terms this is an exceptionally rare event, far less common than a pneumothorax following subclavian vein cannulation. Seneff (1987a) pointed out that during resuscitation, the femoral vein can provide central access without the need to stop chest compressions.

The femoral vein as a site for large-bore renal cannulae in the acute setting has been a popular choice since the 1960s (Seneff 1987a).

The more rare complications of femoral vein cannulation include massive scrotal haemorrhage (Sung et al 1981) and arteriovenous fistula formation (Fuller et al 1976).

The external jugular

The external jugular vein can be used for central vascular access, although its high incidence of anomalous anatomy and its severe angle with the subclavian vein make it an unpopular choice. In its favour is the relatively low risk of pneumothorax and the fact that it is part of the surface anatomy of the neck and therefore easily located. Soni (1989) suggested that its superficial nature may make it more susceptible to sepsis and therefore less suitable as a long-term access route.

The major disadvantage of this access site is the difficulty in threading a catheter into the central circulation. The tight angle with the subclavian can be difficult to negotiate even with the help of a 'J' wire. Soni (1989) emphasized the need for radiographic placement of catheters inserted via the external jugular site in view of the cannulation difficulties.

When this vein is selected, it is not uncommon to find that the operator has used a peripheral cannula to access it, rather than the traditionally longer central catheter. It is important to establish whether this is the case as minimal cannula dislodgement could lead to extravasation, with the associated hazard of haemorrhage, infiltration and loss of systemic effects of the drug being infused.

Complication from external jugular catheterization is rare, however Ghani & Berry (1983) reported four cases of hydrothorax 24–48 hours after external jugular vein cannulation. It was presumed that the catheter tip had rested transversely across the wall of the superior vena cava (SVC) and that this had led to erosion and subsequent infusion of fluids directly into the pleural space.

The internal jugular

The internal jugular vein is probably the most common site for central venous access. Seneff (1987b) stated that its high success rate and low incidence of complications make it an extremely good site for central venous catheterization. He believes that the main complications of this approach are carotid artery puncture and laceration of local neck structures from needle probing. Soni (1989) suggested that the main contraindication to the internal jugular approach is coagulopathy, this being a relatively blind technique which punctures a deeply situated vein in close proximity to the carotid artery. Anatomically the neck is highly innervated and both the insertion procedure and the residual cannula can cause extreme tenderness to the patient.

The vagus nerve lies in a posterior position between the internal jugular vein and the carotid artery, and the sympathetic trunk lies behind the vagus. The phrenic nerve lies lateral and posterior to to the internal jugular vein (Woodburne & Burkel 1994). Damage to the sympathetic chain by either needle puncture or infiltration with local anaesthetic can lead to Horner's syndrome (Soni 1989), which is the term given to a collection of symptoms arising from damage to sympathetic nerves in the cervical region. The syndrome includes a constricted pupil, ptosis and an absence of sweat gland activity over the affected side of the face. Damage to the phrenic nerve results in diaphragmatic palsy.

In practice, catheters in the internal jugular vein can provide a nursing challenge. Beard growth in men, diaphoresis in the febrile patient and poor control of oral secretions in the patient with altered consciousness can all lead to problems with fixation of the catheter and the need for repeated dressing of the site. Invariably the catheter or its associated administration sets and connections are in close proximity to the patient's hair.

Inadequate fixation of the catheter can lead to increased mobility and subsequent mechanical thrombophlebitis. Soni (1989) suggested that head movement may contribute to catheter movement and subsequent contamination of the site. Regular observation of the site for signs of inflammation or infection is required.

The subclavian

This is another popular site for central venous access and Soni (1989) suggested it had certain advantages over other access sites, but stressed the potential hazards of catheter placement and the need for considerable care when undertaking the procedure.

The technique of subclavian vein catheterization was first described by Aubaniac (1952) and there continues to be debate over the advantages of using this site.

Before the introduction of modern, high-specification catheterization kits, this was often considered as a last resort access route and was approached with a great deal of respect. The literature reports a range of complications – some fatal – and by the late 1960s there were calls for this route to be abandoned (Shapira & Stern 1967). There has been a revival in the popularity of the site, perhaps due to the increased amount of long-term access or perhaps because of the realization that no site is perfect. Soni (1989) suggested that, with the recent increase in use of this site, there has also been an increase in the complacency with which the venepuncture is performed. He postulated that the operator who has never experienced a complication from this site has either not performed very many or has been exceptionally lucky.

Sennef (1987b) is rather less cautious and described subclavian venepuncture as 'quick and easy to learn'. Many studies have reported a 90–95% success rate for the first attempt at catheterization of the subclavian vein (Simpson & Aitchison 1982).

Soni (1989) cited coagulopathy as one of the most significant contraindications to the selection of this access route. The subclavian vein is located in close proximity to the artery, and in view of the relatively 'blind' nature of the technique, arterial puncture is a significant complication. Once arterial puncture has occurred, it may be impossible to arrest the bleeding as there is no point at which pressure can be applied to the artery; a surgical repair via thoracotomy may be the only solution.

The subclavian is probably the most popular and convenient site for long-term venous access. It is easy to secure the catheter to the chest wall, and as a result there are fewer incidents of mechanically induced thrombophlebitis and infection.

The commonly acknowledged complications of this route reflect the structures which are in close proximity to the subclavian vein. Soni (1989) noted that the pleura, subclavian artery, phrenic nerve and even the trachea are all within easy reach of 'a misguided needle'. He also noted that a guide wire which has been forced can end up in the mediastinum, as can a catheter.

Pneumothorax is the most common complication of subclavian vein catheterization. Seneff (1987b) reported that pneumothorax accounts for 25–33% of all the reported complications of this access route, and also that the incidence of pneumothorax is inversely proportional to the operator's level of experience.

The presentation of the pneumothorax may be immediate or delayed. Despite the performance of a 'check X-ray', it is not uncommon to discover a small pneumothorax a couple of days after the insertion of the catheter (Soni 1989). The incidence of pneumothorax can increase dramatically if the patient is undergoing positive pressure ventilation and may present as a tension pneumothorax.

Subclavian artery puncture is reported to be as frequent a complication as pneumothorax but the literature comes mainly from the 1970s, prior to the introduction of modern catheterization kits. Soni (1989) believes the incidence to be lower than for pneumothorax. Seneff (1987b) concurs with Soni that in the presence of a coagulopathy, catastrophic haemorrhage may ensue. He suggested that a platelet count less than 50 000 or a PTT ratio greater than 3 predisposes the patient to haemorrhage.

A less widely debated complication is subclavian vein thrombosis. There is much in the literature to support the existence of thrombosis (Hansen & Christensen 1983, McLean-Russ et al 1982, Maurer et al 1984, Weiner et al 1984), but the reports are inconsistent because of the range of criteria used to diagnose the condition. Seneff (1987b) considered this complication to be under-diagnosed.

The literature is more consistent in reporting the thrombogenic nature of the sub-clavian vein when used for large-bore, double-lumen renal catheters (Barton et al 1983, Brady et al 1989, Cimochowski et al 1990, Vanherweghem 1986). Renal catheter manufacturers now actively attempt to promote the jugular vein as the optimal access route.

Seneff (1987b) suggested that the incidence of thrombosis is proportional to the length of time that the catheter remains in situ. However, he acknowledged that the mechanism is inconclusive as there are reports of subclavian thrombosis after unsuccessful attempts at subclavian cannulation (Weiner et al 1984).

The risk of thrombosis also appears high in patients in whom catheters have been inserted for the purpose of PN administration; indeed, much of the literature relating to thrombotic complications comes from this patient group. Seneff (1987b) postulated that the hyperosmolar nature of PN could be a contributive factor and that the risks for critically ill patients, whose access is for a different purpose, may be considerably lower. It would appear that clinical evidence of large vein thrombosis occurs in 1–3% of subclavian catheters inserted for PN administration (Freund 1981, McLean-Russ et al 1982).

Seneff (1987a) suggested that there are no absolute contraindications to CVC placement in patients who require it, although there may be absolute contraindications to specific approaches. For example, subclavian access should be avoided in patients whose baseline respiratory function would not tolerate a pneumothorax.

CATHETER SELECTION

The ideal catheter should fulfil several important criteria. They should:

- carry a low risk of infection
- be non-thrombogenic
- be hypoallergenic
- be atraumatic to the intimal lining of the blood vessel
- have a smooth surface to prevent the attraction of cells and microorganisms
- be easy to insert
- be comfortable for the patient
- have an inherent tensile strength to withstand normal wear and tear, thus preventing catheter embolism
- be radio-opaque.

Given the known complications of CVCs, it is essential that modern catheters are routinely manufactured with luer-lock fittings and, where possible, in-line clamps. Elliot et al (1994) advocated that catheters should have graduated markings to facilitate placement and monitoring of their position, and recommended that they be kink-resistant and have a means by which to secure them to the skin.

An enormous range of CVCs are now available, of varying composition, size and insertion technique. Modern catheters are biocompatible, have innovative designs and have greater versatility (Baranowski 1993). When choosing a catheter for central access, it is important to consider its use and duration of placement in order that the correct catheter is selected.

Even in the short term, if the therapy to be delivered is damaging to blood vessels, e.g. PN, chemotherapy or concentrated inotropes, then central access will be required to facilitate haemodilution and safe administration of the products.

Short-term therapies (less than 3 weeks) usually justify the placement of non-tunnelled, percutaneous CVCs. Several months of therapy may indicate the need for a peripherally inserted central venous catheter (PICC) or other longer term catheter, while prolonged therapies will require the placement of long-term tunnelled catheters or implantable devices (Baranowski 1993).

The selection of a multi-lumen device will depend on the range of therapies required, the compatibility of the therapies and the need for sampling access. Most commonly, multi-lumen catheters have either two, three or four lumens. More complex catheters such as cardiac output catheters may have five or more.

Other considerations for device selection include the general medical history of the patient, their activity level, an evaluation of their vascular access and their psychological needs. The medical team should not be solely responsible for the selection of the device; where appropriate, the patient or their carer should be involved in the decision-making process. This is more of an issue for longer term therapy than for the emergency setting.

Catheter materials

Early catheters were made of rigid materials such as polyethylene, polyvinyl chloride and Teflon. The rigidity of these materials meant that insertion was easy, even over long distances. These materials have largely been superseded as they had a tendency to damage the intimal lining of the vessel, causing platelet aggregation and thrombus formation (Hadaway 1989). There are reported cases of vessel perforation, but they are relatively rare. The more modern polyurethane catheters show less thrombogenicity than their predecessors, are rigid to facilitate insertion, but then become more pliable as they attain body temperature. Baranowski (1993) noted the superior tensile strength of the polyurethane catheter and that this permits the manufacture of thinner-walled catheters, which subsequently reduce the degree of vessel obstruction caused by the catheter. Some catheter manufacturers have further enhanced the biocompatibility of the polyurethane catheter by constructing the tip out of a silicone elastomer (Silastic) material, thus reducing the likelihood of intimal damage to the blood vessel.

Silastic is a lightweight material which floats within the blood vessel, and is therefore less likely to cause damage to the vessel wall (Baranowski 1993). Some short-term catheters are made of this material, but they require specialized insertion techniques and it is more common to see polyurethane catheters for short-term acute care use. The majority of longer term access catheters are designed using this type of material.

Topography

The topography of the catheter surface is of importance. Catheters whose surfaces are roughened usually promote the adherence of platelets and microorganisms. It is thought that a catheter's relative thrombogenicity predisposes the patient to an increased risk of bacterial colonization and subsequent septicaemia (Elliott 1988, Lopez-Lopez et al 1991). Certain bacteria (in particular *coagulase-negative staphylococci*) excrete a carbohydrate-based 'slime' which coats intravascular catheters and helps microorganisms to bond to them. This subsequently reduces the effectiveness of antibiotic therapy (Kamal et al 1991).

A polyurethane catheter has now been developed that has been bonded with antiseptic substances rather than antibiotic substances. Maki et al (1991) performed a randomized prospective study on a novel polyurethane catheter impregnated with silver sulphadiazine and chlorhexidine. The trial took place in a surgical intensive care unit. Their findings were encouraging, with a 50% reduction in catheter colonization and a 75% reduction in catheter-related septicaemia. During their trial there was no evidence of adverse effects of the antiseptic substances, nor could the substances be detected in the blood of the patients tested. The catheter is designed to sustain the release of the antiseptic agents over a 15 day period, although small amounts (< 1%) continue to be released after this period (Farber 1993).

Another concern is the development of a fibrin sheath along the length of the catheter. Within seconds of insertion, intravascular catheters are coated with plasma proteins and subsequently with platelets (Kristinsson 1989). Some catheter materials are more predisposed to platelet attraction than others (Borow & Crowley 1985). Within 5–7 days, this coating will have developed into a fibrin sheath (Baranowski 1993).

In an attempt to address the problems of 'slime' or fibrin development on CVCs, manufacturers now produce catheters which are coated or bonded with substances thought to reduce the incidence of these problems.

Bonded catheters

Heparin-bonded catheters are now available to reduce the thrombogenicity of the catheter and to improve their biocompatibility (Hoar et al 1981). Baranowski (1993) is mindful that even though this technique may be more advantageous than systemic heparinization, the practitioner should consider the risks of heparin allergy or the development of heparin antibodies.

More recent advances include the development of catheters which can be bonded with antibiotics immediately prior to insertion. A catheter can be treated with a type of surfactant at the time of manufacture. This surfactant allows antibiotics such as cephalosporins and penicillins to be ionically bonded to the surface prior to insertion.

Kamal et al (1991) undertook a study of central and arterial catheters in a surgical intensive care unit. Prior to insertion, the catheters were dipped in a solution containing cefazolin sodium which then ionically bonded to the catheter surface. Their study demonstrated a sevenfold reduction in bacterial colonization of the central catheters, and a fivefold reduction in the colonization of the arterial catheters.

Due to the small number of arterial catheters involved in the study, the data were not statistically significant. As with the heparin-bonded catheter, the possibility of sensitivity to the antibiotic should not be forgotten. Microbiologists would also caution us against the development of resistant organisms from the random use of antibiotic therapy.

Cuffs

The attachable cuff made of biodegradeable collagen and impregnated with silver ions is another useful development (Hadaway 1989). The cuff is placed subcutaneously around the intravenous device. The collagen promotes tissue growth which provides a physical barrier to any bacteria that may try to migrate from the skin surface along the catheter and into the circulation. The silver ions produce a chemical barrier against microbial colonization. The use of an implantable cuff is not new. Dacron cuffs have been available on long-term skin tunnelled catheters for many years. This new, attachable cuff allows it to be utilized with short-term catheters in an attempt to reduce the infection rate. Hadaway (1989) considered that the cost of the collagen/silver ion cuff is outweighed by the cost of treating catheter-related septicaemia. The efficacy of the implantable cuff appears undisputed (Babycos et al 1993, Bonawitz et al 1991, Flowers et al 1989, Maki et al 1988).

Catheter design

Many modern catheters are constructed with in-built extensions, which facilitate the manipulation of connections with minimal disturbance of the entry site. The advantage of this is the reduction in the incidence of mechanical thrombophlebitis from movement of the catheter within the vessel. These extensions usually have in-built clamps to reduce the likelihood of air embolism when undertaking tubing changes or any other procedure which opens the CVC to the atmosphere. Some catheter materials are easily damaged by in-line clamps, e.g. Silastic catheters, and these are usually manufactured with a reinforced area where it is safe to clamp.

Multi-lumen catheters have an advantage in the acute care setting where patients require continuous infusions of incompatible products. Multi-lumen catheters for short-term access usually have lumens which exit at different points along the length of the catheter; those for long-term access often have lumens which open at the same place at the tip of the catheter.

Considering that one advantage of a multi-lumen catheter is the ability to co-infuse incompatible products through the same access site, this would appear to be a design fault of some long-term catheters.

Collins & Lutz (1991) undertook an in vitro study of simultaneous infusion of incompatible drugs in multi-lumen catheters. They highlighted the lack of data on the subject and sought to use an in vitro model to investigate the administration of PN and phenytoin, both known to be incompatible, via multi-lumen catheters. The catheters compared were a triple-lumen catheter with staggered openings (the type typically used in the UK for short-term acute access) and a double-lumen catheter with adjacent openings at the tip of the catheter (the type usually associated with long-term catheters or implantable ports). Their findings concluded that the catheter with adjacent openings was inferior to that with staggered openings, as it resulted in drug precipitation.

Concern has been raised over the possible increased infection risk associated with multi-lumen catheters (Kovacevich et al 1988, Powell et al 1988, Gil et al 1989, Horowitz et al 1990). It is difficult, however, to draw conclusions from these studies as the populations vary, their samples sizes are relatively small and the criteria for determining catheter-related sepsis are not the established ones suggested by authors such as Maki et al (1977). In contrast, Gianino et al (1992) were able to demonstrate a low incidence of infection amongst multi-lumen catheters when a specialist team is involved in the management of the venous access.

CATHETER INSERTION

There are three methods of central venous catheter placement:

- over a needle
- through a cannula
- over a guide wire.

Placement over a wire and through a cannula both allow for the introduction of a multi-lumen catheter if required. (It is important when inserting multi-lumen catheters that all of the lumens are flushed with sodium chloride 0.9% prior to insertion, which both ensures patency and prevents air embolism.)

Each insertion method has advantages and disadvantages which need to be considered when selecting the method of choice.

Over a needle

This technique usually involves the use of an extra long cannula, which is inserted in the same way as a standard cannula. This is most commonly associated with the placement of cannulae in the internal jugular vein (Soni 1989). This technique is often favoured by anaesthetists who are placing short-term or emergency cannulae,

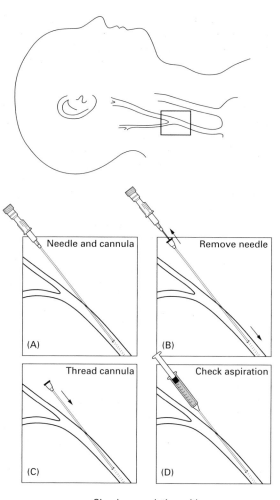

Fig. 10.2 Placing a cannula over a needle. (After Soni 1989, with permission.)

Needle and cannula (A)

Remove needle (B)

Thread cannula (C)

Check aspiration (D)

Simple cannulation with
a long cannula

e.g. at the scene of a cardiac arrest or elective placement prior to thoracic, abdominal or vascular surgery.

As for all central cannulation, the patient is laid flat and, where possible, placed in a head-down position (Trendelenburg). This assists with the filling of the neck veins to facilitate palpation and cannulation (Fig. 10.2).

The head is usually turned away from the insertion site and the vessel is punctured. A flashback is seen when the vessel is entered, and the cannula is advanced and the trochar withdrawn in the same manner as for peripheral cannulation. The cannula is aspirated to ensure free flow of blood, which implies that the cannula has not left the vessel, it is well positioned in the vessel and it is not kinked.

The advantages of this technique are its speed of access, minimal handling and low cost. The disadvantages include the length of the trochar which can cause significant trauma if the operator is inexperienced (Soni 1989), the limitation of a single lumen catheter and the reduced range of catheter material available for this insertion method. Soni also suggests that this minimal handling technique can result in a tendency to 'skimp on aseptic technique'. This technique is usually restricted to the jugular approach.

Through a cannula

This is an established technique whereby a small, wide-bore cannula is inserted into a central vein, in a very similar manner to peripheral cannulation. Having established a flashback, the trochar is withdrawn. It is important to avoid introducing air into the venous system when the trochar is removed, so it is common practice for the operator to occlude the end of the cannula using a sterile gloved finger. A flexible catheter is then threaded through the cannula. The cannula is aspirated to confirm placement and patency. It is usual practice then to flush the catheter with sodium chloride 0.9% or heparinized saline to prevent obstruction from clot formation. This method can be used to place short or long catheters.

The introducing cannula is often removed, although this will depend on the construction of the catheter that has been passed and the risk of bleeding, as the introducer cannula is inevitably of a larger diameter than the catheter that has been passed through it.

This method is employed for the placement of transvenous temporary pacing wires, for the placement of pulmonary artery or cardiac output catheters and to facilitate transvenous biopsies, e.g. myocardial or hepatic biopsy.

Over a guide wire

This method of placement is known as the Seldinger technique. It was first described by Dr Seldinger in 1953 and has continued to gain in popularity ever since (Seldinger 1953). Commercially produced kits for CVC insertion continue to evolve with many labour-saving and hazard-reducing features built into their design.

The basic Seldinger kit comprises a wide-bore hollow needle, a flexible guidewire which will fit through the needle, and a catheter to be threaded over the guide wire. More elaborate kits include smaller needles and wires with a series of dilators which are used to prepare the vessel for the cannula placement. The use of dilators means that flexible, large catheters can be passed into the vein.

The vein is punctured using a needle (or a cannula and trochar depending upon the type of kit selected) and the needle is aspirated to ensure placement in the vein. Avoiding the introduction of air, the syringe is removed and the guide wire is passed down the needle into the vein (see Fig. 10.3). The needle is withdrawn, leaving the wire in the vein. A catheter is now threaded over the wire and fed into the vein. As the catheter is advanced the wire is removed. More advanced catheter kits use a system which enhances continuity of action for the operator. The syringe which is used to aspirate the needle has a central bore down which the wire is passed. This reduces the risk of either air embolism or operator contamination by blood.

If a kit with a dilator is selected, it will be easy to pass the catheter through the skin and into the vessel because the skin hole will have been enlarged by the dilator. If a dilator kit is not selected, it is usually necessary to nick the skin with a blade to facilitate passage of a malleable catheter through the barrier of the skin. Blood is aspirated from the catheter in the usual way to ensure correct placement in the vein. The catheter is then flushed with sodium chloride 0.9%.

Care must be taken not to lose the guide wire as it has been known for operators to push both the catheter and the wire into the circulation.

There are a variety of guide wires on the market, some with different coatings, some with different shaped ends. The 'J' wire has evolved to help placement of catheters which are difficult to thread into the vein. The difficulty in threading a jugular vein can be due to the relative right angle with which the internal jugular enters the subclavian vein, and the 'J' shape to the end of the wire facilitates its passage around such a corner. Most wires, whether 'J' or standard, are usually manu-

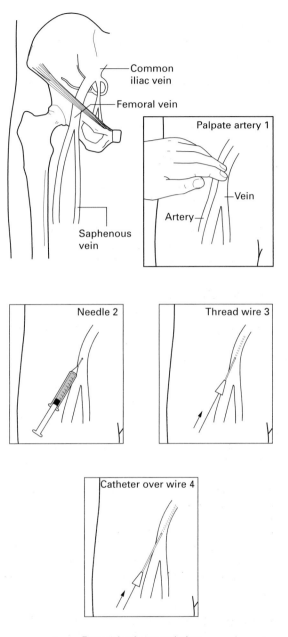

Fig. 10.3 Placing a catheter over a wire. (After Soni 1989, with permission.)

Femoral vein cannulation using Seldinger technique

factured with a flexible end and a rigid end. It is important that it is the flexible end which is inserted into the vein.

An advantage of the Seldinger technique is the small needle puncture allowing the vessel to be dilated up to an exact fit with the cannula size. This reduces the risk of bleeding and the likelihood of air entrainment around the catheter. The use of a dilator removes the need for a surgical nick in the skin and reduces the size of the skin hole. A disadvantage is the complexity of the commercial kit with its inherent cost, possible wire embolus and the risk of contamination of the wire if the environment is inadequately prepared.

PATIENT CONSIDERATIONS

Irrespective of insertion method, it is essential to explain the intended procedure to the patient and to obtain her informed consent to the procedure. Where this is not possible, it is important to explain to a family member the intended actions of the practitioner and the objectives of the treatment. Although consent of one adult for another has no basis in law, keeping family members up to date with treatment is of benefit to promote good relations with the public and to prevent misunderstandings (Medical Defense Union 1996).

During the insertion procedure, it is important that the patient is offered psychological support. The positioning of the patient may be uncomfortable, particularly for those who experience shortness of breath. Cannulation of the neck veins usually requires the placement of sterile towels over the head and face, which can be particularly traumatic for claustrophobic patients.

Despite infiltration of the skin and subcutaneous tissues with local anaesthetic, central vein cannulation can still be an uncomfortable procedure. A significant amount of pressure is usually experienced by the patient as the operator locates, cannulates and dilates the vessel. These experiences are compounded when the operator is inexperienced or when the vessels prove to be difficult to cannulate. It is not uncommon during a prolonged procedure for the local anaesthetic to have worn off by the time the operator is ready to suture the cannula to the skin. It is debatable which is more uncomfortable, repeated infiltration with local anaesthetic or two transient needle pricks to suture the cannula in place.

If the patient is troubled by lying flat, it may be possible to elevate the head of the bed as soon as the catheter is in place. Suturing the catheter and applying the dressing can be done with the patient in an upright position.

MANAGEMENT OF CENTRAL VENOUS ACCESS

Aseptic technique

A strict aseptic technique is required for the placement of central venous catheters, irrespective of the method chosen. Despite the wealth of research into the infective complications of CVCs, aseptic precautions vary between centres and operators. Stringent aseptic technique is considered mandatory for short- or long-term central catheter placement and its importance should not be underestimated.

Elliott et al (1994) recommended that staff should prepare themselves as for theatre – sterile gown and gloves, mask and hat and a full surgical scrub technique performed prior to gowning.

It has often been assumed that catheters inserted in the operating theatre pose a lower risk of infection than those inserted in a ward environment. The results of two recent prospective studies do not support this view and in fact demonstrate that it is the amount of barrier precaution utilized during the insertion process, rather than the environment, which influences the incidence of infection in CVCs (Mermal et al 1991, Raad et al 1994). Maximal barrier precautions are said to be sterile gown and gloves, hat and mask. Sterile gloves and a small fenestrated drape produce a higher incidence of infection than maximal barrier precautions (Pearson 1995).

Skin preparation and site care

In the event that there is gross contamination of the skin, Elliott et al (1994) recommended that it be cleaned with soap and water prior to routine disinfection of the site. What form that disinfection should take has been the subject of much research and debate.

For many years, the use of an alcohol-based iodine solution to clean the insertion site was recommended. This has now been superseded by the work of Maki et al (1991), who demonstrated the efficacy of aqueous chlorhexidine for the management of central access sites. Alcohol-based iodine products are only efficacious for a few minutes and as they dry they lose their activity. By contrast, aqueous chlorhexidine 2% has been shown to remain active on the skin surface for 6 hours after application.

Just as important as the selection of the cleansing solution are the method and duration of the cleansing process. It is recommended that the site be cleaned in concentric circles, moving from the intended site of access out towards the periphery (Baranowski 1993). Elliott et al (1994) emphasized the need to clean beyond the intended site of insertion. As an example, they suggested that for jugular or subclavian access, the skin preparation should include the neck and top of the trunk of the patient. They also recommended that the insertion site be cleaned again after correct placement of the catheter. It is important, when doing this, to avoid further contamination of the site.

The use of antimicrobial ointments to prevent local colonization of CVC sites is controversial. Maki & Band (1981) were unable to demonstrate any effectiveness of antibiotic or iodine-based ointments in the prevention of catheter-related sepsis. Concern has been raised that antibiotic ointments may disrupt normal skin flora and promote the growth of yeasts such as *Candida* (Pearson 1995). The use of mupirocin, an antistaphylococcal agent, in conjunction with tincture of iodine prior to catheter insertion, has been shown to reduce the incidence of internal jugular colonization in cardiac surgical patients (Hill et al 1990). Mupirocin resistance has been reported, however, and its effectiveness for use in catheter site maintenance is yet to be established in controlled trials (Pearson 1995).

Dressings

The type of dressing to use on CVCs provokes perhaps the greatest discussion of all. Gauze and tape or transparent dressings are probably the most common methods employed.

Transparent polyurethane dressings have the obvious benefit of facilitating observation of the entry site without disturbance. The earlier transparent dressings were occlusive in nature, the type now considered appropriate for wound management. The modern transparent dressing is described as moisture-permeable and is reported to produce less moisture build-up at the entry site. The use of these dressings still remains one of the most debated issues in i.v. site care.

There are reports that transparent dressings promote the local growth of *Candida* and contribute to the risk of catheter-related infection (Conly et al 1989, Craven et al 1985). However, other studies have shown no difference between the use of gauze and transparent dressings (Hoffman et al 1988, Ricard et al 1985). Maki (1987) investigated the use of transparent dressings on peripheral devices and could establish no clinical significance between the use of gauze and the transparent moisture-permeable dressing. These authors advocated that the transparent dressing placed on the cannula at the time of insertion be left in place until the cannula is removed, providing the cannula is routinely replaced 48–72 hours post-insertion.

Most of the literature surrounding CVC dressings relates to short-term, non-tunnelled catheters. There is little written about long-term, tunnelled catheters. The length of time that a transparent dressing can be left on a CVC is as yet unknown (Pearson 1995).

Securing the catheter

That the catheter should be secured is undisputed – a mobile catheter is not only prone to mechanical thrombophlebitis but may also become dislodged. Long-term catheters are usually immobilized by their Dacron cuffs, whereas short-term catheters are usually sutured. Sutures are, by default, fixed to the skin and do not always control the entry site of the cannula. It is usually prudent to further secure the catheter using adhesive tape or by the strategic placement of the dressing. Care should be taken to support the weight of administration sets to prevent undue traction on the catheter and unnecessary strain on the sutures (which may either break or pull out of the skin, thus making the catheter vulnerable to dislodgement).

Catheter position

The position of the catheter is often confirmed by X-ray, although many experienced operators are confident of catheter position based on the ease of insertion and free aspiration of blood from all lumens. It is prudent to check whether an X-ray is required prior to using the catheter.

Seneff (1987a) suggested that, with the exception of a femoral cannula, the optimal placement of the cannula tip is in the distal innominate vein or proximal superior vena cava. Fatal complications resulting from misplacement of CVCs have been reported for more than two decades (Adar & Mozes 1971, Brandt et al 1970, McGee et al 1993, Maschke & Rogove 1984). According to Seneff (1987a), catheters positioned in the subclavian vein have a tendency to migrate to an extrathoracic site when the arm is moved. Sheep & Guiney (1982) confirmed earlier reports when they described fatal cardiac tamponade resulting from catheter tip placement in the right atrium. There are also many reports of dysrhythmias resulting from incorrect catheter placement (Daniels et al 1984, Iberti et al 1985, Kasten et al 1985, McGee et al 1993, Seneff 1987a).

Catheter removal

This is an important aspect of the management of CVCs, and perhaps receives the least attention. The risks associated with catheter removal are not new, the most significant of which is perhaps air embolism.

Air embolism has been reported to occur up to 72 hours after the removal of a CVC (Hanley et al 1984, Phifer et al 1991). A survey demonstrated that nurses were more aware of the risks of embolism following catheter removal than were doctors. Nurses were better informed about the preventative strategies which could be employed during and after CVC removal (Mennim et al 1992).

To prevent air embolism, it is recommended that patients who can tolerate lying flat are asked to do so during the catheter removal procedure. Failing this, they may be asked to breathe in and hold their breath for the few seconds required to remove the catheter. Following removal of the CVC and achievement of haemostasis, an occlusive transparent dressing (not moisture-permeable) should be applied and left in place for 72 hours. However, some authors (Elliot et al 1994) fail to address this important issue and recommend the application of a gauze dressing on removal of a central catheter. It is important to inspect the integrity of the catheter after removal. There are reports in the literature of catheter separation from the hub and catheter rupture following high-pressure injectate or excessive negative pressure during catheter aspiration (Scott 1988). Separation of a catheter fragment leads to catheter embolism and may result in the catheter lodging in the right side of the heart (Baranowski 1993). Scott (1988) reported a mortality incidence of 30% if the catheter fragment is not retrieved.

The nurse should be aware of the potential for catheter embolus. If the catheter is not intact on removal, a medical officer should be informed. It is usual practice to perform a chest X-ray to locate the radio-opaque fragment. Retrieval of the fragment is usually performed using transvenous biopsy forceps. The risk of catheter embolus is increased if a stylet (needle) has been reintroduced into a catheter during the insertion procedure.

Microbiological assessment

Following removal of a CVC, it is not uncommon to send the catheter tip to the microbiology department for bacterial culture and sensitivity assessment. If this is clinically indicated, the tip of the catheter should be cut off, using sterile scissors, placed in a sterile container and sent to microbiology. This is usually a routine procedure for high-risk patients, who are generally defined as:

- those who are actively immunosuppressed
- those who are immunocompromised by their disease process, e.g. ITU patients of all ages
- those with pyrexia of unknown origin
- those in whom catheter-associated infection is suspected
- those in whom septicaemia would be potentially life-threatening.

Microbiological assessment can be carried out in two ways. The first method is to roll the catheter tip several times across a bacterial culture plate, incubate the plate and then analyse the number of bacterial colonies. This technique was established by Maki. The second method is to flush the catheter tip with culture broth and to culture the fluid (Cleri et al 1980). These techniques facilitate assessment of extraluminal and intraluminal bacterial colonization, the two most important routes for catheter-related septicaemia (Elliott 1993).

However, as Elliott (1993) stated, the drawback of this method is that diagnosis is made after the catheter has been removed, and therefore some catheter removal may prove to be unnecessary. Markus & Buday (1989) proposed a brush culture technique to facilitate catheter culture in situ. This is rarely used in the UK and may prove inappropriate if the catheter to be sampled contains inotropes or other vasoactive agents.

In acute care, when faced with a septic, critically ill patient, it is often more prudent to presume the CVC to be the cause of the sepsis and to remove it, rather than leave the potential source of infection in situ for 3 days while awaiting the results of the catheter culture.

COMPLICATIONS OF CENTRAL VENOUS CATHETERIZATION

Some complications have already been alluded to in association with particular access routes. This section will discuss the most common hazards of central venous catheterization, the mechanisms by which they occur, and any remedial or preventative action which can be taken to avoid or minimize their impact upon the patient.

Air embolism

This complication is almost exclusively limited to central rather than peripheral access. The veins of the thorax are under the influence of the changing pressures within the thoracic cavity. The pressure changes are due mainly to respiration, but pressure change is also seen in relation to gravity, i.e. lying down vs. sitting up.

Atmospheric air pressure, at sea level, is 760 mmHg. At the end of expiration, the intrathoracic pressure is in equilibrium with atmospheric pressure. As inspiration occurs and the chest expands, the intrathoracic pressure falls, causing a pressure gradient between the atmosphere and the lungs. Air rushes into the lungs until the pressure inside the chest is again in equilibrium with the atmosphere. When an individual begins to exhale, the chest wall compresses the lungs, causing the intrathoracic pressure to rise. Intrathoracic pressure is now greater than atmospheric pressure and this causes air to leave the lungs until the intrathoracic pressure is again in equilibrium with atmospheric pressure. These changes in pressure are only mild; however, the movement of gas along a pressure gradient is very efficient.

The central veins experience these pressure changes, with their internal pressure alternating subtly between being just above or just below atmospheric pressure. If a cannula is inserted into a central vein and left open to the atmosphere, each time the pressure in the vein falls below atmospheric pressure, air will be sucked into the circulation (i.e. during the inspiratory phase of the respiratory cycle). Air can be entrained into the circulation in this way at a rate of 100 ml/s (Phifer et al 1991).

Prevention

Vigilance is essential to prevent air embolism. The individual inserting the catheter will usually require the patient to lie flat, or even head down (Trendelenburg's position). This causes the neck veins to fill, making them easier to palpate, but also making them less likely to experience negative pressure and entrain air. It is usual practice during catheter insertion for the operator to occlude the end of the catheter whenever the syringe or guide wire is removed.

Most catheters include in-line clamps to allow them to be safely disconnected during administration set changes or any other procedure involving disconnection. All staff who handle CVCs must ensure that bungs are replaced correctly, that only luer-lock fittings are employed and that the luer locks are screwed together tightly. When taking over the care of a patient, it is important to check the safety of the connections on a CVC.

All burettes have in-built air inlets to allow the fluid to flow out. When using burettes on CVCs, it is essential that the product selected contains an air occlusion device to prevent air being entrained down the tubing and into the patient.

If an infusion is being delivered from a bottle, e.g. human albumin, antibiotics or clotting agents, an air inlet is usually inserted into the bottle so that the fluid can flow out. If a bottle is used on a CVC, it is essential that the patient and the infusion are constantly observed so that the infusion can be switched off when complete, thus preventing air embolism through the empty bottle.

In both these situations, air embolism is much more likely in a patient whose circulation is reduced, e.g. as a result of dehydration or haemorrhage. A patient whose circulation is empty may experience negative pressure in the central veins throughout the entire respiratory cycle. The more laboured a patient's breathing, the greater the range of pressure change within the chest and the greater the risk of air embolism.

The risk of air entrainment from a bottle or burette is of even greater significance if the infusion is being administered into a pumped extracorporeal circuit, e.g. in haemofiltration or haemodialysis. The pumped circuit has the capability to entrain air in proportion to the pump speed. Most (but not all) of these systems have methods of air detection, but despite these features entrained air can jeopardize the patient's treatment, create delays and increase nursing workload.

The risk of air embolism is often underestimated by health care staff. The longer a catheter remains in situ, the more likely it is that a tract will be established around the catheter into the vessel (Mennim et al 1992). There are reported cases of patients experiencing air embolism through entrainment of air around catheters and transvenous pacing wires whilst the device is still in situ (Johnson et al 1991).

The removal of a CVC is a time of high risk because, for a brief period, the vein is again open to the atmosphere. When patients are able, it is advisable to lie them flat to remove a central catheter (Mennim et al 1992). If this is not possible, an alternative strategy is to ask patients to breathe in and hold their breath. At this point the venous pressure should be either in equilibrium with or higher than atmospheric pressure.

Many staff are unaware of the continued risk of embolism after the cannula has been removed and haemostasis achieved. The literature demonstrates that air embolism is possible up to 72 hours after catheter removal (Hanley et al 1984, Phifer et al 1991) and that the likelihood of embolism is proportional to the length of time during which the catheter was in situ. This would appear to be due to persistency of the skin tract down to the vein (Hanley et al 1984, Phifer et al 1991). It is therefore recommended that an occlusive dressing is applied to the site for 72 hours following removal of a CVC.

Management

An air embolism is a medical emergency and is associated with significant mortality. Nurses who care for patients with CVCs should be aware of this hazard, how to recognize it and the best course of action to deal with the problem.

Patients who experience air embolism may present with a range of symptoms, including:

- shortness of breath
- altered consciousness
- visual disturbance
- hemiparesis
- chest pain
- a low cardiac output state.

Any cause of the embolus should be found and rectified, e.g. by turning off any open three-way taps, replacing missing bungs, closing in-line clamps, applying pressure to any central puncture sites, etc. The patient will require oxygen via a face mask and should be placed on her left side in a steep Trendelenburg position as a matter of urgency. A member of the medical staff should be contacted as an emergency.

The object of the positioning is to facilitate entrapment of the air embolus in the apex of the ventricles. If the air is successfully trapped in the ventricles, it is unlikely to be pumped into the aorta and consequently through the carotid arteries and up to the brain where it may induce ischaemia, blindness or CVA. If the air is successfully trapped in this manner, it can be aspirated from the ventricles under image intensity.

In the event that the air does circulate to the brain, there are case reports of successful treatment with hyperbaric oxygen therapy, which causes the gas bubble to reduce in size and to be forced into solution in the blood (Halliday et al 1994). Few centres, however, have the ability to deliver hyperbaric oxygen therapy.

Throughout this time, the patient will need calm reassurance and prompt decisive action from the practitioner. An emergency call should be put out to obtain assistance as quickly as possible. Emergency equipment should be available.

Pneumothorax

A pneumothorax is diagnosed when air can be detected between the pleural membranes that surround the lungs. This can occur following central vein cannulation, and the mechanism is not dissimilar to that described in air embolism.

During the central venous catheterization process, the operator must locate the vessel which is under the surface of the skin. If, whilst probing with their needle, the operator punctures the pleural membrane it is possible for environmental air to be entrained down the needle and into the pleural space. This is most commonly seen following subclavian vein cannulation, but can also be seen following a low approach to the internal jugular vein (Seneff 1987b).

The pleura experience the pressure changes already described for air embolism. Therefore, during inspiration, the pleural pressure is negative and air can be sucked into the pleura. If air enters the pleural space, it causes the two pleural membranes to separate and the normal mechanics of breathing is impaired. If the air can enter the pleural space (via the needle puncture) but cannot escape again this is termed a tension pneumothorax.

Small pneumothoraces rarely cause complications unless the patient is already compromised by respiratory disease. A small pneumothorax in an asymptomatic patient will usually be left to resolve spontaneously. If the pneumothorax is large or the patient compromised, the condition will be treated by the insertion of a pleural underwater seal drain. It is possible to entrain large quantities of air into the pleural space. This causes lung compression and can, in extreme circumstances, lead to electromechanical dissociation (EMD) of the heart. This is a medical emergency which will require resuscitation. In this situation, the EMD results from the large pneumothorax causing a mediastinal shift, kinking of the SVC and/or IVC and acutely obstructing the venous return to the heart. The lack of venous return causes reduced preload, reduced contractility, reduced stroke volume and subsequently reduced cardiac output.

The patient will usually complain of dyspnoea, will often become agitated or restless and may experience a sense of foreboding. They will usually require oxygen via a face mask, psychological support and positioning to optimize their respiratory function. Help should be summoned and the nurse will need to assist with the insertion of a chest drain, which is connected to an underwater drainage system. It is common practice to check the position of the drain on X-ray.

Hydrothorax

This may occur if the central venous catheterization process results in a catheter being placed in the pleural space. If the cannulation process is traumatic, it is possible for the operator to puncture the pleura and to think that they have located the vessel when really the cannula is in the pleural space. Due to local tissue trauma, the operator may even experience relatively free flow of blood when the cannula is aspirated.

If the placement of the catheter is not checked by X-ray prior to its use, a practitioner may inadvertently infuse intravenous fluids into the pleural space, thus causing a hydrothorax.

There are also reports of hydrothorax formation following erosion of the superior vena cava, although this appears to be a result of poorly positioned external jugular catheters (Ghani & Berry 1983).

The presentation and treatment are the same as for pneumothorax. The speed of presentation may depend on the speed of infusion of intravenous fluids.

Haemorrhage

Most CVCs are large-bore devices. If a patient has a high central venous pressure

(CVP), she will be at risk of bleeding from the catheter should it become dislodged or if a connection is inadvertently left open to the air. This is, in effect, the opposite situation to an air embolism. Air embolism will be a risk for patients with low CVP who experience subatmospheric pressure in their vessels during respiration.

Haemorrhage will be a risk for patients whose CVP is higher than atmospheric pressure. This may occur in a range of patients, e.g. those with:

- chronic obstructive airways disease
- acute pulmonary embolism
- liver failure
- congestive heart failure
- the overhydrated or overtransfused patient.

Due to the diameter of the catheter and its placement in a large, high-flow vessel, it is possible for substantial haemorrhage to occur via a CVC. Nurses must be very wary of this complication – all connections and the security of the catheter must be checked regularly.

MONITORING

Haemodynamic monitoring

Bedside haemodynamic monitoring permits continuous surveillance of the cardio-vascular system and provides the physiological data to guide therapy (Daily & Schroeder 1994).

In order to undertake haemodynamic monitoring, the vascular system must be cannulated and the pressure within the circulation interpreted. All electronic equipment for measuring haemodynamic information has three fundamental components:

- a transducer to detect physiological activity
- an amplifier to increase the size of the signal
- a recording device to display the information, either on a screen or as a paper recording.

Using high-pressure manometer tubing, it is possible to transmit pressure with minimal distortion. In connecting the manometer tubing to a central or arterial catheter, the effect is to artificially increase the length of the vessel so that it can be attached to the monitoring equipment.

By connecting the manometer tubing to a transducer, it is possible to convert mechanical energy (pressure) into electrical energy (the waveform) (Daily & Schroeder 1994).

The electrical signal produced by the transducer is transmitted through a cable to the monitor. The monitor contains an amplifier which modifies the signal by increasing the voltage and filtering the signal. The improved quality signal is then displayed as a waveform on the monitor.

Transduced, electronic information has the advantage of a rapid response time. There is no time lag between a physiology event and the information received on the monitor. Waveforms can be analysed and this may supply the practitioner with additional information. Mean values can also be calculated.

To improve the accuracy of pressure recordings, the weight of air or 'atmospheric pressure' must be eliminated from the recording. Atmospheric pressure will vary with altitude and environmental factors such as humidity and temperature. The elimination of the influence of environmental pressure is achieved by opening the transducer to air and adjusting the display system to read zero (Daily & Schroeder 1994).

Thus atmospheric pressure is described as zero, rather than 760 mmHg, which is the true value at sea level. If the true value was used in medical practice, then any pressure recordings, such as blood pressure, would have to be added to atmospheric pressure. A normal blood pressure would, in truth, be 880/840 mmHg. The normal range for blood pressure would also vary depending upon the altitude at which a person lived. In an attempt to reduce the complexity of reality, medicine adjusts its equipment so that atmospheric pressure is read as zero, and records all pressure values in relation to this.

In order for a transducer to be accurate, the user must ensure that the transducer recognizes atmospheric 'zero'. To test this, the transducer tap is opened to air and if the monitor fails to record zero, the zero button is pressed to reset the monitor.

Purely calibrating a machine to a single value is less accurate than calibrating it to a range of values. Most reusable transducers are recalibrated when they are serviced; the modern transducer is disposable and is precalibrated by the manufacturer. Practitioners who work with reusable transducers should check that they are regularly calibrated to at least two electronically known values, e.g. 50 and 100 mmHg, or 100 and 200 mmHg. Calibration is a quality control measure.

Transducers are very sensitive and easily damaged, and the calibration to zero should be checked regularly throughout the day to ensure accuracy of the equipment.

For accuracy of results, transducers are usually positioned at a standard level in relation to the patient's position. This is traditionally in line with the patient's right atrium. Anatomically this is either the mid-axillary line or the sternal notch. The latter point is more consistent for recordings as it is a geographical reference point which is easy to find. It is, however, only in line with the right atrium when a patient is sitting up. The mid-axillary line is a more universal reference point. The practitioner should make a note of whichever site is selected so that readings are consistent.

Accuracy can only be assumed if the equipment is well maintained and the patient is well positioned. Connections should be tightly luer-locked to ensure that there is no 'leakage' of pressure into the lower pressured environment. The pressure signal from the patient is transmitted through fluid-filled manometer tubing. This fluid is usually heparinized saline, 1 unit/ml, delivered via a pressurized flush device. The flush device is maintained at a constant pressure of 300 mmHg in adults, which produces a continuous flush of approximately 3 ml/h through the system (Daily & Schroeder 1994). Lower pressures and volumes are usually used in paediatrics. It is not uncommon in paediatrics to use volume-controlled pumps and syringes to administer a continuous flush to monitoring devices; this prevents volume overload from uncontrolled in-line flush devices (Daily & Schroeder 1994).

Heparinized saline has traditionally been used to maintain the patency of the system which would otherwise be at risk of clotting. The use of heparin is not without risk and there have been several papers investigating the need for it in a pressurized system (Peterson & Kirchhoff 1991, Taylor et al 1989). Most studies have small sample sizes (Hook et al 1987, Leighton 1994), but their data suggest that heparin is not required to maintain the patency of transduced catheters. Hook et al (1987) concluded that it was probably the consistent pressurized flush that maintained the patency rather than the presence of heparin.

The responsiveness of the system depends on its resonant frequency (Daily & Schroeder 1994), i.e. the speed with which the system oscillates. To ensure the greatest accuracy, the practitioner should consider the following issues.

Tubing length Where possible this should not exceed a metre, as increased tubing length reduces the system's responsiveness.

Tubing material It is essential to use dedicated manometer tubing which is noncompliant. Soft i.v. tubing is distensible and can reduce the quality of the transmitted pressure wave, resulting in a recording of reduced pressure.

Diameter of the catheter The smaller the diameter of the catheter, the more resistance it presents to flow through it. It is best to use the largest catheter possible to obtain accurate results. However, this must be tempered by the risks of large-bore cannulation and the device selected should be the best option for the patient. If, for example, a practitioner uses a multi-lumen catheter to record CVP, it is important that the largest lumen is selected. This creates the least resistance and produces the most accurate recording (Daily & Schroeder 1994).

Prevention of air bubbles The presence of air bubbles in the fluid-filled tubing will cause a reduction in the accuracy of the recordings. Air, like most gases, is compressible. If air bubbles are present in the system they will be compressed by the pressure wave that is being transmitted through the fluid-filled tubing. This will cause the pressure signal to weaken because some of the pressure has been absorbed by the gas bubbles.

A physical property of a liquid is that it is unable to be compressed. It is therefore a good medium to transmit a pressure signal, provided there are no gas bubbles in the liquid to distort the accuracy. Care must be taken when priming the system to eradicate all air bubbles. If a transducer set has been primed and then left to stand before use, many microbubbles will have come out of solution and will be attached to the walls of the tubing. It is essential to eliminate all these and to flush the system prior to use.

Prevention of clots Small clots in the intravascular catheter can also cause a distortion in the transmission of the pressure wave. Regular flushing of the system and the use of a continuous flush device can contribute to reducing this risk (Daily & Schroeder 1994).

Distortions of the pressure wave caused by bubbles, clots, distensible tubing, over-long tubing, etc. is called damping. The features of a damped trace are loss of waveform dynamics, lower peak pressures and higher trough pressures (referred to as a narrow pulse pressure), and rounding of the waveforms with a loss of definition, e.g. loss of the dicrotic notch on an arterial wave.

Staff should be familiar with normal haemodynamic waveforms in order to interpret the abnormal or to detect change in the quality of the information.

Measurement of right atrial or central venous pressure

The central venous pressure is the pressure in the great veins supplying the venous return to the heart. As these vessels are in continuity with the right atrium, CVP is usually the same as right atrial pressure (RAP).

The CVP or RAP usually reflects the filling pressure of the heart, in particular the right atrium. This usually gives an indication of the quality of filling of the right ventricle. In health it is also assumed to be an indication of the filling of the left ventricle. There are certain circumstances when the behaviour of one ventricle may not have any bearing on the function of the other, e.g. in right or left heart failure. CVP is often used to assess the circulating volume. If the CVP is low, the circulating volume may be low. It is not possible, however, to assume this correlation as other factors must be considered, e.g. the patient's vascular tone. A profoundly peripherally dilated patient may have a normal circulating volume despite recording a low CVP. Peripheral dilation is seen in pyrexia, sepsis and anaphylaxis, and in patients in whom vasodilators are being used. The opposite is also true: if a patient is dehydrated, the sympathetic nervous system will increase the vascular tone to maintain the intravascular pressure; thus a hypovolaemic patient may record a normal CVP.

CVP is not therefore a true measurement of intravascular volume, but rather a

Fig. 10.4 A typical central venous pressure waveform. **a**, the increase in venous pressure seen during atrial systole. Because the atria have contracted, the venous return cannot enter the atria and accumulates in the great veins, causing an increase in pressure. **c**, the transient increase in pressure caused by the bulging of the tricuspid valve during the isovolumetric contraction of the ventricles. **v**, the change in pressure seen as the atria fill while the tricuspid valve is closed.

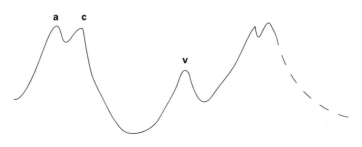

a   The increase in venous pressure seen during atrial systole. Because the atria have contracted, the venous return cannot enter the atria and accumulates in the great veins, causing an increase in pressure.

c   The transient increase in pressure caused by the bulging of the tricuspid valve during the isovolumetric contraction of the ventricles.

v   This is the change in pressure which is seen as the atria fill whilst the tricuspid valve is closed.

measure of the pressure in the central veins, and can only contribute to the assessment of intravascular volume (Soni 1989).

If a CVC is connected to a pressure transducer, it should be possible to record the CVP. A typical CVP waveform is illustrated in Figure 10.4. Alterations in CVP traces are seen in disease. For example, if a patient experiences atrial fibrillation (AF), their CVP trace will not usually demonstrate 'a' waves. Patients who have been overfilled or who have tricuspid valve regurgitation (TVR) will have very dominant 'v' waves, typical of TVR.

Left atrial pressure

Left atrial waveforms are usually similar to right atrial waveforms, but with less definition due to the distensibility of the pulmonary venous system. True left atrial recordings are only obtained by the insertion of a direct left atrial catheter. This is usually restricted to post-cardiac surgical situations because the fine cannula must be placed through the chest wall and into the left atrium. This method of monitoring is not without risk. Gentle traction is placed on the catheter when it is ready to be removed. The catheter is usually removed relatively easily, but there is a risk that a patent hole will remain in the left atrium. This can result in tamponade and the patient must be monitored and observed during and after left atrial catheter removal.

It is more common to pass a pulmonary artery flotation catheter in order to obtain information about the left side of the heart. This is a transvenous system without the inherent risks of bleeding from an atrial puncture site.

Arterial pressure recording

Arteries have forward flow and, as a result, waveforms are usually characterized by systolic waves followed by diastolic waves. Systole of the left ventricle produces a high-velocity ejection of blood through the aortic valve and into the aorta. The aorta slows the pulse wave slightly by the distensibility of the aortic wall and by the curve of the aortic arch. As systole finishes, the aortic valve closes and this generates a second small rise in pressure in the aorta. The closure of the aortic valve can be

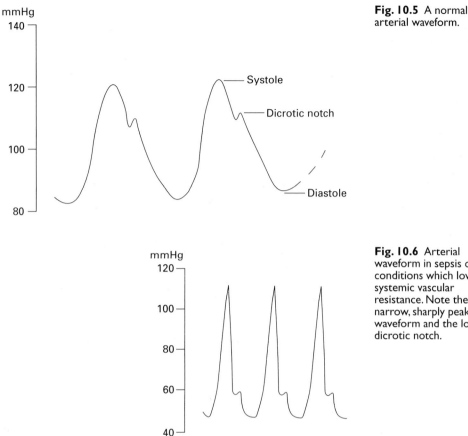

Fig. 10.5 A normal arterial waveform.

Fig. 10.6 Arterial waveform in sepsis or conditions which lower systemic vascular resistance. Note the narrow, sharply peaked waveform and the lower dicrotic notch.

seen on the arterial waveform and is termed the 'dicrotic notch'. Figure 10.5 illustrates an arterial waveform in health.

When systemic vascular tone is normal, the arterioles generate resistance to blood flow and pressure within the arteries is sustained for relatively long periods of time. This creates a large area under the curve of the wave, and the top of the wave, although clearly definable, is not excessively peaked.

In patients whose vascular tone is abnormally dilated, perhaps due to sepsis, the vasculature has less tone, is relatively unresistant and pressure is allowed to dissipate very rapidly. This produces a much narrower pressure wave with less area under its curve, indicating that perfusion pressure has not been sustained for any length of time. This produces an overall reduction in mean pressure. The dicrotic notch is still seen, but appears to be in a different position (Fig. 10.6). Its timing will not have changed (it is still produced by the closure of the aortic valve at the end of systole), however the amount of pressure left in the aorta when the dicrotic notch occurs is much reduced. This means that by the time the aortic valve closes, systolic pressure has already disappeared. The arterial pressure trace also appears much more peaked.

In ill health where vascular tone is altered, arterial waves can appear less consistent and may even appear to be out of sequence. Shock waves of blood can appear to rebound up an artery, giving the appearance of either a double wave or a wave which is back to front, i.e. diastole before systole.

Arterial waveforms which are transduced from positional arterial catheters or

Fig. 10.7 Damped arterial waveform. Note the raised diastolic pressure, the narrowed pulse pressure and the loss of definition to the wave.

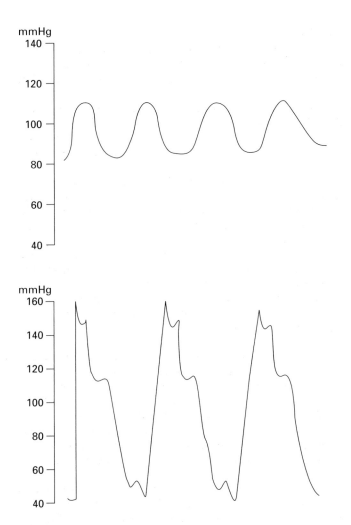

Fig. 10.8 Arterial waveform with 'overshoot'. Note the abnormally high peak pressure, the double peak at the top of the wave and the additional diastolic activity.

from partially occluded arterial catheters can appear damped (Fig. 10.7). This is the term used to describe loss of definition of the waveform. It can also be seen when the manometer tubing contains bubbles.

It is also possible to have a transduced arterial pressure wave which is under-damped. The waveform appears to have an exaggerated peak, and often the systolic wave appears to have two peaks. This is commonly described as 'overshooting' (Fig. 10.8). To reduce the likelihood of overshooting, inaccuracies related to the tubing length and material, the diameter of the cannula, air bubbles and clots should be eliminated (see p. 283). Commercial damping devices are available if the problem cannot be resolved.

Risk factors

Arterial catheters present significant risks to patients and should only be used when the benefits of patient management outweigh the disadvantages of catheter placement. One of the most significant contraindications to arterial cannulation is coagulopathy. However, an arterial catheter placed at first attempt by an experienced practitioner may offer lower risk than numerous puncture sites to monitor gases or chemistry.

Insertion site and procedure

The most popular insertion site is the radial artery. This is one of two arteries which supply the hand, the other being the ulnar artery. By cannulating the radial artery, there is still another artery to guarantee adequate blood supply to the distal limb (Fig. 10.9).

It is good practice to ensure that limb perfusion can be achieved using the other artery. This is called an Allen's test. The artery which is intended to be used is occluded using digital pressure. The hand is observed to determine whether collateral supply is adequate to maintain perfusion to the limb. If it is not it would be prudent to select another site (Soni 1989).

The brachial artery is rarely a first choice because it is the only artery supplying the arm at that point; it divides lower down to form the radial and ulnar arteries. Long-term usage of the brachial artery is not recommended (Daily & Schroeder 1994). The dorsalis pedis and posterior tibial arteries can also be used and both benefit from collateral circulation.

Arterial catheters are usually placed using the Seldinger technique. The difference between an arterial and a venous catheter is the presence of side holes in an arterial catheter. This promotes through-flow to maintain the perfusion of the distal limb. Some operators choose to use small-gauge venous catheters in place of arterial catheters, although this is not recommended by the manufacturers. These venous catheters are positioned using the trochar as for a standard venepuncture.

It is common practice to suture arterial catheters in an attempt to reduce the hazard of exsanguination in the event that the catheter becomes dislodged.

A transparent, moisture-permeable dressing is usually selected to secure the catheter and promote observation of the site. Care must be taken to ensure that luerlock fittings are used and that they are tightly connected. Whilst the arterial catheter is in situ, the practitioner must carefully observe the patient, the catheter site and the distal limb. The catheter should be observed in the same way as a venous cannula, looking for signs of erythema, oedema, leakage, bleeding, discharge or tracking along the arterial route.

The distal limb must be inspected and compared with the other, non-cannulated limb for colour, warmth, sensation, capillary filling and blanching. Deterioration in any of these features is indicative of impaired perfusion to the distal limb. The signs must be reported immediately and it is good practice to electively replace the device.

In the event that a femoral artery site has been used, where there is no collateral supply, any signs of limb ischaemia could have devastating complications. Removal of the catheter is essential and it may be necessary to perform a Fogarty embolectomy to restore circulation to the limb (Daily & Schroeder 1994).

The femoral artery is a common site for paediatric arterial monitoring and is the only site for the placement of intra-aortic balloon pumps. In patients whose femoral arteries have been catheterized, particularly when the catheter is a large-bore device, it is important to monitor pedal pulses in addition to the range of arterial observations previously listed. It may be necessary to utilize a portable Doppler to confirm pulses in a patient whose pulses are difficult to palpate. Many units choose to monitor foot temperatures as an early indication of deterioration in peripheral arterial flow.

Complications

Complications of arterial catheterization include limb ischaemia, haematoma and aneurysm formation. The latter may require surgical repair. A significant complication is disconnection, which can have devastating results if not detected early. It is

Fig. 10.9 Placing an arterial catheter over a needle. (After Soni 1989, with permission.)

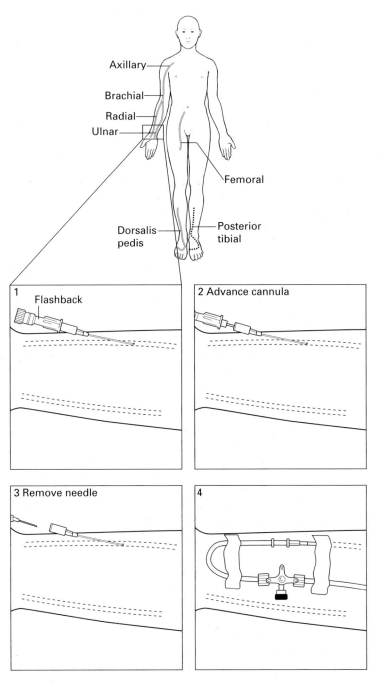

Sites for arterial catheterization

Axillary

Brachial

Radial

Ulnar

Femoral

Dorsalis pedis

Posterior tibial

1 Flashback

2 Advance cannula

3 Remove needle

4

considered good practice to be able to observe at all times a limb containing an arterial catheter. An arm should not, therefore, be left under the bed clothes where haemorrhage could go undetected.

Management

It is considered good practice to clearly label an arterial catheter to prevent unintentional drug administration. Other than heparinized saline, no fluids or drugs should be injected into an arterial catheter. The exception to this rule might be the instillation of a thrombolytic agent to restore perfusion to a thrombosed artery. Eradication of all air from the continuous flush system of an arterial catheter is essential. Even small air bubbles in an arterial system can cause local air embolism and subsequent tissue ischaemia.

Removal As with all intravascular devices, arterial catheters should be removed when they are no longer clinically useful. Care must be taken when removing an arterial catheter; non-sterile gloves should be worn and it would be good risk management to wear goggles to prevent blood splashes to the eye (RCN 1994). The flush device should be switched off, arterial alarms on the monitor disabled, any sutures removed and, using sterile gauze, pressure should be applied to the site while the catheter is gently pulled out. Firm pressure should be applied to the puncture site for at least 3 minutes, or longer if there is a known coagulopathy. After 3 minutes, the edge of the gauze should be tentatively lifted to observe whether the site has stopped bleeding. If it has not, firm pressure must be applied for a further 3 minutes. This process should be repeated until the bleeding is arrested.

A sterile pressure dressing should be applied and left in place for about an hour. The site should be inspected regularly for bleeding or haematoma formation. The distal limb perfusion should also be assessed in case the pressure dressing is too tight. If an arterial catheter has been removed in preparation for discharge of the patient to a ward, it would be prudent to tell the ward nurse where the arterial puncture was, and when any dressings should be removed.

Intra-aortic balloon pump removal is usually a medical task and carries a significant risk of blood contamination. Apron, gloves and eye protection should be worn. Pressure is applied in a similar manner to the removal of an angioplasty catheter (although intra-aortic balloon pump catheters are of a significantly larger gauge), usually for about 20 minutes. Again the site is cautiously inspected and further pressure applied if indicated. A pressure dressing is applied and usually left in situ for 24 hours. Pedal pulses should be checked to ensure that the pressure dressing does not cause reduced perfusion to the distal limb.

Special pressure-controlled devices are available for controlled removal of large-bore femoral catheters, e.g. the 'Femstop'. These reduce the risk of both blood contamination and underperfusion of the limb from inappropriate pressure application. Due to the transparent nature of the device, observation of the site is possible even during the application of continuous pressure.

Pulmonary artery pressure monitoring

Pulmonary artery (PA) flotation catheters can be used to measure pulmonary artery pressures. This was a British invention which allowed a catheter to be floated through the right side of the heart and into the pulmonary circulation. It was first described in the literature by Swan et al (1970).

By attaching the catheter to a pressure transducer it became possible to measure the pressure changes in the pulmonary circulation. An inflatable balloon was incorporated into the design of the catheter tip. By inflating the balloon and wedging the catheter in a small pulmonary artery, the artery could be obstructed, thus preventing blood flow past the catheter. The transducer was then able to record the pressure in the pulmonary vascular bed, which is in direct continuity with the left atrium. Whatever pressure is present in the left atrium is transmitted back through the pulmonary vascular bed and interpreted by the wedged pulmonary artery

Fig. 10.10 Normal pressure values in the heart. (After Soni 1989, with permission.)

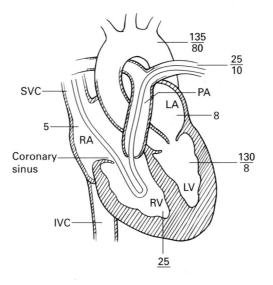

catheter. This technique allows for monitoring of left heart pressure without catheterization of the left side of the heart.

Image intensity is often used to assist with the placement of this type of catheter. Some centres, however, rely solely on pressure changes to identify the placement of the catheter tip. The pressure changes recorded by the monitoring equipment will reflect the pressure changes in the heart as the catheter passes through the various chambers (Fig. 10.10). The pressure waveforms corresponding to these chambers are shown in Figure 10.11.

There are several designs of pulmonary artery catheter:

- *Simple*, incorporating a balloon and a distal lumen through which pulmonary pressure will be measured.
- *Intermediate*, incorporating a balloon, a distal lumen and a proximal lumen through which the CVP may be measured.
- *Complex*, incorporating a balloon, distal and proximal lumens, plus a thermistor and connections for cardiac output studies. This catheter can be used to measure cardiac output, cardiac index, systemic vascular resistance and pulmonary vascular resistance, as well as the traditional pulmonary artery pressure, pulmonary capillary wedge pressure and CVP.

It is also possible to purchase cardiac output catheters which can pace the myocardium, catheters which monitor mixed venous oxygenation as sampled from the pulmonary artery, and catheters with additional lumens for fluid administration. Cardiac output catheters are also being developed with ion electrodes at their tips for in situ measurement of pH.

Despite the increasing popularity of pulmonary artery and cardiac output monitoring, it still carries an intrinsic risk of morbidity. If the information obtained will not improve the management of the patient then the procedure should not be carried out. When the catheter is no longer clinically useful, it should be removed. When using the PA catheter it is important to recognize the unwedged and wedged pressure waveforms. When inflating the balloon to measure a wedge pressure, a section of the pulmonary bed will be deprived of blood flow. Were the catheter to remain wedged for prolonged periods of time, ischaemia would occur. The practitioner at the bedside must be able to recognize the waveform in order to act in the best interest of the patient.

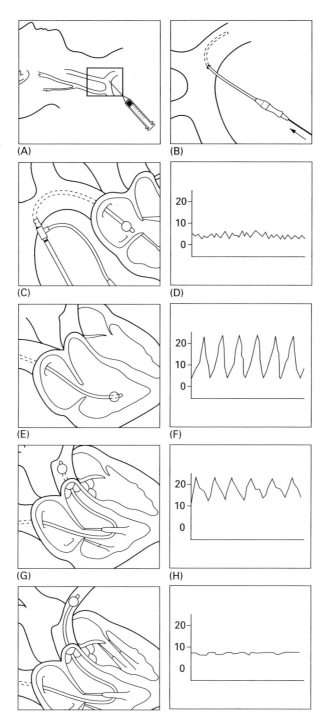

Fig. 10.11 Pressure waveforms corresponding to the chambers of the heart through which the PA catheter is passing. (After Soni 1989, with permission.)

Removal of the PA catheter is similar to removal of other central venous catheters. It must be remembered, however, that this catheter is much longer and less easy to handle. The practitioner should wear gloves and may require a surface on which to place the catheter when it is removed, i.e. a disposable absorbent pad. Prior to removal of the catheter, the practitioner must check that the balloon at the end of the catheter has been deflated. Significant valvular damage could occur if the catheter were removed with the balloon inflated. There are reports of the PA catheter being passed between the chordae tendonae of the tricuspid valve. On occasions, this has led to chordae rupture. As the catheter is removed it will pass through the pulmonary and tricuspid valves. This can often cause electrical irritability, with atrial and ventricular ectopics being seen. In this event it is prudent to continue to remove the catheter rather than to stop pulling and run the risk of leaving the catheter tip positioned in a valve which may cause worse dysrhythmias. The patient's ECG should be observed during catheter removal.

Due to the design of the catheter, it will have been inserted through an introducer cannula. The hole in the vessel may be large and pressure will need to be applied for several minutes. As with other CVCs, an occlusive dressing should be placed on the site and left in situ for 72 hours.

Temporary endocardial pacing

Patients in acute, life-threatening heart block or profound, persistent bradycardia will require a temporary, transvenous pacing wire. Some tachycardias may also be managed with overdrive pacing, although this is less common (Soni 1989).

To pace the heart successfully, a current must be passed through it, and therefore an electrical circuit must be formed (Soni 1989). This is achieved by having two electrodes with heart muscle in between. The electrodes may be built into the same pacing wire, in which case it is termed bipolar, or one electrode may be in the wire whilst the other is placed on or in the skin. This type of wire is classified as unipolar. Modern temporary wires are usually bipolar.

These wires are inserted through an introducer cannula in a central vein, usually under X-ray guidance. In the case of heart blocks, the wire is positioned past the point of block, in the ventricles. In the case of bradycardia, an atrial wire may be used.

It is difficult to secure the wires against the myocardial wall, and atrial wires may be difficult to position. As a result, the majority of temporary pacing wires are ventricular because the wire can be positioned up against the apex of the ventricle. The wire is connected to a pacing box; the battery should have been tested in advance. All pacing boxes are battery-controlled – the patient is never connected to 240 volts!

The entry site at the skin is treated like a cannula site. It is common to see several coils of pacing wire to the entry site. It is hoped that if undue traction is placed on the wire, the coils will tighten, rather than the wire become dislodged. Pacing wires are always sutured in place at the skin entry site.

As pacing wires are more rigid than i.v. catheters, the risk of myocardial perforation is much higher and the patient should be observed for potential tamponade – although this is rare, it is an acknowledged complication (Soni 1989). Pacing wires are removed in the same way as PA catheters with similar attention to dysrhythmias.

VASCULAR ACCESS FOR ACUTE RENAL FAILURE

The human kidney has several functions, the main one of which is excretory. The kidney is responsible for the excretion of water-soluble wastes, excess electrolytes, drugs, hormones and water (Berne & Levy 1993). In the event that the kidneys should fail, the excretory role of the kidney can be mimicked by the artificial filtration of blood through a permeable membrane. This is most commonly achieved through a hollow fibre filter. The filtration which occurs is determined by the pore size of the membrane and the volume of blood passing through the filter.

Small dissolved electrolytes pass across the membrane easily, and as a result clearance of these substances is determined by blood flow and the surface area of the filter.

In haemodialysis, blood and a physiological solution (dialysate) flow in opposite directions through the filter separated by a semi-permeable membrane. Solutes transfer across the membrane down their concentration gradients. This process is termed diffusion. The transfer of small molecules < 200 daltons (Da) is efficient and is determined by the rate of flow of the blood or the dialysate, whichever is slower. Transfer of molecules becomes progressively less as molecular size increases.

In haemofiltration, blood alone flows past one side of the membrane. The hydrostatic pressure gradient across the membrane results in ultrafiltration of water and an accompanying solute loss through convection (solute drag). This system permits the passage of molecules up to 10–20 000 Da almost as freely as water, in a process very similar to glomerular filtration.

The filtrate is discarded and a physiological substitution fluid replaces lost plasma volume. Fluid balance is manipulated by controlling the amount of substitution fluid. Whichever technique is utilized, vascular access will be necessary to deliver blood to the filter and subsequently return the filtered blood to the body.

If the patient is in an intensive care unit, haemofiltration will usually be the treatment of choice. Haemofiltration can be carried out as a slow continuous therapy, avoiding large fluid losses which might make an already sick patient less cardiovascularly stable. Haemofiltration machines are very portable and require no special facilities. They are designed for continuous or intermittent use. Chemistry and fluid balance can be independently manipulated with the modern machines that are currently available. Modern haemofiltration is venovenous, which carries a lower mortality than arteriovenous haemofiltration.

Haemodialysis, in comparison, requires an environment with soft water plumbing, which is not always available outside a renal unit. Dialysis is designed as an intermittent treatment and is only suitable in patients who are cardiovascularly stable and fit enough to be transferred to the renal unit.

In the acute setting a wide-bore double lumen venous catheter will be employed for either haemofiltration or dialysis.

Catheters

There are two designs of catheter lumen in common use. The circumferential lumen is perhaps superior to the staggered lumenal openings. Blood should be able to flow into the catheter irrespective of the position of the catheter within the vessel (Fig. 10.12).

These catheters are traditionally 8 Fg and are inserted using a Seldinger technique. As large vessels are required to tolerate such large catheters, access is usually restricted to the internal jugular, subclavian and femoral veins. Given the known association of venacaval thrombosis, the jugular vein often remains the first-line choice. Special catheters have been designed for the jugular site. They are the same

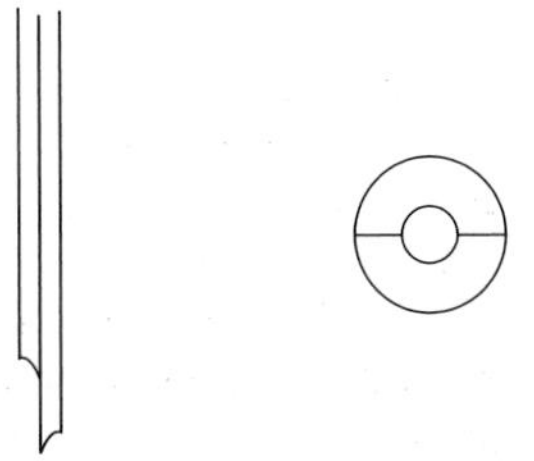

Fig. 10.12 Catheter designs in cross-section.

Fig. 10.13 Haemofiltration catheter modified for the internal jugular site.

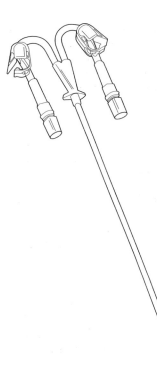

diameter as for the SVC or femoral vein, but their extension ends have been curved back towards the tip of the catheter. This change in direction of the extensions allows the connections to be positioned away from the hair and the side of the face. This is both more comfortable for the patients and should logically offer a lower infection rate (although these data are not yet available) (Fig. 10.13).

In acute ITU or ward settings, these catheters are used as long as the patient's renal failure is deemed to be reversible. As with all CVCs, the catheter will be replaced regularly and, where appropriate, the access site will be rotated. Patients who are ambulatory will prefer not to have femoral vein catheters, both for comfort and for ease of dressing. There is also concern about the risk of vessel perforation. Renal catheters are more rigid than other catheters and are more likely to carry a risk of perforation when a patient starts to mobilize.

Renal catheters are usually dedicated to filtration or dialysis only, rather than being accessed for convenience. If a patient needs a peripheral cannula, it should be inserted rather than using the higher risk renal catheter. Renal catheters are of no use if they are not fully patent. Most renal units maintain patency of their catheters with heparin to ensure that they are available for the next access. A renal catheter with a poorly controlled i.v. infusion will undoubtedly clot off, rendering the access useless. This means not only that renal treatment will be delayed, but also that the patient will have to go through unnecessary recannulation to continue their treatment. Given the diameter of this type of cannula, it is wise not to remove the cannula if the patient is actively heparinized as haemostasis can be difficult to secure. Clotting agents may need to be given to patients with coagulopathies prior to removing this type of catheter.

Management

As with all CVCs, the patient should be correctly positioned, pressure should be applied until haemostasis is achieved and an occlusive dressing should be applied and left in place for 72 hours. If the cannula has been in for 5 days or more, or if catheter-related infection is suspected, the tip of the catheter should be sent for microbiological culture and sensitivity assessment. Catheters used for renal management are associated with an increased risk of septicaemia (Pearson 1995).

Arteriovenous shunts/fistulae

Once acute renal failure appears irreversible, it will be necessary to consider alternative access for continued renal treatment. Medium-term access is usually achieved by the use of an arteriovenous shunt, while long-term access is secured by the formation of an arteriovenous fistula.

Scribner and others pioneered the development of the shunt in the 1960s. This utilized new plastic materials such as Teflon and Silastic. The shunt is a piece of tubing connecting an artery and a vein. It can be clamped and then disconnected to attach the vessels up to the tubing of the dialysis machine. At the end of the treatment the shunt can be reconnected.

Shunts are useful but remain relatively high-risk as a disconnection can lead to massive haemorrhage. Shunts are usually used for in-patients. It is good practice to keep shunt clamps in close proximity in the event of a disconnection (Brundage 1980).

Arteriovenous anastamoses can be surgically created to produce a fistula. A fistula is a direct connection between an artery and a vein. Connecting an artery to a vein creates extreme turbulence within the fistula, which causes the vessel to dilate, producing a reservoir which can be needled to produce a physiological alternative to an implantable port.

Patent fistulae have a characteristic 'thrill', a vibration which is palpable with minimal tactile contact. Observation of the thrill of a fistula is part of the nursing care. Patients with established fistulae know the sensation of their fistula intimately and will be quick to inform the practitioner of any change in the quality of blood flow. Use of the fistula for anything other than dialysis is both unacceptable and dangerous. Care must be taken not to occlude a fistula. Fistulae can be harmed by pressure. Care must be taken not to take blood pressures on an arm containing a fistula; tight clothing should also be avoided (Brundage 1980). With good management, fistulae should last for several years; however, most renal failure patients who are not transplanted will require several fistulae to be formed during their lives.

CONCLUSION

As the range of usage for acute vascular access continues to widen, the complexity of the devices continues to increase. This expansion of i.v. therapy is crossing more boundaries and has a progressively wider implication for the scope of nursing practice than ever before. Once seen as a last resort or reserved only for the critically ill, the central venous catheter has become commonplace in a variety of care settings (Baranowski 1993). The nurse involved in the care of these patients is increasingly challenged to be familiar with the growing range of devices available. In addition, the management of these devices can vary between centres. By the development of a coordinated, national approach to i.v. therapy, based on sound principles rather than anecdotal rituals, nurses will develop the knowledge base from which to expand their individual scope of practice in order to respond to this increasingly challenging discipline.

REFERENCES

Abi-Nader J A 1993 Peripherally inserted central venous catheters in critical care patients. Heart & Lung 22(5): 428–434

Adar R, Mozes M 1971 Fatal complications of central venous catheter. British Medical Journal 3: 746

Aubaniac R 1952 L'injection intraveneuse sousclaviculare advantage et technique. Presse Med 60: 1456

Babycos C, Barrocas A, Webb W 1993 A prospective randomized trial comparing the silver-impregnated collagen cuff with the bedside tunneled subclavian catheter. Journal of Parenteral and Enteral Nutrition 17: 61–63

Baranowski L 1993 Central venous access devices: current technologies, uses, and management strategies. Journal of Intravenous Nursing 16(3): 167–194

Barton B R, Hermann G, Weil R III 1983 Cardiothoracic emergencies associated with subclavian haemodialysis catheters. Journal of the American Medical Association 250: 2600–2662

Berne R M, Levy M N 1993 Physiology, 3rd edn. Mosby-Year Book Inc., St Louis, USA

Bonawitz S, Hammel E, Kirkpatrick J 1991 Prevention of central venous catheter sepsis: a prospective randomised trial. Am Surg 57: 618–623

Borow M, Crowley JG 1985 Evaluation of central venous catheter thrombogenicity. Acta Anaesthesiologica Scandinavica 198: (Suppl) 59–64

Brady H R, Fitzcharles B, Goldberg H et al 1989 Diagnosis and management of subclavian vein thrombosis occurring with subclavian cannulation for haemodialysis. Blood Purif 7: 210–217

Brandt R L, Foley W J, Fink G H et al 1970 Mechanisms of perforation of the heart with production of hydropericardium by a venous catheter and its prevention. American Journal of Surgery 119: 311–316

Brundage D J 1980 Nursing management of renal problems, 2nd edn. Mosby, St Louis, Missouri, USA

Cimochowski G E, Worley E, Rutherford W E, Sartain J, Blondin J, Harter H 1990 Superiority of the internal jugular over the subclavian access for temporary dialysis. Nephron 54: 154–161

Cleri D J, Corrado M L, Seligman S J 1980 Quantitative culture of intravenous catheters and other intravenous inserts. Journal of Infectious Diseases 141: 781–786

Collin J, Collin C, Constable F L, Johnstone I D 1975 Infusion thrombophlebitis and infection with various cannulas. Lancet 2: 150–153

Collins J L, Lutz R J 1991 In vitro study of simultaneous infusion of incompatible drugs in multilumen catheters. Heart & Lung 20(3): 271–277

Conly J M, Grieves K, Peters B 1989 A prospective randomised study comparing transparent and dry gauze dressings for central venous catheters. Journal of Infectious Diseases 158: 310–319

Craven D E, Lichtenberg D A, Kunches LM et al 1985 A randomized study comparing a transparent polyurethane dressing to a dry gauze dressing for peripheral intravenous catheter sites. Infection Control 6: 361–366

Daily E K, Schroeder J S 1994 Techniques in bedside haemodynamic monitoring, 4th edn. Mosby, St Louis, USA

Daniels S R, Hannon D W, Meyer R A et al 1984 Paroxysmal supraventricular tachycardia. American Journal of Cardiovascular Surgery 138: 474

Dennis A R, Leeson-Payne C G, Langham B T, Aitkenhead A R 1995 Local anaesthesia for cannulation; has practice changed? Anaesthesia 50: 400–402

Elliott T S J 1988 Intravascular device infections. Journal of Medical Microbiology 27: 161–167

Elliott T S J 1993 Line-associated bacteraemias. Communicable Diseases Report 3(7): R91–R96

Elliott T S J, Faroqui M H, Armstrong R F, Hanson G C 1994 Guidelines for good practice in central venous catheterization. Journal of Hospital Infection 28: 163–176

Farber T M 1993 ARROWgard blue antiseptic surface: toxicology review. A-76 20M. Arrow International, Inc., USA

Flowers R H, Schwenzer K J, Kopel R F, Fisch M J, Tucker S I, Farr B M 1989 Efficacy of an attachable subcutaneous cuff for the prevention of intravascular catheter-related infection. A randomized controlled trial. Journal of the American Medical Association 261: 878–883

Freund H R 1981 Chemical phlebothrombosis of large veins. Archives of Surgery 116: 1220–1221

Fuller T J, Mahoney J J, Juncos L I et al 1976 Arteriovenous fistula after femoral vein catheterization. Journal of the American Medical Association 236: 2943–2944

Ghani G A, Berry A J 1983 Right hydrothorax after left external jugular vein catheterization. Anaesthesiology 58: 93–94

Gianino M S, Brunt L M, Eisenberg P G 1992 The impact of a nutritional support team on the cost and management of multilumen central venous catheters. Journal of Intravenous Nursing 15(6): 327–332

Gil R T, Kruse J A, Thill-Baharozian M C, Carlson R W 1989 Triple vs single-lumen central venous catheters. A prospective study in a critically ill population. Archives of Internal Medicine 149: 1139–1143

Hadaway L C 1989 Evaluation and use of advanced i.v. technology part 1: central venous access devices. Journal of Intravenous Nursing 12(2): 73–82

Halliday P, Anderson D N, Davidson A I, Page J G 1994 Management of cerebral air embolism secondary to a disconnected central venous catheter. British Journal of Surgery 81: 71

Hanley P C, Click R L, Tancredi R G 1984 Delayed air embolism after removal of venous catheters. Annals of Internal Medicine 101: 401–402

Hansen E K, Christensen KM 1983 Fatal thrombosis after subclavian catheter. Anaesthesia 38: 765–766

Hill R L, Fisher A P, Ware R J, Wilson S, Casewell M W 1990 Mupirocin for the reduction of colonization of internal jugular cannulae – a randomized controlled trial. Journal of Hospital Infection 15: 311–321

Hoar P F, Wilson R M, Mangano D T et al 1981 Heparin bonding reduces thrombogenicity for pulmonary artery catheters. New England Journal of Medicine 305: 993–995

Hoffman K K, Western S A, Kaiser D L, Wenzel R P, Groschel D H M 1988 Bacterial colonization and phlebitis-associated risk with transparent polyurethane film for peripheral intravenous site dressings. American Journal of Infection Control 16: 101–106

Hook M L, Reuling J, Leuttgen M L, Norris S O, Elsesser C C, Leonard M K 1987 Comparison of the patency of arterial lines maintained with heparinized and nonheparinized infusions. Heart & Lung 16: 693–699

Horowitz H W, Dworkin B M, Savino J A, Byrne D W, Pecora N A 1990 Central catheter-related infections: comparison of pulmonary artery catheters and triple lumen catheters for the delivery of hyperalimentation in a critical care setting. Journal of Parenteral and Enteral Nutrition 14: 588–592

Hughes R E, Magovern G J 1959 The relationship between right atrial pressure and blood volume. Archives of Surgery 79: 238–243

Iberti T J, Benjamin E, Gruppi L, Raskin J M 1985 Ventricular arrhythmias during pulmonary artery catheterization in the intensive care unit. American Journal of Medicine 78: 451–454

Johnson C W, Miller D L, Ognibene FP 1991 Acute pulmonary embolism associated with guidewire change of a central venous catheter. Intensive Care Medicine 17(2): 115–117

Kamal G D, Pfaller M A, Rempe L E, Jebson P J 1991 Reduced intravascular catheter infection by antibiotic bonding. A prospective, randomized, controlled trial. Journal of the American Medical Association 265: 2364–2368

Kasten G W, Owens E, Kennedy D 1985 Ventricular tachycardia resulting from central venous catheter tip migration due to arm position changes: report of two cases. Anaesthesiology 62: 185–187

Kovacevich D S, Faubion W C, Braunschweig C L et al 1988 Prevalence of catheter sepsis in parenteral nutrition patients with triple vs. single lumen. Journal of Parenteral and Enteral Nutrition 12(Suppl): 23S

Kristinsson KG 1989 Adherence of staphylococci to intravascular catheters. Journal of Medical Microbiology 28: 249–257

Lam S, Scannell R, Roessler D, Smith M A 1994 Peripherally inserted central catheters in an acute-care hospital. Archives of Internal Medicine 154: 1833–1837

Langham B T, Harrison D A 1992 Local anaesthetic: does it really reduce the pain of insertion of all sizes of venous cannulation? Anaesthesia 47: 890–891

Leighton H 1994 Maintaining the patency of transduced arterial and venous lines using 0.9% sodium chloride. Intensive and Critical Care Nursing 10: 23–25

Lopez-Lopez G, Pascual A, Perea E J 1991 Effect of plastic catheter material on bacterial adherence and viability. Journal of Medical Microbiology 34(6): 349–353

Maki D G, Band J D 1981 A comparative study of polyantibiotic and iodophor ointment in the prevention of vascular catheter-related infection. American Journal of Medicine 70: 739–744

Maki D G, Cobb L, Garman J K, Shapiro J M, Ringer M, Helgerson R B 1988 An attachable silver-impregnated cuff for prevention of infection with central venous catheters: a prospective randomized multicenter trial. American Journal of Medicine 85: 307–314

Maki D G, Ringer M 1987 Evaluation of dressing regimens for prevention of infection with peripheral intravenous catheters. Journal of the American Medical Association 258: 2396–2403

Maki D G, Ringer M, Alvarado C J 1991 Prospective randomized trial of povidone–iodine, alcohol, and chlorhexidine for prevention of infection associated with central venous and arterial catheters. Lancet 338: 339–343

Maki D G, Weise C E, Sarafin H W 1977 A semiquantitative culture method for identifying intravenous catheter-related infection. New England Journal of Medicine 296: 1305–1309

Markus S, Buday S 1989 Culturing indwelling central venous catheters in situ. Infect Surg May: 157–162

Maschke S P, Rogove H J 1984 Cardiac tamponade associated with a multilumen central venous catheter. Critical Care Medicine 12: 611–613

Maurer A H, Au F C, Malmud L S et al 1984 Radionuclide venography in subclavian vein thrombosis complicating parenteral nutrition. Clinical Nuclear Medicine 9: 397–399

McGee W T, Ackerman B L, Rouben L R, Prasad V M, Bandi V, Mallory D L 1993 Accurate placement of central venous catheters: a prospective, randomized, multicenter trial. Critical Care Medicine 21(8): 1118–1123

Mclean-Russ A H, Griffith C D M, Anderson J R et al 1982 Thromboembolic complications with silicone elastomer subclavian catheters. Journal of Parenteral and Enteral Nutrition 6: 61–63

Medical Defense Union 1996 Informed consent. MDU, London

Mennim P, Coyle C F, Taylor J D 1992 Venous air embolism associated with removal of central venous catheter. British Medical Journal 305: 171–172

Mermal L A, McCormick R D, Springman S R, Maki D G 1991 The pathogenesis and epidemiology of catheter-related infection with pulmonary artery Swan–Ganz catheters: a prospective study utilizing molecular subtyping. American Journal of Medicine 91(Suppl. 3B): 197S–205S

Park G R, Manara A R 1994 Intensive care. Oxford Medical Publications, Oxford University Press, Oxford

Pearson M L 1995 Guideline for prevention of intravascular-device-related infections. Infection Control and Hospital Epidemiology 17(7): 438–473

Peterson F Y, Kirchhoff K T 1991 Analysis of the research about heparinized versus nonheparinized intravascular lines. Heart & Lung 20: 6: 631–640

Phifer T J, Bridges M, Conrad S A 1991 The residual central venous catheter track– an occult source of lethal air embolism: a case report. Journal of Trauma 31: 1558–1560

Powell C, Fabri P J, Kudsk K A 1988 Risk of infection accompanying the use of single-lumen vs double-lumen subclavian catheters: a prospective randomized study. Journal of Parenteral and Enteral Nutrition 12: 127–129

Raad I I, Hohn D C, Gilbreath B J et al 1994 Prevention of central venous catheter-related infections by using maximum sterile barrier precautions during insertion. Infection Control and Hospital Epidemiology 15: 231–238

Ricard P, Martin R, Marcoux J A 1985 Protection of indwelling vascular catheters: incidence of bacterial contamination and catheter-related sepsis. Critical Care Medicine 13: 541–543

Royal College of Nursing 1994 Guidance on infection control in hospitals. RCN, London

Scott W L 1988 Complications associated with central venous catheters: a survey. Chest 94(6): 1221–1224

Seldinger S I 1953 Catheter replacement of the needle in percutaneous arteriography: a new technique. Acta Radiologica 39: 368–375

Seneff M G 1987a Central venous catheterization: a comprehensive review, Part 1. Journal of Intensive Care Medicine a 2: 163–175

Seneff M G 1987b Central venous catheterization: a comprehensive review, Part II. Journal of Intensive Care Medicine b 2: 218–232

Shapira M, Stern W Z 1967 Hazard of subclavian vein cannulation for central venous pressure monitoring. Journal of the American Medical Association 201: 327–329

Sheep R E, Guiney W B Jr 1982 Fatal cardiac tamponade. Journal of the American Medical Association 248: 1632–1635

Simpson E T, Aitchison J M 1982 Percutaneous infraclavicular subclavian vein catheterization in shocked patients: a prospective study in 172 patients. Journal of Trauma 22: 781–784

Soni N 1989 Anaesthesia and intensive care: practical procedures, 1st edn. Heinemann, Avon, UK

Sung J P, Bikangaga A W, Abbott J A 1981 Massive hemorrhage to scrotum from laceration of inferior epigastric artery following percutaneous femoral vein catheterization: case report. Milit Med 146: 362–363

Swan H J C, Ganz W, Forrester J et al 1970 Catheterization of the heart in man with use of a flow-directed balloon-tipped catheter. New England Journal of Medicine 283: 447–451

Taylor N, Hutchison E, Milliken W, Larson E 1989 Comparison of normal versus heparinized saline for flushing infusion devices. Journal of Nursing Quality Assurance 3(4): 49–55

Vanherweghem J L, Cabolet P, Dhaene M et al 1986 Complications related to subclavian catheters for haemodialysis. International Journal of Artificial Organs 5: 297–309

Weiner P, Sznajder I, Plavnick L et al 1984 Unusual complications of subclavian vein catheterization. Critical Care Medicine 12: 538–539

Woodburne R T, Burkel W E 1994 Essentials of human anatomy, 9th edn. Oxford University Press, New York, USA

Long-term central venous access

Janice Gabriel

INTRODUCTION

As more patients become recipients of a vascular access device (VAD), especially for intermediate- to long-term parenteral therapies, it is important to ensure that the device selected not only meets their clinical needs, but is also acceptable to them and can become a part of their life (Barbone & Rockledge 1995, Gabriel 1996a).

This chapter will look at the types of central venous access devices (CVAD) available for meeting the individual patient's intermediate- to long-term needs, i.e. skin-tunnelled catheters, implantable ports and peripherally inserted central catheters (PICCs). The indications for each device, placement techniques and management, together with the overall advantages and disadvantages, will be discussed, not only in relation to meeting the patient's clinical needs, but also in relation to how they can affect an individual's lifestyle.

HISTORY OF CENTRAL VENOUS ACCESS DEVICES

Recent years have seen an expansion in the numbers of patients receiving parenteral therapies. Medical research has produced an array of treatments, many of which are required to be administered intravenously (i.v.).

In 1991 it was estimated that 85% of all patients admitted to hospitals in the (USA) were recipients of a VAD (Coulter 1993). However, intravenous therapy is not confined solely to the hospital environment. Increasing numbers of patients who are not acutely ill, e.g. those who have chronic conditions such as cystic fibrosis requiring intermittent parenteral antibiotics or those who have cancer and require the continuous infusion of, or intermittent treatment with, cytotoxic chemotherapy, are successfully being managed away from the hospital environment providing they have a suitable VAD (Earlam 1993).

While a peripheral i.v. device can still meet the clinical requirements of many patients requiring venous access for a few days, there has been an increasing patient population requiring longer-term parenteral therapy and/or the administration of vesicant fluids/drugs (Brovia et al 1973, Barbone & Rockledge 1995). This has led to the development of a range of CVADs.

INDICATIONS FOR A CENTRAL VENOUS ACCESS DEVICE

Goodwin & Carlson (1993) defined a central venous access device (CVAD) as a catheter which has its tip located in the superior vena cava. Other, shorter catheters inserted by similar techniques, but whose tips do not extend as far as the superior vena cava should not be described as CVADs, e.g. peripherally inserted catheters (PICs). A PIC does not extend beyond the axillary vein and should be described as a midline peripherally inserted catheter (Goodwin & Carlson 1993). Some practitioners prefer to place CVADs into the right atrium using fluoroscopy or ultrasound guidance. Gormon & Buzby (1995) suggested this position for long-term catheter placement, especially if the practitioner has easy access to the use of fluoroscopy and/or ultrasound guidance.

The position of all CVADs should be confirmed directly after placement by chest X-ray (Hadaway 1989). CVADs can be used for the administration of blood products, parenteral antibiotics and antiviral agents, cytotoxic drugs and parenteral nutrition. As many of these agents are vesicant, or highly irritant to a patient's veins, their administration directly into the superior vena cava ensures their rapid dilution by the large volume of blood flowing through this vessel (Lowel & Bothe 1995, Richardson & Bruso 1993).

Patients with poor peripheral venous access, requiring parenteral therapy for a short period of time or in an emergency situation, may automatically become recipients of a CVAD because they have no accessible vein for a peripheral cannula. Apart from these patients, Shapiro (1995) identified five other groups of patients who could potentially benefit from the use of a central venous catheter as those requiring:

- continuous infusions of cytotoxic drugs
- prolonged/intermittent parenteral therapies
- prolonged blood product support
- administration of vesicant drugs
- paediatrics requiring parenteral therapies.

VEIN SELECTION

Before discussing the specific devices available, it is important to identify which veins are commonly used for introducing a central venous access catheter (Gormon & Buzby 1995):

- bilateral cephalic veins
- external jugular veins
- saphenous veins
- inferior epigastric vein
- gonadal veins
- lumbar veins
- intrathoracic veins
- femoral veins.

The basilic and median cubital veins can also be used (Fig. 11.1).

Selection of a particular vein is dependent upon the individual patient's anatomy, medical condition and proposed reason for wishing to establish venous access. CVADs can be placed either percutaneously, i.e. by 'puncturing' the patient's skin to obtain access to a blood vessel, or surgically, i.e. by surgical cut-down through the patient's skin to identify the desired blood vessel for introduction of the CVAD.

Bilateral cephalic veins/external jugular veins

The cephalic and external jugular veins can be accessed peripherally or by surgical cut-down. The tip of the CVAD is then threaded into the SVC or right atrium, via the subclavian or innominate veins. Gormon & Buzby (1995) suggested that these are the preferred routes for establishing central venous access by a percutaneous or surgical cut-down approach, as the incidence of pneumothorax is minimal and the risk of subsequent bleeding from arterial injury is greatly reduced.

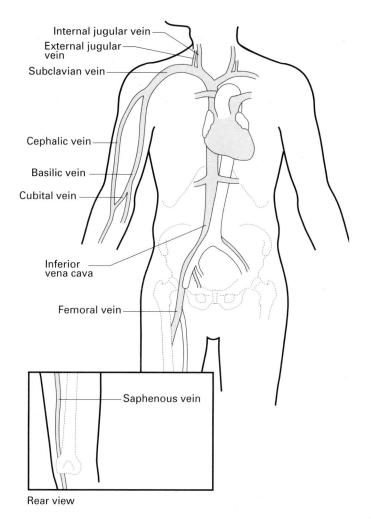

Internal jugular vein

External jugular vein

Subclavian vein

Cephalic vein

Basilic vein

Cubital vein

Inferior vena cava

Femoral vein

Saphenous vein

Rear view

Fig. 11.1 Venous access points for the introduction of central venous catheters.

Saphenous veins

The saphenous veins can be used successfully as a means of establishing central venous access, providing the skin surrounding the surgical cut-down is healthy and free from infection. This will reduce the risk of infection to the patient. First, a surgical cut-down procedure is used to identify the saphenous vein. The catheter is then advanced, under the guidance of fluoroscopy, to the right atrium. Once in position, the catheter is sutured to the patient's skin to prevent it from becoming dislodged (Gormon & Buzby 1995).

While this technique will ensure central venous access for the patient, it is associated with a high risk of infection and is disliked by patients for long-term use due to its position (Gormon & Buzby 1995).

Inferior epigastric vein

The use of the inferior epigastric vein requires an involved surgical cut-down procedure through the patient's abdominal wall into the peritoneum. Once in the peritoneum, the inferior epigastric vein is identified. The CVAD is then tunnelled under the skin to the umbilicus. An incision is made into the inferior epigastric vein, the catheter is passed through it and advanced, under fluoroscopy guidance, to the right atrium. The CVAD is then secured to the blood vessel and the incision closed (Gormon & Buzby 1995). Although this procedure for central venous access is involved it can be relied upon for long-term access. However, its position is associated with a high risk of infection and dissatisfaction by patients for long-term use.

Gonadal and lumbar veins

The technique for placing a CVAD via the gonadal vein requires the patient to be lying supine on the operating table. The patient's flank is then elevated by use of a sandbag or beanbag. An incision is made through the abdominal wall into the retroperitoneum and the gonadal vein identified. As with the inferior epigastric approach, the CVAD is tunnelled under the patient's skin and the catheter is advanced through the gonadal vein, under fluoroscopy guidance, until the right atrium is reached (Gormon & Buzby 1995).

Gormon & Buzby (1995) suggested the lumbar veins be used as an alternative if the gonadal vein is unsuitable. However, if the patient has experienced a central venous thrombosis, the lumbar veins are often enlarged, making them readily identifiable for easier access.

Intrathoracic veins

Gormon & Buzby (1995) discussed how the intrathoracic veins can be used when other options for placing CVADs have been eliminated. Two techniques can be used: a thoracotomy and a transthoracic approach.

Thoracotomy

The thoracotomy approach involves entering the patient's chest through the fourth intercostal space. The surgeon then decides which blood vessel to cannulate, depending upon the patient's anatomy. Once the CVAD has been placed, the device is then secured, a chest drain is inserted and the chest closed. There is a high degree of morbidity associated with this procedure due to the possible complications arising from the insertion procedure (Gormon & Buzby 1995).

Transthoracic approach

The transthoracic approach is considered to be the easiest and safest approach for placing a CVAD into an intrathoracic blood vessel. This technique involves a surgical incision into the parietal pleura to expose an upper intercostal vein. The CVAD is then tunnelled under the skin, on the patient's chest wall, and the catheter advanced through the intercostal vein into the right atrium under fluoroscopy guidance. The incision is closed once the CVAD has been secured and a chest drain is left in situ during the postoperative period (Gormon & Buzby 1995).

Femoral veins

The femoral vein approach can be performed relatively quickly, under local anaesthetic, by a percutaneous or surgical cut-down technique. However, it is associated with an increased incidence of iliofemoral thrombosis (Gormon & Buzby 1995). The procedure involves tunnelling the CVAD under the patient's skin from the umbilicus to the femoral vein. The CVAD is then introduced into the vein and, under fluoroscopy guidance, advanced to the right atrium.

Although this approach can be used for long-term use, it is associated with an increased risk of infection and disliked by many of its recipients due to the position of the catheter.

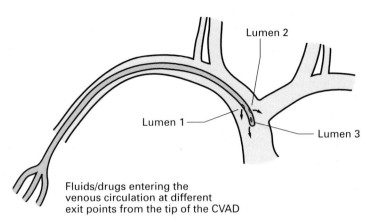

Fig. 11.2 Multi-lumen vascular access devices. Staggering of lumens ensures that fluids/drugs do not mix as they exit the catheter and enter the venous circulation.

Lumen 2

Lumen 1

Lumen 3

Fluids/drugs entering the venous circulation at different exit points from the tip of the CVAD

Table 11.1 External diameter sizes of CVADs (Goodwin & Carlson 1993)

Gauge (ga)	French (Fr)
23 ga	2.0 Fr
20 ga	3.0 Fr
18 ga	4.0 Fr
16 ga	5.0 Fr

TYPES OF CENTRAL VENOUS ACCESS DEVICE

CVADs can be constructed from either polyurethane or silicone rubber. They are available in a variety of gauge sizes and can be single, dual or triple lumen, depending upon the device selected. The multi-lumen devices have their exit points staggered at the proximal end of the CVAD to ensure that there is no mixing of the drugs/fluids as they exit the catheter and enter the venous circulation (Fig. 11.2).

Gauge sizes

The size of the CVAD will be described by the various manufacturers in terms of length and gauge size. The length will be expressed in either millimetres or centimetres, e.g. 36 mm or 60.0 cm, etc. The gauge size will refer to the external diameter of the device and not the internal diameter. The external diameter can be expressed in either 'French' (Fr) or 'gauge' (ga) size, e.g. 4.0 Fr or 18 ga (Table 11.1). With multi-lumen devices it is the overall diameter of the device which is stated, e.g. 5 Fr (16 ga) (Goodwin & Carlson 1993).

For the individual internal lumen size of a CVAD one would need to consult the specific product information supplied by manufacturers.

The flow rate through the CVAD will depend upon the internal diameter of the particular device. Individual manufacturers should be able to provide specific information on their products regarding the gravity flow rates and rates achieved by the use of a pump.

Catheter design and construction material

CVADs are commonly constructed from either polyurethane or silicone rubber (Camp-Sorrell 1992, Ryder 1995, Wickham et al 1992).

Polyurethane

CVADs constructed from polyurethane are more rigid than those constructed from silicone rubber. Consequently, in the longer term, they are more likely to break, due to an inability to recover from kinking and bending. This material does not soften when it comes into contact with body fluids, i.e. blood, and can cause irritation to the wall of the blood vessel, resulting in phlebitis and a higher incidence of thrombosis (Strumpfer 1991, Sansivero 1997).

Higher flow rates can be achieved through polyurethane CVADs than through those constructed from silicone rubber, as the walls of these devices are thinner, resulting in a lumen with a larger internal diameter.

Silicone rubber

Silicone rubber is a very flexible material which has the ability to recover from kinking and bending. Due to the softness of this material, in the majority of cases where the wall of the blood vessel becomes irritated, the degree of phlebitis is not as severe as occurs with polyurethane CVAD; the incidence of thrombosis is also reduced (McCredie & Lawson 1984, Sansivero 1997). However, a disadvantage is that silicone rubber can be easily damaged by sharp instruments, e.g. toothed forceps used for clamping.

'Open-ended' and valved CVADs

Tunnelled catheters, implantable ports (with the exception of the port with a multi-layered septum) and PICCs can be either 'open-ended' or valved. An 'open-ended' CVAD can allow blood to reflux into the lumen(s) of the device (Mayo 1995). When the injection hub is removed, the catheter should be clamped to prevent air entering the patient's venous circulation (Delmore et al 1989). There have been further modifications to the tips of CVADs; for example, Dr Groshong, an American clinician, developed a three-position slit valve as an integral part of the catheter's tip. In the absence of a negative or positive pressure, this valve remains closed, preventing air from entering the lumen(s) of the CVAD or blood refluxing. The design of this valve dispensed with the necessity of having to use a clamp to prevent air entry or the reflux of blood (Delmore et al 1989).

Skin-tunnelled catheters

In the 1970s, J. Broviac, an American clinician, developed a long-term skin-tunnelled catheter for patients requiring prolonged parenteral nutrition (PN) (Broviac et al 1973). These catheters were tunnelled under the patient's skin, on the chest wall, and accessed the central venous system via the external jugular or cephalic veins. These devices had a Dacron cuff attached to the portion of catheter that was tunnelled under the skin (Fig. 11.3). The aim of the Dacron cuff was twofold: firstly, it facilitated the growth of the surrounding tissue around the cuff and therefore stabilize the catheter without the need for suturing; and secondly, the ingrowth of tissue, coupled with the skin tunnelling technique, created additional barriers, thus minimizing the potential for infection (Harris et al 1987).

In the late 1970s, an American haematologist, Dr Hickman, realized the potential of a skin-tunnelled catheter for patients undergoing bone marrow transplantation. By modifying 'Broviac's' catheter, i.e. by increasing the internal diameter and creating a thicker wall, the durability of the device was increased (Harris et al 1987).

All skin-tunnelled catheters are available today, with one, two or three lumens.

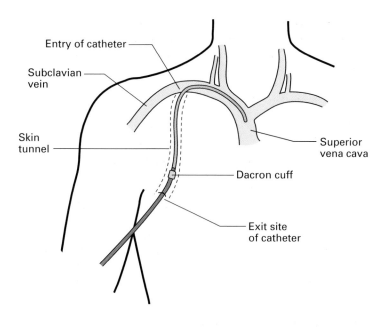

Fig. 11.3 Placement of skin-tunnelled catheter.

Entry of catheter

Subclavian vein

Skin tunnel

Superior vena cava

Dacron cuff

Exit site of catheter

Implantable injection ports

The first implantable injection port was introduced into clinical practice in 1982 (Gullo 1982). This CVAD consisted of a subcutaneous injection port attached to a venous catheter (Boothe et al 1984). Today, these devices are available either with the catheter already attached to the injection port or unassembled, in which case the individual placing the device must securely attach the catheter to the port (Gullo 1993). The unassembled system allows the catheter to be inserted before attaching the injection port. However, this technique can occasionally result in the catheter becoming detached from the injection port (Gullo 1993). These devices are either open-ended or have a valve.

A newer development of the injection port is a device which is designed to accept a conventional i.v. cannula. This device is funnel-shaped and access to the catheter is achieved by passing a cannula through the multilayered self-sealing silicone septum (Fig. 11.4) (Walker & Calzone 1994). These devices are only available with open-ended catheters. Both types of port are available with single or dual lumens. With dual lumen devices, each lumen is attached to a separate injection port.

The original and more widely used implantable injection ports are accessed by palpating the device through the patient's skin and using a 'Huber' needle to puncture the port's silastic membrane (Fig. 11.5). It is vital that the individual accessing the injection port ensures that the needle has passed through the silastic membrane and into the port's reservoir. If the tip of the needle is not in the reservoir, extravasation of fluids/drugs could occur.

The design of the 'Huber' needle minimizes the risk of 'coring' to the silastic membrane and therefore reduces the incidence of leakage (Gullo 1993, Soo et al 1985). However, the life of the port is limited by the overall number of punctures to the silastic membrane. In time, even with the use of a 'Huber' needle, leakage becomes a possibility. 'Huber' needles are available in a variety of gauge sizes and lengths. They can be straight or right-angled. The choice of which to select is dependent upon what is to be administered and the duration of administration. A 'Huber' needle greater than 20 g should be used for the administration of blood products, as

Fig. 11.4 Implantable injection port with multilayered septum.

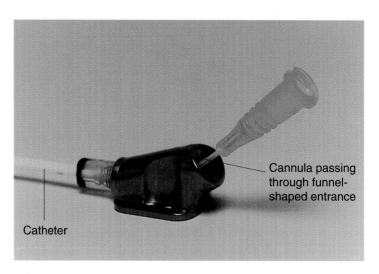

Catheter

Cannula passing through funnel-shaped entrance

Fig. 11.5 Implantable injection port with silastic membrane.

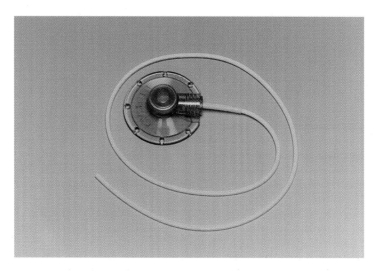

the internal diameter of the needle is large enough not to cause potential damage to the platelets as they are infused. If the patient is to receive an infusion as opposed to a bolus injection, an angled 'Huber' needle will probably be more comfortable and easier to secure when an i.v. administration set is attached to it (Fig. 11.6).

All ports should be well flushed with sodium chloride 0.9% after each use to ensure that no drugs/infusates are retained in the reservoir. This will prevent any drug remaining in the reservoir from being 'flushed' into the venous circulation when the device is next used (Ben-Arush & Berant 1996).

Peripherally inserted central catheters

Peripherally inserted central catheters (PICCs), a group of single and dual lumen CVADs, were developed in the late 1970s in the USA (Hadaway 1989). Venous access is achieved by cannulating a peripheral vein in the arm, i.e. the cephalic,

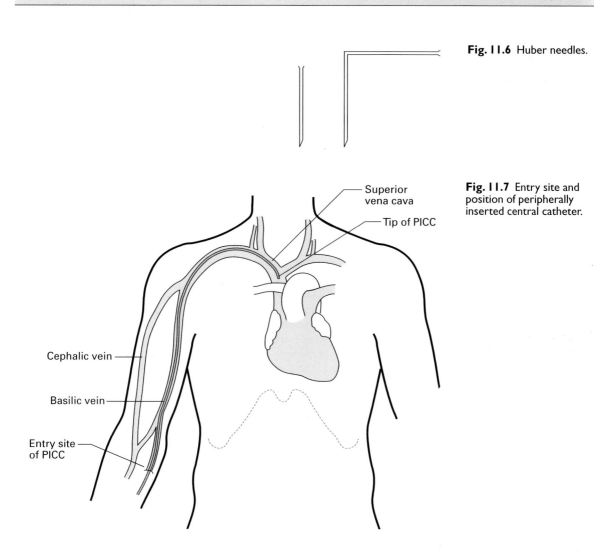

Fig. 11.6 Huber needles.

Fig. 11.7 Entry site and position of peripherally inserted central catheter.

Superior vena cava

Tip of PICC

Cephalic vein

Basilic vein

Entry site of PICC

basilic or median cubital vein. The catheter is then advanced through the cannula, or introducer, until it reaches the superior vena cava/right atrium (Fig. 11.7).

PLACEMENT OF CVADs

Patient assessment

Prior to placing a CVAD, for intermediate- to long-term use, it is important that the patient's clinical condition and lifestyle are assessed. This will help to ensure that the patient will 'accept' the device and complications are minimized (Gabriel 1997, Sansivero 1997). Firstly, the clinical needs of the patient should be assessed to determine which CVAD(s) will meet their needs. Secondly, if the patient is expected to spend time away from the hospital environment, or indeed become actively involved in the care and management of his own CVAD, the selected device should be acceptable to him and he should be able to manage it.

Prior to the placement of the CVAD the patient's blood count should be checked to ensure that the platelet count is adequate for the procedure (Sansivero 1997). If appropriate, a clotting screen should also be undertaken. Where necessary, a thrombocytic patient can have the CVAD placed whilst receiving a platelet infusion. Patients with an elevated INR can have their anticoagulant therapy adjusted accordingly (Richardson & Bruso 1993). For all insertions, except in the case of a PICC, the patient should be placed in the Trendelenburg position. This will ensure that the venous access point is below the level of the heart and therefore minimizes the risk of an air embolus. As PICCs are placed in an arm vein, the Trendelenburg position can be dispensed with, providing the person placing the device ensures that the patient's arm remains below the level of the heart (Richardson & Bruso 1993).

CVADs can be placed under either local or general anaesthetic in order to minimize the discomfort of the procedure for the patient. The exception to this are PICCs, which can be successfully placed using a topical anaesthetic ointment or without any anaesthetic at all. This is because the procedure involves accessing an antecubital fossa vein with a conventional wide gauge cannula or introducer of a similar size.

Skin-tunnelled catheters

Skin-tunnelled catheters can be placed either by a cut-down technique or by a 'percutaneous' approach (Gormon & Buzby 1995). The cut-down procedure involves tunnelling a few centimetres of the catheter under the patient's skin using a trocar. A cut-down is then made into the vein, and the 'tunnelled' catheter threaded through the vessel until the tip of the CVAD reaches the superior vena cava/right atrium (Fig. 11.3). The percutaneous technique involves using a cannula to directly access the vein; no cut-down is used. Similarly to the cut-down approach, a trocar is used to tunnel the catheter under the skin so that its exit point site is away from where it enters the vein (Fig. 11.3).

Implantable injection ports

The implantable injection port is placed by making an incision into the patient's skin and creating a subcutaneous pocket. The device is then anchored, with sutures, to the underlying muscle and the catheter tunnelled under the skin until it reaches the desired venous access point. The skin overlying the port is then surgically closed. The commonest area for siting these devices is on the patient's chest wall (Fig. 11.8). However, they can be placed more peripherally, e.g. on an arm. These devices are available with one or two ports. Each port is attached to a single lumen catheter. If a patient requires more than two lumens to meet their clinical needs, there is no reason why two devices cannot be placed, e.g. a single and a dual lumen (Sansivero 1997).

Peripherally inserted central catheters

As with all CVADs, clinical assessment of the patient is important to minimize problems associated with the insertion procedure. As PICCs are placed by cannulation of the basilic, cephalic or median cubital vein, it is important that the clinical assessment of the patient takes into account any underlying condition which could result in pressure on the venous anatomy of the arm, axilla or supraclavicular fossa, i.e. a previously fractured clavicle, presence of a cardiac pacemaker, previous surgery or radiotherapy to that part of the body, a history of axillary vein thrombosis. If the assessment of the patient does reveal any of these, e.g. left axillary node dissection, then the other arm should be considered, in this example the right arm (Richardson & Bruso 1993).

The basilic vein is the ideal vein as, anatomically, it is the largest of the three and provides the straightest route leading to the superior vena cava (Hadaway 1989,

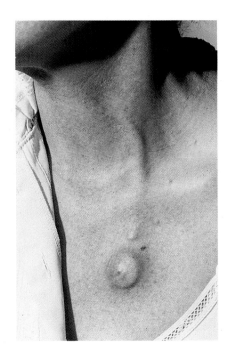

Fig. 11.8 Injection port with silastic membrane in situ.

Sansivero 1997). In the majority of patients, even if this vein cannot be readily visualized, there is usually no problem in palpating it. For the minority of patients who do not have a readily accessible antecubital fossa vein, fluoroscopy and/or ultrasound can be used to identify the vessel and therefore allow cannulation to take place (Andrews 1995, Sansivero 1997).

Once the vein has been selected for the placement of the PICC, the distance from the intended insertion site to the proximal end of the clavicle should be measured (Fig. 11.9). Up to 3 cm should be added to the length of the catheter for placements in the left arm to ensure the device reaches the superior vena cava. This additional length takes into account the position of the superior vena cava (Gabriel 1996a).

When cannulation has been achieved, the PICC should be threaded through the cannula/introducer until the required length has been inserted (some PICCs are available with 'depth' markings printed onto the device to ensure the correct length is placed, whilst others are provided with a sterile tape measure). By asking the patient to place his chin on his shoulder, on the placement side, the passage of the PICC into the subclavian vein is enhanced. The cannula/introducer is then withdrawn and the PICC secured with either sutures or a self-adhesive anchoring device and Steri-Strips (Fig. 11.10). As with all CVADs, a chest X-ray will be required to confirm the position of the PICC if it was not placed under the guidance of fluoroscopy (Hadaway 1989) (see Box 11.1).

Insertion complications

The possible complications, other than infection, that could be encountered during the insertion procedure and in the first 7 days are summarized in Table 11.2.

Air embolus

Air embolus is a potentially preventable complication of CVAD placement and removal. It is a result of air entering the venous circulation and travelling to the pul-

Fig. 11.9 Pre-insertion measurement of peripherally inserted central catheter.

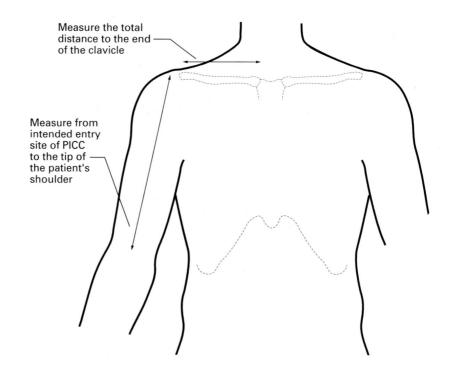

Measure the total distance to the end of the clavicle

Measure from intended entry site of PICC to the tip of the patient's shoulder

Fig. 11.10 Dressing to secure Huber needle in injection port.

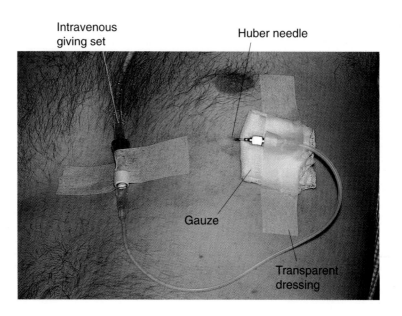

Intravenous giving set

Huber needle

Gauze

Transparent dressing

monary vein. The risk of this complication can be minimized by placing the patient in the Trendelenburg position, or, in the case of PICC placements, by ensuring that the patient's arm is kept below the level of the heart (Richardson & Bruso 1993).

■ **BOX 11.1**

Steps involved in placing a PICC

- Assess the patient's clinical needs and lifestyle:
  — Will a PICC meet the patient's clinical needs?
  — Has the patient had any axillary/supraclavicular fossa surgery/radiotherapy?
  — Does the patient have a history of axillary vein thrombosis?
  — Does the patient have a cardiac pacemaker?
  — Is there a history of a fractured clavicle?
  — Will the patient's lifestyle prevent him from coping with a PICC?
  — Does the patient have inaccessible antecubital fossa veins?
  — Is the patient's blood count satisfactory for a PICC placement?
  — Is the patient on anticoagulants? If yes, what is the clotting screen?
  If the answer to any of the above is 'yes', further assessment will be necessary to ensure that a PICC is the most appropriate CVAD, e.g. can the opposite arm be used if the patient has had axillary/SVF surgery/radiotherapy (see text).
- Select a vein and apply local anaesthetic cream as required prior to commencing the procedure.
- Measure the distance from the intended site of insertion to the proximal end of the clavicle, adding up to 3 cm for insertion on the left hand side (see text).
- Prepare your equipment for the procedure.
- Lie the patient flat on a bed and extend the selected arm for the PICC placement at right angles to the patient's body (a couch may be too narrow to support the patient's arm comfortably during the procedure).
- Wearing sterile gloves and gown, clean the skin around the intended entry site with an appropriate antiseptic.
- Cannulate the selected vein with the cannula or introducer supplied with the PICC to gain venous access and release tourniquet.
- Remove the stylet from the cannula/introducer and begin to thread the PICC.
- Ask the patient to place his chin onto his shoulder on placement side.
- Continue to thread the PICC through the cannula/introducer until the required length has been placed (check with the markings on the PICC or using a sterile tape measure).
- Remove the cannula/introducer.
- Flush with sodium chloride 0.9% for valved PICCs, or heparinized saline for open-ended PICCs.
- Attach the injection hub.
- Stabilize with either sutures or self-adhesive anchoring device and Steri-Strips.
- Apply the dressing.
- Confirm the position of the PICC by chest X-ray if not placed under fluoroscopy guidance.

Clinical features of an air embolus can include:

- chest pain
- dyspnoea
- tachycardia
- hypotension.

Pneumothorax

Pneumothorax occurs if air enters the space between the pleural lining and the lung. Richardson & Bruso (1993) reported that it was a complication in 5% of all patients who have their CVAD placed directly into the subclavian vein.

Table 11.2 Complications (other than infection) of catheter insertion

	Valved skin-tunnelled catheter	Open-ended skin-tunnelled catheter	Open-ended injection port	Valved injection port (chest placement)	Open-ended PICC and injection port (peripheral placement)	Valved PICC
Air embolus	Not once device is in situ	✓	✓	Not once device in situ	✓	×
Pneumothorax	✓	✓	✓	✓	×	×
Catheter malposition	✓	✓	✓	✓	✓	✓
Pinch-off syndrome	✓	✓	✓	✓	×	×
Thrombosis	✓	✓	✓	✓	✓	✓
Chemical phlebitis	Very rare	Very rare	Very rare	Very rare	Very rare	Very rare
Mechanical phlebitis	Very rare	Very rare	Very rare	Very rare	✓	✓
Atrial fibrillation	✓	✓	✓	✓	✓	✓

Clinical features of a pneumothorax can include:

- pain on inspiration and expiration
- dyspnoea.

Haemothorax

Haemothorax can be a result of puncturing the subclavian vein or artery during the insertion procedure. Blood then leaks into the pleural cavity (Richardson & Bruso 1993).

Clinical features of a haemothorax can include:

- dyspnoea
- tachycardia.

Arterial puncture

Arterial puncture will result if an artery is cannulated or punctured during the insertion procedure. This complication is readily identifiable by the pulsation/spurting of bright red blood, i.e. arterial blood, into the syringe or through the cannula/introducer. If the subclavian artery has been punctured, a chest X-ray should be performed to assess whether a mediastinal haematoma has occurred (Richardson & Bruso 1993).

Nerve injury

The ulna and median nerves can be damaged during PICC placement if they accidentally come into contact with the cannula/introducer. Similarly, damage to the radial cords of the brachial plexus can also result from subclavian placements of other types of CVAD (Richardson & Bruso 1993).

Clinical features of nerve injury may include:

- tingling
- loss of movement down part or all of the affected arm.

Catheter malposition

A chest X-ray should be performed after the placement of any CVAD to verify its position, if it was not placed under fluoroscopy guidance (Hadaway 1989). A CVAD may become malpositioned not only as a result of the insertion procedure, but also by spontaneous migration or following a repair procedure (Richardson & Bruso 1993, Sansivero 1997).

Clinical features A malpositioned CVAD may present the patient with no symptoms, but if clinical features are present, they may include:

- continuous backflow of blood into the catheter
- coughing
- ear/neck pain on the side of insertion
- palpitations/arrhythmias
- inability to aspirate blood (or difficulty in doing so).

Atrial fibrillation

Atrial fibrillation can result if the catheter extends beyond the superior vena cava (SVC) and into the heart.

Thrombosis

Wickham et al (1992) reported that the formation of thrombosis following CVAD placement is probably multifactorial. They discussed how the catheterization of the vein causes damage to the wall of the blood vessel. This initial trauma leads to the release of thromboplastic substances which causes platelets to collect at the site of the injury. These initial thrombi can then go onto develop into larger areas, or break away causing occlusion elsewhere in the venous system.

Clinical features can include:

- swelling of the neck, chest or arm/leg
- skin discoloration
- skin temperature changes
- infusion difficulties
- inability to aspirate blood (or difficulty doing so).

Pinch-off syndrome

Hinke et al (1990) described pinch-off syndrome (POS) as a condition which can arise when the CVAD is compressed between the clavicle and the first rib.

Clinical indications of POS can include:

- inability to infuse fluids
- difficulty in aspirating blood.

If these signs are ignored, the catheter can go on to rupture and migrate through the blood vessels and into the heart.

ROUTINE MANAGEMENT

Skin cleansing prior to catheter placement

Elliott (1993) emphasised the importance of appropriate and effective skin cleaning prior to the placement of any vascular access device. He stated that contamination of the intravenous catheter by bacteria on the patient's skin could result in infection of the CVAD. The resulting infection might be confined to the insertion site, with the patient complaining of localized pain, and could be associated with erythema, oedema and even a purulent discharge. A systemic infection resulting from an infected CVAD may be more difficult to diagnose. The patient might present with a low-grade pyrexia and may have only a slightly elevated white cell count (Elliott 1993).

Maki et al (1991) carried out a randomized trial of skin cleansing agents for the prevention of catheter-associated infections. They concluded that aqueous chlorhexidine 2% used for cutaneous disinfection prior to insertion of an i.v. device and for post-insertion site care substantially reduced the incidence of device-related infection, compared with povidone-iodine 10% and alcohol 70%.

Accessing the injection hub

Linares et al (1985) suggested that the commonest cause of catheter-related septicaemia was due to a catheter hub becoming colonized by microorganisms. It is therefore vital to ensure that injection hubs of CVADs are adequately cleaned before they are accessed or removed. This can be achieved by cleaning with chlorhexidine aqueous 0.5% or a presaturated alcohol wipe. The hub should be cleaned for a minimum of 30 seconds and allowed to dry for a further 30 seconds before being accessed/removed (Gabriel 1993). A strict aseptic technique should be used when accessing the CVAD.

Dressings

Skin-tunnelled catheters

With skin-tunnelled catheters, the rationale for applying dressings permanently over the insertion site has been questioned. The reason for this is that after 14 days the skin tunnel has formed in the majority of patients and tissue has begun to grow into the Dacron cuff, thereby creating a barrier against infection (Masoorli 1993).

For dressings over CVADs, Young et al (1988) evaluated four dressing protocols in a total patient population of 168, as follows:

- gauze
- transparent polyurethane (changed twice weekly)
- transparent polyurethane (changed every tenth day)
- transparent polyurethane (changed weekly).

It was concluded that, providing the patient's skin was adequately cleaned with either povidone-iodine or aqueous chlorhexidine at the time of the dressing change, the transparent polyurethane dressing was the more effective barrier against infection. They also concluded that, providing there was no exudate under the dressing, the renewal interval should be every 7 days. If the dressing is left for longer than 7 days, its increasing adherence to the patient's skin can make it difficult to remove and could possibly lead to trauma and damage to the skin, thereby increasing the risk for infection.

Implantable ports

Once the wound overlying the skin incision has healed, there is obviously no need for further dressings, unless the patient requires a continuous infusion. In this latter case, a dressing will be required to stabilize the infusion device while it remains in situ. In the study by Young et al (1988), a transparent occlusive dressing was shown to be more effective in minimizing the risk of infection than conventional gauze dressings. If a patient requires continuous access to the injection port, the needle/cannula can be secured by a transparent dressing with a piece of sterile gauze placed under the needle/cannula. This will prevent movement of the needle/cannula and minimize the possibility of a pressure sore developing on the patient's skin. Unless there is any exudate, the dressing can be left undisturbed for 7 days (Fig. 11.10).

PICCs

As there is usually some slight oozing of blood immediately after the placement of a PICC, a small piece of sterile gauze can be placed over the insertion site. This can then be covered with a transparent, occlusive polyurethane dressing. The following day the whole dressing should be removed and the patient's skin cleaned with either povidone-iodine or aqueous chlorhexidine (Young et al 1988, Maki et al 1991). The PICC should then be secured with sterile Steri-Strips, and a transparent, occlusive dressing applied (Fig. 11.11). If the patient does not require access to the PICC continuously, e.g. for intermittent cytotoxic drug therapy, the injection hub can be wrapped in sterile gauze, to prevent it causing a pressure sore on the forearm, and a second transparent dressing can be applied, to overlap with the first. This will create a waterproof barrier to allow the patient to shower. Unlike skin-tunnelled catheters and implantable injection ports, PICCs require to be continually dressed while they are in situ. Following the first dressing change, 24 hours after insertion, a weekly dressing change interval is recommended (Young et al 1988).

Maintaining patency

Goodwin & Carlson (1993) drew attention to the importance of the flushing tech-

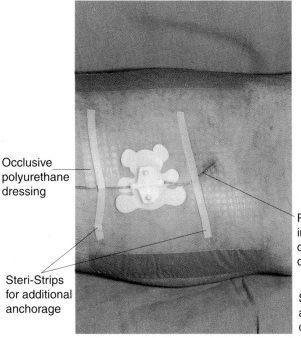

Fig. 11.11 Peripherally inserted central catheter in situ.

Occlusive polyurethane dressing

Peripherally inserted central catheter (PICC)

Steri-Strips for additional anchorage

Self-adhesive anchoring device

nique in preventing occlusion of all CVADs. They recommended a rapid push–pause or pulsated flushing technique. This creates turbulence within the lumen(s) of the catheter, thereby decreasing the risk of fibrin and platelets becoming adhered to the internal wall(s) of the CVAD and minimizing the risk of occlusion. If the CVAD has more than one lumen, each one should be flushed separately, i.e. treated as if it were a separate device (Masoorli 1993).

There has been great debate over the flushing frequencies and flushing solutions for all CVADs (Masoorli 1993). The general concensus is that CVADs with a valve should be flushed with sodium chloride 0.9%. Despite the results of a study by Barbone & Rockledge (1995) suggesting that sodium chloride 0.9% is as effective as heparinized saline in maintaining the patency of 'open-ended' CVADs, there is no uniformly agreed protocol. Whether to use sodium chloride 0.9% or varying strengths of heparinized saline, and at what intervals, appears to be very much dictated by individual departments and hospitals (Dunn 1987, Geritz 1992, Kelly 1992, Masoorli 1993). If the CVAD is open-ended and has a lumen smaller than a 21g, it will require more frequent flushing than a wider gauge device to ensure that it remains patent (Masoorli 1993). (Individual catheter manufacturers will provide guidance relating to their specific product range.)

There is a uniform opinion that injection ports should be flushed monthly with heparinized saline. However, the strength of the heparinized saline still varies among individual departments and hospitals (Moore et al 1986). Studies have shown that 1 mg/day of warfarin can reduce the incidence of thrombosis in recipients of CVADs (Bern et al 1986, Wickham et al 1992). Some centres also add heparin to the infusion bags of patients receiving ambulatory treatment to minimize the risk of thrombosis (Lokich et al 1985).

Blood samples should not be taken through the lumen of a CVAD which has recently been used for the administration of drugs or fluids, as this could result in inaccurate biochemistry results or drug level analysis. If this is the only route available for obtaining such blood samples, infusions should be stopped for a minimum of 20 minutes (RCN 1992).

Blood sampling

Blood samples can be obtained from CVADs providing the lumen of the device is greater than 22g. Withdrawing blood through a CVAD with a lumen smaller than 21g can potentially damage the platelets and result in altered laboratory results (Scott 1995).

To obtain a blood sample, it is important to ensure that all the materials are prepared in advance and are within easy reach. A delay in flushing the CVAD directly after obtaining a blood sample can lead to occlusion. It is also important to ensure that a strict aseptic technique is maintained at all times to minimize the risk of infection to the patient (Linares et al 1985). The injection hub should be removed for blood sampling. Attempting to aspirate blood through an injection hub can leave traces of blood around the hub, which can potentially lead to infection (RCN 1992).

Individual hospital policies and procedures may vary, but the general principles of obtaining a blood sample from a CVAD are presented in Box 11.2.

Aspiration of blood from a PICC is a much slower procedure than from other types of CVAD, due to the length of the device and the size of the lumen. Providing the individual is aware of this, and flushed the PICC as soon as the blood sample is obtained, there is no reason why PICCs cannot be used successfully for this purpose (Scott 1995). A syringe smaller than 10 ml, and vacuum blood collection systems, should not be used on PICCs without consulting individual manufacturers, as there is the potential for the pressure that they create to lead to rupture of the catheter (Conn 1993, Richardson & Bruso 1993, Sansivero 1997).

Conn (1993) highlighted that the smaller the syringe size, the higher the pressure

---

■ **BOX 11.2**

Blood sampling

- Following a strict aseptic technique, remove the injection hub and aspirate twice the prime volume of the lumen of the CVAD and discard. This will ensure that the stagnant contents of the CVAD lumen do not contaminate the blood sample and possibly lead to an inaccurate laboratory analysis.
- Aspirate the required amount of blood and decant into the relevant collection tube(s)/bottle(s). Do not use vacuum collection bottles directly onto the CVAD, or syringes smaller than 10 ml, without consulting the advisory literature for the individual catheter's manufacturer, as there is a potential for the pressure to be too high and rupture of the device could result (Conn 1993, Richardson & Bruso 1993).
- Using a rapid push–pause method, flush the CVAD with 10–20 ml of sodium chloride 0.9% to minimize the risk of occlusion (Goodwin & Carlson 1993, Masoorli 1993). Open-ended CVADs should then be flushed with heparinized saline according to individual department/hospital's policies, finishing with positive pressure.

---

generated. She demonstrated that the average person injecting a 1 ml syringe can exert a pressure in excess of 300 pounds/square inch (psi), which can result in catheter rupture.

MANAGEMENT OF COMPLICATIONS

Occlusion

Occlusion of a CVAD may be either intraluminal or extraluminal (Wickham et al 1992). Both intraluminal and extraluminal occlusions prevent blood from being aspirated back from the CVAD. However, with an extraluminal occlusion it is sometimes possible to continue with the infusion of drugs/fluids without realizing that there is a problem (Mayo & Pearson 1995).

Intraluminal occlusion

Intraluminal occlusions are more commonly a consequence of clotted blood. A CVAD can become occluded by a blood clot in a relatively short period of time, especially if it has a small lumen, e.g. smaller than a 21g. Total occlusion can also develop over several days as a result of a clot of blood gradually increasing in size, resulting in progressively slower infusion of fluids/drugs (Wickham et al 1992). Precipitation of incompatible drugs and of PN can result in sudden occlusion of the CVAD.

Extraluminal occlusion

Extraluminal occlusion should be considered when it is possible to infuse drugs/fluids into a CVAD, but impossible or difficult to aspirate blood. This condition has been described by Mayo & Pearson (1995) as 'persistent withdrawal occlusion' (PWO). PWO can be a result of malposition of the CVAD, an anatomical obstruction or fibrin sheath formation (Tschirhart & Rao 1988).

A chest X-ray to confirm the correct positioning of the CVAD at the time of placement will minimize the risk of PWO as a result of malpositioning. However, subsequent migration of the tip of the CVAD into a smaller vessel or perforation of the SVC/endocardium can occasionally occur (Wickham et al 1992). Malposition of CVAD can also result if the device is shortened during a repair procedure.

An anatomical obstruction (e.g. a fractured clavicle), presence of a cardiac pace-

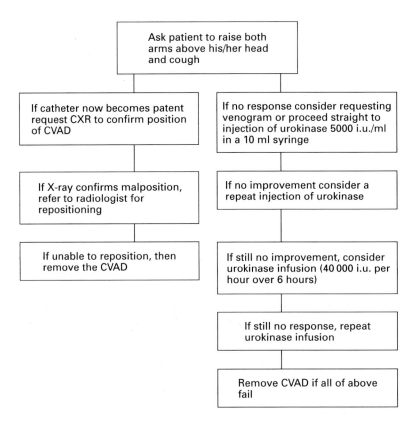

Fig. 11.12 Procedure to follow in the event of extraluminal occlusion.

maker, enlarged/removed axillary nodes or previous radiotherapy to the axilla/supraclavicular fossa can all result in pressure on the venous system and possibly lead to PWO, especially if a CVAD was placed through a vessel underlying one of these conditions (Tschirhart & Rao 1988).

Fibrin sheath formation is the commonest cause of PWO and has been reported in the majority of CVADs left in situ for more than 7 days (Mayo & Pearson 1995, Wickham et al 1992). Fibrin sheath formation occurs as a result of fibrin and platelets being deposited along the external wall of the CVAD. When this sheath reaches the tip of the CVAD, it can act as a 'one-way' valve, allowing drugs/fluids to be infused, but preventing the withdrawal of blood (Mayo & Pearson 1995). Sometimes this fibrin sheath can totally envelope the CVAD, i.e. from tip to entry site, resulting in extravasation of drugs/fluids (Wickham et al 1992).

If precipitation has been excluded as a possible cause of the occlusion, the pathway in Figure 11.12 could be used to assess whether the CVAD is malpositioned, or, if occluded, to restore it to patency.

A venogram can be useful, depending upon an individual hospital's policies and procedures, to confirm or exclude the presence of a fibrin sheath if PWO is experienced. If fibrin sheath formation is suspected, it can be treated initially in the same manner as if the CVAD was occluded by blood, i.e. instillation of 5000 i.u./ml of urokinase, and left for between 10 and 60 minutes before being aspirated back (Stewart 1993). A syringe smaller than 10 ml should never be used for this purpose, as the potential pressure is too high and could lead to rupture of the CVAD (Conn 1993). If difficulty is encountered with injecting the urokinase, a three-way tap can be attached to the end of the CVAD. Two syringes, one empty and one containing the urokinase, are then attached to the tap (Fig. 11.13). A gentle rocking

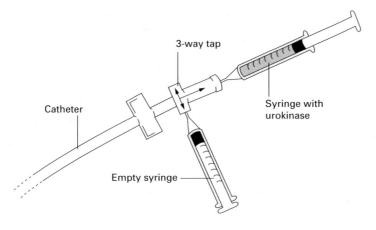

Fig. 11.13 Three-way tap and two syringes used to overcome difficulty with injection of urokinase in the event of a fibrin sheath formation.

action between the two syringes will then ensure that the urokinase is instilled into the lumen of the CVAD.

If the bolus injection of urokinase is unsuccessful in restoring the patency of the CVAD, Haire & Leiberman (1991) suggest that a urokinase infusion of 40 000 i.u./h over 6 hours can be used. Out of 19 CVADs in which Haire & Leiberman used a urokinase infusion, 15 responded and patency was restored. Of the four devices that remained occluded, two were malpositioned and the patency was restored in the remaining two after they responded to a further 6-hourly infusion of urokinase.

Thrombosis

Patients with certain types of malignancies, i.e. mucin-secreting adenocarcinomas, promyelocytic leukaemia and myeloproliferative disorders, are more at risk of thrombosis as a result of CVAD placement than other groups (Brothers et al 1988, Wickham et al 1992). Camp-Sorrell (1992) highlighted a study which recorded a 40% risk of thrombosis in patients with adenocarcinoma of the lung who had a CVAD, compared with 17% in patients with small-cell lung cancer or squamous cell carcinoma.

However, the process of developing a thrombosis related to CVADs is believed to be linked to a series of events (Ryder 1995, Wickham et al 1992). The process of introducing the catheter into the vein causes trauma, which results in thromboplastic substances and platelets collecting at the site of venepuncture. Obviously, the larger the size of the puncture or cut-down, the greater the injury to the vein. This trauma to the vein may result in the development of small thrombi which can adhere to the wall of the damaged vein, or possibly migrate, increasing in size and leading to occlusion of a larger vessel (Camp-Sorrell 1992, Moore et al 1986, Wickham et al 1992).

The size and rigidity of the CVAD can also cause further trauma to the vein. Large, rigid catheters are associated with a higher risk of thrombosis than finer, more supple devices (Camp-Sorrell 1992, Ryder 1995, Wickham et al 1992).

The rapid administration of vesicant/highly irritant drugs or infusates can lead to chemical phlebitis, which may result in the development of thrombosis (Ryder 1995, Wickhman et al 1992).

The clinical features of thrombosis formation are variable and may not become apparent until there is total occlusion of the blood vessel. Early symptoms may include erythema of the skin overlying the CVAD, oedema, discomfort, pyrexia and pain radiating down the arm on the side the device has been placed. Later symptoms tend to be more indicative of the underlying problem, with facial swelling, neck vein distension and arm swelling. Diagnosis is usually confirmed by venogram or Doppler examination (Moore et al 1992, Wickham et al 1992).

It is possible to treat a patient's thrombosis without removing the CVAD, but this depends upon the severity of the symptoms and the patient's general condition (Wickham et al 1992, Sansivero 1997). Management of the thrombosis is more effective if treatment is initiated early. Treatment can include the surgical removal of the clot, but more commonly streptokinase, urokinase or heparin is administered as a continuous infusion through the CVAD. A review of the literature has identified that although these agents have been used with varying degrees of success, there are no uniform doses or lengths of infusion (Brothers et al 1988, Moore et al 1986, Wickham et al 1992). Brothers et al (1988) highlighted that the use of streptokinase or urokinase is so effective that, once the patient's thrombosis has resolved, parenteral therapy can be resumed through the original CVAD.

Phlebitis

Richardson & Bruso (1993) identified three types of phlebitis: chemical, mechanical and infective.

Chemical phlebitis

As the tip of a CVAD terminates in a large blood vessel, i.e. the superior vena cava, it would be rare to see this type of phlebitis in recipients of skin-tunnelled catheters, implantable ports or PICCs. This is because the drugs or fluids infused are quickly diluted by the volume of blood flowing through the vessel, so they have little opportunity to irritate the lining of the vein's wall.

Mechanical phlebitis

Mechanical phlebitis is more likely to occur within the first 7 days following insertion of the CVAD. It commonly results from too large a device being placed into an individual with small blood vessels. As the blood is restricted from flowing around the catheter, phlebitis results. This type of phlebitis is more obvious in recipients of PICCs and peripheral implantable ports, where too large a device has been placed in a small cephalic, basilic or median cubital vein. It can usually be resolved within 48 hours by the application of heat to the upper arm, for 20 minutes three times a day (Richardson & Bruso 1993).

Goodwin & Carlson (1993) investigated the incidence of mechanical phlebitis in male and female recipients of PICCs and concluded that women were almost twice as likely to be affected as men. They reasoned that this was because women had smaller blood vessels, resulting in a decreased blood flow around the catheter.

Infective phlebitis

If phlebitis presents more than 7 days after insertion of the CVAD, or if a suspected case of mechanical phlebitis is not resolved by the application of heat, infection could be the cause (Richardson & Bruso 1993). A swab should be taken from the insertion site and sent to microbiology for culture and sensitivity. If considered appropriate, blood should also be aspirated from the lumen(s) of the CVAD and sent for culture and sensitivity.

Management of infection

CVAD-related infection is probably very much underestimated in its associated morbidity and mortality (Elliott 1993). Press et al (1984) investigated the incidence of infections in 922 patients with skin-tunnelled catheters and identified that 14.4% had a catheter-related infection of whom four died, i.e. four out of 922 patients.

Maki (1993) suggested that the incidence of infection from catheters inserted via the antecubital fossa was far lower than that from catheters inserted via the chest and trunk areas. The reason he identified was the lower number of skin commensal organisms present on the arm, (10 colony-forming units (CFUs per site) compared with the chest (10 000 CFUs) per site). The skin temperature is also lower on the arm, thus presenting a less hospitable environment for bacteria to multiply.

If there is redness and/or discharge around the insertion site, a swab should be taken and sent to microbiology for culture and sensitivity. The site should then be cleaned with an appropriate skin cleansing agent, e.g. chlorhexidine or povidone-iodine, and dressed daily (Maki et al 1991). When the results of the swab culture are known, an antibiotic may be prescribed, depending upon the infection and the individual clinician's preference.

The development of an unexplained pyrexia in a patient with a CVAD is not an indication for removing the device (Goodwin & Carlson 1993). To confirm, or indeed eliminate, the CVAD as the cause of the infection, blood cultures should be taken from both the CVAD and a peripheral vein. The microbiology results of both cultures should then be compared. The decision to remove an infected CVAD very much depends upon what the infection is, how ill the patient is, and the individual hospital's policies and procedures. If the CVAD is removed as a proven or suspected focus of infection, its tip should be sent for microbiological culture and sensitivity.

Brothers et al (1988) reported that, in a study of 300 patients with implantable injection ports, 26 experienced an infection resulting in tissue necrosis in the skin overlying the port. Of these 26 patients, 23 were successfully treated with either parenteral or enteral antibiotics. The three patients who did not respond to anti–biotic therapy had their devices removed.

Damaged catheters

Rupture of a CVAD can be prevented by ensuring that high-pressure methods of drug/fluid administration are avoided, i.e. needles smaller than 21g, syringes smaller than 10 ml (Conn 1993). Vacuumed blood collection bottles and infusion pumps should not be used without consulting the manufacturer's literature for each individual CVAD (Conn 1993).

A condition known as pinch-off syndrome (POS) can occur as a result of a CVAD placed via the subclavian vein becoming compressed between the clavicle and the first rib. This can lead to fracture and migration of the catheter's tip. POS can be prevented by ensuring that the CVAD is placed correctly and that a post-insertion X-ray is undertaken to confirm the position of the device (Hinke et al 1990).

More commonly, damage or complete rupture of skin-tunnelled catheters or PICCs occurs in the length of catheter exiting from the patient (Sansivero 1997).

With open-ended CVADs, care should be used when clamping the catheter to minimize the risk of damage. 'Non-toothed' clamps should be used on the catheter when removing the injection hub. Valved CVADs do not necessitate the use of clamps when removing the injection hub, because the absence of either a negative or positive pressure will prevent the opening of the three position slit valve (Delmore et al 1989). However, if the catheter is not securely anchored to the patient's skin when connected to an infusion, the device can twist. The increasing stress from the twisting can result in damage and possibly a complete rupture of the CVAD. The location of the damage will determine whether it is possible to repair the catheter. If the damage is to the injection hub, this can easily be replaced, as all CVADs accept standard luer-lock connections. If the damage is to the length of catheter from the insertion site to the injection hub, its repairability will depend upon whether the individual manufacturer provides a repair kit.

Generally speaking, single-lumen CVADs are the easier to repair. Due to the complexity of the construction of multi-lumen CVADs, repair is more difficult.

> ### ■ BOX 11.3
>
> *Procedure for replacing a PICC (Sansivero, 1997)*
> - Following a strict aseptic technique, clean the catheter and surrounding skin with an appropriate antiseptic.
> - Using a pair of sterile scissors, cut off the length of PICC attached to the injection hub of the catheter.
> - Pass a wire through the remaining PICC.
> - Gently pull on the PICC to facilitate its removal over the wire.
> - Place a new PICC over the wire.
> - Remove the wire.
> - Secure and dress the PICC as if it were a primary insertion.
> - Request a chest X-ray to confirm the position of the PICC.

(Individual manufacturers will be able to provide specific information relating to their products.) If damage to the CVAD has occurred in the portion of the catheter that is actually in situ, it may not be possible to repair it without shortening the device.

The manufacturer of the valved device does supply repair kits. The procedure involves removing the damaged part of the device, which necessitates shortening the exposed length of catheter containing the damage, and replacing the injection hub. If it is suspected that the tip of the catheter could have moved during the repair procedure, a chest X-ray should be performed before use of the device is resumed.

Many of the manufacturers of the open-ended CVADs also supply repair kits with comprehensive instructions. Some of these kits involve the use of sterile glue to mend the CVAD, so the catheter cannot be used until the glue has thoroughly dried.

With PICCs, it may be possible to attempt to replace the catheter by adopting the procedure outlined in Box 11.3.

REMOVAL OF CVADs

Prior to removal of a CVAD, the patient should have a full blood count and, if appropriate, a clotting screen performed, to ensure there is no increased potential for haemorrhage. Similarly to the insertion procedure, CVADs can be removed under a local or general anaesthetic to minimize the discomfort of the procedure for the patient. The exception to this are PICCs, which can easily be removed without anaesthesia (Gabriel 1993).

PICCs

PICCs can easily be removed by applying gentle traction to the device once the Steri-Strips, self-adhesive anchoring device or sutures have been removed. If difficulty is encountered, the application of heat to the patient's upper arm will increase the blood flow and the diameter of the vein, and therefore aid the removal of the PICC. An alternative to this approach is to apply gentle traction to the PICC and use a piece of adhesive tape to secure it to the patient's forearm. This should be left for approximately 30 minutes before a further attempt is made to remove the catheter (Sansivero 1997).

Skin-tunnelled catheters

Whether these devices have been placed by a surgical cut-down technique or by a percutaneous approach, the removal procedure is the same (Gabriel 1993). It is common practice to use a local anaesthetic to infiltrate the area around the Dacron cuff, usually 5 cm along the skin tunnel (Fig. 11.3). The skin can then be incised and the Dacron cuff identified. Once the cuff has been located, the surrounding tissue is dissected until the cuff is 'free'. Gentle traction is then applied to the catheter to remove it. An alternative approach involves applying gentle but firm traction to the catheter. In some instances this will prove sufficient to 'free' the Dacron cuff and therefore release the catheter without dissecting the cuff. There is, however, a risk of applying too much traction and snapping the catheter, which may then result in its migration (Sansivero 1997). A pressure dressing should be applied to the skin overlying the site where the catheter enters the vein. Sutures or Steri-Strips are commonly used to close the skin after the catheter has been removed, and a dressing applied.

Implantable injection ports

Either a general anaesthetic or local anaesthetic is used for the removal of injection ports. The procedure involves locating the injection port and making an incision into the overlying skin. Once the device is identified, the sutures securing it to the underlying tissue are removed. Gentle traction is then applied to remove the port and catheter. The skin is usually closed with sutures and a dressing applied (Gabriel 1993).

ADVANTAGES AND DISADVANTAGES OF EACH TYPE OF CVAD

The main advantages and disadvantages of each device are summarised in Table 11.3.

THE NURSE'S ROLE IN PLACING CVADs

The introduction of PICCs into clinical practice in the USA has resulted in all States now allowing nurses to place these catheters, provided that i.v. therapy is an integral part of their practice and they have the necessary skills (Coulter 1993). In the UK, PICCs are a new introduction which appears to be nurse-driven (Gabriel 1996b). The usual scenario by which nurses in the UK augment their area of practice is either when their medical colleagues delegate tasks/procedures or when technological advancements have simplified procedures previously undertaken by medical staff, e.g. venesection, electrocardiogram recording, administration of cytotoxic chemotherapy, etc. (Devine 1991, Maule 1994, Wright 1991).

Since its establishment, the UKCC, the regulating body for nurses in the UK, has produced a number of documents to provide professional guidance to nurses. *The Scope of Professional Practice* (UKCC 1992) emphasizes that it is the individual nurse who is professionally accountable for her clinical practice. There is no reason why an individual nurse cannot develop her own area of practice, providing she has the necessary skills and knowledge to be of benefit to an individual patient.

The nurse concerned must be prepared to be accountable for her own practice to the patient, her employer and the UKCC. With more nurses now taking on specialist roles, it is inevitable that they will encounter new developments which could be of potential benefit to individual patients (Moloney 1986). The UKCC has clearly indicated that there is no objection to nurses specializing and broadening their indi-

Table 11.3 Advantages and disadvantages of CVADs

Type	Features	Advantages	Disadvantages
Skin-tunnelled catheters	*Lumens available:* one, two or three, either open-ended or valved *Insertion technique:* surgical cut-down or percutaneous approach *Anaesthetic required:* either local or general *Dressings:* only required while incision and skin tunnel are healing *Limitations on patient's lifestyle:* some, e.g. swimming and bathing unless waterproof dressing is worn *Removal technique:* surgical cut-down or gentle but firm traction *Long-term scarring:* some, i.e. from skin tunnel and insertion site	• Available with one, two or three lumens • Ideal for patients who are needle-phobic • Can be used long-term	• Increased infection risk compared with ports and PICCs • Some limitations on patient's lifestyle
Implantable injection ports	*Lumens available:* one or two, either open-ended or valved (open-ended only available with multilayered septum) *Insertion technique:* surgical cut-down *Anaesthetic required:* either local or general *Dressings:* only required while skin incision is healing and to secure needle/cannula when in situ *Limitations on patient's lifestyle:* none *Removal technique:* minor surgical procedure *Long-term scarring:* from incision for placement/removal of reservoir	• Suitable for long-term use for individuals requiring intermittent venous access	• Not ideal for patients who are needle-phobic • Only available with two lumens, unless more than one device is placed, e.g. a single + a dual • Huber needles required for all types except the port with multilayered septum
PICCs	*Lumens available:* one or two, either open-ended or valved *Insertion technique:* cannulation of a peripheral vein *Anaesthetic required:* not always, but topical anaesthetic cream is usually applied *Dressings:* required to be changed weekly while PICC is in situ *Limitations on patient's lifestyle:* some, e.g. swimming and soaking in bath *Removal technique:* gentle traction *Long-term scarring:* no	• Quick and easy to place with minimal discomfort to the patient • Can be used long-term • Lower rate of infection and associated insertion complications than other CVADs	• Only available with two lumens, unless more than one device is placed, e.g. a single + a dual • Dressing required the whole time the PICC remains in situ • Some limitations on lifestyle

vidual area of practice, providing the nurse concerned possesses the necessary knowledge and skills, and is accountable for her own actions.

In the USA, Mansell (1983) reported that the introduction of a nurse-led PICC insertion programme into his hospital resulted in increased numbers of patients becoming recipients of a CVAD. On the surface this may appear to have been a negative aspect of the programme, but the nurses' assessment and education of the individual patients not only ensured that they received the appropriate i.v. catheter for their clinical needs and lifestyle at the outset of treatment, but also decreased the incidence of problems associated with the management of the CVADs, e.g. catheter malposition, infection, etc. The need for constantly resiting peripheral cannulae was greatly reduced, as was the incidence of chemical phlebitis associated with the inappropriate use of peripheral cannulae for some parenteral therapies.

In the UK, Hamilton et al (1995) have shown that suitably skilled nurses assuming responsibility for the placement of skin-tunnelled catheters has improved the service to their patients. These nurses not only achieve a lower rate of insertion complications than their medical colleagues, e.g. catheter malposition, infection, etc., but also provide a quick response time for the placement of CVADs. The nurses also undertake an assessment of the patient's needs before placing the CVAD, and provide the necessary education and training for both patients and staff.

There are also financial savings in nurses assuming responsibility for the placement of CVADs (Hamilton et al 1995, Mansell 1983). A nurse's time may be less expensive than a senior medical colleague. A quick response time and adequate assessment of the patient ensure that he receives the most appropriate CVAD from the earliest opportunity, with minimal complications (Hamilton et al 1995). Financial savings are also realized by a reduction in complications associated with i.v. therapy and by placing the most appropriate CVAD at the earliest opportunity.

Where i.v. therapy is an integral part of a nurse's practice, she has the opportunity to augment her knowledge and skills to assume responsibility for placing a patient's CVAD. Not only is this financially attractive to health service managers, but it also provides continuity of care for individual patients. The patient has the opportunity to discuss the implications of life with a CVAD with a nurse who knows him. The nurse can then use her knowledge of the patient (e.g. the patient's underlying medical condition, proposed treatment and lifestyle), to suggest the most suitable CVAD.

QUALITY OF LIFE

Safe, simple and reliable venous access has to be beneficial for any patient requiring intermediate- to long-term parenteral therapy. In recent years, developments in technology have increased the range of CVADs able to meet the clinical needs of individual patients. There are now implantable injection ports which can be sited on the chest wall or placed peripherally in an arm, skin-tunnelled catheters and PICCs, as discussed earlier in this chapter. These devices are available in a range of sizes and can be open-ended or valved. Whichever catheter is selected, it will become a part of that patient's life for the foreseeable future (Loughran & Borzatta 1994, Wickham et al 1992).

It is also the case that the range of treatments is increasing, and so, in future, more and more patients will require a vascular access device.

CVADs are now becoming necessary devices for the treatment and management of patients with chronic disease (Ryder 1995). Patients who are recipients of such devices will be expected to 'live' with their CVAD, and in many instances will assume responsibility for its care and management. In this situation, it is important not only to match the clinical needs of the individual to the CVADs available, but also to consider the impact such a device could have on the patient's lifestyle (Earlam 1993). If the patient will not psychologically accept the CVAD that has been placed, he will be less likely to accept it as part of his life. This potential problem can be overcome by involving the patient in the decision-making process as to which catheter will be placed and by ensuring that he is provided with knowledge and training to manage the CVAD selected (Bruner 1990).

The placement of a CVAD for intermediate- to long-term parenteral therapy is rarely an emergency procedure. Assessment of the individual patient's clinical needs, and assessment and understanding of his lifestyle will often yield more than one suitable CVAD. If there is such a choice, the final decision as to which catheter to place should rest with the patient. If the patient is aware of the care and mainte-nance of any proposed CVADs, and any restrictions that could be imposed on his lifestyle, he will be able to decide which device is preferable. This will help to ensure that he can safely 'live' with his device, with the minimum of disruption to his lifestyle (Gabriel 1997).

As long ago as 1966, Henderson believed that health education was an essential part of a nurse's role if she was to become a health promoter. With the delivery methods of health care changing, especially in relation to parenteral therapies, the role of the nurse is becoming more complex (DOH 1989). With more nurses assum-ing greater responsibility for establishing venous access, they must ensure that they are able to advise their patients appropriately, so that all patients receive a CVAD that is acceptable to them (Gabriel 1996b, 1997).

A cystic fibrosis patient requiring intermittent courses of parenteral antibiotics may prefer to opt for a PICC each time he has a chest infection. This would ensure that there were no visual reminders of his underlying medical condition during periods of good health and no necessity to maintain the patency of the CVAD when it was not in continual use. Another patient with cystic fibrosis may prefer an implantable injection port, to provide 'peace of mind' by knowing that he had ready venous access when required. A third patient may opt for a skin-tunnelled catheter, because he has a dislike of needles and is not prepared to undergo a PICC insertion each time parenteral antibiotics are required.

Fallowfield (1990) identified that disruption to an individual's life can cause depression and anxiety, which may result in a decline in overall quality of life. What an individual perceives as a 'disruption' is obviously open to debate (Thompson et al 1989). For example, does an implantable injection port which is noticeable when wearing certain clothes constitute a disruption? or a PICC preventing the individual from swimming; or a skin-tunnelled catheter acting as a visual reminder to the patient and his partner that there is an underlying medical condition? Nurses special-izing in caring for patients who require a CVAD have the opportunity to know them over a long period of time. They should be able to use their knowledge of the patient to ensure that the most suitable CVAD is selected. However, once a CVAD is selected, its positioning can also have an effect on the acceptability of the device to the patient.

Thompson et al (1989) undertook a survey of 24 recipients of skin-tunnelled catheters and implantable injection ports. Part of the questionnaire dealt with the effects of the CVAD on clothing, personal hygiene, body image, relationships, employment and leisure activities. Many of the recipients of skin-tunnelled catheters considered the device and its integral clamp to be bulky. This caused prob-lems with clothing, especially for the female recipients who stated that the device caught on their bras. Nine of the 24 patients would have preferred a lower insertion site. None of the patients was prevented from driving because of their CVAD, although it was found that right-sided placements were more comfortable. Only five out of the 24 patients in the study perceived their CVAD as having an adverse effect on body image, a proportion similar to that found by Daniels (1996). Both studies highlighted that recipients of CVADs viewed them as part of their treatment process. Thompson et al (1989) cautioned against health care professions becoming complacent about CVADs. Nurses must be aware of the developments in this area which could potentially benefit patients, especially as more become recipients of CVADs (Coulter 1993).

CONCLUSION

In recent years, the range of reliable CVADs has been expanding and it is anticipated that the number of patients using such devices will continue to grow. Nurses are becoming increasingly familiar with these devices both in relation to their management and in relation to their placement. Through education of health care professionals, we can work towards ensuring that each recipient of a CVAD receives the most appropriate device for him as an individual. Education and assessment must be an ongoing commitment.

REFERENCES

Barbone M, Rockledge P A 1995 VAD patency. Paper presented at 9th National Association of Vascular Access Networks (NAVAN) Conference, Salt Lake City. NAVAN Program no. 9506

Ben-Arush M, Berant M 1996 Retention of drugs in venous access port chamber: a note of caution. British Medical Journal 312: 496–497

Bern M M, Bothe A, Bristrain B 1986 Prophylaxis against central venous thrombosis with low-dose warfarin. Surgery 99: 216–221

Boothe A, Piccione W, Ambrosino J, Benotti P N, Lokich J J 1984 Implantable central venous access system. The American Journal of Surgery 147: 565–569

Brothers T E, Von Moll L K, Arbor A, Niederhuber J E, Roberts J A, Walker-Andrews S, Ensminger W D 1988 Experience with subcutaneous infusion ports in three hundred patients 1988. Surgery, Gynaecology & Obstetrics 6(4): 295–301

Broviac J, Cole J J, Scribner B H 1973 A silicone rubber atrial catheter for prolonged parenteral alimentation. Surgery, Gynaecology & Obstetrics 136(4): 602–606

Bruner D W 1990 Model quality assurance program for radiation oncology nursing. Cancer Nursing 13(6): 335–338

Camp-Sorrell D 1992 Implantable ports: everything you always wanted to know. Journal of Intravenous Nursing 15(5): 262–272

Conn C 1993 The importance of syringe size when using implanted vascular access devices. Journal Vascular Access Network 3(1): 11–18

Coulter K 1993 PICC lines, line management – a general overview. Paper presented at the 7th National Association of Vascular Access Networks (NAVAN), Washington, DC. NAVAN, Draper, UT

Daniels L E 1996 Exploring the physical and psychosocial implications of central venous devices in cancer patients – interviews with patients. Journal of Cancer Care 5: 45–48

Delmore J, Horbett D V, Jack B L 1989 Experience with the Groshong long-term venous catheter. Gynaecologic Oncology 2(34): 216–218

Department of Health 1989 Working for patients. HMSO, London

Devine J 1991 Points of view. Nursing Standard 5(42): 43

Dunn D L 1987 The case for the saline flush. American Journal of Nursing 6: 798–799

Earlam 1993 Quality of life. At Home: The Newsletter for Homecare Therapy Initiatives 6: 2–4

Elliott T S J 1993 Line-associated bacteraemias. Communicable Diseases Report 3(7): R91–96

Fallowfield L 1990 The quality of life – the missing measurement in health care. Souvenir Press (E & A) Ltd, London

Gabriel J 1993 Long term vascular access devices – education for patients to choose and care for their own venous catheters. National Florence Nightingale Memorial Committee Scholarship, RCN Library, London

Gabriel J 1996a Care and management of peripherally inserted catheters. British Journal of Nursing 5(10): 594–599

Gabriel J 1996b Peripherally inserted central catheters: expanding UK nurses' practice. Surgical Nurse 5(2): 71–74

Gabriel J 1997 Individual patients' perceptions of life with a PICC. Unpublished MPhil thesis, University of Portsmouth

Geritz M A 1992 Saline versus heparin in intermittent infuser patency maintenance. Western Journal of Nursing Research 14(2): 131–141

Goodwin M, Carlson I 1993 The peripherally inserted catheter: a retrospective look at 3 years of insertions. Journal of Intravenous Nursing 12(2): 92–103

Gormon C, Buzby G 1995 Difficult access problems. Surgical Oncology Clinics of North America 4(3): 453–473

Gullo S M 1982 Implanted ports. Technologic advances and nursing care issues: Nursing Clinics of North America 28(4): 850–871

Gullo S M 1993 Implanted ports. Technologic advances and nursing care issues: Nursing Clinics of North America 28(4): 850–871

Hadaway L C 1989 An overview of vascular access devices inserted via the antecubital area. Journal of Intravenous Nursing 13(5): 297–306

Haire W, Lieberman R 1991 Thrombosed central venous catheters: restoring function with six hour urokinase infusion after failure of bolus urokinase. Journal of Parenteral and Enteral Nutrition 16: 129–132

Hamilton H, O'Byrne M, Nicholai L 1995 Central lines inserted by clinical nurse specialists. Nursing Times 91(17): 38–39

Harris L C, Rushton C H, Hale S J 1987 Implantable infusion devices in the paediatric patient: a viable alternative. Journal of Paediatric Nursing 2(2): 174–179

Henderson V 1966 The nature of nursing – a definition and its implication for practice, research and education. MacMillan, New York

Hinke D H, Zandt-Stastny M D, Goodman L R, Quebbeman E J, Kyzywda E A, Andris D A 1990 Pinch-off syndrome: a complication of implantable subclavian venous access devices. Radiology 177: 353–356

Kelly C 1992 A change in flushing protocols of central venous catheters. Oncology Nursing Forum 19(4): 599

Linares J, Sitges-Serra A, Garau J 1985 Pathogenesis of catheter sepsis: a prospective study with quantitative and semi-quantitative cultures of catheter hub and segments. Journal of Clinical Microbiology 21(3): 357–360

Lokich J, Bothe A, Benotti P, Moore C 1985 Complications and management of implanted venous access catheters. Journal of Clinical Oncology 3(5): 710–717

Loughran S C, Borzatta M 1994 Peripherally inserted central catheters: a report of 2506 catheter days. Journal of Parenteral and Enteral Nutrition 19(2): 133–136

Lowel J A, Bothe A Jr 1995 Central venous catheter related thrombosis. Surgical Oncology Clinics of North America 4(3): 479–491

McCredie K, Lawson M 1984 Percutaneous insertion of silicone central venous catheters for long-term intravenous access in cancer patients. Internal Medicine for the Specialist 5(4): 100–105

Maki D G 1993 Complications associated with intravenous therapy. Paper presented at the 7th NAVAN Conference. Washington, DC

Maki D G, Ringer M, Alvarado C J 1991 Prospective randomised trial of povidone-iodine, alcohol, and chlorhexidine for prevention of infection with central venous and arterial catheters. Lancet 338: 339–343

Mansell C 1983 Peripherally inserted central venous catheterization by IV nurses – establishing a procedure. National Intravenous Therapy Association 6: 355–356

Masoorli S 1993 Cost containment program for IV nursing. Paper presented at 7th NAVAN Conference, Washington, DC

Maule W 1994 Screening for colorectal cancer by nurse endoscopists. New England Journal of Medicine 330(3): 183–188

Mayo D, Pearson D 1995 Chemotherapy extravasation: a consequence of fibrin sheath formation around venous access devices. Oncology Nursing Forum 22(4): 675–680

Moloney M 1986 Professionalization of nursing, 2nd edn J B Lippincott, Philadelphia

Moore C L, Erikson K A, Yanes L B, Franklin M, Gonsalves L 1986 Nursing care and management of venous access ports. Oncology Nursing Forum 3: 35–39

Press O W, Ramsey P G, Larson E B, Fefer A, Hickman R O 1984 Hickman catheter infections in patients with malignancies. Medicine 63: 189–200

Reed W 1991 Intravenous access devices for supportive care of patients with cancer. Current Opinion in Oncology 3: 634–642

Richardson D, Bruso P 1993 Vascular access devices – management of common complications. Journal of Intravenous Nursing 16(1): 44–49

Royal College of Nursing (RCN) 1992 Skin tunnelled catheters – guidelines for care. Scutari Projects, Harrow

Ryder M A 1995 Peripheral access options. Surgical Oncology Clinics of North America 4(3): 395–427

Sansivero G E 1997 Update on advanced PICC placement. Paper given at Bard PICC Workshop, London

Scott W L 1995 Central venous catheters: an overview of food and drug administration activities. Surgical Oncology Clinics of North America 4(3): 377–390

Shapiro C L 1995 Central venous access catheters. Surgical Oncology Clinics of North America 4(3): 443–451

Soo K C, Davidson T I, Selby P, Westbury G 1985 Long-term venous access using a subcutaneous implantable delivery system. Annals of the Royal College of Surgeons of England 67: 263–265

Stewart N 1993 CVC Complications. Paper presented at National Association of Vascular Access Networks Conference, Washington, DC

Strumpfer A 1991 Lower incidence of peripheral catheter complications by the use of elastomeric hydrogel catheters in home intravenous therapy patients. Journal of Intravenous Nursing 14(4): 261–267

Thompson A M, Kidd E, McKenzie M, Parker A S, Nixon S J 1989 Long term central venous access: the patient's view. Intensive Therapy and Clinical Monitoring May: 142–144

Tschirhart J, Rao M 1988 Mechanism and management of persistent withdrawal occlusion. The American Surgeon 54: 326–328

United Kingdom Central Council for Nursing, Midwifery and Health Visiting 1992 The scope of professional practice. UKCC, London

Walker S, Calzone K 1994 Trial results of a new peripherally placed implantable venous access port, Bard Cath-Link 20™. Oral presentation 9th NAVAN Conference, Salt Lake City. NAVAN 1(2)

Wickham R, Purl S, Welker D 1992 Long-term central venous catheters: issues for care. Seminars in Oncology Nursing 2(8): 133–147

Wright S 1991 Nursing development? Nursing Standard 5(38): 52

Young G P, Alexeyeff M, Russell D R 1988 Catheter sepsis during parenteral nutrition: the safety of long-term opsite dressings. Journal of Parenteral and Enteral Nutrition 12(4): 365–370

Intravenous therapy in the community

Jill Kayley

CHAPTER 12

INTRODUCTION

Intravenous therapy is routine practice within hospitals and has been for many years. As technology has changed, new forms of mechanical equipment and more manageable therapy have been developed which enable some of the treatments to become less specialized and therefore manageable in the community by less highly trained personnel.

In the context of increasing demand for acute hospital bed spaces and lengthening waiting lists, combined with sufficient resources and skills within the community, it is a natural development for i.v. therapy to take place outside the hospital setting. Patients now have a greater influence on the choice of treatment and location of the various options available, and in many circumstances prefer the comfort, familiarity and relaxation of their own home environment.

To carry out this form of treatment safely and effectively within the community requires comprehensive organization, multidisciplinary working and refinement of technical skills to ensure that all the coordination required takes place smoothly and efficiently.

Definition of intravenous therapy in the community

It is important to define what is understood by the phrase 'intravenous therapy in the community'. In the context of this chapter, it is classified as any intravenous treatment administered at home, in GP surgeries, community hospitals, outpatient clinics, day units and nursing or residential homes.

'Patient' is used consistently throughout this text for convenience to mean any of the following: client, user, consumer, person or individual. 'Carer' is used to identify any individual who is involved in the administration of the i.v. therapy and support of the patient in a non-professional capacity, and could be a family member, friend or neighbour.

BACKGROUND

Intravenous therapy in the community is not a totally new concept, but has been a well established practice for a very small number of chronic conditions that require long-term i.v. therapy. These programmes have developed because it is impractical both socially and economically for them to be carried out in hospital or on an outpatient basis (see Table 12.1). In the USA, i.v. therapy in the community has been established for 10–15 years and is generally referred to as non-inpatient i.v. therapy, home i.v. therapy or outpatient i.v. therapy. The driving force in the USA for developing a community i.v. therapy service was a desire to reduce the costs of hospital in-patient episodes and for patients to return home and to work or school.

Compared with the USA, there is little published data on community i.v. therapy related to the UK experience, although the last 7 years have seen an increase in pub-

Table 12.1 Established intravenous therapies

Conditions	Treatment	Started
Haemophilia A & B	Factor VIII + IX	1971
Intestinal failure	Parenteral nutrition	Late 1970s
Primary antibody deficiency	Immunoglobulin	Mid-1980s
Cystic fibrosis	Antibiotics	Mid-1980s

lished papers. The majority of papers do not address i.v. therapy in the community in a broad sense, but relate to specific conditions and their treatments.

The home treatment programme of factor VIII or IX for haemophiliacs was started in 1971 in Oxford, Newcastle and the Royal Free Hospital, London. The first group of patients admitted to the programme were those with severe haemophilia who made the heaviest call on the centres for 'on-demand' treatment (Rizza & Spooner 1977). Prior to this, patients requiring factor VIII or IX had to travel to the centre to receive treatment, often in considerable discomfort and pain, if they had had a bleed. For home treatment, patients and carers were taught to perform venepuncture using a steel winged infusion device for administering the factor VIII or IX.

Home parenteral nutrition (PN) was started in the late 1970s and early 1980s for patients with intestinal failure, and the few patients having PN at home at this time had tunnelled central venous catheters in situ. Patients and carers were taught to administer their treatment at home and there are still a few patients currently having PN who started with the early programme. There are now approximately 250 patients having home PN in this country and the majority are either self-administering or a carer is involved.

The home programme for immunoglobulin therapy for the treatment of primary antibody deficiency was first established in Oxford and Northwick Park, Harrow (Brennan 1987, Chapel & Brennan 1988, Webster et al 1988). Prior to this, most patients had intramuscular (i.m.) immunoglobulin but this caused quite severe reactions in a number of them. Currently, patients eligible for joining the home programme are taught at one of the 10 specialist centres in the UK. The training programmes are well established and patients/carers are taught to cannulate in order to administer the immunoglobulin therapy. Rapid subcutaneous immunoglobulin therapy infusions are starting to be used in the UK instead of i.v. immunoglobulin (Gardulf et al 1991).

Patients with cystic fibrosis require intermittent courses of i.v. antibiotics for infections and this treatment was started in the community in the mid-1980s (David 1989, Ellis 1989). Prior to this, patients were admitted to hospital for the full course of treatment. Many patients with cystic fibrosis have long-term central venous catheters (CVCs) or implantable ports; others have peripherally inserted central catheters (PICCs) or midline catheters inserted when treatment is needed; and some just have a peripheral cannula inserted for the course of treatment. Patients and carers are usually taught to administer the i.v. antibiotic therapy and may only have the first or second dose of treatment in hospital before going home.

Current intravenous therapies in the community

The current situation in the UK is that i.v. therapy in the community is expanding to cover a wider range of treatments and conditions (see Table 12.2). However, the overall management of the therapy in terms of who delivers, where, and how, for these patients, is still fragmented and varied.

Table 12.2 Current i.v. therapies (see also Daniels 1996, Kayley 1996, Kayley et al 1996, Low 1994, Roberts & Seaby 1994, Watters 1997, Williams 1995)

Condition	Treatment	Duration of treatment
Acute or chronic infection	Antibiotics	6–8 weeks or less
Cytomegalovirus	Antivirals	Short or long term
Serious fungal infection	Antifungals	Short or long term
Haematological disorders	Blood/platelets	Intermittent/long term
Cancer	Chemotherapy	Intermittent courses
		Short or long term
Nausea/vomiting	Anti-emetic	Short term
Acute/chronic pain	Analgesia	Short or long term
Thalassaemia	Desferal	Long term/life
Sickle cell disease		
Gaucher disease	Ceredase	Long term/life
Heart failure	Dobutamine	Short term
Dehydration	Intravenous fluid	Short term
Patients having nephrotoxic drugs who cannot maintain an adequate oral intake of fluid		

VASCULAR ACCESS

Vascular access can be either peripherally or centrally placed. The choice of vascular access for i.v. therapy in the community is dependent on the nature and duration of the treatment, the patient and her lifestyle, who is administering the treatment, and how it is managed in the community. Currently, the majority of i.v. therapy suitable for management in the community is longer-term, and therefore patients require appropriate venous access.

Peripheral cannulae

Peripheral cannulae are not usually appropriate for longer-term i.v. therapy administered outside the hospital setting for the following reasons:

- They are primarily designed for short-term use.
- It is recommended that they should be resited every 48–72 hours to reduce the risk of phlebitis (Goodinson 1990). Therefore, someone in the community would have to take on that responsibility or patients would need to travel back to the hospital to have the cannula resited each time.
- There is a higher risk of thrombophlebitis, extravasation than with centrally placed vascular access devices.
- Vesicant drugs should not be administered via a peripheral cannula unless under very close and constant supervision because of the risk of extravasation (Chrystal 1997).
- They are not suitable for the administration of hyperosmolar solutions, e.g. parenteral nutrition.
- They are not user-friendly for patients who are administering their own i.v. therapy.
- Some of the pre-filled self-regulating devices used for i.v. drug administration in the community may continue infusing even if the peripheral cannula has become displaced, causing infiltration.

Peripheral cannulae or winged infusion devices are, however, often used for patients who administer their own intermittent therapy, e.g. haemophiliacs who have factor VIII and IX treatment, and patients with primary antibody deficiency who have immunoglobulin therapy. Individuals or their carers are taught to perform the cannulation/venepuncture and the cannula/winged infusion device is inserted for the administration of the treatment and then removed.

Central vascular access

Centrally placed vascular access devices are generally more suitable for the majority of community-based i.v. therapy. These can be divided into three groups:

- skin-tunnelled cuffed/uncuffed catheters
- peripherally inserted central catheters (PICCs)
- implantable ports (central and peripheral).

For a detailed description of, and information about each vascular access device, see Chapter 11.

The choice of device for use in the community is dependent on several factors:

- general condition of the patient
- any relevant past medical history
- type of treatment
- frequency of treatment
- duration of treatment
- who is administering the therapy and how
- lifestyle of the patient
- patient choice.

The choice of vascular access should be discussed with patients prior to insertion so that they are aware of the different types of vascular access device that are suitable, what they look like, and where the device would be positioned once inserted, thus enabling them to make an informed choice (Wainstock 1987) (see Box 12.1).

Many of the aspects to be considered for patients in the community are set out in Table 12.3.

METHODS OF ADMINISTRATION

The method of administration of any i.v. therapy falls into three categories:

- *Continuous infusion* – the infusion of a volume of drug/fluid continuously, over a given period of time. A pump or pre-filled device is required to ensure the safe and correct administration rate. The volume of actual drug/fluid can be anything from small volume to large depending on the treatment. Examples of continuous infusions administered in the community are parenteral nutrition (PN), chemotherapy, analgesia and rehydration fluid.
- *Intermittent infusion* – the infusion of drug/fluid over a relatively short period of time which is then stopped until the next dose is due. The frequency of administration could be daily or more often. Examples of this method of administration are antibiotics, antivirals, antifungals, chemotherapy, immunoglobulin, factor VIII/IX, blood and blood products.
- *Direct intermittent injection* – the administration of a smaller volume of drug/fluid using a syringe and needle, or syringe and cannula, over a short period of time. Examples of this method of administration are antibiotics, chemotherapy, analgesics, anti-emetics and catheter flushes.

■ BOX 12.1

Case histories: Choosing a device

Consultation with the patient

Katie needed long-term venous access for administration of an antiviral drug for the treatment of cytomegalovirus. The different types of venous access that would be suitable for long-term use were discussed with and shown to Katie. She wanted to have an implantable port as she did not want a tube visible on the outside of her body because people would see it, she wouldn't be able to swim and it would alter her body image. A close friend of Katie's had a skin-tunnelled cuffed central catheter inserted not long before she died. Katie felt that if she were to have the same type, it would be a constant reminder of her friend when she was so ill.

Lack of consultation

Barbara had been having i.v. therapy in the community for a number of months via a peripheral implantable port. The port had become blocked and a temporary triple-lumen central catheter was inserted. Barbara's i.v. therapy was long-term so it was arranged for her to have a skin-tunnelled cuffed central catheter inserted, with the peripheral implantable port and temporary central catheter removed. No-one discussed the catheter insertion with Barbara and when she came round after the general anaesthetic she found the skin-tunnelled central catheter had been inserted via the femoral vein in her groin and tunnelled up to her belly button. She was devastated as she had had no idea that this site could be used and it would mean that she could no longer wear the tight skirts she enjoyed wearing as it would be too uncomfortable.

Careful consideration should be given to the method of administration of any i.v. drug in the community as this has implications for the amount and cost of equipment, the time involved and how manageable the process is in the community.

The main items of equipment required for the three methods of administration are as follows:

- For a *continuous infusion*:
  — pump to regulate infusion (portable, ambulatory or volumetric)
  — designated administration set
  — drip stand (if volumetric pump used)
  — closed system connectors
  — large sharps bin.
- For an *intermittent infusion*:
  — pre-filled device, or
  — small ambulatory pump with designated administration set, or
  — infusion bags, drip stand and administration sets
  — closed system connectors
  — large sharps bin.
- For a *direct intermittent injection*:
  — syringe and needle, or
  — syringe and cannula
  — small sharps bin.

The equipment and supplies required for a direct intermittent injection are considerably cheaper and easier to obtain and organize than those required for a continuous or intermittent infusion. This should therefore be an important consideration when planning to discharge a patient into the community for i.v. ther-

Table 12.3 Advantages and disadvantages of alternative central vascular access devices*

Vascular access device	Advantages	Disadvantages
Tunnelled cuffed catheter	More secure – Dacron cuff anchors catheter in place No discomfort with use Easily accessible Can be used for blood sampling	Altered body image Can get caught in clothing and bedding May require a minor surgical procedure to remove Discomfort with car seat belts Requires good waterproof covering for swimming Vulnerable to activities that may catch or pull on catheter
Tunnelled uncuffed catheter	Easy to remove No discomfort with use Easily accessible Can be used for blood sampling	Less secure – can be dislodged/pulled out Exit site suture must remain in place Altered body image Can get caught in clothing and bedding Discomfort with car seatbelts Requires good waterproof covering for swimming Vulnerable to activities that may catch or pull on catheter
Peripherally inserted central catheter	Easy to remove No discomfort with use Easy to conceal under clothing No scar once removed	Less secure – can be dislodged/pulled out Not recommended for water activities, particularly swimming Need to avoid heavy lifting and excessive movement of arm Difficult for self-administration without use of extension tubing More liable to occlude than wider lumen catheters
Implantable port	Concealed under skin – only small, raised area visible No restrictions on physical activities Suitable for bathing, showering and swimming Monthly flush required when not in use No dressing required	Requires surgical procedure to remove Each use requires a needle puncture More difficult to access, particularly to oneself Skin can become sore with frequent accessing

*Vascular access devices vary between different manufacturers. The above table is a general guide only, and not an exhaustive or inclusive list.

■ BOX 12.2

Ensuring the correct infusion rate

John was discharged from hospital on vancomycin 1 g twice daily. The community nurses were visiting to set up the infusion via a volumetric pump. John said the infusion had been running over 75 minutes in hospital, but when one of the community nurses checked the package insert of the drug, it stated that the infusion should run at a rate of 10 mg/min. Therefore, John's dose of vancomycin should be infused over 100 minutes.

---

apy – the aim should be to find the safest and most straightforward method of administration regardless of who is administering it.

The method and rate of administration of any i.v. drug is dictated by the manufacturer's recommendations. Generally, patients having i.v. therapy in the community start the treatment whilst in hospital. The rate and method of administration should therefore be decided and commenced in hospital. However, if for any reason the administration method in hospital does not comply with the manufacturer's recommendations, it is the responsibility of those involved in the community to ensure that these recommendations are adhered to (see Box 12.2). If a patient suffers a reaction because a drug is given too quickly, there may be no support from the company that manufactured the drug if their recommendations were not followed.

EQUIPMENT

Ambulatory infusion devices

In the USA there is a wide range of ambulatory infusion devices which are used particularly for home and outpatient i.v. therapy (Schleis & Tice 1996).

There is a fast-growing demand for ambulatory infusion devices, with new products and variations to existing devices being developed all the time. A number of these are now available in the UK and are used more commonly, though not solely, for home i.v. therapy such as antimicrobials, analgesia, PN and chemotherapy (Woollens 1996).

The two types currently available in the UK are:

- non-electrically powered ambulatory infusion devices, e.g. elastomeric devices or mechanical single-dose infusors
- electrically powered ambulatory infusion devices.

For detailed description and information about each of the above ambulatory infusion devices, see Chapter 8.

Ambulatory infusion devices are ideal for patients having i.v. therapy in the community as they are lighter and smaller than the large volumetric pumps and designed specifically to be worn by the patient usually in a carry case or pouch.

Specific factors to be considered for patients in the community relating to the two types of ambulatory infusion device are discussed below (Medical Devices Agency 1997).

Non-electrically powered devices

Advantages

- Portability allows greater freedom and independence for the patient.

- They are easy and straightforward to use which reduces teaching time for user and trainer.
- No pre-programming is required, and therefore there is a reduced risk of user error.
- The majority are pre-filled with the drug and diluent, thus eliminating the need for reconstitution by the user.

Disadvantages

- There are no alarm or alert facilities.
- Some pre-filled devices need to be removed from the fridge for a period of time prior to use to allow them to reach room temperature.
- Infusion time can be affected by changes in temperature, and condition and patency of the vascular access device.

Electrically powered devices

Advantages

- Portability allows greater freedom and independence for the patient.
- Some are multifunctional with a range of infusion facilities.
- There is a locking system to prevent tampering or misuse.
- Devices have alarm and alert facilities.

Disadvantages

- They are complicated to operate for a user unfamiliar with the device, and therefore increased teaching time is required.
- The multifunctional infusion facility may increase the risk of user error.
- They require designated administration sets.

Availability of 'high-tech' equipment and training

The provision and availability of 'high-tech' equipment, e.g. pumps, for community i.v. therapy is a difficult and not easily resolved issue. All i.v. therapy in the community requires equipment – the amount, complexity and cost depend on the drug or treatment and how it is to be administered.

Community trusts do not generally have resources to purchase pumps for i.v. therapy, especially when the demand for them is low and infrequent. Acute hospitals have pumps for use on the wards, but they do not generally have a surplus available to loan to the community. Pumps can be hired from commercial companies, and some of the pump manufacturers are beginning to offer more flexible options other than outright purchase.

For some i.v. therapies administered in the community, e.g. PN and chemotherapy, a pump is a prerequisite for safe and accurate administration, and one is therefore provided as part of the whole package. However, as a general rule in the community, unless the patient or carer is particularly capable and confident to regulate a gravity infusion, then a pump or pre-filled device should always be used. The hospital may or may not have used a pump but in the hospital there is always nursing and medical cover 24 hours a day.

The Medical Devices Agency database has over 900 reports (current figure to 1997) concerned with incidents involving infusion devices. A large proportion of these reports have been identified as due to user error and not failure of the infusion pumps (Richardson 1995).

If pumps are to be used for the administration of i.v. therapy in the community then the provision of training related to these pumps for all those involved, especially the operators, must feature as a very high priority (MDA 1995). Any pump, whether battery or electrically operated, must be maintained and serviced by a medical engineering department at defined intervals. Community trusts need to make arrangements to ensure that all equipment is maintained and serviced on a regular basis, and these are often made through acute hospitals which all have a medical engineering department (MDA 1995).

Any pump used should be as simple as possible whilst being fit for the purpose, have good safety features and intelligible alarms (MDA 1995, 1997, Morling & Ford 1997). All operators of pumps must be well trained and fully understand all aspects and workings of the pump. Pump manufacturers will provide training for operators and there should always be a product user manual available. If patients or carers are going to be responsible for operating the pump, they should be well trained before discharge into the community takes place. If community nurses are involved in the administration, they should have the opportunity to undertake training before the patient is discharged, or training should be provided in the community. If patients are to be left with an infusion running, they should be taught, at the very least, how to switch the pump off and who to call for help (MDA 1995).

PATIENT ASSESSMENT AND DISCHARGE PLANNING

Early assessment of any patient being considered for i.v. therapy in the community is of paramount importance. It will help to ascertain at an early stage whether the treatment is manageable in and appropriate for the community. The assessment should involve a multidisciplinary team, including someone from the community or at least someone with a knowledge of working in the community. The multidisciplinary team should comprise of the following people (Sheldon & Bender 1994):

- physician
- hospital nurse
- pharmacist
- social worker
- liaison nurse
- general practitioner
- patient and carer.

When assessing patients for i.v. therapy in the community, it is important to ascertain whether they are suitable to have this treatment at home. Each patient should be considered on an individual basis in relation to the assessment criteria in Box 12.3 balanced against the treatment options available in order to form a judgement of suitability.

It is impossible to safeguard against every eventuality and once patients are discharged into the community they do not have anyone looking over their shoulder. However, the majority of patients who self-administer i.v. therapy are generally highly motivated, understand the importance of the treatment and have a sense of self-control and autonomy. It is important to provide good, regular ongoing support to monitor how they are coping in the community.

Discharge planning begins with the initial assessment of the patient and is an ongoing process until the point of discharge from hospital. It should ideally be coordinated by one person as this encourages continuity, avoids duplication, minimizes the likelihood of problems occurring and ensures all the necessary aspects are considered and dealt with as appropriate. It should involve the following:

■ BOX 12.3

Assessment criteria for treatment at home

- Is the patient able to comply with the treatment regimen? Consider the following: age; physical disability; pain; disease; side-effects of medication; poor vision; poor manual dexterity; exhaustion.
- Does the treatment need to be given i.v. rather than via another route?
- Are there any implications in relation to allergies/anaphylaxis?
- Does the patient/carer/family understand the implications of the treatment, the venous access, how to recognize and deal with any complications and who to contact throughout the day or night?
- Who will administer the i.v. therapy, what training will they require, where will that training be done, and by whom?
- Is the treatment appropriate and manageable for the community?
- What equipment supplies are required and where will they come from?
- Is the patient medically and psychologically fit for discharge?
- Will any blood monitoring be required? If so, what, how often, and who will assimilate the results?
- Is the patient's home situation suitable, do they have a telephone and is there anyone else in the house?
- Are there any wider family issues and responsibilities?
- What ongoing support is available, from whom and what are the follow-up arrangements?
- Is the GP happy to accept the patient home for this treatment?
- What level of support and involvement are the community nurses and GPs able to provide?

Circumstances where patients may not be suitable

- Patient is confused/has dementia.
- Patient is elderly/frail and lives alone.
- Patient may abuse venous access, e.g. intravenous drug user.
- Patient's home situation is unsuitable, e.g. no telephone; no running water; no electricity; isolated; or dirty.
- Patient has no insight/comprehension of the treatment.
- Patient is not suitable to administer the therapy and no-one else is able to do it.
- Patient cannot give informed written or verbal consent.

- communication and liaison with:
  — patient/carer
  — members of the multidisciplinary team
  — GP, community nurse and primary health care team (PHCT)
- documentation of all plans and decisions made
- organization of drugs, equipment and ancillary items
- a treatment plan – duration of treatment, review date and/or completion date
- follow-up arrangements
- planning a realistic discharge date that is satisfactory to all those involved.

Good communication and careful discharge planning are an integral part of the whole process and essential for a smooth trouble-free transition from hospital to home.

WHO DELIVERS?

The decision as to who will administer the i.v. therapy in the community should

Table 12.4 Who delivers?

	Pros	Cons
Patient/carer	Patient autonomy/control Available 24 hours/day Technique good Methodical and thorough	Training is time-consuming, therefore possible delayed discharge from hospital More difficult to monitor patient/carer technique
Community nurse	Works in the community Able to monitor patient Works 7 days a week Flexible hours (a.m./p.m.) in some areas	Requires training and support Several nurses are involved in the administration
Private home i.v. company	Flexible service Experienced nurses Able to monitor patient 24-hour back-up support	Cost Patient could have care from several different agencies
Practice nurse	Limited number of nurses involved (one or two) Able to monitor patient	Requires training and support 5-day service during daytime
Outpatient nurse	Medical back-up available Able to monitor patient	Patient has to travel 5-day service, 9 a.m. to 5 p.m.
Hospital outreach/specialist nurse	Experienced nurses Able to monitor patient	Not feasible for long distances, large numbers of patients and frequent dosing
General Practitioner	Would have to get involved and learn	Requires training and support for all GPs in the practice Limited up-to-date knowledge about i.v. drug administration Not enough time or resources

involve the patient/carer. There are a range of people listed in Table 12.4 who could be involved in the administration, subject to the following considerations:

- availability of resources
- i.v. trained community nurses
- regimen of i.v. therapy – frequency/duration
- dexterity of patient/carer
- age of patient
- compliance and understanding
- ease of administration
- type of venous access
- wider picture of home situation and condition of patient.

Patient/carer administration

If it is appropriate for the patient/carer to administer the i.v. therapy then training will be required. In most circumstances, it is preferable that this is carried out in the hospital prior to discharge so that the patient/carer is fully trained and competent upon final discharge into the community. It is not realistic or acceptable to start the training in hospital and then to expect a community nurse, who may not have been involved, to continue the training and supervision. Training a layperson is time-consuming, requires patience and consistency, and should be provided by a limited number of trainers (see Box 12.4 for training guidelines) (Lowry 1995).

■ BOX 12.4

Guidelines for training patients/carers (Redman 1997)

- Limit the number of trainers to two or three.
- Draw up written guidelines (step by step) of how to administer the therapy and be very specific, starting with a list of equipment and supplies required.
- The trainers should go through the guidelines thoroughly together so they are all teaching the same method.
- Give the patient/carer a copy of the guidelines to read before starting the training.
- Find a suitable environment which is comfortable, with room for all persons involved.
- Set aside plenty of time.
- Ensure no distractions and a calm environment.
- Start with the basics – handling equipment, connecting needles to syringes, drawing up sodium chloride 0.9% for flushing.
- Demonstrate each stage, then let the patient/carer try.
- Keep explanations simple and short. Emphasize what to do rather than what not to do.
- Encourage the patient/carer to write her own additional instructions on the guidelines.
- Give feedback and allow plenty of time for questions.
- Do not suggest alternative procedures or short-cuts. Stick rigidly to the guidelines until a routine is established.
- Cover side-effects and complications, and what to do and who to contact.
- Move slowly from dependence to independence and appreciate that it may take a number of teaching sessions.
- Observe the patient/carer doing the whole procedure from start to finish, without intervention, before discharge.
- Ensure the patient/carer feels confident about the administration.
- Document all training undertaken.
- Try to arrange for someone competent to be with the patient/carer the first time she administers the i.v. therapy in the community.

The following should be borne in mind when arranging the training of patients/carers:

- The trainers need to feel confident about their own skills/knowledge about the therapy/treatment.
- The trainers must be able to present the information in an orderly and understandable manner.
- The trainers must be able to work on the same level as the patient/carer.
- The patient/carer must be able to learn.
- It is important to recognize that not all patients/carers want to take on the administration of their i.v. therapy, not all are suitable and not all can be taught.

The role of community nurses

The extent and involvement of community nurses in i.v. therapy in the community will vary depending on the duration and frequency of treatment, who is administering it and the community nurse's knowledge, ability and skills.

There is a clear need for community nurses to acquire and develop their skills in relation to i.v. therapy within the scope of their professional competence and development. These responsibilities are clearly stated within the UKCC's *Code of Professional Conduct* (UKCC 1992a) and *Scope of Professional Practice* (UKCC 1992b). The *Code of Professional Conduct* states:

> 'As a registered nurse, midwife or health visitor, you are personally accountable for your practice and, in the exercise of your professional accountability, must:
>
> 1. act always in such a manner as to promote and safeguard the interests and well being of patient and clients;
>
> 2. ensure that no action or omission on your part, or within your sphere of responsibility, is detrimental to the interests, condition or safety of patients and clients;
>
> 3. maintain and improve your professional knowledge and competence.'

Community nurses are ideally placed to provide i.v. therapy as well as support to patients/carers in the community, and may have many of the skills required, but may require access to a community-based theoretical i.v. training programme, supervised practice and ongoing support.

Currently, the provision of i.v. training for community nurses is very fragmented, even non-existent in some areas, and many community nurses only have access to hospital-based i.v. training programmes (Corbett et al 1993). These are good in their own right but do not generally address any relevant community issues. A community-based i.v. training programme should address the following (Kayley 1995):

- types of venous access, especially centrally placed
- management of central venous access
- complications of central venous access
- management of i.v. therapy in the community
- pharmaceutical aspects
- legal aspects and scope of professional practice
- management of anaphylaxis
- practical training
- management, safe handling and disposal of cytotoxic drugs.

It can be difficult for community nurses to gain and maintain sufficient practical skills in i.v. therapy to enable them to cope with the full variety of different therapies and venous access devices that they may encounter. Although a community nurse may learn about particular i.v. therapies and the venous access relevant to the expected need, some patients referred may have completely different requirements. Until i.v. therapy in the community becomes routine practice, which at this stage is still a long way off, community nurses will only see these patients infrequently, which makes it very difficult for them to maintain particular skills and have the confidence to use them.

It must therefore be recognized that community nurses will need to keep updating their practical skills and theoretical knowledge. This may be achieved by visiting the relevant unit each time a new patient is referred or by having a specialist/liaison nurse who is able to meet with community nurses when required for practical training and updating (Kayley 1995, Oliver 1991).

Community nurses are accountable for their own practice and once they accept a patient for i.v. therapy in the community, they are accepting accountability for the treatment and care they provide to that patient (see Box 12.5).

The UKCC *Standards for the Administration of Medicines* (UKCC 1992c) provides clear guidelines in relation to the prescription of medication. Therefore, if community nurses are involved in the administration of the i.v. therapy, the treatment should be clearly written on a community drug chart stating the drug name, dose, route, frequency, timing of administration and the review or completion date of the

■ **BOX 12.5**

Questions that need to be answered before accepting a patient for intravenous therapy

- What is the name of the drug/treatment?
- What is the drug/treatment for?
- What are the side-effects?
- How should it be administered?
- At what rate should it be administered?
- Is the dose prescribed the correct dose for that patient (weight, height, etc.)?
- Does the patient have any allergies?
- Does the patient have any relevant past medical history?
- Has the patient had any problems/side-effects with the treatment so far?
- How many doses of drug treatment has the patient had?
- Is any blood monitoring required; if so, how often?
- Is there a finish or review date for the drug/treatment?
- What type of venous access does the patient have?
- When was the venous access placed/inserted?
- When will the venous access need changing and by whom (peripheral cannula)?
- If centrally placed, where is the tip positioned?
- What are the complications of this type of venous access?
- What are the signs and symptoms of the complication?
- Who should be contacted if any problems occur?

treatment (Scales 1996). The patient's name must be clear and the drug chart should be signed and dated by the prescribing doctor, but countersigned by the GP once the patient is home.

Private home intravenous companies

There are a number of private home i.v. companies in the independent sector which can provide a range of services for patients requiring i.v. therapy in the community, including:

- assessment and discharge planning
- specialist nurses to administer i.v. therapy, monitor and support the patient
- cannulation and venepuncture
- 24 hour access for specialist advice
- policy for the management of anaphylaxis
- policy for the management of extravasation
- liaison with hospital
- training and support for community nurses and other members of the primary health care team (PHCT)
- liaison with GPs
- reconstitution or preparation of i.v. therapy in device/pump of choice
- delivery of drugs plus all ancillary equipment to patient on a regular basis
- collection of sharps bins and clinical waste.

There is an immediate and identifiable cost involved with the use of private companies and, as more companies have developed, pricing has had to become more competitive. It is difficult to predict how these companies will develop and expand, but currently the number of companies is small, the range of services offered varies, and the ways in which they operate differ. However, in some areas there is no existing system within the community to maintain patients on i.v. therapy, so using private companies is a way of enabling these patients to be supported in the community.

Practice nurses

Practice nurses are based in the health centre/surgery and therefore patients have to go to them for treatment. This encourages ambulant patients to get out of the house and be more independent. The service that practice nurses provide is generally Monday to Friday during the daytime with some early evening cover. In this situation, appropriate i.v. therapies would be intermittent, require minimal equipment and could be administered over a relatively short period of time.

Outpatient nurses

Attending an outpatient department is an option for patients who may need regular monitoring and those who are unable or unsuitable to administer their own therapy and where there is no carer or nurse available to carry this out. Outpatient departments provide a Monday to Friday service, usually between the hours of 9 a.m. and 5 p.m., and therefore other arrangements would need to be made at the weekends. Patients have to travel to the department and they may spend long periods of time there, waiting and receiving treatment.

Specialist nurses

Specialist nurses may be available to administer i.v. therapy to patients under their care, but as specialist nurses are few in number this is not sustainable or feasible in the following circumstances:

- long-term treatment
- frequent dosing
- if large numbers of patients are involved
- if there are long distances to travel.

General practitioners

The majority of GPs are keen for patients to be in the community, but their workload is ever increasing with no additional resources. GPs' involvement in the administration of i.v. therapy in the community is only realistic for infrequent, short-term, pre-agreed therapy that could be shared with other professionals.

Practice nurses and GPs, like community nurses, may not be familiar with or experienced in i.v. therapy and therefore require training, supervised practice and ongoing support, all of which require time and resources.

PRESCRIBING

In April 1995, a UK Department of Health executive letter, *EL (95) 5: Purchasing High Tech Healthcare for Patients at Home*, was implemented (DOH 1995). This document shifted the funding of high-tech packages of care from the FP10 prescribing system to the purchasers. The NHS Executive identified the amount that was currently being spent on these high-tech packages of care through GP prescribing, and these funds were shifted to the purchasers. The responsibility for patient care has not been affected, but GPs are no longer able to prescribe certain drugs/treatments on FP10 prescription forms.

The document listed the main groups of patients who were receiving high-tech packages of care at home via the GP FP10 prescribing system:

- patients with renal failure receiving continuous ambulatory peritoneal dialysis (CAPD)
- cystic fibrosis patients receiving intravenous or nebulized antibiotics
- cancer patients receiving i.v. chemotherapy agents
- HIV patients receiving i.v. or nebulized anti-infectives
- patients receiving PN or various types of specialized enteral feeding
- thallassaemics receiving desferrioxamine
- patients receiving continuous anticoagulant treatment.

The document also listed the drug preparations likely to have been prescribed as part of packages, recognizing that the list was not inclusive of all the drugs.

The *EL* (*95*) *5* is now well established and many of the initial teething problems have been ironed out, but the exact interpretation of a 'package of care' still varies from area to area. A package of care was understood to mean that the drug and any necessary delivery systems, additional equipment and delivery were provided by a single supplier. This is very clear in the case of well established and recognized high-tech treatments such as PN and CAPD, where a true package cost can be identified which includes all the equipment and ancillary items. However, for some i.v. therapies, e.g. i.v. antibiotics, where the drug may be provided in powder form and the ancillary equipment requirement is not excessive or complex, it could be argued that this is not a package of care and therefore does not fall under the *EL* (*95*) *5* directive.

The GP FP10 prescribing system works in the following way:

1. GP writes a prescription.
2. Prescription goes to a chemist.
3. Chemist dispenses drug.
4. Prescription goes to Prescription Pricing Authority.
5. Chemist is reimbursed.

If the drug/treatment is not allowed to be prescribed via the FP10 system then the chemist will not be reimbursed for dispensing that drug. It is therefore essential that there are clear guidelines at local level for prescribing of drugs and provision of all equipment for any i.v. therapies that are administered in the community.

ALLERGIC/ANAPHYLACTIC REACTIONS

All drugs possess the potential to cause hypersensitivity reactions and, although not common, they do occur. Therefore, the prevention and treatment of such reactions should be an important consideration for i.v. therapy in the community (RCN 1988). Hypersensitivity reactions can range from a mild rash to a severe anaphylactic reaction. The intensity and severity of the response are thought to be related to administration, the rate of absorption of the drug and the patient's degree of hypersensitivity (Moeser 1991).

Community nurses should carry particular drugs for use in the event of an allergic/anaphylactic reaction. Anaphylaxis kits and related policies/guidelines are generally available in relation to the administration of i.m. or subcutaneous injections in the community, but these policies and guidelines should be modified to enable them to be used in the event of an allergic/anaphylactic reaction in a patient receiving an i.v. drug.

Teaching patients/carers who are administering i.v. therapy in the community about the signs of an allergic/anaphylactic reaction and the appropriate action or

■ BOX 12.6

Case history: Teaching about anaphylaxis

Susan was discharged home to complete her course of i.v. antibiotics, which had to be given three times a day. She was keen to be at home as she had two small children and had already spent over 2 weeks in hospital. The community nurses were able to administer the two doses in the daytime but there was no-one to give the evening dose. Susan's husband was taking her to the hospital in the evening for her dose of antibiotic and she often had to wait over an hour before it was given. Her husband was prepared to learn how to administer the antibiotic. Anaphylaxis was discussed with him at length and the appropriate treatment, should it be necessary, explained. He was so overwhelmed by the prospect of learning how to give the antibiotic and by the fear of anaphylaxis, and what he would have to do if this happened, that he felt he could not take this on. Susan completed her course of antibiotic with no reaction but had to continue going to the hospital each evening.

treatment to take is a difficult and unresolved issue (see Box 12.6). For many patients/carers in the community, possible drug reactions are not even discussed.

The current situation in the UK is that first doses of i.v. drugs are rarely, if ever, given in the community and most patients are well established on treatment before discharge. Therefore, the likelihood of them experiencing a severe reaction is very rare and, if it did occur, it would most likely be of a mild to moderate nature (Conlon 1996, Nathwani et al 1997).

Patients who have immunoglobulin therapy in the community are taught about allergic/anaphylactic reactions as part of their training programme. They are issued with a pre-filled syringe of adrenaline, e.g. EpiPen, and taught to give it in the event of a reaction, then to seek medical help (Chapel 1994).

It is important to get into perspective the rarity of a severe anaphylactic reaction and to concentrate on educating patients and carers about early signs and symptoms of an allergic reaction, and the importance of seeking advice immediately.

As part of the hospital assessment and discharge planning process, the following should be considered:

- Does the patient have any relevant past medical history?
- Does the patient have any allergies?
- How long has the patient had this treatment?
- Has the patient experienced any problems with the treatment so far?
- Has the treatment been given in the same way in hospital as it will be given at home?

It is important to document all this information even if there is nothing of note to report as it provides evidence of careful and thorough assessment.

Once the patient is discharged into the community, it is essential that she is monitored closely and assessed on a regular basis. She should be encouraged to report anything, however insignificant it may seem. Always listen to the patient and if in doubt seek advice.

DRUG STORAGE AND TRANSPORTATION

Intravenous drugs for administration in the community come in a range of preparations, from dry powder in vials to ready prepared syringes, cassettes, bags and pre-filled devices. Any drug preparation should be labelled by the pharmacy department, compounding unit or the drug manufacturer and this label should state:

- the name and dose of the drug
- the expiry date of the drug
- how it should be stored
- temperature at which it should be stored
- any reconstitution directions
- any administration directions.

If drugs do not require refrigeration then the label states the temperature at which they should be stored, which is usually below 25°C. A good guide is to suggest that drugs are stored in a cool room away from direct heat and sunlight and out of reach of children.

The majority of drugs that require refrigeration are those that have been reconstituted and prepared in an aseptic services department or compounding unit. The recommended storage temperature in the fridge is usually between 2 and 5°C. For many of these drugs, a refrigerator is provided as part of the package of care, especially when the patient has considerable stock which would be unreasonable or impractical to store in a domestic refrigerator. The drug refrigerators supplied are regularly maintained and checked by the provider and usually contain a thermometer so that the correct temperature can be maintained; some have a door locking system.

Some prepared i.v. drugs require storage in a frozen form, generally at –2°C, and the pharmaceutical companies who prepare/reconstitute the drug will provide a temperature-controlled freezer with the drugs.

If drugs are to be stored in a domestic refrigerator, it is important to consider the following before the patient is discharged:

- Is there room in the patient's refrigerator for the drugs?
- Is the refrigerator working properly?
- Does the patient have a refrigerator thermometer? If not, suggest she buys one.
- Do children have access to the refrigerator?
- Does the patient have a hard container with a lid in which the drug(s) could be stored?
- Is there a tray on which the drug(s) could be stored?

Drugs that are stored in a refrigerator may need to be removed prior to administration for a period of time varying from 30 minutes to 4 hours. If the drug is going to be removed from the refrigerator for longer than the recommended 'warming up' period, then the length of time for which the drug remains stable should be checked with a pharmacist. It is also useful to know this information in case there is a power cut.

Prior to discharge the following considerations should be discussed with, explained to, and understood by the patient/carer:

- how and where the drug should be stored
- the temperature at which the drug should be stored
- how the drug will be kept out of reach of children and animals, if appropriate
- where to dispose of the drug/device/equipment once used
- what to do in the event of a spillage of drug
- who to contact if there are any problems or queries.

If private home i.v. companies are used, they will usually provide all the ancillary equipment required, as well as the drug, and take responsibility for ensuring that the patient has sufficient stock at all times. If drugs and ancillary equipment are provided by the hospital, the patient needs to know when more supplies will be needed and where to obtain these.

Private home i.v. or pharmaceutical companies which prepare or reconstitute drugs transport and deliver them directly to the patient's home in an appropriate container – often in a cool box. They always check that someone is at the property and able to receive the drugs and transfer them to the refrigerator as soon as possible.

If patients are transporting their own drugs home from hospital, in whatever form, they should be advised to bring a cool box or rigid container for transportation and they must not leave the drugs in a hot car or in direct sunlight. Patient-ready cytotoxic drugs must be transported in a sealed, labelled, rigid container and handled in accordance with local policy (RCN 1989).

Some drugs (but not cytotoxic drugs; RCN 1989) may require reconstituting in the home setting. This should be done in a clean, well ventilated room with sufficient space to organize and prepare the drug. Care must be taken not to spill or splash any drug on surfaces that may be damaged, e.g. varnished or polished wood. Using a melamine tray is helpful as this can easily be wiped and cleaned before and after each use. The drugs can be prepared on the tray and carried to the patient.

DISPOSAL OF WASTE

Patients and carers should be aware of the correct disposal procedure for the equipment and drugs they are using. They should have sharps bins and clinical waste bags and know how and where these are to be disposed of safely once full. Any unused drugs or solutions should ideally be returned to the hospital pharmacy department so they can be dealt with appropriately.

Cytotoxic drug waste and sharps should be incinerated at a temperature of 1000°C (RCN 1989). Local policies must identify systems for the collection and disposal of cytotoxic drug waste and sharps in the community (Daniels 1996). Community personnel must be aware of and informed about these policies and the relevant documentation required.

BENEFITS AND PROBLEMS WITH COMMUNITY INTRAVENOUS THERAPY

There is little doubt that most patients would prefer to be at home rather than in hospital. The experience in the US in relation to community i.v. therapy has proved that patients having a wide range of i.v. therapies can be managed in the community safely and effectively (Sheldon & Bender 1994). Patients are now wanting and expecting to go home to have their i.v. treatment, especially when they are aware of patients in other areas having similar treatments at home. However, systems must be in place to support this type of service or the problems that may arise outweigh the benefits to the patient (see below and Table 12.5).

Benefits

- Care and support takes place in the home environment with its stability and familiarity.
- The patient has a degree of autonomy and a better quality of life in the context of treatment.
- The patient has the ability to be able to return to work/school/family life.
- Less time is spent in hospital, which in turn releases acute beds for other patients.

Table 12.5 Problems of intravenous therapy

Problem	Example	Consequence
Inappropriate referral Unsuitable patient	Treatment not manageable, i.e. q.d.s. dosing Patient not medically or psychologically stable	Sleep deprivation/decreased socialization from frequent dosing Readmitted to hospital as unable to cope
Poor communication	GP and community nurse not aware of patient's discharge	Isolation/no support for patient/carer
Poor discharge planning	Patient discharged on Friday afternoon with no back-up support	Isolation/anxiety for patient/carer
Inadequate equipment/ supplies	Antibiotic powder but no reconstitution fluid No administration sets and sharps bins	Anxiety for patient/carer Unable to administer therapy Further journey to hospital for missing supplies/ equipment
Inappropriate or impractical equipment	Heavy drip stand and pump that won't move on carpet; no drip stand therefore not able to be mobile during therapy	Reinforcing sick role Immobility for patient Compromising safety
Inadequate practical training/no written instructions	Patient not competent to administer therapy; nothing to refer to as back-up	Intravenous therapy may not be administered safely and properly; possible associated risk, i.e. infection
No support/back-up	No telephone access for specialist advice	Isolation/anxiety for patient/ carer. Risk of problems/ complications not being dealt with immediately
Variations in management of venous access	Patient advised by one nurse to flush venous access with 5 ml sodium chloride 0.9% after treatment, and by another to flush with 5 ml heparinized saline	Confusion/anxiety for patient/carer Compromising good practice
No organised follow-up	Patient discharged into the community for 6-week course of i.v. antimicrobial therapy with no follow-up appointment until completion of the course	Problems/complications may not be picked up and dealt with promptly No ongoing monitoring of patient's condition

- There is a reduced risk of developing nosocomial infections, e.g. methicillin-resistant *Staphylococcus aureus* (MRSA) and *Clostridium difficile* (Allwood et al 1997).

Problems

When problems occur, these can cause untold anxiety, confusion, isolation and anger for patients/carers and their families in addition to coping with an illness, its treatment and a new skill. This reinforces the importance of planning community i.v. therapy with a multidisciplinary approach, so that all aspects are covered with a key person coordinating the whole package of care. If this is done carefully and thoroughly then the problems listed in Table 12.5 should not occur.

■ **BOX 12.7**

Case history: Drug reaction

Brian had been at home for 2 weeks having a once daily i.v. antibiotic via a central venous catheter which the community nurse was administering. His course of treatment was for 6 weeks overall and he had 2 weeks of this treatment whilst in hospital. Brian complained of wanting to cough when the antibiotic was given and this was reported to the hospital. He was seen by the consultant and nothing abnormal could be detected. A sodium chloride 0.9% flush was given i.v. with no problem, but as soon as the antibiotic was administered Brian started coughing again. It was felt that this was a drug reaction which had manifested itself in an unusual way and the treatment was stopped.

QUALITY ASSURANCE

There need to be agreed standards to ensure that good-quality community i.v. therapy is provided for each individual patient. Intravenous therapies that are already well established in the community have developed their own standards, although these should be reviewed and evaluated on a regular, ongoing basis.

Intravenous therapies that are new to the community or in the development stage need to learn from the more established practice and develop quality assurance models which incorporate standards for the following:

- patient selection, screening and assessment
- discharge planning
- education and training for patients/carers and community nurses
- the role of the multidisciplinary team – physician, nurse, pharmacist, social worker, liaison nurse
- involvement of GP, primary health care team and other agencies
- provision of drugs and equipment
- follow-up and ongoing support
- outcome monitoring.

For these standards to be effective, there must be good documentation of each stage.

If standards for measuring quality assurance are not developed then i.v. therapies in the community that are not yet well established will fail, and patients and others involved will experience the problems listed in Table 12.5 and this is not acceptable practice.

CONCLUSION

The administration of i.v. therapy in the community is a viable and manageable concept. Increased demand on the acute sector for beds, pressure from patient groups, and advances in technology and treatments all mean that i.v. therapy in the community is going to increase.

There is still an enormous amount of work that needs to be done nationally within both the acute and the community setting to ensure that this type of treatment is organized and managed safely and effectively. Improved communication between the hospital and community is essential, as well as a wider understanding of the types of i.v. therapy that are manageable in the community.

Intravenous therapy in the community must be respected as an important process and should be carefully planned and documented. There needs to be an established procedure for outcome monitoring, feedback and quality assurance in order to ensure a high level of service and patient care.

Realistically, there is unlikely to be the funding to use private home i.v. companies on a widespread basis, and therefore community nurses are going to be increasingly called upon to administer i.v. therapy and support patients/carers. Community trusts need to take this issue on board and make the commitment to provide education, training and ongoing support for community nurses.

Funding is often the critical issue for such services and at some stage in the further development of i.v. therapy in the community, the source, allocation and distribution of funding need to be addressed.

REFERENCES

Allwood M, Stanley A, Wright P 1997 Administration of chemotherapy. In: Allwood M, Stanley A, Wright P (eds) The cytotoxics handbook. Radcliffe Medical Press, Oxford, ch 5

Brennan V 1987 Home therapy for antibody deficient patients. Nursing Times 83(31): 24–26

Chapel H M 1994 Consensus on diagnosis and management of primary antibody deficiencies. British Medical Journal 308: 581–585

Chapel H M, Brennan V 1988 Immunoglobulin replacement therapy for self infusion at home. Clinical and Experimental Immunology 73: 160–162

Chrystal C 1997 Administering continuous vesicant chemotherapy in the ambulatory setting. Journal of Intravenous Nursing 20(2): 78–88

Conlon C P 1996 Outpatient intravenous antibiotic therapy. Journal of Antimicrobial Chemotherapy 38(4): 557–559

Corbett K, Meehan L, Sackey V 1993 A strategy to enhance skills. Developing intravenous therapy skills for community nursing. Professional Nurse 9(1): 60–63

Daniels L E 1996 Innovations in cancer care in the community: home therapy. British Journal of Community Health Nursing 1(3): 163–168

David T J 1989 Intravenous antibiotics at home in children with cystic fibrosis. Journal of the Royal Society of Medicine 89(82): 130–131

Department of Health 1995 Executive letter EL (95) 5. Purchasing high-tech healthcare for patients at home. HMSO, London

Ellis J M 1989 Let parents give the care: i.v. therapy at home in cystic fibrosis. Professional Nurse 4(12): 587–592

Gardulf A, Hammarstrom L, Smith C I E 1991 Home treatment of hypogammaglobulinaemia with subcutaneous gammaglobulin by rapid infusion. Lancet 338: 162–166

Goodinson S M 1990 Good practice minimum risk factors. Complications of peripheral venous cannulation and infusion therapy. Professional Nurse 6(3): 175–177

Kayley J 1995 Home intravenous therapy. Primary Health Care 5(8): 39–46

Kayley J 1996 IV therapies in practice. Journal of Community Nursing 10(4): 4–6

Kayley J, Berendt A R, Snelling M J M et al 1996 Safe intravenous antibiotic therapy at home: experience of a UK based programme. Journal of Antimicrobial Chemotherapy 37(5): 1023–1029

Low C 1994 Intravenous therapy : Community care in HIV-related CMV disease. British Journal of Sexual Medicine 21: 24–26

Lowry M 1995 Evaluating a patient teaching programme. Professional Nurse 11(2): 116–119

Medical Devices Agency 1995 Device bulletin. Infusion systems. MDA, London

Medical Devices Agency 1997 Device bulletin. Selection and use of infusion devices for ambulatory applications. MDA, London

Moeser L C 1991 Anaphylaxis. A preventable complication of home infusion therapy. Journal of Intravenous Nursing 14(2): 108–112

Morling S, Ford L 1997 IV therapy: selection, use and management of infusion pumps. British Journal of Nursing 6(19): 1094–1100

Nathwani D, Seaton A, Davey P 1997 Key issues in the development of a non-inpatient intravenous antibiotic therapy programme – a European perspective. Reviews in Medical Microbiology 8(30): 137–147

Oliver G 1991 Intravenous line care at home. Primary Health Care 1(5): 12–16

Redman B K 1997 Evaluation and research in patient education. In: Redman B K (ed) The practice of patient education, 8th edn. Mosby, St Louis, ch 4, p 69–90

Richardson N 1995 A review of drug infusion incidents. The situation from the national perspective. British Journal of Intensive Care (suppl.): 8–10

Rizza C R, Spooner R J D 1977 Home treatment of haemophilia and Christmas disease: five years' experience. British Journal of Haematology 37: 53–66

Roberts K, Seaby L 1994 Use of the Baxter PCA infusor in the community. British Journal of Nursing 3(18): 960–963

Royal College of Nursing (RCN) 1988 Anaphylaxis. Guidance for all nurses and health visitors working in community settings. RCN, London

Royal College of Nursing/Oncology Nursing Society 1989 Safe practice with cytotoxics. Scutari Projects, Middlesex

Scales K 1996 Legal and professional aspects of intravenous therapy. Nursing Standard 11(3): 41–48

Schleis T G, Tice A D 1996 Selecting infusion devices for use in ambulatory care. American Journal of Health-System Pharmacists 53: 868–877

Sheldon P, Bender M 1994 High technology in home care. An overview of intravenous therapy. Nursing Clinics of North America 29(3): 507–519

United Kingdom Central Council for Nursing, Midwifery and Health Visiting 1992a Code of professional conduct. UKCC, London

United Kingdom Central Council for Nursing, Midwifery and Health Visiting 1992b The scope of professional practice. UKCC, London

United Kingdom Central Council for Nursing, Midwifery and Health Visiting 1992c Standards for the administration of medicines. UKCC, London

Wainstock J M 1987 Making a choice: the vein access method you prefer. Oncology Nursing Forum 14(1): 79–82

Watters C 1997 The benefits of providing chemotherapy at home. Professional Nurse 12(5): 367–370

Webster A, Ryan A, Thomson B 1988 Home intravenous immunoglobulin therapy for patients with primary hypogammaglobulinaemia. Lancet 2: 793

Williams D N 1995 Home intravenous antibiotic therapy (HIVAT): indications, patients and antimicrobial agents. International Journal of Antimicrobial Agents 5(1): 3–8

Woollens S 1996 Infusion devices for ambulatory use. Professional Nurse 11(10): 689–695

FURTHER READING

Alexander H R, Lucas A B 1994 Long term venous access catheters and implantable ports. In: Alexander H R (ed) Vascular access in the cancer patient. JB Lippincott, Philadelphia, ch 1, p 3–16

Auty B 1995 Types of infusion pump and their risks. Classifying infusion pumps into risk categories. British Journal of Intensive Care (suppl.): 11–16

Brown J 1988 Peripherally inserted central catheters: use in home care. Journal of Intravenous Nursing 13(3): 144–147

Cochrane S 1994 A mark of approval – patient satisfaction with an IV self infusion teaching programme. Professional Nurse 10(2): 106–108, 110–111

Conway A 1996 Home intravenous therapy for bronchiectasis patients. Nursing Times 92(45): 33–35

Finnegan S 1989 Home parenteral nutrition. Professional Nurse 5(2): 79–81

Friend B 1992 Self-service. Nursing Times 88(44): 26–28

Gabriel J 1994 An intravenous alternative. Nursing Times 90(31): 39–41

Kendrick R 1993 Teaching children with cystic fibrosis and their families to give IV therapy. Paediatric Nursing 5(1): 22–24

Kayley J 1996 Use of IV antibiotics at home. Community Nurse 2(7): 15–16

Neiderpruem M S 1989 Factors affecting compliance in the home IV antibiotic therapy client. Journal of Intravenous Nursing 12(3): 136–142

Royal College of Nursing Leukaemia and Bone Marrow Transplant Nursing Forum 1995 Skin tunnelled catheters. Guidelines for care, 2nd edn. Scutari Projects, Middlesex

Sheldon P, Bender M 1994 High technology in home care. An overview of intravenous therapy. Nursing Clinics of North America 29(3): 507–519

Stephenson K 1989 Giving antibiotics at home. Nursing Standard 40(3): 24–25

Tice A D 1995 The importance of teamwork for outpatient parenteral antibiotic therapy. International Journal of Antimicrobial Agents 5(1): 13–17

Wood S 1991 A life saving technique (home parenteral nutrition). Primary Health Care 1(7): 20–21, 23

Wood S 1991 Extending the principle of self care: intravenous therapy in the community. Professional Nurse 6(9): 543–549

Specialities

Blood transfusion therapy

Helen Porter

INTRODUCTION

A blood transfusion consists of the administration of whole blood or any of its components to correct or treat a clinical abnormality (Porter 1996). The first documented blood transfusion took place in 1492 when Pope Innocent VII was given blood taken from three young men. All four subsequently died (Harmening-Pittiglio et al 1989). Other uses of blood through history have included bathing in it and drinking it. In 1667, Samuel Pepys reported that a man had received a transfusion of 12 oz of sheep's blood without apparent ill effect. The early 1900s saw an increase in the documented use of transfusion in medicine (Mandelfield 1993).

With advances in medical practice, there are increasing numbers of indications for blood transfusion therapy, including organ transplantation, cardiac surgery and myelosuppressive therapies such as intensive chemotherapy and bone marrow transplantation. Many of these therapies would not be possible without the use of blood. Along with this increase in therapeutic use there has been an increase in knowledge of the complications experienced and their management.

The nurse plays a vital role through all the stages of blood transfusion therapy: initial venesection, the identification of clinical need, the blood delivery to the patient, with monitoring and assessment. The actions of the nurse are dependent on an in-depth knowledge of all aspects of transfusion therapy to ensure safe and effective delivery of care.

The National Blood Transfusion Service

The National Blood Transfusion Service was founded in 1945 and until 1994 was organized on a regional basis. Since 1995, following reorganization, the activities of the re-named National Blood Service (NBS) have been organized into five entities: the three zones, the Bio Products laboratory and the International Blood Group Reference Laboratory. Services provided include (Gibson & Ouwehand 1997):

- collection, processing and issuing of blood and blood components
- tissue bank and cord blood stem cell services
- diagnostic reference services
- clinical and scientific advice
- research and development
- teaching and training.

COMPONENTS OF BLOOD

Blood transfusion therapy involves the use of whole blood and its individual components. The 1960s saw the development of technology that could separate blood into its components (Kay & Huehns 1985). Whole blood contains cellular, plasma and electrolyte components. The cellular component consists of erythrocytes, leucocytes and platelets. Plasma contains proteins, antibodies and water. There is a wide range of blood products available for many clinical indications (see Table 13.1).

Table 13.1 Range and features of blood products

Type of transfusion	ABO/Rh cross-matching	Administration	Shelf-life/storage
Red cell transfusion	Required	Administer through a blood administration set containing an integral filter (usually 170 microns). The set should be changed at least 12-hourly	Following donation, red blood cell storage is 35 days if kept at 4°C (Mims 1994). Within a few hours of storage, fibrin particles, clumps of white blood cells, disintegrating platelets and small clots can be detected (Fantus & Schirmir 1938). These may lead to non-haemolytic febrile reactions and respiratory impairment (Porter 1996). The longer the blood has been stored, the greater the amount of microaggregates
Platelet concentrates	Platelet transfusions do not require cross-matching although ABO and rhesus compatibility are preferred	Administer through a platelet administration set or as a bolus	Following donation the shelf-life is 96 hours for platelets at room temperature
Fresh frozen plasma	ABO compatibility required, rhesus compatibility preferred	Administer through a blood administration set containing an integral filter. The set should be changed every 12 hours	After donation and separation from the red blood cell component, the plasma is frozen and stored at −20°C. Administration should be immediately after thawing
Granulocytes	ABO and HLA human leucocyte antigen required	Administer through a blood administration set containing an integral filter. The set should be changed every 12 hours	Transfuse within 24 hours of collection
Cryoprecipitate	ABO compatibility between donor plasma and recipient's red blood cells	Administer through a blood administration set containing an integral filter or a platelet administration set. The set should be changed every 12 hours	Stored at −30°C for 1 year

Red cell transfusions

There is a variety of red cell preparations available for different clinical indications. Each unit will increase haemoglobin by 1 g/dl and the haematocrit by 3% in a 70 kg adult.

Whole blood The use of whole blood is uncommon and is usually indicated when acute, massive blood loss has occurred.

Packed red cells Platelet-rich plasma is removed from the whole blood, leaving the same red cell concentration as whole blood. This is used to correct red blood cell deficiency.

Modified packed red blood cells Leucocyte-depleted red blood cell transfusions can be achieved at source or at the bedside. They are used for patients who have previously experienced febrile reactions and who may have developed antibodies to donor leucocytes. In particular, they may be used where patients require multiple transfusions.

Washed red blood cells Plasma is removed and the cells are suspended in saline. This preparation is indicated where expansion of blood volume is not tolerated or where there is a history of non-haemolytic transfusion reactions to plasma proteins.

Frozen red blood cells These may be used in cases of rare blood groups or autologous blood donations. Although there is a shelf-life of 3 years while frozen, they must be transfused within 12 hours of thawing.

Platelet concentrates

These are used to treat platelet disorders such as (Hows & Brozovic 1990):

- bone marrow failure due to disease or secondary to myelosuppressive therapy
- platelet dysfunction
- autoimmune thrombocytic purpura
- dilutional thrombocytopenia.

Clotting disorders such as disseminated intravascular coagulation (DIC) may also require platelet support. Platelet transfusions may come from random donors, single donors or from individual pheresis sessions at source from specific identified donors. Where allo-immunization develops following multiple transfusions, HLA-matched platelets may be indicated.

Fresh frozen plasma

This is indicated in the following cases:

- microvascular bleeding with abnormal coagulation
- DIC
- thrombotic thrombocytopenic purpura
- liver damage
- dilution of clotting factors following massive haemorrhage.

Plasma is separated from whole blood and all coagulation factors are preserved. Uses include correcting clotting deficiencies where the cause is unknown or where specific clotting factors are unavailable. Plasma pooling enhances the potential of several infectious agents such as hepatitis B, hepatitis C, HIV and parvovirus for dissemination by transfusion (Barbara 1990). Improved purification and viral inactivation techniques are being developed where cloned products are unavailable.

Granulocytes

These are used in the treatment of infection in neutropenic patients, particularly if there is a focus of infection and patients are unresponsive to empirical antibiotic therapy.

Cryoprecipitate

This is the component of plasma containing factor VIII. It is used to correct bleeding disorders associated with deficiency of factor VIII or fibrinogen and clotting defects induced by massive transfusion (Mims 1994).

HUMAN PLASMA FRACTIONS

Immunoglobulin

Intravenous immunoglobulin is used to treat immunological disorders, such as autoimmune thrombocytopenic purpura (AITP), primary hypogammaglobulinaemia, haematological malignancies (including chronic lymphocytic leukaemia and myeloma) and HIV. Immunoglobulin is also used to prevent infections such as hepatitis A, measles, rubella, tetanus, hepatitis B and varicella zoster (McClelland 1996) where specific immunoglobulins are obtained from specific donors with high-titre IgG antibodies.

Human albumin

Intravenous human albumin is available in 5 or 20% solutions. It is used to treat hypoproteinaemic oedema with nephrotic syndrome (20%), ascites in chronic liver disease (20%) and acute fluid volume replacement (5%) (McClelland 1996).

Clotting factor concentrates

Factor VIII is used to treat haemophilia A, factor IX is used to treat haemophilia B, and prothrombin complex concentrate is used for replacement of multiple clotting factor deficiencies and rapid correction of oral anticoagulant effect (McClelland 1996).

FACTORS RELATED TO TRANSFUSION THERAPY

Donor issues

Blood donors can give 450 ml of whole blood up to three times a year. Plasma can be donated via apheresis up to 15 times a year and platelets via apheresis up to 24 times a year. Selection criteria are applied to potential donors to minimize harm to both the donor and the recipient, and include:

- age between 18 and 65 years (60 for plasma)
- in good health
- questioning donors on risk factors
- blood tests for evidence of infection with hepatitis B, hepatitis C, HIV-1, HIV-2 and syphilis (*Treponema pallidum*)
- current medications/drugs.

Donor selection is paramount in minimizing the risks associated with blood transfusion-related viral infection such as hepatitis and HIV. Alter (1987) showed that, before the ability to detect hepatitis B surface antigen (HBsAg), eliminating commercial donors motivated by cash payment significantly decreased the risk of hepatitis B virus infection in recipients. Pre-donation information to potential donors on the activities that increase the risk of becoming HIV-positive has recently had a major impact on the safety of blood (Polesky 1989). The identification of 'high-risk' activities such as intravenous drug usage and male homosexuality allows the identification of a minority group of donors who can be asked to exclude themselves from donation (Barbara 1990). The exclusion of male homosexuals as donors has seen a decrease in the number of donors found to be HBsAg-positive (Barbara 1990). The importance of self-rejection is stressed to potential donors at selection interviews. Leaflets prepared by the Department of Health which specify risk groups are given to each donor. Donor selection includes (Polesky 1989):

- recent exposure to individuals with a transfusion-transmitted viral disease
- past history of hepatitis, signs of hepatitis or AIDS
- having been implicated as a donor in a case of transfusion-transmitted viral disease.

Reliance is placed on the donor to answer truthfully questions on general health, medical history and any drugs taken (Hewitt et al 1990). Donor education has been calculated to be more than 95% successful in excluding HIV-positive donors (Barbara 1990). Routine screening for HIV commenced in October 1985.

ABO and Rh

Karl Landsteiner in 1901 was the first to label the blood groups A and B followed by group O. AB was discovered the following year (Kay & Huehns 1985). In 1940, the rhesus groups were recognized by Stetson and Levine. The ABO system is the most important system for transfusions, with rhesus being the second most important. Approximately 15% of the UK population do not express the rhesus antigen on their red blood cells (Mims 1994).

The ABO antigens are located on the surface of the red blood cells on the red cell membrane. The genes controlling the antigens are inherited and determine the patient's blood group. There is racial variation in the frequency of ABO blood groups within a population (Waters 1991). A and B may be present together, as in the group AB, or independently, as in groups A and B. If the antigen is not present, it is group O. IgM antibodies, found in the plasma, are associated with the ABO system (Cook 1997a). Activation of these antibodies mediates cell lysis. The commonest cause of transfusion-related death in the United States is the transfusion of ABO-incompatible blood (Williamson et al 1996). A survey in the UK (McClelland & Phillips 1994) showed that episodes where patients received the wrong blood as a result of poor patient identification may complicate as many as 1 in 30 000 transfusions. However, mortality is minimized due to the distribution of blood groups in the UK, which means that the misidentified patient is likely to receive ABO-compatible blood (Williamson et al 1996) (see Table 13.2).

Transmissible disease screening

Many agents are transmittable by blood transfusion, including:

- bacteria – syphilis (*Treponema pallidum*), brucellosis

Table 13.2 ABO groups and serology (Mims 1994)

	A	B	AB	O
Plasma antibodies	Anti-B	Anti-A	No A or B	Anti-A and anti-B
Frequency in the UK (%)	42	8	3	47

- parasites – malaria, *Trypanasoma cruzi* (Chagas' disease), *Toxoplasma gondii*, *Babesia microti*
- plasma-borne viruses – hepatitis B, hepatitis A, hepatitis C, serum parvovirus, HIV-1 and -2
- cell-associated viruses – cytomegalovirus, Epstein–Barr virus, HTLV-1.

Rarely, the Colorado tick fever virus and *Coxiella burnetii* (Q fever) can cause transfusion complications. Barbara (1990) identified the main concerns of transfusion microbiology to be:

- maintaining a safe supply in relation to infectious agents
- selection of donors
- research.

American reports suggest that the risk of transfusion-transmitted infection from a donor who is infectious but not yet seropositive is about 1 in 500 000 for HIV, 1 in 100 000 for hepatitis C virus and 1 in 60 000 for hepatitis B virus (Schreiber et al 1996). Between 1985 and 1993, almost 6000 cases of AIDS associated with transfusions were registered in 14 countries (Franceschi et al 1995). In the Franceschi study, the number of cases reported in the UK was 542, with an annual incidence of 1.02/million. The majority of these cases were haemophiliac patients. This rate of blood-borne AIDS is lower than that registered in the US, which has an annual incidence of 3.61/million. AIDS transmission through blood transfusions was recognized before the identification of the virus as the causative agent (Franceschi et al 1995). Since 1984, there has been evidence of the favourable impact of control procedures such as donor selection and screening and the treatment of blood and blood products (Franceschi et al 1995).

In 1990 the Expert Advisory Group on AIDS (EAGA) reviewed its advice on testing of tissue and organ donors for HIV antibodies. This confirmed that it is essential that blood from donors is tested and found to be negative before transplantation is confirmed.

HIV testing

HIV is a lentivirus belonging to the family Retroviridae which causes chronic infection and is slow-growing. The mean incubation period between the transfusion of infected blood and a diagnosis of AIDS has been estimated at 4.5 years (Polesky 1989).

The UK health departments recommend that named testing for evidence of HIV infection should only be done with informed consent and that confidential pre-test discussion should be offered to all those who have the test done (Department of Health 1996). The time from infection to the development of the antibody is known as the 'window period'. During this period the test result will show as negative, as the patient has yet to seroconvert and produce antibodies; however, the person may be highly infectious. It is imperative when potential blood donors are counselled that any risk activities are highlighted.

The two forms of HIV antibody testing are the ELISA and the Western Blot method (Alcorn 1995). The ELISA test, which is highly accurate, uses antigens which capture viral antibodies in the blood. A colour reaction is triggered by a chemical added to an enzyme attached to the antibody. The Western Blot method relies on HIV proteins together with an antibody–antigen binding mechanism.

Legge (1997) stated that the introduction of a polymerase chain reaction (PCR) test for HIV is inevitable and that, with testing directly for the virus rather than antibody, the window period would be reduced from around 3 weeks to days. However, Legge cited Dr John Barbara, consultant microbiologist at the National Blood Authority, who reported that there would be a 'minimal reduction in risk' as we already have a safe system.

Hepatitis testing

Viruses have been associated with hepatitis following transfusion but the frequency is difficult to establish (Polesky 1989). In the rare occurrence of fulminant hepatitis, about 70% of patients will die. This is particularly a problem in chronically transfused patients.

Hepatitis A belongs to the family Picornaviridae. It replicates in infected liver cells and its transmission is usually via the oral–faecal route as the virus may be shed in the stools of acutely ill patients. This is usually linked to water or food contamination or with poor hygiene. It is rare for hepatitis A to be transmitted via blood transfusion. Infection can be prevented by giving intramuscular immunoglobulin within 2 weeks of exposure.

Hepatitis B belongs to the family Hepadnaviridae. When an individual is infected with the virus, antibodies and antigens can be detected in the serum. Transmission occurs via blood and body fluids, including vertical transmission (transplacentally).

Hepatitis C is a single-stranded RNA virus discovered in 1989. It is primarily transmitted via blood. Testing was introduced in 1991. As the test has been improved, the incidence of post-transfusion hepatitis C has decreased. Hepatitis C screening using PCR will be introduced next year as part of European legislation.

Cytomegalovirus testing

Cytomegalovirus belongs to the family Herpesviridae. It can persist in the host and cause latent infection. Many recipients are already carriers of the virus. Approximately 50% of UK blood donors have an antibody to CMV, as it is a common virus that causes asymptomatic infection in most individuals (Pomeroy & Englund 1987). Polesky (1989) stated that transfusion may not be a significant route of infection. It is, however, a significant problem in neonates and immunosuppressed patients, particularly allogeneic bone marrow transplant recipients. In these immunocompromised patients, serious infection can occur. CMV disease may be caused by reactivation of the virus or by acquisition of the virus from blood products or transplanted organs (Pomeroy & Englund 1987).

Common clinical manifestations of CMV are fever, pneumonia, hepatitis, pancreatitis, colitis and retinitis. CMV is a common cause of death in bone marrow transplant patients (Pomeroy & Englund 1987). Transmission via blood transfusion is well documented. In these at-risk patient groups, prevention is dependent on the use of seronegative blood in seronegative recipients.

Screening for antibodies

As well as directly screening for the virus, infections can be detected by the presence of antibodies. These include hepatitis, HIV and HTLV-1 and -2. Other clinically significant blood cell antibodies, such as Rh D, Rh E, Rh C and Kell, are also tested for.

The recipient

Before any transfusion, the recipient is tested for ABO, rhesus factor and screened for antibodies. The blood is then cross-matched with the donors to test for serological compatibility (Weinstein 1997). Full laboratory compatibility testing for cross-matching of red blood cell transfusion can usually be done within 1 hour (Mims 1994).

The decision to transfuse must be based on weighing the therapeutic benefit to the recipient against the potential risks (Polesky 1989). This reflects the tenet of the UKCC's *Code of Professional Conduct* to 'act always in such a way as to promote and safeguard the wellbeing and interests of patients and clients' (UKCC 1992). The use of blood products is dependent on carefully considered clinical criteria as transfusions can be both beneficial and harmful to the patient (McClelland 1996). Serious causes of harm include acute haemolytic reactions, the rare immunological complications such as graft-versus-host disease and transfusion-associated lung injury which can cause death (Williamson et al 1996).

The UK has no system for comprehensive monitoring of transfusion hazards. A voluntary and confidential system of reporting transfusion-related deaths and other serious complications has filled this gap (Williamson et al 1996). The SHOT (serious hazards of transfusion) initiative covers the whole of the UK and the Republic of Ireland. The aim is to improve transfusion safety and to develop policy, clinical guidelines and training.

ADMINISTRATION, MONITORING AND OBSERVATION

Blood product transfusion therapy carries a significant risk. The incorrect transfusion of incompatible ABO grouping is associated with significant mortality. The nurse involved in transfusion therapy needs to develop the appropriate knowledge and skills to ensure safe and effective care. Local blood transfusion policy will determine procedures to guide nursing practice and will cover prescription, issue of blood products, checking procedure, use of equipment, and monitoring and observation for both immediate and delayed reactions.

Checking procedure

The checking procedure involves ensuring that there are no discrepancies between the information on the patient's identity label, the compatibility label and the compatibility report; the ABO and Rh D group on the blood pack, on the compatibility label and the compatibility report; and the donation number given on the blood pack, on the compatibility label and the compatibility report. This should be done by two people, one of whom should be a registered nurse or doctor (McClelland 1996). The pack is also checked for signs of leakage and for its expiry date. The Blood Transfusion Services of the United Kingdom advise that before starting the transfusion, the patient's temperature and pulse are recorded and then re-checked every 15 minutes for the first half hour of each pack, and then hourly until completion. Patient information and support are essential to ensure informed consent and to allay fears as the general public becomes more aware of the risks associated with the transmission of viral infection.

Monitoring

Throughout the transfusion, the patient must be monitored closely for any clinical features of a transfusion reaction. These include flushing, urticaria, vomiting, diarrhoea, fever, itching, headache, haemoglobinuria, pain at or near the transfusion site, rigor, severe backache, collapse and circulatory failure (McClelland 1996). When blood components are kept at room temperature, there is an increased risk of bacterial proliferation. Blood transfusions must therefore be started within 30 minutes of removing the pack from the refrigerator and be completed within 5 hours of commencement (McClelland 1996). Within these criteria, the speed of the transfusion will be dependent on the patient's clinical need and condition. The low temperature of the blood being infused can also lead to venospasm, which may result in an aching pain at the site and lead to slowing or cessation of flow via the administration set. A warm pack placed over the cannula site will relieve the venospasm and increase vasodilation, allowing better flow rates. Flow rate can also be influenced by size and location of cannula. No drugs or infusion solutions should be added to any blood component.

Safe handling of body fluids

As highlighted by the requirement of screening blood for infectious organisms, blood has the potential to carry and transmit infection. It is therefore paramount that health care professionals handling blood products take appropriate precautions for their own safety (Box 13.1).

Use of equipment

Within a few hours of storage of blood, particulate matter such as fibrin, clumps of white blood cells, disintegrating platelets and small clots can be detected (Fantus & Schirmir 1938) which can lead to clinical problems such as non-haemolytic febrile reactions and respiratory impairment following transfusion (Porter 1996). Standard blood administration sets contain in-line filters of (usually) 170 microns. Microaggregate and leucocyte depletion filters are available from 10 to 200 microns.

Leucocyte depletion of blood and blood components

Transfusion with leucocytes can sensitize the patient as a result of the white blood cells or HLA antigens causing adverse effects. Leucodepletion will reduce the incidence of adverse effects of transfusion such as non-haemolytic febrile transfusion reactions in transfusion-dependent patients.

Leucocyte depletion techniques aim to prevent or delay the onset of non-haemolytic febrile transfusion reactions. They may also abolish or ameliorate recurring non-haemolytic febrile transfusion reactions for transfusion of cellular blood components, particularly in newly diagnosed patients with aplastic anaemia and patients who are potential bone marrow transplant recipients. They may also be used as an alternative to CMV antibody-negative blood and for intrauterine transfusions (Royal College of Physicians 1993), as leucodepletion to less than 5×10^6 residual white cells per unit is effective in preventing CMV transmission. However, leucocyte-depleted red cells and platelets can only reduce the development of anti-leucocyte antibodies in multiple transfused patients if all transfused units are filtered (McClelland 1996).

Methods of leucocyte depletion include:

- microaggregate filters

- centrifugation followed by removal of the buffy coat
- leucocyte depletion filters
- apheresis techniques at the time of platelet pheresis.

Microaggregate filters also aim to remove red cell debris, platelets and fibrin strands. Pre-storage filtration at source rather than at the bedside has the benefit of removing the white blood cells which may otherwise release damaging cytokines during storage.

Blood warmers

Rapid infusion of cold blood can cause cardiac arrest. The use of a blood warmer is advised if the rate of transfusion in an adult is greater than 50 ml/kg per hour, or in children if the rate is greater than 15 ml/kg per hour (McClelland 1996). Blood warmers may also be indicated in patients with cold agglutination disease. Care should be taken with the use of blood warmers as heating of blood may damage the cellular component, causing haemolysis, and there may be an increased risk of bacterial contamination where a water-filled bath is used.

TRANSFUSION REACTIONS

The transfusion of any blood product carries with it the potential of a transfusion reaction (Cook 1997b), and this reaction may be immediate or delayed.

Immediate reactions

Acute haemolytic reaction

This may occur after as little as 5–10 ml of blood have been transfused into the recipient and can be fatal. This acute intravascular haemolysis is classified as a transfusion reaction involving an immune response (Cook 1997a). The basic element of an immune response is an antigen–antibody reaction.

The haemolysis occurs within the vasculature. Red blood cell destruction occurs as a result of the binding of an antibody to a red blood cell. The complement cascade, triggered by IgM, results in the rupture of the cell. If the cascade sequence is completed, total cell lysis will result (Cook 1997a). The most common cause is the transfusion of ABO-incompatible blood, and it may be fatal. Free haemoglobin released from the haemolysis filters through the kidneys leading to haemoglobinuria. This is associated with disseminated intravascular coagulation (DIC), hypotension, fever, chills, agitation, pain at cannula site, oozing from wound sites, haemoglobinaemia, haemoglobinuria, lumbar pain (often severe) and facial flushing. A sense of 'impending doom' may be associated with cytokine release (Weir 1995). Immediate action is required, preventing any further transfusion of incompatible red blood cells. Treatment of organ failure, such as maintenance of the haemodynamic state by treatment of hypotension and renal support, is essential. Appropriate therapy for DIC is also required.

Extravascular haemolysis

Haemolysis may be triggered by the response of IgG to a foreign antigen (Weir 1995). This results from previous exposure to an antigen such as bacteria or fungi. Red cells are removed into the extravascular space for destruction. Extravascular haemolysis is usually self-limiting (Cook 1997a) and treatment is symptomatic.

Anaphylaxis

Anaphylaxis, although rare, may occur when only a small volume of blood has been transfused. The typical signs of anaphylactic shock include bronchospasm, respiratory difficulties and shock with widespread peripheral vasodilation. Appropriate resuscitation procedures are required.

Febrile non-haemolytic reaction

This occurs where the recipient mounts an antibody response to the donor's white blood cells and accounts for 30% of all transfusion reactions (Beutler et al 1995). Patients may experience symptoms shortly after commencement of the transfusion or up to some hours later. Patients may be sensitized by multiple transfusions. The allergic response is characterized by pyrexia, flushing, palpitations, dyspnoea and tachycardia. The onset of symptoms usually occurs 30–60 minutes after commencement of the transfusion. This may be prevented by the use of leucocyte filters and may be treated with antipyretics.

Transfusion-related acute lung injury (TRALI)

Antibodies in the donor plasma can mount an immune response against the recipient's leucocytes. Infiltration of the lower lung fields gives rise to chills, fever, non-productive cough and dyspnoea.

Adult respiratory distress syndrome (ARDS)

Where massive transfusions are given, microaggregate debris consisting of platelets, leucocytes and fibrin formed during red cell storage may lead to pulmonary insufficiency, which is potentially fatal.

Circulatory overload

Increased transfused volume, particularly with whole blood, may lead to circulatory overload. Children and small adults are at an increased risk, as are patients with pre-existing cardiac or pulmonary function disorders (Cook 1997b). Where blood transfusions are given to compensate for anaemia, there may not be a requirement for fluid volume as there is in cases of massive haemorrhage. This sudden increase in blood volume due to the transfusion may cause problems of pulmonary venous engorgement, leading to pulmonary oedema, congestive cardiac failure and acute respiratory failure.

Clinical features of circulatory overload include the sudden onset of dyspnoea, headache, tachycardia and tachypnoea. Fluid balance should be monitored and diuretics administered as clinically indicated.

Hypothermia

This may be caused by the rapid transfusion of blood products directly from the blood bank refrigerator. Blood administered by a central venous catheter carries a higher risk as the cold blood enters the central circulation, potentially reducing the body's core temperature. Where large volumes of blood are required to be transfused rapidly, e.g. following trauma and haemorrhage, the use of a blood warmer is indicated. Care must be taken not to warm the blood above 38°C as overheating may cause haemolysis (Cook 1997b).

Pulmonary oedema

Pulmonary oedema may also be initiated as the result of an immune response. It is initiated by the stimulation of recipient antibody against donor antigen. Respiratory distress may progress to hypoxia which can become fatal.

Anticoagulants

Citrate is a commonly used anticoagulant in blood transfusions. It binds with calcium in the blood to interrupt the clotting cascade (Cook 1997b). Where multiple units are transfused, the citrate infusion may lead to hypocalcaemia. Risk groups include:

- patients with pre-existing liver damage
- patients with osteoporosis
- cytopheresis with large volumes of citrated plasma infused (Cook 1997b)
- exchange transfusions in neonates.

The resultant hypocalcaemia may give rise to symptoms of nausea and vomiting, numbness and tingling, muscle cramps, convulsions and tetany. Physical assessment may exhibit positive Trousseau's and Chvostek's signs. Prolonged QT interval may be seen on ECG recordings. Slowing the infusion rate may relieve symptoms but in some cases calcium therapy may be required; however, caution is needed as calcium therapy may give rise to hypercalcaemia due to the additive effect with the body's release of calcium from the skeletal stores.

Potassium changes

During storage, red blood cells disintegrate and potassium leaks from the cells into the plasma. As the length of storage increases, so does the level of potassium. Clinical problems are only likely where the patient has pre-existing renal problems or excessive potassium release such as large wounds.

Symptoms of hyperkalaemia include irritability, anxiety, abdominal cramping, diarrhoea and weakness of lower extremities. Physical assessment may exhibit an irregular pulse with the possibility of cardiac arrest if the potassium level exceeds 8.5 mmol/L.

Hypokalaemia may also occur as a result of metabolic acidosis arising from citrate metabolism. Donor red cells also try to correct potassium leakage once transfused, transporting plasma potassium into the cells and therefore out of the plasma (Cook 1997a).

Symptoms of hypokalaemia include fatigue, muscle weakness, leg cramps, nausea and vomiting, paraesthesia and gastrointestinal ileus. Physical assessment may exhibit decreased bowel sounds, decreased muscle reflexes and a weak and irregular pulse.

Sepsis

Bacteria may enter the blood transfusion from a number of sources, including the following:

- the donor
- the collection/venepuncture equipment
- manipulation of blood into its components
- damage to the container during storage
- the infusion administration equipment
- the hands of the nurse
- the patient's own skin flora.

Where the organisms, particularly Gram-negative organisms such as *Pseudomonas*, have been able to proliferate, a build-up of endotoxins may occur. Infusion of organism and endotoxins may lead to sepsis, septic shock and potentially multisystem organ failure and associated syndromes such as DIC.

Delayed reactions

Graft-versus-host disease

Graft-versus-host disease is most commonly identified with allogeneic bone marrow transplant recipients and is associated with incompatible donor leucocytes. In immunosuppressed patients, functioning donor leucocytes may engraft and mount an immune response against the host. Clinical features include fever, skin rash leading to desquamation, liver and gastrointestinal tract disturbance. Graft-versus-host disease associated with transfusions carries a significant mortality rate of 75–90% (Weir 1995). The risk of transfusion-associated graft-versus-host disease may be minimized by irradiation of 25 gray (Gy) of the transfused blood products. This damages the chromosomes of the transfused white blood cells, thereby preventing them from proliferating.

Delayed haemolysis

This occurs in patients who have been immunized to a red cell antigen. Haemolysis may be delayed up to 2–10 days post-transfusion and may be indicated by no rise in haematocrit (Cook 1997a). The patient may present with fever, falling haemoglobin, jaundice and haemoglobinuria (McClelland 1996).

Infections

Contamination of blood from infectious organisms may occur at any stage from its donation to transfusion. Infection may also arise from reactivation of a latent virus within the host.

In immunocompromised patients, such as allogeneic bone marrow recipients, cytomegalovirus infection is a significant cause of mortality. Infection may follow transfusion of cellular blood components. In the case of seronegative recipients, CMV-negative blood products should be used. Leucodepletion by filtration is an alternative.

Malaria

Plasmodium falciparum is the most dangerous of the four human malarial parasites. The incidence of malaria infection following blood transfusion is increasing as blood donors undertake more exotic foreign travel. Careful history-taking from donors regarding foreign travel will minimize the risk of transmission. Note should be taken of persistent fevers post-transfusion (Barbara & Contreras 1990).

Iron overload

Each unit of blood contains 250 mg of iron that the body is unable to excrete (Davis & Brozovic 1990). Patients who are chronically dependent on blood transfusions may become overloaded with iron, resulting in pigmentation, impaired growth, liver cirrhosis, cardiac failure, diabetes and hypothyroidism. Chelating agents such as desferrioxamine will minimize iron accumulation.

Alloimmunization

Multiple transfusion may lead to repeated stimulation of human leucocyte antibody production. The responsible antigen is primarily the white blood cell and the class 1 HLA antibodies. This may lead to platelet refractoriness, which is the failure to increment following platelet transfusions on more than one consecutive occasion. Screening for identified antigens may be required together with the use of leucocyte filters.

Biochemical changes in stored blood

When blood is stored, biochemical changes occur due to metabolism and cell death. Alterations of the cell wall during storage may result in electrolyte shifts (Cook 1997). These include potassium leaking from the cell into the plasma and the accumulation of cell debris. The released potassium in blood products that have been irradiated is double that of non-irradiated blood products. Other biochemical changes include raised ATP and plasma haemoglobin and lowered plasma sodium and pH.

REFUSAL OF TRANSFUSION THERAPY

Blood transfusion therapy is becoming increasingly important in modern medicine and surgery. However, this option may not be acceptable to all patients. For example, the Jehovah's Witnesses are a sect who refuse to take blood or blood products because they believe they must obey Jehovah's commands along with various passages in the Old Testament which prohibit the eating of blood, e.g. Leviticus 7:26. A blood transfusion is seen as the equivalent of eating blood and a devout Jehovah's Witness would rather die than be cut off from his own community and be denied the prospect of eternal life (Mir, 1997, personal communication). The health care professional may be confronted with difficult ethical problems when faced with the dilemma of a Jehovah's Witness refusing blood for himself or his family. However, it must be remembered that although a transfusion may be life-saving, to a Jehovah's Witness it may mean death in terms of the afterlife.

It must also be remembered that with recent media hype, patients are generally more anxious about receiving blood transfusions. Kaberry (1991) described the panic she felt concerning the risk that the blood she was to receive might be incompatible or that she might get HIV from the transfusion. In a study by Dougherty (1994), a patient described how she felt regarding her blood transfusion and how surprised she was at her reaction to receiving someone else's blood:

> 'I didn't think about the cannula, the blood was going in and I found the blood quite disturbing. I didn't think I would .... Now I know what Jehovah's Witnesses mean, this body fluid from someone else coming into me, whether or not I would have thought that before AIDS and stuff, I don't know.'

This highlights the importance of reassurance and understanding in order to alleviate anxiety that may appear irrational but that nevertheless causes concern for patients.

OTHER TECHNIQUES USED IN BLOOD TRANSFUSION

Autologous transfusions

Blood conservation is now an important issue in hospital medicine (Chernow et al 1996). This has developed as there has been an increased awareness of the risks involved in blood transfusions. The developing technologies such as continuous intra-arterial monitoring devices, microchemical technologies, new drug development and intraoperative salvage techniques have made blood conservation techniques possible (Chernow et al 1996). The theoretical advantages of using autologous blood are the reduction in the risk of immunological incompatibility and transmission of some infectious agents (McClelland 1996), although the risks of viral transmission by allogeneic transfusion in the UK are very small (Voak et al 1993).

Autologous blood can be derived from:

- pre-deposit donation
- intraoperative red cell salvage
- acute normovolaemic haemodilution (ANH) involving immediate pre-operative venesection and haemodilution with a plasma expander.

Pre-deposit donation

Autologous red cells can be stored for up to 5 weeks (McClelland 1996) following donation of 2–4 units. The risks associated with preoperative autologous blood donation (PABD), which the patient seeks to avoid, may exceed those of allogeneic transfusion (AuBochon 1996). The risk of sepsis associated with preoperative autologous donation and subsequent transfusion should not be underestimated (Dinse & Deusch 1996).

Roberts et al (1996) showed that autologous pre-donation is less expensive than allogeneic packed red cells; however, preoperative blood donation may not be cost-effective if blood is collected when it is not likely to be needed or if autologous blood is used just because it is available (AuBochon 1996).

Subcutaneous low-dose recombinant human erythropoietin (rHuEPO) at doses of 100 IU/kg twice a week for 2 weeks has been shown to be effective in facilitating autologous blood donation (Sans et al 1996).

Intraoperative salvage

Blood shed at the time of surgery can be collected, washed and anticoagulated before reinfusing into the patient. This should not be considered where the patient has evidence of systemic sepsis, infected surgery site or malignant disease.

Postoperative infusion of shed blood may lead to a delayed increase in bleeding. It can cause a delayed coagulopathy and other harmful effects that can be damaging to the postoperative patient (Vertrees et al 1996).

Hedstrom et al's (1996) study of autologous blood transfusion in hip replacements showed an increase in plasminogen activator inhibitor 1 (PAI-1), which is a possible risk perimeter for thromboembolism in their control group of patients receiving allogeneic blood. They concluded that, although autologous blood may not reduce blood loss in total hip replacement surgery, the increase in PAI-1 after allogeneic transfusion is avoided.

Strict medical indications for retransfusion are indispensable (Dinse & Deusch 1996). Collection of wound drainage blood is associated with inflammatory mediators such as the activation of complement, and release of PMN elastase and cytokines (Arnold et al 1995).

In 1993, the British Committee for Standards in Haematology Blood Transfusion Task Force published revised guidelines for autologous transfusion (Voak 1993). These were revised to keep pace with the increasing experience with autologous blood. These guidelines outline:

- general considerations
- selection of patients
- practical aspects of collection
- storage and transfusion
- pre-transfusion tests
- disposal of unused blood
- record-keeping
- quality control and audit.

Red cell rejuvenation

Red cell rejuvenation procedures are reserved for salvaging rare or O type units that are close to their expiry (Harmening-Pittiglio et al 1989). These procedures are time-consuming and intricate. Red cells are incubated at 37°C for 1 hour in solutions containing inosine, pyruvate, phosphate, adenine and sometimes glucose (Weir 1995). Due to the manipulation of the blood and the associated risk of bacterial contamination, it should be transfused within 24 hours although it can be glycerolized and frozen.

Blood substitutes

Substances other than blood have been developed with the capacity to pick up oxygen from the lungs and transport it to the tissues. These include modified haemoglobin solutions, perfluorochemicals and microencapsulated haemoglobin. Red cell substitutes need to be immunologically inert, isotonic and safe (Odling-Smee 1990).

Apheresis

The term apheresis comes from the Greek meaning 'to take away'. Apheresis was first developed in the early 1900s (Culotta 1989). Methods of apheresis have been developed and refined and techniques are available to remove individual blood cell components.

Leucopheresis

This is the removal of white blood cells. It may be done to reduce the number of circulating cells in patients with leukaemia, to provide donation of white blood cells for immunocompromised patients with severe infection and to provide functioning lymphocytes for immunotherapy.

Plateletpheresis

This is the removal of platelets to treat thrombocytopenic patients. This may be required when HLA-compatible transfusions are needed for the patient to increment. Patients with elevated platelet counts such as polycythaemia vera may benefit from a reduction in platelet levels following therapeutic plateletpheresis.

Stem cell harvesting

Immature cells are removed from the circulating peripheral blood following mobilization with growth factors such as granulocyte colony stimulating factor (G-CSF) plus or minus chemotherapy. These are then used for autologous transplantation following myeloablative chemoradiation.

Plasmapheresis

Plasma is removed and exchanged in disorders such as Waldenstrom's macroglobulinaemia, multiple myeloma, Guillain–Barré syndrome and thrombotic thrombocytopenic purpura (TTP). Plasma may be removed for donation to increase the supply of frozen plasma for specific blood groups or to supply immune plasma to immunocompromised patients.

Apheresis is performed by centrifugation of the blood and relies on the different weights of the blood components. Centrifugation can be performed by either intermittent or continuous flow.

CONCLUSION

Blood transfusion is probably safer now than it has ever been (Williamson et al 1996). However, any hospital that is involved in the use of blood products for transfusion should have policies and procedures to ensure safe practice (Cook 1997b). The use of therapeutic blood transfusion is increasing as advances are made in medicine and surgery. Along with this has come an increased knowledge of the risks involved and their optimal management. Future developments include refinement of viral testing techniques, development of autologous transfusion techniques and development of red cell substitutes. Nurses need to keep up to date with these practices to ensure safe and effective care through the formulation of optimum policies and procedures.

REFERENCES

Alcorn K (ed) 1995 The scientific basis to HIV antibody testing. The national AIDS manual. NAM Charitable Trust, London

Alter H J 1987 You'll wonder where the yellow went: a 15 year retrospective of post transfusion hepatitis. In: Moore S B (ed) Transfusion transmitted viral disease. American Association of Blood Banks, Arlington, VA, p 53–86

Arnold J P, Haeger M, Bengtsson J P, Bengtsson A, Lisander B 1995 Release of inflammatory mediators in association with collection of wound drainage blood during orthopaedic surgery. Anaesthesia in Intensive Care 23(6): 683–686

AuBochen J P 1996 Cost effectiveness of preoperative autologous blood donation for orthopedic and cardiac surgeries. American Journal of Medicine 101(2a): 38s–42s

Barbara J 1990 Microbiology in the national blood transfusion service. PHLS Microbiology Digest 7(1): 4–7

Barbara J A J, Contreras M 1990 Infectious complications of blood transfusion: bacteria and parasites. In: Contreras M (ed) ABC of transfusion. British Medical Journal, London

Beutler E, Lichtman M, Coller B et al 1995 Williams hematology, 5th edn. McGraw-Hill, New York

Chernow B, Jackson E, Miller J A, Wiese J 1996 Blood conservation in acute care and critical care. American Association of Critical Care Nurses 7(2): 191–197

Cook L S 1997a Blood transfusion reactions involving an immune response. Journal of Intravenous Nursing 20(1): 5–14

Cook L S 1997b Non-immune transfusion reactions: when type and cross match aren't enough. Journal of Intravenous Nursing 20(1): 15–22

Culotta E 1989 Apheresis. In: Harmening D (ed) Modern blood banking and transfusion practices, 2nd edn. F A Davis, Philadelphia

Davies S C 1995 Reforming England's blood transfusion service. British Medical Journal 311: 1383–1384

Davis S A, Brozovic M 1990 Transfusion of red cells. In: Contreras M (ed) ABC of transfusion. British Medical Journal, London

Dinse H, Deusch H 1996 Sepsis following autologous blood transfusion. Anaesthetist 45(5): 460–463

Dougherty L 1994 A study to discover how cancer patients perceive the cannulation expereince. Unpublished MSc thesis, University of Surrey, Guildford

Fantus B, Schirmir E H 1938 The therapy of the Cook County Hospital – blood preservation technique. Journal of the American Medical Association 111: 317

Franceschi S, Dal-Maso L, La Vecchia C 1995 Trends in incidence of AIDS associated with transfusion of blood and blood products in Europe and the United States, 1985–1993. British Medical Journal 311: 1534–1536

Gibson P, Ouwehand W (eds) 1997 London and South East zone. Diagnostic services user guide. National Blood Service, London

Harmening-Pittiglio D, Harrison C R, Wright N E 1989 Blood preservation: historical perspectives, review of metabolism, and current trends. In: Harmening D. Modern blood banking and transfusion practices, 2nd edn. F A Davis, Philadelphia

Hedstrom M, Flordal P A, Ahl T, Svensson J, Dalen N 1996 Autologous blood transfusion in hip replacement. No effect on blood loss but less increase of plasminogen activator inhibitor in a randomised series of 80 patients. Acta Orthopaedica Scandinavica 67(4): 317–320

Hewitt P E et al 1990 The blood donor and tests on donor blood In: Contreras M (ed) ABC of transfusion. British Medical Journal, London, p 1–4

Hows J M, Brozovic B 1990 Platelet and granulocyte transfusions. In: Contreras M (ed) ABC of transfusion. British Medical Journal, London

Kaberry S 1991 Blood simple? Nursing Times 87(20): 56

Kay L A, Huehns E R 1985 The development of blood transfusion. Clinical Blood Transfusion. Pitman, London

Legge A 1997 Direct HIV testing of donated blood is inevitable. British Medical Journal 31(4): 7

McClelland B (ed) 1996 Handbook of transfusion medicine, 2nd edn. HMSO, London

McClelland D B L, Phillips P 1994 Errors in blood transfusion: survey of hospital haematology departments. British Medical Journal 308: 1205–1206

Mandefield H 1993 Tissue of progress. Nursing Times 89(1): 626–628

Mims Handbook of Haematology 1994 Haymarket Medical, London

Olding-Smee W 1990 Red cell substitutes. In: Contreras M (ed) ABC of transfusion. British Medical Journal, London

Polesky H F 1989 Transfusion-transmitted viruses. In: Harmening D (ed) Modern blood banking and transfusion practices, 2nd edn. F A Davis, Philadelphia

Pomeroy C, Englund J A 1987 Cytomegalovirus: epidemiology and infection control. American Journal of Infection Control 15(3): 107–119

Porter H 1996 Transfusion of blood and blood products. In: Mallett J, Bailey C (eds) Manual of clinical nursing procedures, 4th edn. Blackwell Science, Oxford

Roberts W A, Kirkley S A, Newby M 1996 A cost comparison of allogeneic and preoperatively or intraoperatively donated autologous blood. Anesthesia and Analgesia 83(1): 129–133

Royal College of Physicians of Edinburgh 1993 Consensus conference. Leucocyte depletion of blood and blood components. Royal College of Physicians, Edinburgh

Sans T, Bofil C, Joven J, Cliville X, Simo J M, Llobet X, Pero A, Galbany J 1996 Effectiveness of very low doses of subcutaneous recombitant human erythropoietin in facilitating autologous blood donation before orthopedic surgery. Transfusion 36(9): 822–826

Schreiber G B, Busch M P, Kleinman S H, Korelitz J J 1996 The risk of transfusion-transmitted viral infections. New England Journal of Medicine 334: 1685–1690

United Kingdom Central Council for Nursing, Midwifery and Health Visiting 1992 Code of professional conduct for the nurse, midwife and health visitor, 3rd edn. UKCC, London

Vertrees R A, Conti V R, Lick S D, Zwischenberger J B, McDaniel L B, Shulman G 1996 Adverse effects of post operative infusion of shed mediastinal blood. Annals of Thoracic Surgery 62(3): 717–723

Voak D, Finney R D, Forman K et al 1993 Guidelines for autologous transfusion. I. Pre-operative autologous donation. Transfusion Medicine 3: 307–316

Waters A H 1991 Platelet and granulocyte antigens and antibodies. In: Dacie J, Lewis S M (eds) Practical haematology, 7th edn. Churchill Livingstone, Edinburgh, p 441–454

Weinstein S H 1997 Plumer's principles and practice of intravenous therapy, 6th edn. JB Lippincott, Philadelphia, New York, ch 17

Weir J 1995 Blood component therapy. In: Terry J, Baranowski L, Lonsawy R A, Hedrick C (eds) Intravenous therapy – clinical principles and practice. WB Saunders, Philadelphia, p 165–187

Williamson L M, Heptonstall J, Soldan K 1996 A SHOT in the arm for safer blood transfusion. British Medical Journal 31(3): 1221–1222

Parenteral nutrition

Pearl Burnham

CHAPTER 14

INTRODUCTION

Parenteral nutrition (PN) is the infusion of nourishing fluids, commonly containing dextrose, amino acids, fat, electrolytes, vitamins, minerals and trace elements, through a catheter into the venous circulation. The most common route of administration is via the subclavian vein, with the catheter tip placed at the distal end of the superior vena cava. Parenteral nutrition may also be infused via a peripheral vein, most commonly the cephalic or basilic vein. The solutions used for peripheral infusion have a lower osmolarity than those used in central administration, to help avoid phlebitis and thrombosis.

HISTORY OF PARENTERAL NUTRITION

William Harvey's description of the circulatory system in 1616 allowed scientists to consider the possibility of infusion into the veins as an active management measure. Sir Christopher Wren, who injected opium, wine and oils into dogs by using a goose quill attached to a pig's bladder (Grant 1992), performed the first recorded intravenous infusion of substances into the venous circulation in 1656.

During the 1800s, scientists began to experiment with infusing different 'foods' into the bloodstream, fresh cow's milk being one of them. This idea was further developed in the early 1900s, when Henriques and Anderson hydrolysed goat muscle with a pancreatic extract to form a non-allergenic solution containing a mixture of amino acids and di- and tripeptides. They added glucose, sodium and potassium and successfully infused the solution into goats over 16 days as a continuous drip. This is thought to be the first successful intravenous feeding procedure in animals.

In 1891, Matas infused saline intravenously into a man. Sodium chloride and dextrose solutions were infused into the peripheral veins of soldiers during World War I, and it is around this time that the first experiments in central venous cannulation were being conducted (Grant 1992). Two of the most serious problems of early experimentation in nutrient infusion in humans were the high volume of fluid needed to hydrate (which put patients at risk of developing pulmonary oedema), and the hyperosmolarity of the fluids due to the high glucose load. These were gradually overcome with the development of central venous cannulation, which enabled introduction and infusion of low-volume feeds.

In 1920, Yamakawa infused emulsified fat solution into a human, and by 1945 fat emulsion was advocated routinely as an energy source, although the fat emulsions used (derived from castor oil and cotton seed oil) produced serious side-effects, such as fever, coagulation defects and jaundice. By 1967, fat emulsion derived from soybean oil stabilized with egg-yolk phosphatides had been developed.

A year later, Dudrick et al (1968) became the first researchers to describe successful long-term parenteral nutrition. At this time, the three main ingredients (glucose, fat and amino acids) were infused from separate bottles on a rotating basis due to fears that the solutions would become unstable if mixed. During the latter part of the 1970s, experiments demonstrated the stability of the 'All-in-One' system which, as the name implies, combined the main ingredients in a single infusate, and clinicians began using this routinely for adults. The demand in the 1980s and 1990s has been for ongoing refinements to the solutions and a longer 'shelf-life' of solutions once compounded.

A recent development (1997) has been the introduction of the prefilled triple chamber bag for parenteral nutrition. This system stores the solutions separately and in a stable condition until needed, thus providing a shelf-life of up to 12 months. When the feed is required for use, the operator squeezes and rolls the bag on a work surface, breaking the seals between the compartments and allowing the fat emulsion and solutions to mix. A multilayer bag, which minimizes the problems of tiny air bubbles forming in the solution during refrigeration, and which are responsible for triggering the sensitive detection mechanisms of infusion pumps, has also been introduced. It has proved particularly successful with patients receiving infusions overnight at home, who previously had their sleep patterns disturbed due to frequent pump alarm activation (Wood 1991).

INDICATIONS FOR PARENTERAL NUTRITION

Parenteral nutrition is required when the intestine is unavailable or unable to absorb or digest an adequate amount of nutrients on a temporary or permanent basis. In general terms, patients who have minimal or no nourishment for 5–7 days and who fail to demonstrate any progress towards resuming oral intake of nutrients should be considered for parenteral nutrition. However, it is important to encourage the oral ingestion of foods whenever possible; food helps to preserve gut integrity and may prevent bacterial translocation (Hadfield et al 1995).

There is evidence that 40% of hospital in-patients are malnourished, and that their malnourishment increases during their hospital stay (McWhirter & Pennington 1994). Therefore, it is important to identify these patients early and plan interventions to improve their nutritional status. Careful screening and assessment of nutritional status on or before admission to hospital can identify problems which, if left unchecked, would increase morbidity. Commonly, simple actions such as introducing oral supplements like nutrient-dense foods and commercially available sip feeds to at-risk surgical patients preoperatively can act as prophylaxis against significant malnutrition after surgery. Parenteral nutrition is therefore not an intervention which is introduced without careful assessment of patient needs and equally careful assessment of the risks involved. Inevitably, however, it may be the treatment of choice for some severely compromised patients. The following are common conditions or indications for parenteral nutrition (Colagiovanni 1997a):

- as an adjunct to perioperative support, when undernutrition is already suspected
- short bowel syndrome
- inflammatory bowel disease (such as severe Crohn's disease or ulcerative colitis)
- acute pancreatitis
- prolonged paralytic ileus
- major sepsis
- severe burns
- enterocutaneous fistulae
- some malignant diseases
- acquired immunodeficiency syndrome.

ASSESSMENT

Patients admitted to hospital should have height and weight recorded in the appropriate nursing admission documentation. This is a key component of nutritional assessment, and acts as a baseline against which to assess subsequent interventions. To help ensure consistency across institutions in admission nutritional assessments, the British Association for Parenteral and Enteral Nutrition (BAPEN) (see 'Additional information', p. 397) recommends that all patients should be asked the following questions (BAPEN 1996):

- Have you unintentionally lost weight recently?
- Have you been eating less than usual?
- What is your normal weight?
- How tall are you?

Answers to these questions can then be added to the information on signs and symptoms, underlying disease and planned actions (see Fig. 14.1) to provide the basic information from which the clinician will make his decision on the next course of action. Patients considered to be malnourished or at risk following this initial assessment should be referred to the nutrition support team for comprehensive nutritional assessment.

DETERMINING NUTRITIONAL REQUIREMENTS

Healthy adults have basic daily requirements of essential nutrients such as protein, fats, carbohydrate, water, electrolytes, minerals and vitamins. The approximate requirements of calories, protein and water for an adult are shown in Box 14.1.

In sickness, these requirements are often increased. For every 1°C rise in body temperature, for example, there is a 10% increase in energy requirements (Elia 1990). It is therefore important to be alert to the signs of new ill-health in patients, and to monitor physiological and biochemical status.

■ **BOX 14.1**

Approximate daily nutritional requirements for an adult (Payne-James & Wicks 1994)

Kilocalories	25–35 non-protein kcal/kg
Protein	0.8–1.2 g/kg
Water	30–35 ml/kg

THE NUTRITION SUPPORT TEAM

The delivery of parenteral nutrition is a complex process and is best managed by a multidisciplinary nutrition support team. There is strong evidence from research conducted throughout the world that complications are minimized and satisfactory outcomes reached when such a team manages parenteral nutrition (BAPEN 1994, Burnham 1995, Colagiovanni 1997a, Grant 1992, Keohane et al 1983, Nehme 1980). The team will usually consist of:

- clinician
- nutrition nurse specialist
- dietitian
- pharmacist
- biochemist.

Fig. 14.1 Summary of indications for nutrition support (Payne-James & Wicks 1994).

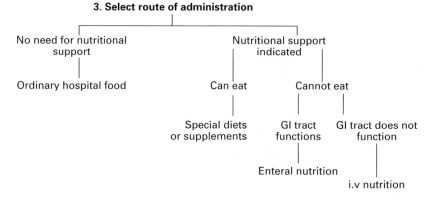

1. Screening

Signs and symptoms of malnutrition	Underlying disease		Planned interventions
Weight loss 5-10% (last 2-3 months)	Low nutritional intake	Increased requirements	Surgery
Serum albumin <35g/l	Inflammatory bowel disease	Burns	Repeated investigations or x-rays
Muscle wasting and fatigue		Mutiple trauma	
Anorexia	Chronic pain	Pyrexia (1°C)	Cytotoxic drug therapy
Vomiting and diarrhoea	Pancreatitis	Infection	Radiotherapy
Chewing or swallowing difficulties	Depression	Fistulae	
Oedema or skin lesions	Cancer	Cancer	

2. Calculate requirements

3. Select route of administration

No need for nutritional support — Ordinary hospital food

Nutritional support indicated

Can eat — Special diets or supplements

Cannot eat

GI tract functions — Enteral nutrition

GI tract does not function — i.v nutrition

In a well-functioning team, these disciplines interlink with each other to provide the support needed to administer parenteral nutrition safely. The dynamics of each team, however, vary considerably. Within some teams the clinician takes the lead, in others it may be the pharmacist or the dietitian, but in the majority the nurse is the only full-time dedicated member and is therefore best placed to coordinate the day-to-day work.

Members of the nutrition support team will make their assessment through a variety of means (Springett & Murrey 1994):

- the patient's clinical history
- dietary history

- physical examination
- body mass index (weight/height^2, kg/m^2)
- anthropometric measurements
- biochemical status
- immunological status
- muscle function.

Many centres use standard tables when estimating patients' requirements for PN (for example, Tables 14.1 and 14.2 and Box 14.2). From these assessments, a composite picture of the patient's nutritional status emerges. No single assessment is viewed in isolation; rather, it is the total view which provides the assessment. From these data, a basic regimen for an individual patient can be designed, a formula for which is shown in Box 14.3.

Careful liaison with pharmacy staff is important at this stage, as they can comment and advise on the suitability and stability of suggested regimens. The prescription should be written clearly and precisely, and it is probably advisable to utilize a standardized pre-printed prescription chart (Fig. 14.3).

PREPARING THE PATIENT

Once the need for parenteral nutrition has been established, an important function of the nurse specialist is to explain to the patient why the therapy is necessary, how it will be administered, and where and how the catheter is to be inserted. The nurse may also be able to give an estimate of the length of the therapy. Once he is satisfied that the patient understands the need for the treatment and how it will be managed, a consent is obtained.

It may be appropriate to introduce the patient to another recipient of parenteral

Table 14.1 Equations for estimating basal metabolic rate (reproduced with kind permission from Schofield 1985)

Age group	Basal metabolic rate (kcal/day)	
	Females	**Males**
15–18 years	13.3 W + 690	17.6 W + 656
18–30 years	14.8 W + 485	15.0 W + 690
30–60 years	8.1 W + 842	11.4 W + 870
Over 60 years	9.0 W + 656	11.7 W + 585

W = weight in kg.

Table 14.2 Estimate of nitrogen requirements (reproduced with kind permission from Elia 1990)

Metabolic status	Nitrogen (g/kg per day)
Normal	0.17 (0.14–0.20)
Hypermetabolic	
5–25%	0.20 (0.17–0.25)
25–50%	0.25 (0.20–0.30)
> 50%	0.30 (0.25–0.35)
Depleted	0.30 (0.20–0.40)

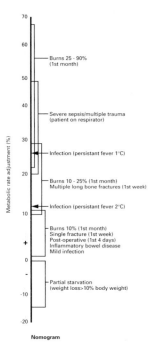

Fig. 14.2 Method of estimating approximate energy and nitrogen requirements in adults receiving artificial nutritional support (Elia 1990).

■ **BOX 14.2**

The process of nutritional assessment (PEN Group 1997)

Energy

1. Determine approximate basal metabolic rate using Table 14.1.
2. Adjust for stress using nomogram (Fig. 14.2).
3. Add a combined factor for activity and diet-induced thermogenesis:
   — bed-bound immobile: +10%
   — bed-bound mobile/sitting: +15%
   — mobile on the ward: +25%.
4. If increase in energy stores is required, add 400–1000 kcal/day. If decrease in energy stores is required, reduce energy intake.

Nitrogen

1. Estimate nitrogen requirements using Table 14.2.
2. For obese individuals with a body mass index of 30–40 kg/m², use approximately 75% of the value estimated from body weight. For those with a body mass index > 50 kg/m², use approximately 65% of value estimated from weight.

■ **BOX 14.3**

Formula for designing a basic PN regimen for an individual patient (Prior 1992)

1. Calculate the baseline daily energy and nitrogen requirements (basal metabolic rate).
2. Other baseline requirements:
   Water 30 ml/kg per day
   Sodium (mmol) = $2 \times$ wt (kg)
   Potassium (mmol) = $1 \times$ wt (kg)
   Calcium (mmol) = $0.11 \times$ wt (kg)
   Magnesium (mmol) = $0.04 \times$ wt (kg)
   Phosphate (mmol) = $0.5 \times$ wt (kg).
3. Correct the baseline requirements so that they meet the individual's specific needs.

NB: If a patient is receiving angiotensin-converting enzyme inhibitors or diuretics, the daily sodium intake should be kept below 1.0 mmol/kg per day to avoid fluid retention and oedema.

nutrition; this can help to ease many of the fears patients hold, and allows them to talk through their anxieties with someone in a similar position.

The next stage is to prepare the patient for the catheter insertion procedure. It is crucial to check the clotting time and take a specimen for full blood count beforehand, particularly if there is a history of anticoagulant treatment or abnormal clotting results.

Some institutions prefer to use theatre facilities for catheter insertion, while others use a designated treatment room. Whichever is chosen, the procedure should be carried out in a clean, undisturbed area using strict aseptic technique (Elliott et al 1994, Hehir et al 1992, Raad et al 1994).

ADULT INTRAVENOUS NUTRITION PRESCRIPTION

	Period of Admin	Infusion Rate	Pharmacist Sig.	Batch No. Total Vol	Time Started	Sig. Witness	Time Completed	Vol. Infused
HOSPITAL								
WARD								
UNIT NO.								
SURNAME								
FORENAMES								
CONSULTANT								

DATE REQ'D .... TIME REQ'D

MATERIAL — PRESCRIBED AMOUNT

Vamin .... % .... ml

Glucose .... % .... ml

Intralipid .... % .... ml

Sodium (as chloride) .... to .... mmol total

Potassium (as chloride) .... to .... mmol total

Addiphos { 2 mmol Phosphate / 1.5 mmol Potassium / ml / 1.5 mmol Sodium } .... ml

Additrace .... ml

Solivito N .... vials

Vitlipid Adult N .... ml

Magnesium (as sulphate) .... to .... mmol total

Calcium (as chloride) .... to .... mmol total

Prescriber's Signature .... Date: ....

ADDITRACE CONTAINS IN 10 ml
Fe   20 micromol
Zn   100 micromol
Mn   5 micromol
Cu   20 micromol
F   50 micromol
I   1 micromol
Cr   0.2 micromol
Se   0.4 micromol
Mo   0.2 micromol

SOLVITO N CONTAINS IN 1 VIAL
VitaminB1   3 mg
Vitamin B2   3.6 mg
Nicotinamide   40 mg
Vitamin B6   4 mg
Pantothenic Acid   15 mg
Biotin   0.6 mg
Folic Acid   0.4 mg
Vitamin B12   0.5 mg
Vitamin C   100 mg

VITLIPID N ADULT CONTAINS IN 10 ml
Vitamin A   3300 i.u.
Vitamin D2   200 i.u.
Phytomenadione   150 mcg
Vitamin E   10 i.u.
1000 ml → Intralipid 20% contains 2000 kCal
1000 ml → Glucose 10% contains 400 kCal
1000 ml → Viamin 9 Glucose contains 400 non protein kCal

The nutritional status of a stable adult patient can be maintained by using the following formula:

Vamin 9 Glucose   1500 ml
Glucose 10%   1000 ml
Intralipid 20%   500 ml
Additrace   10 ml
Addiphos   15 ml
Solivito N   1 vial
Vitlipid Adult N   10 ml
Potassium chloride   40 mmol
This provides 2000 non protein kCal & 14.1g Nitrogen

Caution: Expert advice should be sought prior to initiating intravenous nutrition.

Fig. 14.3 An example of a parenteral prescription chart.

CATHETERIZATION OF THE SUBCLAVIAN VEIN

If the patient has hair on the chest area, the insertion site should be clipped before the procedure begins (Elliott et al 1994, Murphy & Lipman 1987). If shaving is requested, it should only be performed immediately prior to insertion (Elliott et al 1994). A semi-permeable occlusive dressing covers the site when the catheter is in situ, and this will adhere properly if the chest is free of hair. Dressing removal will also be less painful for the patient.

The patient lies on her back, and a rolled towel or other bolster may be placed between the shoulder blades. This improves venous access by relaxing the shoulder muscles. The patient is then placed in the Trendelenburg position with head down 20°. This manoeuvre facilitates venous filling and reduces the risk of air embolism. The patient may also be asked to turn her head to the opposite side. It is useful if the assistant is able to talk to the patient and offer support and encouragement at this time.

The person inserting the catheter needs to be a well-practised and skilled operator as the procedure carries significant risk, including pneumothorax, haemothorax, brachial plexus injury and artery puncture. Some nurse practitioners are now trained in central catheter placement, but although this remains rare there are many advantages to having specialist nurses insert central venous catheters (see Box 14.4) (Hamilton 1993, Hamilton et al 1995). The procedure is most likely to be carried out by the senior registrar on the nutrition support team or by the physician, surgeon or anaesthetist who directs the team (see Box 14.5).

Mechanical complications

The procedure carries significant risks. Some of the most common problems are shown in Table 14.3 (Colagiovanni 1997a, Michie 1988).

PERIPHERAL PN

Feeding via a peripheral vein is now becoming regarded as a viable option to central venous feeding (Colagiovanni 1997a, Palmer & MacFie 1997), particularly for patients requiring short-term PN of less than 14 days or when insertion of a central

---

■ **BOX 14.4**

Advantages of a CNS catheter insertion service (Hamilton et al 1995)

- Short response time
- Experience gained by frequent placement – reduces complications
- Reduces infections and length of stay
- Protocols for the management of CVCs ensure a high-quality service
- Liaises and advises on the management of CVCs
- Costs reduced by avoiding anaesthetic/theatre time
- Junior doctors are offered training opportunities for central venous catheterization
- The procedure is explained in detail and the patient counselled prior to the start of invasive therapy
- Educational support of ward staff

■ **BOX 14.5**

Procedure for catheterization of the subclavian vein

- The equipment is assembled and placed on a sterile towel on a dressing trolley.
- Wearing a sterile gown and gloves (Elliott et al 1994, Raad et al 1994), the operator will carefully prepare the patient's skin. Normally, a cleansing lotion such as chlorhexidine in 70% spirit is used to clean the area (Maki et al 1991). The vein to be cannulated is then identified. The field is draped, leaving the patient's face exposed.
- The skin, subcutaneous tissues and surrounding muscle are infiltrated with a local anaesthetic, such as 2% lignocaine, which takes 1–2 minutes to begin to have effect.
- A 10 ml syringe, half-filled with heparinized saline, is attached to the needle and hollow introducer, which is used to puncture the skin. The needle and introducer are then advanced along to the subclavian vein. The needle is withdrawn slowly while the introducer is advanced into the vein. The syringe is then used to flush the introducer.
- The syringe is removed and the catheter, which has been primed with heparinized saline, is advanced down the introducer to the pre-measured point determined by measuring from the insertion site to the sternal angle. A port is fixed to the end, and the catheter is aspirated and flushed with heparinized saline.
- The second phase of the procedure is to create a skin tunnel. The skin is infiltrated with local anaesthetic in a line down from the entry site for about 3 inches. A tiny incision is made at the bottom of this tract so that the catheter can exit at the lower end.
- The needle is then guided down the tract subcutaneously, exiting at the lower end. The hollow introducer is then threaded up the needle, the needle is removed and the port is removed from the end of the catheter. The catheter is then fed down through the hollow introducer, exiting the skin at the lower end of the tunnel. The port is reattached to the end of the catheter and the catheter is flushed.
- The next step is to secure the catheter to the chest wall. This is done by placing two tiny sutures in the hub either side of the catheter. The site is thoroughly cleaned and dried and an occlusive dressing is placed over the entire area. (Placement of catheters will vary according to individual manufacturer's recommendations.)
- A chest X-ray is always taken to confirm the position of the catheter and to exclude pneumothorax before feeding begins.

Table 14.3 Common mechanical problems associated with catheter insertion

Problem	Comment
Subclavian artery puncture	Arterial blood shoots back into the syringe
Catheter misplacement	Check position by chest X-ray before starting feed
Catheter damage/fracture	Retrieval of fragments under X-ray guidance
Hydromediastinum	Observe for chest pain and arrhythmias
Air embolism	Observe for breathlessness
Pneumothorax	Observe for chest pain and breathlessness
Haemothorax	Observe for chest pain and breathlessness
Brachial plexus injury	Patient complains of shooting pain in the arm and pins and needles or numbness in the fingers

Table 14.4 Advantages and disadvantages of peripheral and central venous rates for PN

Type	Advantages	Disadvantages
Central venous catheter	• Reliable long-term access to central venous system • Allows the infusion of high-osmolarity feeds	• Insertion associated with complications • Needs experienced practitioner to insert • Risk of catheter-related sepsis • Central veins may not be available in critically ill patients because they are already in use
Peripheral venous catheter	• Few insertion-related risks • Less traumatic for patient • Can be inserted by suitably trained staff • Less risk of infection • No chest X-ray	• Suitable peripheral veins may not be available • Possibility for development of phlebitis • Requires routine re-siting and rotation of venous sites • Not suitable for those with high nutritional requirements

venous catheter is inadvisable or impossible (Henry 1997). The main problems have been related to volume (usually 2–2.5 litres) and composition (osmolarity and pH) which has resulted in chemical phlebitis. The type and size of catheter can also cause trauma of the vein, resulting in mechanical phlebitis (Colagiovanni 1997a). However, peripheral PN avoids the risks associated with central venous catheterization, reduces cost, simplifies nursing care and prevents delay of initiation of therapy (Palmer & MacFie 1997) (see Table 14.4).

In order to reduce the development of phlebitis, the device should be placed into the largest available forearm vein (Palmer & MacFie 1997). The use of a fine-bore catheter made of silicone or polyurethane (22g being the most commonly used) allows good blood flow around the catheter and rapid circulation of the irritant solution. Many centres also advise the use of a 5 mg glyceryl trinitrate patch placed just under the insertion site to aid vasodilation (Pennington et al 1996). Another method is to alter the solution by giving fewer calories in total, and a significant proportion as fat can reduce the overall osmolarity and further reduce the risk (Colagiovanni 1997a). The use of filters has been shown to reduce the particulate matter and endotoxins, thereby reducing the risk of infection (Colagiovanni 1997b). It may be necessary to rotate venous access sites regularly and this has been shown to reduce the incidence of phlebitis (Palmer & MacFie 1997). All peripheral devices should be inserted with strict attention to aseptic technique and inspected at least once a day and removed at the first signs of phlebitis.

Nutrition nurse specialists are routinely placing peripheral devices and many now also place peripherally inserted central catheters (PICCs). These devices bypass the problems associated with peripheral PN administration as well as allowing access to the central veins (Colagiovanni 1997a).

METABOLIC COMPLICATIONS

A variety of metabolic problems can arise if proper monitoring of patient response

Table 14.5 Common metabolic problems associated with parenteral nutrition

Problem	Clinical features
Hypoglycaemia	Sweaty, clammy, disorientated, drowsy tremor, palpitations, visual disturbance, blood sugar > 2.5 mmol, loss of consciousness
Hyperglycaemia	Hyperosmolar diuresis, polyuria, dehydration
Hypophosphataemia	Neuromuscular changes, tremor, ataxia, slurred speech, irritability, apprehension, stupor, coma
Hypocalcaemia	Tetany, neuromuscular irritability manifested by paraesthesia around the mouth and extremities, muscle spasms, cramps, hyperflexion
Hypernatraemia	Excess sodium. Dry, sticky mucous membranes, oliguria, agitation, loss of skin tone
Hyponatraemia	Low sodium. Mental confusion, muscle twitching, seizures
Hypomagnesaemia	Impairs calcium and potassium metabolism. Signs of tetany, tremor, muscle twitching, nystagmus, convulsions, coma
Hyperkalaemia	Excess potassium. Muscle weakness, colic, diarrhoea, arrhythmias
Hypokalaemia	Low potassium. Muscle weakness, reflexes decreased, arrhythmias, apnoea, respiratory arrest
Hepatobiliary dysfunction	Deranged liver function tests, jaundice, nausea, drowsiness, short attention span, pruritus, raised alkaline phosphatase
Micronutrient deficiencies	Poor skin condition, hair loss, brittle nails
Nitrogen imbalance	Low protein stores eventually lead to muscle wasting, exhaustion, poor cardiorespiratory function, poor concentration, oedema, depression
Metabolic acidosis	Low bicarbonate concentration in the blood. Deep rapid respirations, shortness of breath, weakness, disorientation

to the parenteral nutrition regimen is not followed. Some of these are shown in Table 14.5 (Henry 1997, Roberts 1993).

MONITORING

Biochemical monitoring

It is advisable to establish a programme of routine blood monitoring in order to recognize and treat any metabolic complications, and the biochemistry department plays a crucial role in helping to detect these changes quickly. Figure 14.4 illustrates some of the tests required and the frequency of testing.

Nursing care and monitoring

Ongoing assessment of the patient's response to treatment is part of the nurse's responsibility. Specific interventions are discussed below, and an example of a monitoring regimen is presented in Box 14.6 (Finnegan & Oldfield 1989, Henry 1997, Michie 1988, Stilwell 1992).

Daily weight

This is a crucial part of monitoring, but results can be deceptive. Weight gains of

Fig. 14.4 Tests required and frequency of tests.

Name... Hospital No. ....

Week No. ....

PN patients - biochemical testing

This is a summary of the *minimum* biochemical testing required in stable patients undergoing PN

Analyte	First week	Following weeks as clinically indicated	Weekends as required

Serum tests

Analyte	First week		
Sodium	daily		
Potassium	daily		
Urea	daily		
Creatinine	daily		
Bone profile	twice weekly		
Magnesium	weekly		
Bilirubin	weekly		
AST	weekly		
Gamma GT	weekly		

Heparinised syringe

Bicarbonate	as clinically indicated

Plasma tests

Glucose	daily	BM Stix twice weekly	

Plasma tests - special heparin tubes from Lab.

Zinc	weekly		
Copper			
Selenium			

24 hour urines
Sodium, potassium and urea

Specimen 1 on the day the PN commences.
Specimen 2 on day 3
Specimen 3 on day 6
Twice weekly thereafter as clinically indicated

■ **BOX 14.6**

Nursing monitoring of patients receiving parenteral nutrition

- Daily weight, which is recorded with the patient wearing similar weight clothing, at the same time of day, on the same weighing scales
- 4-hourly temperature, pulse, respirations and blood pressure
- 4-hourly capillary blood glucose estimation (using, for example, BM Stix) for the first 48 hours, then twice daily urinalysis if glucose level is satisfactory
- 24-hour urine collection, twice weekly, for urea and electrolytes, to calculate nitrogen balance
- Accurate assessment of fluid balance and cumulative fluid balance
- Mouth care
- Pressure area care
- Mobilizing exercises

■ BOX 14.7

Formula to calculate nitrogen balance

$$\text{mmol urea/24 hours} \times \frac{28}{60} \times \frac{60}{1000} \times \frac{5}{4} = \text{grams of nitrogen/24 hours}$$

Explanation

Two nitrogen atoms in urea (2 × atomic weight = 28)
Molecular weight urea = 60
1 mole = molecular weight in grams (÷ by 1000 to convert from mmol)
5/4 allows for non-urinary urea nitrogen excretion.

---

more than 0.5–1.0 kg/day might seem to be predictable and desirable outcomes, but in fact may indicate problems. Such dramatic weight changes can only be attributed to unwanted accumulation of fluid, as it is not physiologically possible to gain lean body mass in such short time periods. Weight gain of this type signals a need to reassess the volume and rate of infusion, and may require immediate medical assessment and diuretic therapy.

Four-hourly vital signs monitoring

Temperature, pulse, respirations and blood pressure would normally be recorded 4-hourly for the first 48 hours, and then if the patient's condition is stable they could be recorded twice daily. Any pyrexia, tachycardia or dyspnoea should be reported to the nutrition team immediately as this may herald infection, embolism or a metabolic complication.

Four-hourly blood glucose monitoring

Glucose intolerance in the first few days of receiving parenteral nutrition is not uncommon. If the blood glucose becomes raised, it is usual for the team to recommend the administration of insulin on a sliding scale to re-establish stability. In most cases, however, blood sugar levels remain within normal limits and monitoring can be reduced to twice daily urinalysis. Identifying glycosuria can be of value in the early detection of impending sepsis.

Twice weekly 24-hour urine collection

Twenty-four-hour urine samples are collected to measure sodium, potassium and urea levels as indicators of electrolyte and nitrogen excretion. Infusate levels of electrolytes and proteins are adjusted accordingly. The formula to calculate nitrogen balance is shown in Box 14.7.

Some centres have found that accurate collection of urine over 24 hours is almost impossible unless the patient is catheterized, and the procedure has therefore been abandoned. Others continue to find it an accurate and useful test in estimating electrolyte and nitrogen balance.

Fluid balance

All losses from urine, stoma, fistulae, vomit/nasogastric aspirate and diarrhoea must be recorded. The electrolyte content of each is different and knowing volumes can help in planning replacement. Controlled infusion of parenteral nutrition is vital and a volumetric infusion pump should always be used. For a full discussion of the importance of monitoring fluid balance, see Chapter 3.

Mouth care

Patients receiving parenteral nutrition are commonly unable to take food or fluids by the oral route. Oral hygiene is therefore an important part of nursing assessment and care (Henry 1997). Regular brushing of teeth is encouraged, refreshing mouth-washes are offered regularly, and an artificial saliva spray may be used to retain moisture in the mouth.

Malnutrition causes sore mouth and gums with cracking of the angles of the lips (cheilosis), all of which are distressing for the patient. Such problems are exacerbated when oral hygiene is poor. Aggressive *Candida* infections can be a particular problem which often leads to angular cheilitis. Halitosis is also common and may be unpleasant for the patient. Competent assessment and regular attention to oral hygiene can prevent many of these unpleasant and uncomfortable sequelae of treatment.

Pressure area care

Skin and subcutaneous tissue are at risk of breaking down and becoming damaged when the patient is undernourished, so regular assessment of skin integrity and correct positioning of the patient are essential (Finnegan & Oldfield 1989).

Mobilizing exercises

Patients receiving parenteral nutrition are often lethargic and reluctant to mobilize, but there is good evidence that nitrogen balance can be enhanced by exercise (Millward et al 1994). The aim of parenteral nutrition is to build back lean body mass; if the patient is immobile, the nourishment is more likely to be deposited as fat. A programme of regular exercises should be suggested by the physiotherapist.

RECORDING CARE

It is vitally important that nurse specialists establish a partnership in care with patients from the outset to achieve the most satisfactory outcome. Daily progress should be documented and the care plan regularly referred to and evaluated (see Box 14.8). A carefully designed care plan, if adhered to by all members of the nursing and medical staff, can almost completely eliminate the administrative problems associated with parenteral nutrition. It is therefore important to have written guidelines and policies on catheter management readily available (Clark 1994, Finnegan & Oldfield 1989, Roberts 1993). These would include protocols for:

- catheter insertion
- setting up the nutrient infusion using a volumetric pump
- changing the bag and administration set
- care of the exit site and dressing changes
- removing the catheter.

Procedures should also be available for management of the following:

- air in the administration set
- catheter occlusion
- catheter damage
- catheter sepsis
- obtaining blood cultures.

■ **BOX 14.8**

Daily patient assessments
- Assess temperature and record any pyrexia
- Check the fluid balance chart and record balance and cumulative balance
- Observe the patient for signs of dehydration and presence or absence of oedema
- Check the mouth for signs of *Candida*, cheilosis and other problems
- Record the daily weight
- Observe the catheter insertion site for any redness, discharge or leaking of fluid
- Check the occlusive dressing for signs of peeling or breaks in the surface
- Check the amount of fluid infused and note how much is left in the bag

CARE OF CATHETER AND INTRAVENOUS INFUSION SYSTEM

Despite precautions taken during administration, most contamination occurs during manipulations of intravenous systems, changing bags and drug administration and additives (Colagiovanni 1997b). It is now recognized that the catheter junction and hub are the major sources of catheter infection, particularly in patients receiving PN (Colagiovanni 1997a). Insertion and any intervention should always be performed using good aseptic technique. Handling of the catheter by a minimum of carefully selected and specifically designated staff minimizes the risk of infection (Colagiovanni 1997a, Elliott et al 1994, Michie 1988, Murphy & Lipman 1987). It is not always possible to ensure this in every unit, but it should be possible to identify, train, assess and empower a group of nurses in each unit so that they are competent to manage the daily care of patients receiving parenteral nutrition, and are able to identify common problems as they arise. As a further preventative measure, it is advisable to use a dedicated single-lumen catheter whenever possible; multi-lumen catheters tend to be handled more often and are therefore potentially more liable to introduce infection (Elliott 1993, Roberts 1993, Yeung et al 1988). Many hospitals now use closed luer-lock needleless connection devices. These devices allow access to the catheter while maintaining a closed system, reducing the risk of air embolism, bleeding and infection.

ORGANIZATION OF PARENTERAL NUTRITION

The administration of a sophisticated and potentially hazardous treatment (Michie 1988) such as parenteral nutrition requires a high degree of organization to ensure that no procedures or assessments are unintentionally omitted. Nurse specialists are commonly responsible for initiating the organization of care, and an example of a programme of care is presented in Box 14.8. Any changes in treatment felt necessary on the basis of these assessments should be discussed with the patient, and then communicated verbally to appropriate colleagues in the team and written in the patient's notes.

SUSPECTED CATHETER INFECTION

Catheter-related sepsis is the most common complication of parenteral nutrition. However, this can be reduced when the patient's care is managed by an appropriately trained Nutrition Nurse Specialist (Colagiovanni 1997a, Elliott et al 1994, Hamilton 1993, Hamilton et al 1995, Keohane et al 1983, Murphy & Lipman 1987, Nehme 1980, Springett & Murphy 1994, Wood 1991). It was found in one Trust (Havering Hospital) that once strict protocols for handling catheters and equipment were introduced to the wards, and once the number of people handling parenteral nutrition apparatus was minimized to a designated well-instructed and trained few, the incidence of infection was reduced from 33 to 11% after 1 year. Infections were further reduced when it was decided that the team of four nutrition sisters should handle the catheters exclusively (see Fig. 14.5). A standardized protocol for the treatment of suspected central venous catheter infection was also found to be useful (Fig. 14.6).

When a patient does develop a catheter-related infection, immediate treatment with antibiotics is essential. This may include the following (Havering Hospitals):

- three 12-hourly loading doses of teicoplanin 400 mg instilled into the catheter
- daily dose of teicoplanin 200 mg instilled slowly into the lumen of the catheter to remain and therefore lock the catheter
- after a period of 3 or 4 days of antibiotic therapy, some centres may recommence parenteral nutrition, using a protocol of alternating 12 hours antibiotic lock, then flushing the catheter with saline and continuing the feed for 12 hours
- the antibiotic therapy may continue for up to 12 days.

Such treatment is costly to pursue. An estimate of the treatment costs and potential savings to a trust are shown in Figure 14.7. Clearly, for the patient's comfort and well-being and in the interests of financial prudence, prevention is much better than cure.

DISCONTINUING PARENTERAL NUTRITION

It is unwise to cease parenteral nutrition abruptly, as the patient may experience symptoms of hypoglycaemia. It is more common to wean the patient off more gradually in order to allow the gut time to adapt to the reception of oral food again

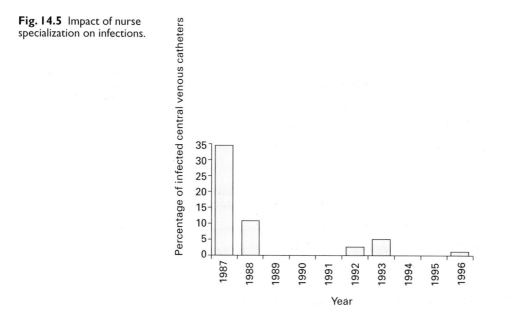

Fig. 14.5 Impact of nurse specialization on infections.

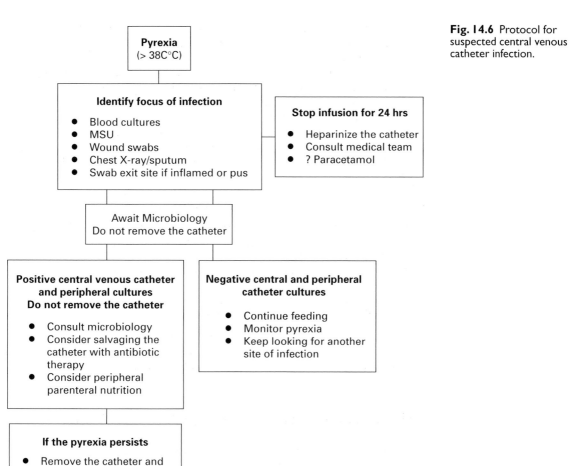

Fig. 14.6 Protocol for suspected central venous catheter infection.

The cost of an infected catheter (1996)

- 12 days drug therapy   £   442.85
- 7 days hospital stay   £ 1950.00
- Replacement catheter   £   25.00
                          £ 2417.85

On average, without a Nurse Specialist, 30% of catheters become infected. 1
On average, 42 patients per year are cared for by the Nurse Specialist. 2

(ITU not included)

THEREFORE ELIMINATION OF INFECTED CATHETERS SAVES

£30 461.91

This does not include Nursing, Medical or Laboratory time

Fig. 14.7 Estimate of cost of an infected central venous catheter.

(Finnegan & Oldfield 1989, Henry 1997). To do this, the nutrient infusion is administered over 48 hours and oral nourishment is reintroduced simultaneously. While the patient is receiving only parenteral nutrition, the gut atrophies, the villi flatten, gastric motility decreases, enzymes become less active, and release of gastric, intestinal, biliary and pancreatic secretions slows down. When oral nutrition is restored, the patient will experience feelings of fullness, altered taste and, on some occasions, diarrhoea. Nurses may find encouraging patients to eat a considerable challenge. It is advisable not to stop the parenteral nutrition completely until the patient is eating sufficient food to maintain weight. An accurate food record chart must be maintained so that intake can be assessed and monitored.

REMOVING THE CATHETER

During weaning the catheter should be kept patent with heparinized saline (Cottee 1995). Cuffed catheters may be removed by gentle traction or surgical dissection by either a nurse or a doctor (Mallett & Bailey 1996). Removal of a non-cuffed catheter is usually a nursing procedure and must be carried out using aseptic technique. The procedure involves the following steps:

- Reassure patients that the procedure is not painful.
- The patient lies flat on her back, with the head lowered 20°.
- The dressing over the entry site is removed and the area is cleaned with a cleansing solution such as chlorhexidine in 70% spirit. This is allowed to dry.
- The sutures retaining the catheter are removed.
- Ask the patient to a perform the Valsalva manoeuvre. Using sterile forceps, the catheter is withdrawn using slow, steady traction to avoid damage to the vessel and to minimize the risk of the tiny valves in the vessel clamping down.
- Apply pressure to the site with a thick pad of swabs for about 5 minutes.
- Examine the catheter to make sure it is complete. Any evidence of missing catheter material could denote a serious problem as the fragments may be acting as emboli.
- Using sterile scissors, cut off the tip and place in a sterile specimen container to be sent to microbiology for culture.
- Cover the entry site with a small occlusive dressing.

HOME PARENTERAL NUTRITION

Home PN can offer patients greater mobility, improve quality of life and reduce hepatic abnormalities (Henry 1997). However, it requires considerable psychological adjustment by both patients and their families (Stilwell 1992). Depression and grief have been expressed by patients who have had to adjust to permanent loss of normal sleeping patterns, and marital and sexual relationships may be strained due to altered body image and feelings (Price & Levine 1979). Patients must be carefully assessed for their suitability before any decision on home therapy is taken (Box 14.9). Those who are suitable should be referred to specialist centres with the experience and back-up facilities to support such high-tech health care at home (Price & Levine 1979, Stilwell 1992, Wood 1991). The therapy is not without risk, so it is wise to check certain basic criteria before embarking on such a treatment:

- Do the patient and carer understand the reasons for long-term parenteral nutrition, and have they accepted that it is necessary?
- Are the patient and carer willing to receive this care in the home?

BOX 14.9

Psychological considerations for home parenteral nutrition (Stilwell 1992)

- Interrupted sleep patterns
  - nocturnal polyuria
  - alarms from pumps
- Depression/grief
  - not being able to eat
  - altered body image from central venous catheters
  - bowel surgery patients who have lost most of their bowel may no longer feel whole people
- Impairment of sexual functions
  - fear of dislodgement of catheter
- Issues related to communication with family/friends; anger

- Have they the mental and physical ability to learn and apply basic principles and techniques of care?
- Is there an appropriate long-term venous access device in place?
- Has appropriate health authority funding been agreed?
- Is there an on-call system for providing expert advice to the patient by telephone day and night?

Some common conditions which may require home parenteral nutrition are

- short bowel syndrome
- enterocutaneous fistulae
- radiotherapy enteritis
- malignancies (very occasionally)
- gut motility disorders
- acquired immunodeficiency syndrome.

Prior to 1995, the provision of parenteral nutrition at home was a joint venture between the hospital, the general practitioner and community nursing services, with the hospital recommending the parenteral regimen and the general practitioner prescribing the necessary fluids/additives. Ancillary items were often funded from the community nurses' medical/surgical budget. In early 1995, the Department of Health issued a new directive (EL(95)5) on the purchasing of high-tech health care at home. The aim was to prevent inappropriate funding of complete packages of care on GP prescription. The Department of Health required health authorities to arrange for certain treatments to be provided as a complete package of care through their contracts. Today, health authorities may choose to purchase the entire package of care from a home care company or they may wish to use the local 'in-house' service from the hospital (Wood & Charles 1997).

To protect the best interests of the patient, BAPEN has published a document which aims to:

- help purchasers understand the scope of clinical and logistical problems associated with home parenteral nutrition
- define quality criteria against which purchased services can be measured.

The document also refers to guidelines and standards in the preparation for discharge of patients requiring home parenteral nutrition (BAPEN 1995). It generally takes between 4 and 6 weeks to teach and prepare a patient for home parenteral nutrition. It is useful to plan this teaching programme by setting a series of well defined learning goals for the patient to achieve (Elia 1994, Henry 1997, Stilwell 1992, Wood 1991). Before commencing the practical teaching, the nurse specialist should discuss the following services with the patient: delivery and storage of feed and equipment; disposal of waste and sharps; overnight feeding; daytime activities; holidays and restrictions; regular monitoring and clinic follow-up; and the involvement of the GP. It may be necessary to enlist the support of social services at this stage to ensure that suitable home arrangements are in place and that the patient is aware of any benefits to which she may be entitled.

Teaching should take place in a quiet, undisturbed area, where the patient and carer have ample opportunity to express fears and concerns. The learning goals set earlier become the basis of the partnership between teacher and patient and, once achieved, should give the patient and carer confidence that they are able to cope independently.

At the end of the programme of teaching, the patient/carer should be able to

- connect the administration set to the bag of parenteral nutrition and in turn to the catheter
- programme the volumetric infusion pump
- disconnect the infusion and flush the catheter
- irrigate a blocked catheter
- make additions to the solution
- change the dressing
- recognize the symptoms and signs of venous thrombosis
- recognize catheter-related sepsis
- recognize symptoms and signs of hyper/hypoglycaemia
- deal with 'first aid' of a catheter fracture
- contact the hospital team when in difficulties.

Each patient should be given the details of the local branch of a patient support group such as PINNT (Patients on Intravenous and Nasogastric Nutrition Therapy), or the paediatric branch (half PINNT) if appropriate. Many patients find great value in the services offered by such groups, and may also become keen to contribute to their development (Wood 1991).

Before discharge, it is useful to present the patient with a folder containing instructions on procedures, the learning goals and when they were achieved, useful names and telephone numbers, the date and time of the next clinic appointment and the help line number for 24-hour advice.

Currently there are only 250–300 patients in the UK receiving home PN; it is a very expensive therapy (Wood & Charles 1997). The annual cost of home parenteral nutrition therapy in 1997 was between £35000 and £45000 per patient (Wood & Charles 1997). This money is well spent, however, when education, planning and support ensure the patient is able to manage in the home.

BANS

In 1995, BAPEN formally launched the British Artificial Nutrition Survey (BANS). The aim of BANS is to invite all acute hospitals to register and provide information on patients receiving artificial nutritional support in the hospital and home settings. The data form a national database of patients receiving nutritional support via the parenteral and enteral routes. This information assists in monitoring patient numbers and assessing treatment outcomes. It helps to establish whether standards of care are adequately met and, more importantly, provides a framework for improvement where standards are not met.

The registering centres are sent an analysis of the local and national data on a regular basis, so health planners and economists benefit from accurate data about the prevalence and growth of home nutritional support and associated costs.

During 1996, a BANS survey was carried out to establish the national database. Over 500 centres were approached in the UK, and by the end of the year, over 300 hospital trusts had registered. Analysis of data from the first 208 trusts (approximately 120 000 beds) showed that only 39% had a nutrition support team, with only 70% of these teams having a specialist nutrition nurse. The survey estimated that the point prevalence for home parenteral nutrition was 270 during 1996. As data are not yet complete, it is not possible to estimate the total number of patients who received parenteral nutrition in hospital. It is hoped that BANS will be able to advise the Department of Health on the use of parenteral nutrition, the diagnosis distribution, the success or failure rate and cost implications, so that this high-tech health care can be adequately monitored and funded.

CONCLUSION

Illness which causes gut failure or malabsorption of nutrients is potentially catastrophic and must be recognized promptly and treated before the patient can begin to recover. Parenteral nutrition, if managed by a multidisciplinary team and administered safely observing strict protocols, is life-saving and capable of shortening recovery time. For those patients who need bowel resection or whose gut failure is irreversible, there is now the option of using self-administered parenteral nutrition at home. This facility enables many home patients to enjoy a very satisfactory quality of life, fully participating in employment and social activities.

ADDITIONAL INFORMATION

British Association for Parenteral and Enteral Nutrition

BAPEN (PO Box 922, Maidenhead, Berks SL6 4SH) was formed in 1992 as a result of recommendations made by the King's Fund report 'A positive approach to nutrition as treatment'. The association's aim is to improve the nutritional treatment of all sufferers from illness who have become, or are likely to become, malnourished and who are unable to consume or absorb normal food in sufficient quantities to effect recovery.

The association comprises five founder groups:

- The Pharmacist's National Total Parenteral Nutrition Group (NTPNG)
- National Nurses Nutrition Group (NNNG)
- Clinical Metabolism and Nutrition Support Group of the Nutrition Society (CMNSG)
- Parenteral and Enteral Group of the British Dietetic Association (PENG)
- Patients on Intravenous and Nasogastric Nutrition Therapy (PINNT).

Reports available from BAPEN include:

- Organisation of nutritional support in hospitals (1994)
- Home parenteral nutrition (1995)
- Enteral and parenteral nutrition in the community (1994)
- Standards and guidelines for nutritional support of patients in hospitals (1996)
- Current perspectives on parenteral nutrition in adults (1996).

Useful names and addresses

PINNT

Chairperson – Mrs Carolyn Wheatley
PINNT
PO Box 3126
Christchurch
Dorset BH23 2 X 5
E-mail:pinnt@dial.pipex.con

Half PINNT

Coordinator – Mrs Gillian Norris
Riverside Lodge
London Road
Whitehouses
Retford
Nottinghamshire DN22 7JG

National Nurses Nutrition Group

Membership Secretary – Ms Ann Marie Daniels
c/o BAPEN
P O Box 922
Maidenhead
Berks SL6 4SH

REFERENCES

British Association for Parenteral and Enteral Nutrition 1994 Organisation of nutritional support in hospitals. BAPEN, Maidenhead
British Association for Parenteral and Enteral Nutrition 1995 Home parenteral nutrition. BAPEN, Maidenhead
British Association for Parenteral and Enteral Nutrition 1996 Standards and guidelines for nutritional support of patients in hospitals. BAPEN, Maidenhead
Burnham W R 1995 The role of a nutrition support team. Artificial nutrition support in clinical practice. Edward Arnold, London
Clark L 1994 Safety first. Nursing Times 90(5): 64–68
Colagiovanni L 1997a Parenteral nutrition. Nursing Standard 12(9): 39–45
Colagiovanni L 1997b Parenteral nutrition and in line filtration. Nursing Times 93(34): 76–78
Cottee S 1995 Heparin lock practice in total parenteral nutrition. Professional Nurse 11(1): 25–29
Dudrick S J, Wilmore D W, Vars H M 1968 Long term total parenteral nutrition with growth, development and positive nitrogen balance. Surgery 64: 134–142
Elia M 1990a Enteral and parenteral nutrition in the community. BAPEN, Maidenhead
Elia M 1990b Artificial nutritional support. Medicine International 82: 3394
Elliott T S J 1993 Line associated bacteraemias. CDR Review 3(7): R91–R95
Elliott T S J, Faroqui M H, Armstrong R F, Hanson G C 1994 Guidelines for good practice in central venous catheterization. Journal of Hospital Infection 28: 163–176
Finnegan S, Oldfield K 1989 When eating is impossible – TPN in maintaining nutritional status. Professional Nurse 83(31): 58–59
Grant J P 1992 Handbook of total parenteral nutrition, 2nd edn. WB Saunders, Philadelphia
Hadfield R J, Sinclair D G, Houldsworth P E, Evans T W 1995 Effects of enteral and parenteral nutrition on gut mucosal permeability in the critically ill. American Journal of Respiratory Critical Care Medicine 152: 1545–1548
Hamilton H C 1993 Care improves while cost reduces. Professional Nurse 608: 592–596
Hamilton H C, O'Byrne M, Nicholai L 1995 Central lines inserted by CNS. Nursing Times 91(17): 38–39

Hehir D J, Stansby R C, Stuart R C, Dawson K J 1992 Catheterization of the subclavian vein. Hospital Update April: 295–299

Henry L 1997 Parenteral nutrition. Professional Nurse 13(1): 39–42

Keohane P, Atrill H, Northover J 1983 Effects of catheter tunnelling and nutrition nurse on reduced catheter sepsis during parenteral nutrition. Lancet 1: 1390

McWhirter J P, Pennington C R 1994 Incidence and recognition of malnutrition in hospital. British Medical Journal 308(6934): 945–948

Maki D G, Ringer M, Alvarado C J 1991 Prospective randomized trial of povidone-iodine, alcohol and chlorhexidine for prevention of infection associated with central venous and arterial catheters. Lancet 338: 339–343

Mallett J, Bailey C 1996 The Royal Marsden NHS Trust manual of clinical nursing procedures, 4th edn. Blackwell Science, London

Michie B 1988 Making sense of TPN. Nursing Times 84(20): 46–47

Millward D J, Bowtell J T, Pary P, Rennie M J 1994 Physical activity, protein metabolism and protein requirements. Proceedings of the Nutrition Society 53: 223–240

Murphy L M, Lipman T O 1987 CVC care in parenteral nutrition: a review. Journal of Parenteral & Enteral Nutrition 11(2): 190–201

Nehme A 1980 Nutritional support of the hospital patients: the team concept. Journal of American Medical Association 243(19): 1906–1908

Palmer D, MacFie J 1997 Alternative intake. Nursing Times 93(49): 62–66

Payne-James J, Wicks C 1994 Key facts in clinical nutrition. Churchill Medical Communications

PEN Group 1997 A pocket guide to clinical nutrition. British Dietetic Association

Pennington C R, Fawcett H, Macfie J, McWhirter J, Sizer T, Whitney S 1996 Current perspectives on parenteral nutrition in adults. BAPEN, Maidenhead

Price B, Levine E 1979 Permanent TPN: psychological and social response of the early stages. Journal of Parenteral & Enteral Nutrition 3(2): 48–52

Prior F 1992 Designing basic TPN regimes. A practical guide. Eastern General Hospital, Edinburgh

Raad, Holn D C, Gilbreath B J et al 1994 Prevention of CVC related infection by using maximal sterile barrier precautions during insertion. Infection Control and Hospital Epidemiology 15(4): 231–238

Roberts P H 1993 Simply a case of good practice. Professional Nurse 8(12): 775–779

Schofield W N 1985 Predicting basal metabolic rate. Clinical Nutrition 44: 1–19

Springett J, Murrey C 1994 Direct input. Nursing Times 90(17): 48–52

Stilwell B 1992 TPN at home. Community Outlook August 2: 18–19

Wood S 1991 A life saving technique. Primary Health Care July: 20–23

Wood S, Charles K 1997 Demanding supply. Nursing Times 93(34): 70–71

Yeung C, May J, Hughes R 1988 Infection rates for single lumen vs triple lumen subclavian catheters. Infection Control and Hospital Epidemiology 9(4): 154–158

Paediatric intravenous therapy in practice

Karen Bravery

CHAPTER 15

INTRODUCTION

The aim of this chapter is to identify aspects of intravenous (i.v.) therapy that relate specifically to paediatrics. A variety of i.v. therapies are administered to children, including i.v. fluids, drugs, chemotherapy, parenteral nutrition, blood and blood product administration. Many of the basic principles for the safe administration of i.v. therapy apply irrespective of age and are covered elsewhere in this book. However, the child has unique developmental and emotional needs, anatomical and physiological differences, and there are specific factors to be considered to safeguard the child receiving i.v. therapy. The nurse administering this type of therapy should be skilled and knowledgeable in basic i.v. techniques and child development (Wheeler & Frey 1995).

PAEDIATRIC FLUID BALANCE

This section will highlight the differences between adults and children in relation to infusion therapy. Children have unique physical characteristics that affect their ability to cope with environmental stresses and to manage the metabolism, absorption, distribution and excretion of drugs and solutions (Wheeler & Frey 1995). The child, especially when ill, is dependent on his care-giver (parent or nurse) to supply his fluid needs either orally or intravenously. Even a relatively minor illness such as diarrhoea and vomiting can lead to a severe fluid imbalance. Furthermore, the detrimental effects of vomiting, diarrhoea and reduced fluid intake appear more rapidly in children (Styne 1994).

The younger the child, the greater is the risk of fluid and electrolyte imbalance, fluid overload and congestive cardiac failure. Even the smallest error in i.v. fluid administration can have serious consequences (Frey 1993).

Physical characteristics of children

Compared with adults, children have:

- a greater fluid requirement per kg of body weight
- an increased basal metabolic rate
- increased fluid in the extracellular fluid space
- increased insensible fluid and evaporative losses
- increased total body sodium and chloride
- decreased total body potassium, magnesium and phosphate
- a higher turnover of fluid
- immature kidney function
- greater circulating blood volume per kg of body weight and smaller absolute blood volume
- increased body surface area and different distribution
- increased caloric requirements
- a smaller cardiovascular system.

The body requires a constant supply of water to sustain life. In the healthy child, the body's requirement for water is met by a normal intake of fluid and food. The child's intake is regulated by thirst and hunger. In health, body fluid loss is achieved via the lungs, skin, urine and faeces. Homeostasis, a balance between fluid intake and output, is maintained by the movement of fluid and electrolytes across the cellular membrane and the excretion of the products of metabolism and excess electrolytes (also see Ch. 3). Imbalance or failure to maintain homeostasis may occur as a result of illness in the child, e.g. fever, diarrhoea, vomiting or burns. Dehydration ensues more rapidly in children due to the higher fluid turnover, increased metabolic rate and greater ratio of skin surface area to body fluid volume (Marks 1994).

At birth, 75–80% of the infant's total body weight comprises water (Livesley 1996). The percentage of body fluid decreases to an adult level of 60% at 1–2 years of age (Marks 1994). In the infant, most of this body fluid is contained in the extracellular compartment (Hazinski 1992). Consequently, the infant has greater levels of total body sodium and chloride and lower levels of potassium, magnesium and phosphate in comparision with an adult (Wheeler & Frey 1995). Approximately half of this fluid is exchanged daily (Hazinski 1988). Extracellular fluid is situated outside the cells and may be either blood plasma (intravascular) or the fluid that bathes the cells (interstitial fluid) (McVicar & Clancy 1992). A decrease in intravascular volume in an infant as a consequence of reduced intake or increased output may rapidly lead to dehydration and reduced systemic perfusion. Conversely, the older child has more body fluid in the intracellular compartment (fluid within the body cells). Reduced fluid intake or increased fluid loss will not compromise intravascular fluid volume or systemic perfusion significantly (Hazinski 1988).

The basal metabolic rate of an infant is double that of an adult in relation to body weight. The increased metabolic rate combined with rapid growth rate results in a greater daily caloric requirement in children. The need for calories increases in the presence of fever and illness (Wheeler & Frey 1995).

The daily fluid requirement per kg of body weight of an infant is three times greater than that of an adult. The child's fluid requirement will increase in the presence of stress and fever.

The body surface area (BSA) of a child is proportionally greater than that of an adult. The head comprises 20% of BSA in an infant compared with 7–9% in an adult. This results in increased surface heat and water loss and greater fluid losses from injuries (Davenport 1996).

Assessment of hydration in paediatrics

History

Assessment of hydration begins with a history from the parent or care-giver. The pre-illness weight should be noted as this will be used to calculate the child's fluid requirements. The history from the parents will aid the determination of the child's current hydration status. The following should be discussed and recorded in the nursing care plan:

- the child's symptoms prior to admission, including the presence of any diarrhoea, vomiting or nausea
- fluid intake and urine output prior to admission
- the child's dietary and fluid preferences and any cultural or religious observances
- the child's normal pattern of elimination.

Physical assessment

This should include assessment of:

- weight and height
- vital signs
- skin condition and turgor
- cutaneous perfusion
- moistness of mucous membranes
- the presence or absence of tears when crying; whether the eyes are sunken
- whether the fontanelles, if present, are flat or bulging
- presence or absence of palpable pulses
- urine output
- neurological status
- capillary refill.

Weight and height Both the weight and height will be needed to determine the child's fluid requirements. Calculations for fluid requirements are based on either weight or surface area. The child's actual weight is subtracted from the child's pre-illness weight. This will highlight either a deficit or an excess of fluid as 1 g of weight lost or gained equals 1 ml of fluid.

The child should be weighed daily, preferably at the same time of day using the same scales, without clothing. Any subsequent change in weight should be documented in the child's record. A gain or loss of 50 g in an infant, 200 g in a child and 500 g in an adolescent should be reported to the medical staff (Wheeler & Frey 1995).

Vital signs Evaluation of vital signs (see Table 15.1) should be based on 'resting' information and measurements. The vital signs of the child 'at rest' can then be compared with those when active. It is normal for a child's heart and respiratory rate to increase when upset and decrease when asleep. It is important to remember that hypotension is frequently a late sign of shock in children, and a normal heart and respiratory rate in a critically ill child may herald cardiorespiratory arrest (Hazinski 1992).

Table 15.2 presents alterations in vital signs associated with fluid volume deficit, fluid overload or electrolyte imbalance.

Signs of dehydration in children These are presented in Table 15.3.

Fluid volume deficit (dehydration)

Dehydration occurs when the total output of all fluids and electrolytes exceeds the

Table 15.1 Normal values of vital signs (Testerman 1989)

Age group	Heart rate (beats/min)	Respiratory (rate/min)	Blood pressure Systolic	Blood pressure Diastolic	Normal temperature (all ages) (°C) Oral	Normal temperature (all ages) (°C) Axillary
Infants	120–160	30–60	74–100	50–70	36.4–37.4	35.6–36.6
Toddlers	90–140	24–40	80–112	50–80		
Pre-schoolers	80–110	22–34	82–110	50–78		
School-aged	75–100	18–30	84–120	54–80		
Adolescent	60–90	12–16	94–140	62–88		

Table 15.2 Alterations in vital signs associated with fluid volume deficit, fluid overload or electrolyte imbalance (Wheeler & Frey 1995, Styne 1994, Hazinski 1988)

Vital sign	Alteration
Temperature	↑ initially, ↓ as dehydration progresses
Pulse/heart rate	Change in rate or rhythm may indicate alteration in circulating blood volume or electrolyte imbalance
	Weak, thready pulse = fluid volume depletion
	Bounding pulse = fluid overload
	Mild dehydration = normal
	↑ = moderate/severe dehydration
Respiratory rate	↑ rate = fluid depletion or overload
	Mild dehydration = normal
	↑ deep and rapid = moderate/severe dehydration
	↑ = acidosis, ↓ = alkalosis
Blood pressure	↓ = fluid volume depletion
	↑ = fluid overload
	Mild dehydration = normal
	Orthostatic hypotension = moderate dehydration
	↓ = severe dehydration

total fluid intake (Hazinski 1988). There are two components for assessment of dehydration: the severity or degree and the type (Davenport 1996). The severity is determined by the percentage of total body weight lost (Table 15.4) and the type of dehydration is classified according to the plasma sodium (Table 15.5).

Hypertonic/hypernatraemic dehydration

This form of dehydration arises when the loss of free water exceeds the loss of sodium. In this instance, fluid moves from the interstitial and cellular compartments into the intravascular compartment. As the intravascular volume is maintained, there are no signs of circulatory failure unless accompanied by large fluid losses (Hazinski 1988). The causes of this type of dehydration include diabetes insipidus, fever, hyperventilation and the administration of high-sodium-content oral fluids to an infant with diarrhoea (Wheeler & Frey 1995).

The child will appear dehydrated, but the signs will not be obvious and the severity of dehydration may be underestimated (Styne 1994). Additional signs include doughy skin, irritability, high-pitched cry and seizures. Hypertonic dehydration may be accompanied by hyperglycaemia and hypocalcaemia (Wheeler & Frey 1995).

Treatment Rapid rehydration may cause cerebral oedema and seizures. A rapid fall in serum sodium will precipitate a fall in serum osmolarity and a consequent shift of fluid from the intravascular compartment into the interstitial and cellular compartments (Hazinski 1988, Styne 1994). The serum sodium should be reduced at a rate of not more than 10 mEq/L per 24 hours (Styne 1994). The fluid deficit should be replaced slowly over 48 hours (Wheeler & Frey 1995).

Isotonic/isonatraemic dehydration

Isotonic dehydration occurs when the losses of sodium and water are proportional. There is no movement of fluid between the intracellular and extracellular compartments. There will be a corresponding fall in plasma volume as the total loss is from the extracellular compartment (Wheeler & Frey 1995). Causes of isotonic dehydra-

Table 15.3 Signs of dehydration in children (Hazinski 1988, 1992, Styne 1994, Wheeler & Frey 1995)

| Sign | Degree of dehydration | | | Comment |
	Mild	Moderate	Severe	
Skin condition	Normal	Cool	Cool or cold	
Skin turgor	Normal	↓ slightly	↓	Assess skin turgor on abdomen or inner thigh
Cutaneous perfusion	Normal	Normal	↓ Skin cyanosed and mottled	
Mucous membranes	Moist	Dry	Very dry	Longitudinal fissure on tongue
Tears	Present	Present/absent	Absent	Infant > 3 months
Eyes	Sunken	Sunken	Sunken	Dark circles around the eyes
Fontanelles	Normal	Slightly depressed	Sunken	Open until 2 years of age. Assess with infant sitting
Palpable pulses	Present	Present/weak	↓	
Urine output	Normal	Oliguria	Anuria or severe oliguria	Normal urine output Infant = 2 ml/kg body weight Child = 1–2 ml/kg body weight Adolescent = 0.5–1 ml/kg body weight
Neurological status				Difficult to assess as unable to answer questions re. orientation
Infant/young child	Alert, restless	Restless or lethargic – but irritable or drowsy	Drowsy May be comatose Usually conscious	
Older child	Alert, restless	Alert (usually)	↓ Level of consciousness	
Capillary refill	Normal	Delayed	Sluggish	

Table 15.4 The degree of dehydration as a percentage of total body weight lost (Hazinski 1988, Wheeler & Frey 1995)

Degree of dehydration	Percentage of total body weight lost
Mild	5% or 50 ml/kg of body weight lost
Moderate	5–10% or 100 ml/kg of body weight lost
Severe	> 10% or 150 ml/kg of body weight lost

tion include diarrhoea and vomiting, intestinal obstruction and reduced fluid intake. The child will appear clinically dehydrated.

Treatment An initial bolus of sodium chloride 0.9% or Ringer's lactate solution may be given at 20 ml/kg of body weight followed by maintenance fluids. The

Table 15.5 Type of dehydration vs. plasma sodium level (Davenport 1996)

Type of dehydration	Plasma sodium level
Hypertonic/hypernatraemic	> 150 mmol/L
Isotonic/isonatraemic	130–150 mmol/L
Hypotonic/hyponatraemic	< 130 mmol/L

deficit should be replaced over 24 hours – 50% over 8 hours and 50% over 16 hours. (Wheeler & Frey 1995).

Hypotonic/hyponatraemic dehydration

Hypotonic dehydration occurs when the loss of sodium is greater than the loss of water. The extracellular fluid shifts into the intracellular compartment in this situation. As the fluid loss is primarily from the intravascular space, the signs of inadequate intravascular volume will be more pronounced even with a mild fluid deficit (Hazinski 1988). This type of dehydration may occur in response to the administration of an oral hypotonic solution to replace fluid loss from diarrhoea and vomiting (Wheeler & Frey 1995). Other causes include inappropriate antidiuretic hormone secretion and excessive dilution of milk feeds in infants (Styne 1994). The clinical signs of dehydration will be present. Additional signs include lethargy, coma and seizures (Wheeler & Frey 1995).

Treatment Treat as for isotonic dehydration with the addition of sodium. If hyponatraemia is severe, sodium chloride 3% may be administered until the plasma sodium level reaches 120 mEq/L (Styne 1994, Wheeler & Frey 1995). The serum sodium should not rise more than 2 mEq/L per hour.

Replacement (deficit) therapy

The goal of replacement or deficit therapy is:

- to maintain intravascular volume and systemic perfusion
- to replace volume deficit and ongoing losses
- to provide maintenance requirements (Hazinski 1988).

Maintenance of intravascular volume and systemic perfusion

The intravascular volume may be restored using a crystalline (sodium chloride 0.9% or Ringer's solution) or a colloid solution (human albumin). A fluid bolus of either solution of 15–20 ml/kg is administered over 20–30 minutes. Additional boluses may be required if the child's condition does not improve. Sodium chloride 0.9% or Ringer's solution are widely used in the USA. In the UK the use of colloids in the form of human albumin solution 4.5% is advocated. There is little data to support the use of either solution (Davenport 1996).

Emergency venous access In an emergency situation, significant delays can occur in the administration of drugs and fluids in the shocked child. Ideally two large-bore peripheral cannulae should be placed. This is difficult if the child is well-covered, with collapsed, barely visible or palpable veins. There are three options to obtain emergency venous access (Davenport 1996):

Percutaneous central venous access Obtaining access via the subclavian, internal jugular or femoral veins is more difficult in children and associated with a risk of increased complications (Manley 1988). Although a quick method of establishing venous access the technique is dependent on the availability of staff experienced in this technique.

Peripheral venous cut-down The most commonly used cut-down sites in children are the saphenous vein of the foot and the radial vein of the forearm (Frey 1993). This method of establishing emergency venous access is utilized infrequently, due to the increasing use of percutaneous central venous access. However, this is a simple and reliable means of venous access in an emergency situation (Davenport 1996).

Intraosseous infusion This is the infusion of drugs, fluids or blood directly into the bone marrow. It is accomplished by the use of an intraosseous needle, bone marrow aspiration needle or a lumbar puncture needle in infants. This method is a quick, simple means of establishing venous access in children (Manley 1988).

The proximal tibia is the usual site of insertion for an intraosseous infusion. Other sites include the distal tibial and distal femoral marrow. Intraosseous infusion should be instituted early in an emergency situation, not after multiple attempts at peripheral venous access. This wastes valuable time during resuscitation. Intraosseous infusion should be utilized after two failed attempts at peripheral venous cannulation (Manley 1988).

Replacement of volume deficit and ongoing losses

Replacement of volume deficit is combined with maintenance requirements (see Table 15.6). The amount of fluid used to restore the intravascular volume should be subtracted and ongoing losses added (Wheeler & Frey 1995).

Ongoing losses The presence of fever will increase the insensible water loss by 10 ml/kg per degree elevation above 37°C. Hyperventilation, diaphoresis, phototherapy and radiant warmers may increase insensible losses by 50–70% (Hazinski 1988). Normal insensible losses are 300 ml/m^2 body surface area per day plus urine output in a child (Hazinski 1992). All fluid losses should be accounted for, measured and recorded on a fluid balance chart. Fluid losses may include diarrhoea, nasogastric aspirate, pleural or wound drainage and blood used during sampling. Losses should be replaced like for like (Davenport 1996).

Fluid requirements will be reduced in cardiorespiratory failure, renal failure and raised intracranial pressure, as these conditions may cause fluid retention. In renal failure, fluid is restricted to insensible losses plus urine and other measured output to maintain fluid balance (Hazinski 1988).

Urine output A relatively small decrease in urine output in a child may be significant and may indicate compromised renal function or perfusion (Hazinski 1992). Infants have a limited ability to concentrate urine and a reduced glomerular filtration rate – 30 ml/min per m^2 at birth and 100 ml/min per m^2 at 9 months of age. This affects their ability to cope with large volumes of water and solutes and affects conservation of the former in deficit (Davenport 1996). Measurement of specific gravity in infants is inaccurate and should not be used to assess hydration.

The collection and measurement of urine pose unique problems in children, especially if they are not toilet-trained. Urine collection devices that adhere to the skin can be used. These are difficult to apply and keep in place in children. If the child is

Table 15.6 Maintenance requirements (Wheeler & Frey 1995)

Amount of deficit	Formula for calculation of fluid required
Mild (5%)	Maintenance + (maintenance × 0.5)
Moderate (10%)	Maintenance + (maintenance × 1.0)
Severe (15%)	Maintenance + (maintenance × 1.5)

Table 15.7 Maintenance requirements based on body weight (Davenport 1996)

Body weight (kg)	Fluid requirement per 24 hours
3–10	100 ml/kg
10–20	1000 ml + 50 ml per extra kg over 10
>20	1500 ml + 20 ml per extra kg over 20

in nappies, the weight of the dry nappy can be subtracted from the weight of the wet nappy to obtain the volume of urine passed. The amount in grams will equal the amount of urine voided in millilitres. The seriously ill child will be catheterized.

All intake and output must be recorded on a fluid balance chart. This chart is a valuable tool in the assessment of fluid requirements (Frey 1993).

Provision of maintenance requirements

Maintenance requirements are calculated using the child's body weight in kilograms or the body surface area (Davenport 1996, Hazinski 1988). A third method also used is based on the actual calories that the child metabolizes. Most units utilize body weight (see Table 15.7) or surface area to calculate maintenance requirements.

Using body weight to calculate maintenance requirements may overestimate the fluid needed for an infant and underestimate that required for an adolescent (Hazinski 1988).

Maintenance requirements based on body surface are calculated using the following formula: $1500 \, \text{ml/m}^2$ per day (Davenport 1996, Hazinski 1988). This method may overestimate the fluid necessary for a small infant or child (Hazinski 1988).

Neonatal fluid requirements The maintenance fluid needs of newborn, low-birthweight and premature infants differ. The smaller, more immature infant has a greater total body water content. The total body water of a term infant is 70%, while a 28-week gestation infant has a total body water content of 85%. This must be accounted for when calculating the fluid requirements of neonates (Frey 1993).

Glucose 5 or 10% is frequently used for maintenance fluids in neonates, as they are at risk of developing hypoglycaemia as a result of decreased glycogen stores and impaired gluconeogenesis (Davenport 1996).

Flow control

Administration of intravenous fluids and drugs to children necessitates precision and flow at a constant rate. Even the smallest error can have serious consequences. Children require controlled administration to avoid overinfusion of solutions or overdose of drugs. An electronic infusion device is essential in paediatric i.v. therapy (Livesley 1996).

An electronic infusion device for use in paediatrics should incorporate the following features (Livesley 1996, Wheeler & Frey 1995):

- greater than 95% accuracy
- capability to be programmed in ml/h or multiples of 0.1 ml/h
- volume limit facility to reduce the risk of overinfusion
- alarms to indicate end of infusion, pump malfunction and absence of flow
- low occlusion pressure alarm to detect extravasation
- variable pressure facility that can be set by the operator with the ability to take

account of the length and diameter of the administration set, viscosity of the solution and flow rate
- childproof characteristics: lockable and tamper-proof programming pads.

Volume control infusion devices

These devices are not recommended for use in paediatric infusion therapy. They regulate flow rate and alarm when the delivery of fluid is interrupted. Use of this device will lead to frequent occlusion alarms generated by the activity of the child and by the additional pressure required to overcome the higher intravascular pressure of small veins and the resistance exerted by small-gauge cannulae and microbore tubing. If there is no variable pressure facility, these pumps may allow high pressures and infiltration may ensue without alarm (Wheeler & Frey 1995).

Variable pressure infusion devices

These pumps exert varying degrees of pressure when resistance is met during an infusion. The pressure can be set by the operator to alarm if pressure rises. This feature will identify small rises in pressure that may indicate an extravasation (Livesley 1996).

Syringe pumps

Syringe pumps are often used in paediatrics for the administration of intermittent doses of drugs. The syringe pump used for this purpose should have a variable pressure facility and accommodate different sized syringes required for accuracy of drug dose in children. One advantage of this infusion device is that the tubing has a lower prime volume. A conventional paediatric i.v. administration set will require fluid volumes of 20–30 ml to flush the set after drug administration (Axton & Hall 1994, Axton & Fugate 1987, Wink 1991). Use of a syringe pump will reduce the amount of fluid administered to the child from frequent drug administration (Axton & Hall 1994).

A potential disadvantage of this system is the risk of free flow or siphonage leading to overdosage of the drug infusing (Southern & Read 1994). This will occur if the syringe pump is more than 80 cm above the infusion site or if the syringe is incorrectly loaded into the pump. Anti-siphon tubing is recommended to guard against free flow from syringe pumps (Southern & Read 1994).

Paediatric intravenous administration sets

Administration sets for use in children should incorporate an in-line calibrated volume control chamber (Wheeler & Frey 1995). This will minimize the amount of fluid administered to the child if free flow of fluid occurs (Hazinski 1992). All administration sets should be used with an infusion pump to prevent free flow of infusion fluid and potential overinfusion.

INTRAVENOUS DRUG ADMINISTRATION IN PAEDIATRICS

Safe administration of intravenous drugs to children requires careful calculation of dosage. The priming volume of the access device and all tubing required should be accounted for to ensure safe delivery of the drug. In addition, the method of administration should be carefully chosen to avoid excessive administration of fluid.

Drug dosage calculation

Drug dosage in children is commonly calculated in milligrams or micrograms per kilogram of body weight (mg/kg or mcg/kg) (Ellis 1995, Frey 1993). The calculation of drug dosage based on age is inaccurate as there are wide variations in children of similar ages as regards body weight. Use of this method should be restricted to life-threatening situations where there is little time available for more accurate calculation (Ellis 1995). Weight is the most frequently used method employed to calculate drug dosage. In contrast to age, this will take account of the child's body mass (Ellis 1995). An alternative method involves the use of body surface area, and this is used to calculate cytotoxic drug doses.

The following formula is commonly used to calculate the amount of drug to be administered to a child:

$$Amount\ to\ be\ given = \frac{dose\ desired}{dose\ available} \times vehicle\ (amount\ diluted\ in)$$

For example, if the dose of amikacin to be administered is 80 mg and the drug is available in a vial containing 100 mg in 2 ml, then the amount to be given is:

$$\frac{80}{100} \times 2 = 1.6\ ml$$

Paediatric nurses are frequently required to convert grams (g) to milligrams (mg) and milligrams to micrograms (mcg). Care should be taken to ensure that no mistakes are made during conversions. Giving a dose of 100 mg when 100 mcg is what is required can have grave consequences.

Displacement volumes

This must be accounted for when reconstituting drugs for administration to children. Failure to account for the displacement volume will lead to an incorrect dose of the drug being given (Ellis 1995).

The displacement volume of a chloramphenicol 1 g vial is 0.8 ml. To reconstitute the drug, 9.2 ml of water is added to a 1 g vial of chloramphenicol. A volume of 10 ml of solution will be present in the vial after reconstitution. Conversely, if 10 ml is added to the vial and 10 ml of the reconstituted solution is given to the child, 0.8 ml will remain in the vial. The child will not have received the dose of 1 g (Ellis 1995).

In adults, it is common practice to administer a complete ampoule or vial of a drug. Only a portion of an ampoule or vial is required in paediatrics (Ellis 1995). If the dose to be administered to a child exceeds 1 ampoule or vial, it should be confirmed by consulting the medical staff or pharmacy department.

Method of administration

Intravenous drugs may be administered to children by direct bolus injection or by means of intermittent or continuous infusion. When administering i.v. drugs, the catheter volume of the access device should be accounted for to avoid retention of the drug within the device. Failure to clear a drug from the access device may have serious consequences if the retained drug is inadvertently flushed into the child at a later date. Ben-Arush & Berant (1996) reported the retention of an anaesthetic drug cocktail within an implantable port in a 2-year-old child following sedation for radiotherapy. Failure to flush the device led to collapse of the child when the device was reheparinized on return to the ward.

All i.v. drugs should be followed immediately with a sodium chloride 0.9% flush or any other compatible solution to clear the drug from the access device. The priming volume of any additional tubing that the drug is administered through should be considered when calculating the amount of sodium chloride 0.9% required to ensure that the whole drug dose is administered to the child.

Small volumes of i.v. drugs (< 3 ml) may require further dilution with a compatible solution according to the manufacturer's recommendations. This will prevent retention of the drug within the i.v. tubing.

Intravenous drugs for infusion may be added to a burette of an administration set or given in a syringe by means of a syringe pump. A burette can be used in older children able to tolerate the extra 20–30 ml needed to clear the administration set of drug. Once added to the burette, the drug should be further diluted in accordance with the manufacturer's instructions. When calculating the rate of the infusion, the flush volume should be added to the drug volume after dilution to give the total amount to be infused.

The flush must be administered at the same rate as the drug, as some of the drug will be retained in the infusion tubing (Axton & Hall 1994). If the flush rate is increased, the retained drug will be given rapidly and may result in speed shock and increased risk of side-effects (Hicks-Keen 1995, Whitman 1995).

A syringe pump should be used for drug administration in infants, toddlers and older children who are fluid-restricted. The tubing used with a syringe pump has a lower prime volume. The syringe containing the drug may be 'piggy-backed' via an extension tubing to the primary set. Luer-lock connections must be used to achieve this connection to avoid disconnection. If the drug is incompatible with the primary solution, a flush of compatible solution will be given before the drug.

PERIPHERAL VENOUS ACCESS

The age and developmental level of the child will often dictate which site is used for peripheral venous access, which is more difficult to achieve in children as the veins are smaller and often obscured by subcutaneous fat. This is complicated by the fact that the child will resist attempts to establish venous access and will not understand the need for a cannula. The main goal of peripheral i.v. access is to provide the treatment with maximum safety and efficiency whilst promoting the child's developmental tasks (Wheeler & Frey 1995). This section covers the management of peripheral venous access and potential problems specific to children.

Intravenous sites used in children

The ideal site for peripheral venous access in children is the one that interferes least with the child's developmental level (O'Brien 1991) (see Table 15.8 and Fig. 15.1 for details of intravenous sites used in children).

Scalp

One advantage of this particular site is that the scalp veins are superficial and easily visualized, especially in the newborn (Wilson 1992). These are readily accessible until the age of 12–18 months when the hair follicles mature and the skin thickens (Frey 1993). Use of this site leaves the hands free. This is important for the child who sucks his fingers or thumb for comfort. However, there are several disadvantages associated with the use of scalp veins. The arteries of the scalp are located in close proximity to the veins and may be hidden within suture lines. This makes pulsation difficult to feel (Wheeler & Frey 1995). Peripheral venous access devices placed in the scalp are difficult to secure and are associated with an increased risk of dislodgement and subsequent infiltration (Frey 1993, Wheeler & Frey 1995). Use of this site can be distressing to parents as the scalp is shaved. Without adequate explanation, parents may think that the infusion enters the brain (Wheeler & Frey 1995).

Table 15.8 Intravenous sites used in children (Wheeler & Frey 1995)

Site	Age	Veins used
Scalp	Infant, toddler	Superficial temporal, frontal, occipital, postauricular, supraorbital, posterior facial
Foot	Infant, toddler	Saphenous, median, marginal, dorsal arch
Hand	Toddler through adolescent	Metacarpal, dorsal venous arch, tributaries of cephalic and basilic
Forearm	All ages	Cephalic, basilic, median, antebrachial
Antecubital	All ages	Cephalic, basilic, median

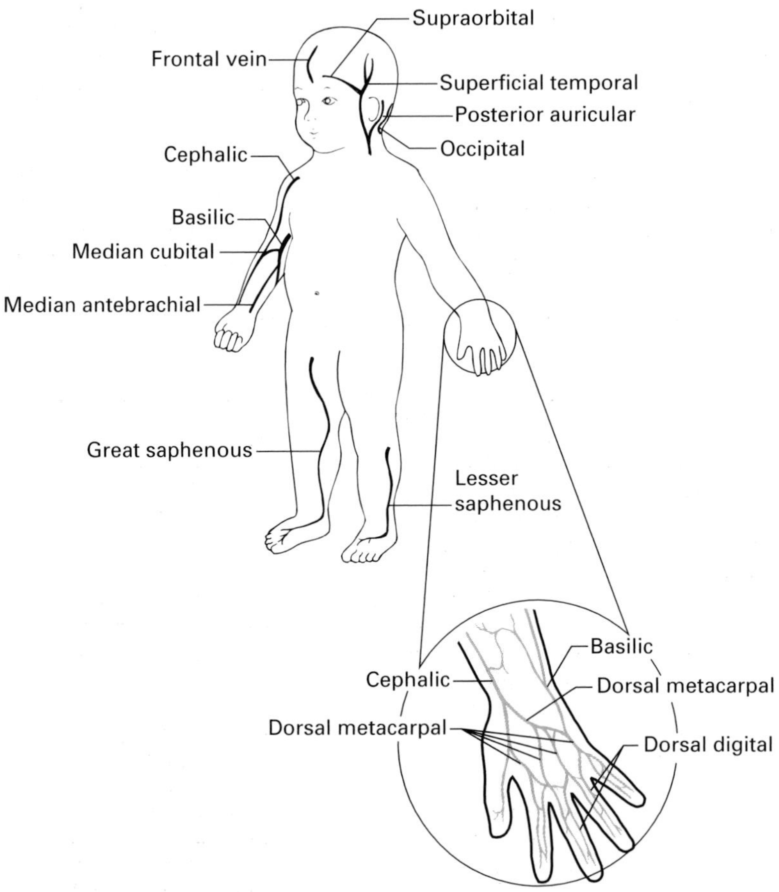

Fig. 15.1 Intravenous sites used in children.

Foot

This site can be used until the child is able to walk. A cannula placed in the foot of an active, mobile toddler may be difficult to maintain. Although the large veins of the foot are visible and accessible, the curve of the foot may make venous entry and catheter advancement problematic, especially at the ankle (Wheeler & Frey 1995). The foot can be used if other sites are not available, e.g. burns or trauma (Tietjen 1990).

Hand and arm

These are the most commonly used sites for peripheral venous access in children. The non-dominant arm should be used where possible and the thumb-sucking hand of an infant avoided (O'Brien 1991). The antecubital veins can be difficult to access in chubby babies and toddlers, whereas the veins located on the hand are often easier to cannulate (Wheeler & Frey 1995). The veins of the inner wrist are easily visible and not obscured by fat but difficult to stabilize across the wrist joint. In addition, cannulation of this site is more painful (Tietjen 1990).

Additional sites

The external jugular or femoral vein can be utilized for venous access if there are no peripheral sites available (Murdoch & Bingham 1990). These sites may be used for emergency venous access.

Peripheral venous access devices (Table 15.9)

The device of choice in the 1970s was the steel winged infusion needle. This device has largely been replaced by plastic, over-the-needle cannulae which can remain in situ for longer periods (Frey 1993). Winged infusion needles are easily dislodged and are best reserved for blood sampling or for an infusion of short duration (Wheeler & Frey 1995).

The most commonly used device for peripheral infusion therapy is the over-the-needle cannula. Some cannulae have wings to aid insertion and taping of the device. Current practice dictates that the smallest gauge, shortest length cannula capable of administering the prescribed therapy should be used (Weinstein 1993). Viscous fluids such as blood may need to be infused via syringe pump or infusion pump designed to deliver blood to overcome the resistance of small cannulae (Frey 1993).

Table 15.9 Peripheral venous access devices used in children (Frey 1993, Wheeler & Frey 1995)

Device	Uses	Comments
Winged infusion set Butterfly needle Scalp vein needle 27–19 gauge (steel)	Infusions of short duration Blood sampling and single bolus drug administration	Easily dislodged Increased risk of infiltration/extravasation
Cannula 26–14 gauge (e.g. Teflon, Vialon)	Neonates: 26 and 24 gauge Child: 24 and 22 gauge Older child: 20 gauge + i.v. fluid and drug administration	Can remain in situ longer than winged infusion device Less risk of infiltration/ extravasation
Midline over-the-needle catheter (polyurethane or silicone)	Used for i.v. therapies of 2–6 weeks' duration i.v. fluid and drug administration	Only suitable for isotonic and slightly hypertonic solutions and drugs NB: If vesicant/hypertonic solutions are to be infused, a central venous access device is recommended

A midline over-the-needle catheter should be considered if therapy will last between 2 and 6 weeks (Wheeler & Frey 1995). A midline catheter is commonly inserted via the basilic, cephalic or median cubital veins in the antecubital fossa in the arm. The catheter tip is in the upper arm in the axilla, distal to the shoulder. In neonates and children, the lower limbs may be used with the tip terminating in the mid- to upper thigh (Hadaway 1995). This type of venous access has been mainly used in neonates (BeVier & Rice 1994). The midline catheter can be used for the administration of i.v. fluids and medications suitable for infusion via a peripheral vein. However, vesicant infusions or solutions > dextrose 10% should not be infused through this device (Hadaway 1995).

Obtaining peripheral venous access in children

The principles of cannulation and venepuncture are detailed in Chapter 9. Specific considerations for achieving successful cannulation in children are discussed in the following section. The ability to cannulate children demands patience and practice.

Environment

The child's bed or room should be considered a 'safe' place and painful procedures performed elsewhere, e.g. the treatment room (Frey 1993, Wheeler & Frey 1995). Babies, especially premature infants, should be kept warm throughout the procedure. The infant's large surface area and thin layer of subcutaneous fat predispose to excessive heat loss. Cold stress can be life-threatening for premature infants (Duck 1997). This can be prevented by the use of an overhead heater or blankets or by working through the portholes of an incubator when establishing peripheral venous access (Tietjen 1990).

Restraining the child

Adequate assistance is vital for successful venepuncture in children. Two people are needed to immobilize the site and secure the device once inserted. The parents should be involved but should not restrain their child. The parents' role should be one of comfort and support throughout the procedure (O'Brien 1991). An infant or toddler can be wrapped in a blanket to aid immobilization and facilitate the procedure. Venepuncture is distressing for both the child and person performing the procedure and number of attempts should be limited to two.

Scalp vein insertion

The scalp around the vein insertion site will need to be shaved prior to placing the cannula. Some parents may like to keep the hair (French 1995). A rubber band placed around an infant's head will aid distension of the scalp veins (Frey 1993). Attach a piece of tape to the band to allow for easy removal (French 1995). Alternatively, the vein may be occluded distally using a finger (Murdoch & Bingham 1990). The access device should be inserted in the direction of venous flow, towards the heart (Wheeler & Frey 1995).

Hand, arm and foot

There are various methods that will aid visibility and distension of the child's veins. The extremities may be warmed by encouraging the child to play in warm water prior to the procedure, as warming causes the vein to dilate. Other methods to increase visibility include positioning the limb lower than the rest of the body and the use of a transilluminator placed beneath the limb (O'Brien 1991, Wheeler & Frey 1995).

Difficulty in advancing the catheter

The presence of valves or venous spasm may prevent advancement of the cannula into the vein. Venous spasm occurs frequently in small veins (Wheeler & Frey 1995). If flashback of blood ceases, wait for the child to calm down and venous spasm to decrease, then flush with sodium chloride 0.9% as the cannula is advanced (Murdoch & Bingham 1990). Flushing will be facilitated by attaching a T-connector or low prime extension set to the cannula. If blood return is absent, often as a result of the small size of the vein and small gauge of cannula, the device can then be flushed with sodium chloride 0.9% to confirm correct placement. This method also reduces the risk of clotting of the device during the procedure (Wheeler & Frey 1995).

Stabilization of the cannula

Once the cannula has been placed, it is essential to secure it to prevent dislodgement (Livesley 1996). The device must also be protected from the child's attempts to manipulate or remove it. The child will be unable to comprehend the importance of not manipulating the device.

Scalp

A cotton wool ball placed under the T-connector and around the cannula may help to stabilize the device on the rounded shape of the head (French 1995). An open-ended paper cup or medicine cup cut in half is often used to protect the catheter from dislodgement (French 1995, Wilson 1992). Any sharp cut edges require covering with gauze to protect the child's skin.

Dressings and tape

The ideal dressing should allow for observation of the site for signs of phlebitis and infiltration and should minimize the risk of dislodgement of the peripheral cannula (Livesley 1996). Dressings used should be sterile, as the use of non-sterile tape over the insertion site may increase the risk of infection (Oldman 1991). A sterile protective dressing with high moisture permeability that keeps the insertion site dry and free of contamination is recommended to prevent proliferation of skin flora under the dressing (Livesley 1993, Wheeler et al 1991b). An important consideration when choosing a dressing is whether paediatric sizes are available. The dressing used should be easy to apply, remove and conform to the shape of the limb and peripheral cannula. A gauze dressing offers less protection from manipulation by the child. Children are naturally inquisitive and a gauze dressing may be easily removed along with the cannula! A low prime extension set attached to the cannula will reduce direct manipulation of the cannula during drug administration and flushing procedures. Either the extension tubing or the infusion tubing should be coiled and taped to the child's limb to reduce tension on the cannula site by inadvertent tugging and movement by the child.

Splints

If the cannula is at a point of flexion, the limb should be splinted to provide additional security and aid immobilization of the limb. The splint used should allow for frequent inspection of the site and be easily removed to aid detection of pressure points (Livesley 1993). The use of a splint will restrict the child's movement, minimize the risk of dislodgement of the cannula and help to prevent undue manipulation of the site and dressing by the child. The splint should be shaped to maintain joint configuration. If bandages are used to apply the splint, the child's fingers and toes should remain visible to allow checks of circulation. The use of bandages will reduce the visibility of the site.

Maintaining patency of peripheral cannuale

Whether sodium chloride 0.9% or heparinized saline should be used to maintain patency of peripheral venous access devices remains controversial. There have been many studies in adults comparing the two flush solutions (Goode et al 1991). However, it remains questionable whether these results can be generalized to paediatric populations. Four paediatric studies found sodium chloride 0.9% to be as effective as heparinized saline and found no difference in the duration of use and complication rates (Hanrahan et al 1994, Kleiber et al 1993, Lombardi et al 1998, McMullen et al 1993). Kleiber et al (1993) maintained that the technique is as important as the flush solution and advocated the use of positive pressure whilst clamping the extension tubing or T-connector. By contrast, a more recent study found that there was more patency and less tenderness associated with the use of heparinized saline (Gyr et al 1995). Pain and discomfort may be a feature of use of heparinized saline (Kleiber et al 1993, McMullen et al 1993). In addition, sodium chloride 0.9% may be less effective in maintaining patency if 24 gauge cannulae are used (Danek & Noris 1992).

A survey of children's hospitals in the USA found that 75% used heparinized saline (10 units/ml) to flush peripheral cannulae. In addition, 55.6% used a 1 ml flush volume (range 0.5–2.5 ml) (Bossert & Beecroft 1994). More research is needed to confirm the optimal flush solution and volume.

Complications of peripheral intravenous therapy in children

Phlebitis

Phlebitis or venous inflammation can result from mechanical or chemical irritation, infection, or a combination of these factors (Livesley 1996).

Mechanical phlebitis Mechanical phlebitis is caused by movement of the cannula within the vein and may also be associated with the material from which the device is constructed (Goodinson 1990a). The movement and activity of the child or manipulation by the child may contribute to the development of phlebitis. To reduce the occurrence of mechanical phlebitis, the cannula should be secured adequately and the limb immobilized with a splint. A low prime extension set will allow manipulation of the device away from the insertion site and reduce movement of the cannula within the vein (Livesley 1996).

Chemical phlebitis Chemical irritation is associated with the composition, i.e high osmolarity, low pH and particulate load of the infusate or drug administered via the cannula (Goodinson 1990b). Small veins may become inflamed when used for the infusion of irritating solutions. In this instance, the cannula occludes the lumen of the vein, obstructs the flow of blood and reduces the dilution of the infusate (Weinstein 1993). Children may be more at risk of chemical phlebitis as their veins are smaller and subject to reduced blood flow around the device.

Septic phlebitis This is associated with contamination of the cannula or infusate or haematogenous spread of bacteria (Goodinson 1990a).

Rotation of cannula sites It is recommended that cannula sites are changed every 72 hours in adult patients to reduce the risk of bacterial sepsis (Maki & Ringer 1991). However, infection of i.v. sites and phlebitis are an infrequent occurrence in children (Hecker 1988, Nelson & Garland 1987). Infusion sites in babies and children usually fail because of infiltration (Hecker 1988). It is common practice in paediatrics to leave cannulae in situ until electively discontinued or until infiltration occurs (Phelps & Helms 1987). In a survey of 100 paediatric units in the USA, 71.9% changed the cannula site when necessary even in the presence of a policy recommendation to change every 48 hours (Bossert & Beecroft 1994). This may reflect the efforts of staff to reduce the number of invasive procedures inflicted on children.

Extravasation injury in children

Early detection and prompt treatment are essential to minimize the complications of extravasation injury in children. Extravasation is defined as the leakage of a vesicant (a drug or solution capable of causing tissue necrosis on contact) out of a vein into the surrounding tissue (San Angel 1995). The incidence of serious extravasation injury in children has been reported as 80–90 per annum in one institution (Flemmer & Chan 1993). Children may be more at risk as a result of their inability to verbalize the pain of extravasation. Neonates in particular may be at greater risk as they often require infusions of high concentrations of glucose and calcium for growth and maintenance of normal levels (Duck 1997). The child or infant is therefore dependent on the nurse to detect and prevent extravasation injuries. In addition, the child's activity and inability to comprehend the importance of not manipulating or tugging the infusion tubing increase the potential for cannula dislodgement. It is essential that nurses are aware of the drugs or solutions that are capable of causing tissue damage and that policies are in place for the prevention and management of extravasation injury in children.

Recognition Signs of extravasation include:

- swelling of the tissues surrounding the infusion/cannula site
- discomfort or burning pain at the infusion/cannula site – observe the child for facial expressions, crying and reluctance to use the affected limb which may indicate an extravasation
- taut, stretched skin over the affected area
- cool, blanched skin (Millam 1988).

It should be remembered that, apart from swelling, the visual signs of tissue damage may be delayed for 24 hours or more (Pettit & Hughes 1993).

Management Early identification and prompt action can significantly reduce the complications associated with extravasation injury (Pettit & Hughes 1993). If extravasation is suspected, it is imperative that the infusion is stopped. This should be followed by an attempt to aspirate the extravasated fluid via the cannula (Banta 1992, Flemmer & Chan 1993, Pettit & Hughes 1993). The affected extremity may be elevated to facilitate fluid reabsorption (Zenk et al 1981). The injection of hyaluronidase 15 units/ml either via the cannula or subcutaneously in a circular pattern around the affected area has been shown to reduce the severity of tissue damage (Banta 1992, Flemmer & Chan 1993, Few 1987). This should be carried out within 1 hour of injury to maximize the beneficial effect (Few 1987). Hyaluronidase is contraindicated if the cause of the extravasation injury is a vasopressor, e.g. dopamine, dobutamine (Pettit & Hughes 1993).

Other methods of treating extravasation injury in children include the use of glyceryl trinitrate patches placed over ischaemic areas following extravasation involving dopamine and concentrated solutions of dextrose and calcium (Denkler & Cohen 1989, O'Reilly et al 1988). Gault (1993) described a technique called 'saline flush-out'. First, the area of extravasation is infiltrated with hyaluronidase, which reduces the viscosity of the connective tissue, making it more permeable to the sodium chloride 0.9% that is flushed through the subcutaneous space. Following this, four small exit incisions are made around the periphery of the extravasation and a large volume of sodium chloride 0.9% (500 ml) is flushed through the subcutaneous space. This technique removes the damaged tissue and conserves the integrity of the overlying skin. In his study, 86% of patients treated with saline flush-out following extravasation injury healed without any subsequent skin loss.

Prevention

- There should be hourly observation and palpation of the i.v. insertion site for signs of extravasation. More frequent observation of the site is advised during vesicant infusions.
- Consideration should be given to the appropriateness of administering vesicant solutions and drugs via peripheral venous access devices. It is recommended that these infusions are administered using a central venous catheter as this will ensure a high rate of blood flow to rapidly dilute the infusate (Banta 1992, Hecker 1988).
- Use an electronic infusion pump that incorporates a variable pressure setting to monitor any rise in pressure. Limiting the occlusion pressure will not prevent extravasation. However, regular recording of pressure may identify a gradual increase, similar to slowing of flow reported in adult gravity infusions (Livesley 1993).
- Cannulae should be used in preference to steel needles to avoid the inherent risk of infiltration associated with the use of these devices (Few 1987, Phelps & Helms 1987).
- Ensure that the cannula is adequately secured and the limb immobilized with a splint. Any dressing, tape, splint or bandage used should facilitate visual inspection and palpation of the site and not obscure the insertion site.
- Act promptly if the child exhibits signs of pain or discomfort, i.e. crying or holding the affected limb. Frequent observation of the site is paramount as children cannot be relied upon to communicate pain effectively.
- Assess blood return and patency of the cannula by flushing with sodium chloride 0.9% prior to administration of vesicant drugs or infusions.

CENTRAL VENOUS ACCESS IN CHILDREN

Central venous access devices (CVADs) are now utilized for many children with chronic diseases who require long-term venous access (Hollis 1992, Marcoux et al 1990) (see Table 15.10). These devices are used for children who require frequent drug administration, parenteral nutrition, blood or blood product transfusion, haemodialysis, peripheral blood stem cell collection and frequent blood sampling (Hollis 1992). The wide range of CVADs currently available has greatly improved the quality of life and ease of administration of many i.v. therapies in paediatrics, particularly paediatric oncology patients (Hollis 1992, Leese 1989). Their use has led to a reduction of the trauma associated with venepuncture. The skin-tunnelled catheter offers the child a virtually needle-free experience of i.v. therapy (Bagnall & Ruccione 1987, Hollis 1992, Leese 1989, Marcoux et al 1990). CVADs have enabled children to receive treatment at home and avoid repeated hospitalization. It is the intention of this section to provide an overview of the use of CVADs and to highlight the differences in maintenance care and management of complications specific to paediatrics.

Types of central venous access device used in children

The following CVADs are used in paediatric i.v. therapy:

- percutaneous, non-tunnelled central venous catheter (single-, dual- and triple-lumen)

Table 15.10 Uses of central venous access devices in children (long term)

Condition	Intravenous therapies
Leukaemia and solid tumours	Administration of chemotherapy and supportive care, e.g. parenteral nutrition, blood and blood products, antibiotics, peripheral blood stem cell collection
Immune deficiency diseases	Administration of i.v. immunoglobulin
Haemophilia, thalassaemia, sickle cell disease, aplastic anaemia	Administration of blood and blood products
Cystic fibrosis	Administration of antibiotics
Gastrointestinal failure	Administration of parenteral nutrition
Acute and chronic renal failure	To facilitate haemodialysis

- peripherally inserted central venous catheter
- skin-tunnelled, cuffed central venous catheter (single-, dual- and triple-lumen)
- implantable port
- haemodialysis/apheresis catheters.

A central venous access device is a device with the catheter tip in a central vein, i.e. superior vena cava (SVC) or inferior vena cava (IVC) in children (Wheeler & Frey 1995).

Percutaneous, non-tunnelled central venous catheter

Percutaneously placed catheters are the most commonly used CVADs in critical care situations (Decker & Edwards 1988). These catheters may be placed directly into the SVC via the right or left subclavian vein or internal/external jugular. The femoral vein may be used in children with the catheter tip ending in the IVC. The internal/external jugular veins are the most frequently used veins in neonates and infants, whereas the subclavian vein can be utilized for older children (Wheeler & Frey 1995). These catheters may be placed under a local anaesthetic or sedative in children (Frey 1993).

Peripherally inserted central catheters (PICCs)

These small-gauge catheters were originally developed for use in neonates in the 1970s (Wiltgen-Trotter 1996). A PICC is defined as a catheter inserted via a peripheral vein with the tip located in the vena cava (Intravenous Nurses Society 1997). Additional insertion sites in neonates and children include the external jugular, axillary, long and short saphenous, temporal and posterior auricular veins. The catheter tip position must be confirmed radiologically prior to use (Intravenous Nurses Society 1997). Sedation may be required for children who are anxious or uncooperative to enable PICC placement (BeVier & Rice 1994, Frey 1995). However, chloral hydrate 50–100 mg/kg given orally has been demonstrated as inadequate for PICC placement (Frey 1995). The use of midazolam may provide more effective sedation for PICC placement in children (BeVier & Rice 1994).

In the USA these catheters are placed by specially trained nurses in both adults (Egan-Sansivero 1995, Rountree 1991, Viall 1990) and paediatrics (Bevier & Rice 1994, Frey 1995, Miller & Dietrick 1997, Wiltgen-Trotter 1996). Currently, there is some interest in the UK in nurse placement of PICCs in adults (Oakley 1997, Gabriel 1996). Nurses able to establish short-term venous access should be able to place PICCs (Gabriel 1996). However, despite the increasing popularity among nurses in the UK of nurse placement of PICCs in adults, this is yet to be mirrored in paediatrics. This may reflect the fact that few paediatric nurses cannulate or perform venepuncture.

PICCs are available in both single- and dual-lumen configurations and the catheter tip may be open-ended or valved. The following sizes have been successfully placed in children: 2, 3 and 4 French (Frey 1995, Miller & Dietrick 1997). The large introducer and catheter size makes the insertion of dual-lumen PICCs problematic in children (Frey 1993). In the USA, PICCs are used in neonates and older children for the treatment of cystic fibrosis, osteomyelitis, AIDS, meningitis, prematurity, congenital heart disease, ruptured appendix, endocarditis and Hirschsprung's disease (Frey 1995, Miller & Dietrick 1997, Stovroff et al 1994).

Tunnelled cuffed central venous catheters (TCVCs)

In children, TCVCs are usually placed in the operating theatre under general anaesthesia, using the subclavian, internal or external jugular, long saphenous or femoral vein (Kiely 1988). Several procedures may be scheduled to coincide with CVC insertion to avoid unnecessary trauma for the child, e.g biopsy, bone marrow aspiration and lumbar puncture (Frey 1993). TCVCs may be placed by surgical cut-down or percutaneous insertion. Placement technique is dictated by surgical preference. Chathas & Paton (1996), in a review of 250 studies, found that the rate of sepsis was 3.5 times greater for surgical than for percutaneous placement. Future clinical studies involving randomization of the two techniques are needed to confirm that this is not the result of differences in patient characteristics. The extremely small size of the subclavian vein in infants and neonates limits the use of the percutaneous approach. Percutaneous insertion is generally used in older children (Wiener et al 1992). An alternative site for CVC insertion in children is the femoral vein with the catheter tunnelled under the skin of the abdomen. This site is useful for children with numerous previous CVCs or thrombosis in the superior vena cava (Frey 1993).

Paediatric-sized TCVCs are available in single- and dual-lumen varieties. Alternatively, adult-sized catheters may be placed to take advantage of larger internal diameters. If an adult-sized catheter is used, it will be cut prior to placement in a child. It is important to know what size of TCVC is placed in a child as catheter volumes may vary if both adult and paediatric sizes are used.

Valved catheters

These catheters are beginning to be used in paediatric patients in the UK (Lucas & Attard-Montalto 1996). However, there is little reference to this in the literature. This may reflect the fact that paediatric sizes have only recently been available in the UK.

Implantable ports

Low profile and adult-sized ports may be used in children. Low profile ports should be used in babies and small children, as lack of subcutaneous fat may cause the larger device to erode through the skin (De Backer et al 1993, Frey 1993). They are ideal for children requiring intermittent venous access who can tolerate the needle access. Implantable ports have been used successfully in paediatrics for the treatment of malignant disease, cystic fibrosis and haemophilia (Bagnall & Ruccione 1987, Becton et al 1988, Essex-Carter et al 1989, Harris et al 1987, Liesner et al 1995, Mirro et al 1990, Sidey 1989, Vidler 1994, Wiener et al 1992, Wurzel et al 1988).

Haemodialysis/apheresis catheters

These catheters are used in the treatment of acute and chronic renal failure and for apheresis procedures, e.g. peripheral blood stem cell harvest. A wide-bore, rigid, dual-lumen catheter is needed to tolerate the high flow rates necessary to perform haemodialysis and apheresis procedures (Asquith et al 1993, Secola 1997). Neither procedure can be performed successfully in children using a conventional tunnelled CVC, as reliable access to the circulation is necessary to take and return flow rates of up to 200 ml/min (Asquith et al 1993) These catheters may be either short-term, uncuffed and non-tunnelled or long-term, cuffed and tunnelled and are inserted in the same manner as a conventional CVC. If the child has no CVAD in situ prior to stem cell harvest, a long-term, dual-lumen apheresis catheter may be placed and used post-harvest for supportive care after the peripheral blood stem cell transplant. Alternatively, if the child has a CVAD in situ, a short-term device may be placed in a femoral vein and removed post-harvest (Secola 1997).

Selection of the appropriate central venous access device

Parents and children should be offered a choice of CVAD where appropriate (Hollis 1992). The nurse involved in preparing the child and family for insertion of a CVAD must be familiar with the wide range of devices available. In addition, she should be aware of the advantages and disadvantages associated with each type (Baranowski 1993, Winslow et al 1995). Some centres may have a specialist nurse to assist families in the selection of the most appropriate device (Bagnall & Ruccione 1987, Frey 1993). In the UK, specialist nurses in the areas of paediatric oncology, intravenous therapy, haemophilia and cystic fibrosis may fulfil this role. The following concerns should be addressed during the selection (see Fig. 15.2):

- duration of the planned intravenous therapy
- type of therapy to be administered via the CVAD
- frequency of venous access
- child/family preference.

Short- and intermediate-term intravenous therapy

Short-term i.v. therapy indicates the use of either a non-tunnelled CVC or a PICC. As these catheters are centrally placed, both are suitable for the administration of vesicant and irritant solutions. PICCs are advocated for intermediate-term i.v. therapy of greater than 2 weeks' duration. To date, no upper limit has been established for the length of time a PICC may remain in situ (Frey 1995). The small gauge of some PICCs may lead to collapse on aspiration (Frey 1995). If frequent blood sampling is a priority, a 3 or 4 French PICC or a non-tunnelled CVC is recommended.

Percutaneous non-tunnelled CVCs are made of PVC and their rigidity, combined with a high incidence of thrombosis and increased risk of dislodgement, limits their use to between a few days and 4 weeks (Viall 1990). The advantage of these catheters is that they are available in dual- or triple-lumen configurations. In paediatrics, these catheters are often used in high-dependency settings where several weeks of i.v. access are required that may include parenteral nutrition (Frey 1993). A potential problem associated with the use of these catheters placed in jugular and femoral veins is their occlusion by the movement of the baby's head or legs (Frey 1993). In addition, femoral vein placement in a child in nappies may result in an increased risk of infection (Wheeler & Frey 1995).

Long-term intravenous therapy

Long-term intravenous therapy (> 6 months) mandates a long-term CVAD. Some decisions regarding the most appropriate device are straightforward and are dictated by the type of therapy to be administered, frequency of venous access and whether a multi-lumen device is necessary. Other factors to be considered are

Fig. 15.2 Selecting the central venous access device in paediatrics.

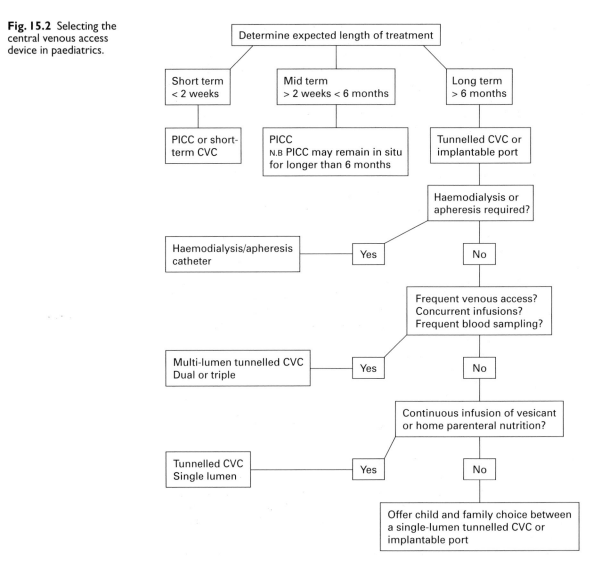

Determine expected length of treatment

Short term < 2 weeks

Mid term > 2 weeks < 6 months

Long term > 6 months

PICC or short-term CVC

PICC
N.B PICC may remain in situ for longer than 6 months

Tunnelled CVC or implantable port

Haemodialysis or apheresis required?

Haemodialysis/apheresis catheter — Yes

No

Frequent venous access?
Concurrent infusions?
Frequent blood sampling?

Multi-lumen tunnelled CVC
Dual or triple — Yes

No

Continuous infusion of vesicant or home parenteral nutrition?

Tunnelled CVC
Single lumen — Yes

No

Offer child and family choice between a single-lumen tunnelled CVC or implantable port

whether the child requires continuous infusions of vesicant drugs or solutions. A dual- or triple-lumen tunnelled CVC will be required to deliver multiple therapies that may incorporate concurrent infusions of incompatible solutions and accommodate the frequent blood sampling necessitated by a bone marrow transplant or intensive chemotherapy (Bagnall & Ruccione 1987, Harris et al 1987, Hollis 1992). A tunnelled CVC is not rigid enough to withstand the high flow rates necessary for haemodialysis or apheresis. These procedures necessitate a haemodialysis or apheresis catheter.

Continuous vesicant infusions, e.g. parenteral nutrition or chemotherapy, should be administered via a tunnelled CVC (Bagnall & Ruccione 1987, Baranowski 1993, Freedman & Bosserman 1995, Harris et al 1987). Extravasation is a potentially devastating complication of continuous vesicant infusions. Implantable ports are associated with an increased risk of extravasation and may not be appropriate for this type of therapy. Incorrect placement, rocking or dislodgement of the needle during infusion may result in extravasation (Schulmeister 1992). Babies and small children cannot be relied upon to remember that they are attached to an infusion and the needle may dislodge during active play or movement.

The child who does not require frequent venous access, haemodialysis, apheresis or continuous vesicant infusions may be offered a choice between a tunnelled CVC or an implantable port. This is dependent on the availability of both devices and a surgeon willing to place either. Much of the routine care and detection of problems associated with the use of CVADs is now the responsibility of parents. It is vital that they receive adequate information to make an informed decision if a choice of CVAD is offered.

Choosing between a tunnelled CVC and an implantable port

Implantable ports have lower overall complication rates, and less risk of dislodgement and occlusion when compared with tunnelled CVCs (Mirro et al 1990, Wiener et al 1992). Significantly lower rates of infection have also been reported (La Quaglia et al 1992, Mirro et al 1990). Other studies have demonstrated lower infection rates in implantable ports, but these did not reach statistical significance (McGovern et al 1985, Ross et al 1988, Soucy 1987, Wurzel et al 1988). Conversely, Wiener (1992) found no difference in infection as a cause of removal when comparing the two devices. It should be noted that all of the above studies represent paediatric oncology patients and may not be applicable to other conditions. When parents are offered a choice, it may be pertinent to consider child and family preference, as evidence of differences in complication rates is inconclusive. Quality-of-life issues and the impact of CVAD on the child and family may be more appropriate factors to guide parents in their choice of device.

The advantages and disadvantages of implantable ports and tunnelled CVCs should be discussed with the child and family to facilitate an informed choice (Baranowski 1993, Marcoux et al 1990, Winslow et al 1995). An explanation of the main care required may be useful to aid decision-making (Table 15.11).

Care and maintenance of central venous access devices

There are many different catheter types and protocols for care. Sound policies and training for the handling of different catheter types will help to minimize potential problems (Hollis 1992). Protocols for the care of CVADs should be based on manufacturers' guidelines, current research, catheter type and volume (Wheeler & Frey 1995). Protocols for use in children should take into account the developmental level of the child and the unique problems associated with the use of CVADs.

Catheter volume in children

The catheter volume of a paediatric-sized tunnelled CVC is 1 ml or less (Wheeler & Frey 1995). This should be accounted for when compiling protocols for flushing, blood sampling and drug administration (see Table 15.12). However, adult-sized tunnelled CVCs and implantable ports may be placed in children to take advantage of the larger internal diameter of the lumen for blood administration and sampling. The catheter will be cut to size during placement and the catheter volume will be reduced accordingly. For example, a 10 French dual-lumen tunnelled catheter cut during insertion will result in a catheter volume of approximately 1 ml (MacGeorge et al 1988). The manufacturers should be consulted if the catheter volume is unknown.

Drug administration

When administering i.v. drugs via CVADs, it is important that the device is flushed

Table 15.11 A comparison of the advantages and disadvantages of implantable ports and tunnelled CVCs (Bagnall & Ruccione 1987, Harris et al 1987, Hollis 1992, Marcoux et al 1990)

Tunnelled CVC	Implantable port
Easier to use in home i.v. therapy	More difficult to use in home i.v. therapy
Easily removed on completion of therapy	Removal more complicated; larger scar
No needles required to access the device	Needles required to access device
Can be repaired if damaged	Cannot be repaired if damaged
Frequent maintenance	Minimal maintenance
Family must learn care	Family need not learn care
Clamps needed at all times	Clamps not required
Some activity restrictions, e.g. swimming, contact sports	Few activity restrictions – child can swim, bath freely; vigorous contact sports and direct pressure on device should be avoided
Outside the body	Under the skin
Visible reminder of disease	Less impact on body image
Increased risk of damage	Less risk of damage
Increased risk of dislodgement as it can be pulled out	Less risk of dislodgement; cannot be pulled out
Increased risk of infection	Less risk of infection
Dressing required	No dressing required
Less risk of extravasation	Risk of extravasation secondary to needle dislodgement

with sufficent amounts of sodium chloride 0.9% to effectively clear the device of drug (see Table 15.12). It is recommended that 10 ml syringes are used routinely for all procedures. A syringe size of less than 10 ml will exert pressures greater than 25 psi (Bard Access Systems 1994a), which may precipitate catheter rupture, catheter embolus or septum rupture, especially if occluded (Conn 1993). Small syringes are often necessary to ensure accuracy of drug dosage in children. It is recommended that the patency of the device is established using a 10 ml syringe before a smaller syringe is used to avoid the risk of damaging the CVAD (Bravery & Hannan 1997).

Blood sampling

When obtaining blood samples from CVADs, care should be taken to ensure that blood loss is minimal, the potential for infection is minimized and an accurate sample is obtained.

Minimizing blood loss A child's circulating blood volume is larger per kilogram of body weight than that of an adult. In addition, the absolute blood volume is small (Hazinski 1992). Neonates, infants and children requiring frequent blood sampling from CVADs are particularly at risk of blood loss. Anaemia and bleeding are common complications of bone marrow transplant, and paediatric bone marrow transplant patients may have blood samples drawn daily or more often (MacGeorge et al 1988). It is essential to minimize blood loss in these patients.

A small loss of blood in a child may significantly affect blood volume and perfusion. For example, a 25 ml blood loss in a 7 kg infant represents almost 5% of the infant's circulating blood volume. Blood replacement may be necessary if blood loss exceeds 5–10% of the circulating blood volume (Hazinski 1992). Doran (1983) recommended that not greater than 5 ml/kg of the child's body weight be with-

Table 15.12 Flushing and heparinization of CVADs (Bard Access Systems 1994a, 1994b, 1995, Camp-Sorrell 1990, Frey 1995, Fry 1992, MacGeorge et al 1988, Wheeler and Frey 1995)

CVAD type	Catheter volume (ml)	Heparin			Sodium chloride 0.9% (ml)	
		Routine heparinization (ml)	Heparinized saline (U/ml)	Frequency	After blood sampling	Drug administration
Skin-tunnelled catheter: small bore	0.15–0.7	1.5	10	Weekly	3	1–2
Skin-tunnelled catheter: large bore	1 ml or less	2–5	10	Weekly	5–10	2–3
Implantable port		3–5	100	Monthly	5–20	2–5
Reservoir	0.2–0.6					
Catheter	0.6–1.5 (uncut)					
PICC	0.04–0.15	1–2	10	12-hourly	3–10	2–3
Short-term CVC	0.3–0.5	0.6–1	10	after use	3–10	1–2

This table should be used as a guide only. It is based on the references listed above. Where a range is specified, it is intended to reflect the variations in flushing protocols. More research is needed to establish the optimum flush volumes required to maintain patency of the wide range of CVADs in current use. Always consult the manufacturers of the device for information on catheter volumes.

Table 15.13 Calculating circulating blood volume in children (Hazinski 1992)

Age	Blood volume (ml/kg)
Neonate	85–90
Infant	75–80
Child	70–75

drawn in a 24-hour period. Blood sampling should be coordinated and limited to once daily in high-risk patients. A running total should be kept if the child is less than 10 kg and the doctor informed if blood loss is greater than 5–10% of the child's circulating blood volume (Hazinski 1992). Table 15.13 will help you to calculate a child's circulating blood volume.

Minimizing the risk of infection Frequent blood sampling from CVADs may be associated with an increased risk of infection (Keller 1994, Long et al 1996). This may be a particular concern in immunocompromised paediatric patients.

Obtaining accurate blood samples To obtain an accurate sample for laboratory analysis, the catheter must be cleared of heparinized saline and infusion fluid (Keller 1994, MacGeorge et al 1988). The amount of blood withdrawn from the CVAD to obtain accurate samples will reflect the smaller catheter volume – 3 ml is sufficient for tunnelled CVCs and implantable ports (Doran 1983, Keller 1994, MacGeorge et al 1988). The smallest possible amount required for each test should be established in hospitals treating children. With microanalytical methods of laboratory analysis, smaller volumes of blood are required and it is often possible to perform multiple tests on one sample (Rutledge 1989).

Methods of blood sampling There are three methods currently utilized for blood sampling. In practice, there appear to be variations both in the techniques for obtaining blood samples and in the rationale for each method. In a survey of 34 paediatric bone marrow transplant units in the USA, Keller (1994) found that 75% used the discard method, 14% used the reinfusion method and only one unit used the mixing method. There were wide variations in the volume of blood discarded: 61%, 4–6 ml; 29%, 7–10 ml; and 32%, 0.5–3 ml. Only four of the units surveyed cited catheter volume as the rationale for the discard volume.

Discard method Using this method, 3 ml of blood is withdrawn and discarded before the sample is taken. If this method is used, care should be taken to minimize blood loss.

Reinfusion method A volume of 3 ml is withdrawn from the CVAD, the sample taken and the withdrawn fluid replaced. This method reduces the amount of blood withdrawn from the child. However, there is a risk of contamination through manipulation of the syringe (Doran 1983, MacGeorge et al 1988). In addition, it is questionable as to how much blood is present in the syringe as it is mixed with heparinized saline. No research to date has been carried out to confirm that reinfusion of the waste blood actually minimizes blood loss.

Mixing method A syringe is attached to the catheter, 4 ml is withdrawn and immediately reinfused into the patient. This procedure is repeated four times without disconnecting the syringe. A new syringe is then attached and the sample taken. MacGeorge et al (1988) compared the mixing and reinfusion methods and found no difference in the accuracy of potassium and haematocrit levels. This method requires good blood flow on aspiration to be effective. Small-lumen silicone catheters may collapse on aspiration and will not be appropriate for this method of blood sampling. The mixing method may eliminate the potential blood loss from frequent blood sampling in high-risk patients, i.e. neonates or bone marrow patients. Further research is required to confirm the accuracy of blood samples obtained by this method.

Exit site care

There is a tendency to utilize the research based on adult populations when devising protocols for the care of exit sites in children. These may not always be appropriate for use in paediatrics.

Dressings are usually necessary for the first 3–4 weeks after insertion of tunnelled CVCs to allow tissue ingrowth into the cuff. The risk of accidental dislodgement may be increased in children with sealed gauze dressings and other means of fixation during the first month after insertion. During this period, an occlusive dressing may offer a more effective means of securing the catheter (Hindley 1997). Once the cuff is securely fixed in the tunnel, dressings may not be necessary (Lucas & Attard-Montalto 1996, Marcoux et al 1990, Sepion 1990). If there is bleeding postoperatively, the dressing should be changed the day after insertion to minimize the risk of subsequent infection (Hindley 1997, Marcoux et al 1990).

The type of dressing, or indeed whether dressings are used at all, is often a reflection of local policy (Hollis 1992). Lucas & Attard-Montalto (1996), in a study of paediatric oncology patients, randomized children 3 weeks after insertion into two different methods of exit site care. One group had a dry sealed gauze dressing and the site was cleaned with chlorhexidine 0.5% once a week. The other group were able to bathe and shower normally with the hubs kept in a plastic bag. The site was dried with a clean towel and sprayed with chlorhexidine 0.5% and alcohol 70%. There were fewer exit site infections in the 'no dressing' group (2/1000 catheter days vs. 4/1000 catheter days). However, this was not statistically significant. The 'no dressing' method was cheaper and needed less teaching time from the nurse.

Taylor et al (1996) advocated the use of occlusive dressings in children. She showed that the use of occlusive dressings does not increase the incidence of site infections during prolonged hospitalization in children > 1800 kg. She maintained that occlusive dressings are useful in children as a means of securing the catheter and providing protection from the child's body fluids, respiratory secretions and food!

Whatever dressing technique is employed when caring for children with central venous access devices, it is vital to ensure that the catheter is adequately secured, especially when attached to infusion devices.

Accidental dislodgement of central venous catheters

Accidental dislodgement of tunnelled CVCs has been described as a major and frequent problem in paediatric oncology patients (Mirro et al 1990, Wiener et al 1992). This may reflect poor tissue ingrowth into the cuff due to poor nutritional status and delayed healing in this group of patients (Alfieris et al 1987, Wiener et al 1992). The incidence of dislodgement is greater in children less than 3 years of age and significantly associated with a cuff to exit site distance of less than 2 cm (Wiener et al 1992). A unique consideration in toddlers and babies is that they may tug at the catheter and unintentionally subject it to traction, thus increasing the likelihood of dislodgement.

Various methods have been described that attempt to overcome this problem – a suture around the cuff, Marlex mesh glued to the skin and retrograde tunnelling (Alfieris et al 1986, Goolishan & Konefal 1989, Vasquez & Racenstein 1987, Wheeler et al 1991a). Simpler measures may be adopted, such as looping and taping the catheter securely to the chest wall using an adherent tape (Frey 1993). Other measures include keeping the catheter out of reach of the baby / toddler by taping it over the shoulder, or around the side or the torso to the back. Ensuring that the catheter remains under clothing may help to deter inquisitive fingers. Babygros and vests that are fastened between the legs are useful in babies. It is recommended that a baby or toddler with the catheter free should never be left unattended. Education of the child and family to avoid traction on the catheter and exercise caution when infusions are in progress is vital.

A problem unique to children is that of rapid growth. The growth of the torso may pull the catheter upwards out of the SVC (Cameron 1987, Reed & Philips 1996). This will be identified by a chest X-ray. If this situation arises, the catheter will require surgical replacement.

Catheter occlusion

Catheter occlusions occur frequently with the long-term usage of CVADs. In children, slower infusion rates may cause back-up of blood in the catheter and subsequent catheter occlusion. In addition, parenteral nutrition solutions used may contain more calcium and phosphorus which may lead to precipitate occlusions, particularly in neonates (Reed & Philips 1996). Other causes of catheter occlusion are mechanical problems, thrombus formation, lipid deposition, drug, mineral or electrolyte precipitate and fibrin sheath formation (Holcombe et al 1992).

Management Once the position of the catheter has been confirmed by chest X-ray or dye studies, attempts can be made to relieve the occlusion using an appropriate agent (Reed & Philips 1996, Wachs 1990). Dye studies are advocated in preference to chest X-ray as they will identify fibrin sheath formation which may result in extravasation if undiagnosed (Mayo & Pearson 1995). When instilling medications to relieve catheter obstruction, the use of syringes less than 10 ml is contraindicated to avoid the risk of catheter rupture (Reed & Philips 1996).

Agents used to relieve catheter occlusion It is important to ascertain the cause of the catheter occlusion to enable the appropriate agent to be used to relieve the obstruction. Clues as to the cause of the obstruction can be elicited from the history of the occlusion. Lipid occlusion generally takes several weeks or days for the catheter to become totally obstructed (Pennington & Pithie 1987), whereas an occlusion caused by a drug precipitate often occurs suddenly and may be caused by insufficient flush volumes in between drugs or drugs and parenteral nutrition (Holcombe et al 1992). Precipitate may be visible in the infusion tubing or catheter (Duffy et al 1989). In practice, it may be difficult to identify the cause of the catheter occlusion. If unsure, urokinase should be tried first to relieve the occlusion before trying other means (Holcombe et al 1992). (See Table 15.14 for more information on agents used to relieve catheter occlusion.)

Catheter damage

Children can and invariably do damage central venous catheters. Catheters can be bitten or even cut with scissors. The incidence of catheter damage in children has been reported to be 6.2–27.5% (Bagnall-Reeb & Ruccione 1990, Cameron 1987). Catheter damage may occur above the bifurcation as a result of catheter fatigue and persistent twisting, or below the bifurcation in the lower portion of the catheter due to wear and tear (Bagnall-Reeb & Ruccione 1990). Education of staff and parents caring for children is vital to prevent catheter damage. If damage occurs at home, parents should be taught to clamp the catheter above the damaged portion and return to the hospital for repair. Atraumatic, non-toothed clamps should always be available wherever the child is cared for.

Table 15.14 Agents used in children to relieve catheter occlusion (Bagnall et al 1989, Duffy et al 1989, Holcombe et al 1992, Levy et al 1991, Pennington & Pithie 1987, Shulman et al 1988, Wachs 1990)

Cause of occlusion	Agent/method of administration
Blood	Urokinase bolus: 5000 units/ml Use amount equivalent to catheter volume (1 ml, tunnelled CVCs; 0.2–0.5 ml, Broviac type CVC; 2 ml, implantable port to accommodate larger priming volume and extension tubing). Leave in situ for 30–120 min. May be repeated to a total of three doses
Fibrin sheath resistant to bolus urokinase	Urokinase infusion: 200 units/kg per hour for 24 hours
Thrombosis	Tissue plasminogen activator: 0.1–0.5 mg/kg per hour
Drug precipitate	Sodium bicarbonate 8.4%: dose equivalent to catheter volume Leave in situ for 60 min 0.1 N solution of hydrochloric acid: dose equivalent to catheter volume; 0.2–1.0 ml has been used. Leave in situ for 20–60 min. Aspirate to avoid adverse reactions May be repeated to a total of three doses
Lipid	Ethyl alcohol 70%: dose equivalent to catheter volume Up to 1 ml has been used. Leave in situ for 60–120 min

Air embolism and haemorrhage

The child with a central venous access device is at risk of air embolism and haemorrhage if the integrity of the i.v. system is interrupted (Marcoux et al 1990). Children are curious and may fiddle with i.v. tubing and caps attached to the catheter. Luer-lock connections and caps should be used and all connections checked at intervals. Currently there is no child-proof connection system or cap available!

Swimming and central venous catheters

Swimming is an important part of normal life for a child. Although some centres do restrict swimming in children with CVCs, there is little research to support this approach. A recent study found no increased risk of catheter-related infection if swimming is allowed (Cromwell et al 1997). The exit site should be healed and the cuff firmly fixed before allowing the child to swim. An adherent, waterproof occlusive dressing is advised to protect the exit site (Frey 1993). The dressing should be changed, the site cleaned and a new dressing applied immediately after swimming.

Needle dislodgement from implanted ports

Needle dislodgement has been identified as the most common cause of extravasation associated with the use of implantable ports (Bothe et al 1984, Brothers et al 1988, Ingle 1995, Moore et al 1986, Ramirez et al 1993, Reed et al 1985, Schulmeister 1989,

Strum et al 1986). Although the potential for needle dislodgement would seem greater in active children, there are few published reports of occurrence of this problem. In a series of 230 paediatric oncology patients, there were 10 episodes of needle dislodgement and subsequent extravasation (Bravery 1998). Recognition of needle dislodgement is compounded by the fact that the needle may dislodge from the port and remain under the skin, giving the illusion that the needle is still in situ (Cunningham & Bonam-Crawford 1993).

Prevention

- When placing the needle do not rock or tilt the needle after insertion as this may cause fluid leakage (Gullo 1993).
- Always use the correct length of needle, 0.75 inches (20 mm) is appropriate for most children. If the needle is too short, it will compress the tissue over the port; as the tissue expands the needle may be pushed out of the port reservoir when the patient moves (Wood & Gullo 1993).
- Insert the needle with the bevel up, facing the shoulder, and tape the tubing to the shoulder. This will reduce traction on the tubing (Bagnall & Ruccione 1987).
- Secure the needle with Steri-Strips and a clear occlusive dressing to allow visualization of the site during infusion.
- Loop and tape the infusion tubing to the child's chest and ensure there is sufficient length to allow movement (Schulmeister 1989, Wickham 1990). This is vital to prevent direct traction on the needle.

Before administration of vesicant drugs and infusions

- Confirm the correct needle position by aspiration of blood (Schulmeister 1992, Wood & Gullo 1993).
- If blood return is absent, flush the port with 20–30 ml of sodium chloride 0.9%. No swelling will indicate correct needle placement (Wood & Gullo 1993).
- Dye studies may be indicated if blood return is absent (Mayo & Pearson 1995). This will confirm the position of the catheter tip and the presence of thrombosis or fibrin sheath, either of which may cause extravasation (Lokich et al 1985, Mayo & Pearson 1995, Moore et al 1986).

During infusion of vesicant infusions

- Frequent assessment of needle position is advised, especially during vesicant infusions. This can be achieved by gently pressing on the needle or by aspiration of blood every 4 hours (Cunningham & Bonam-Crawford 1993, Wood & Gullo 1993).
- Observe the port and chest wall for any signs of swelling.
- Check dressing for leakage as this may indicate extravasation (Schulmeister 1992).
- If extravasation occurs, follow the hospital's extravasation policy.

HOME INTRAVENOUS THERAPY IN PAEDIATRICS

Sidey (1995) commented that paediatric care in the 1990s will consist of short hospital admissions and increasing numbers of acute and chronically sick children needing home care. Indeed, many of these children will require a variety of i.v. therapies on either a short- or long-term basis. Parents have been administering antibiotics, blood products and home parenteral nutrition (HPN) since the mid-1980s (Bisset et al 1991, Cluroe 1989, Ellis 1989, Liesner et al 1996, Ljung et al 1992, Sidey 1990). These home i.v. therapy schemes were initiated by specialist hospital-based nurses and have enabled many children with chronic diseases such as cystic fibrosis, haemophilia and gastrointestinal failure to lead a more 'normal' lifestyle. In turn, this has allowed some children to be cared for at home and avoid long periods of hospitalization.

Home intravenous therapies may be administered by either paediatric community nurses (PCNs) or parents. Central venous access devices to facilitate these therapies are frequently placed in a specialist, tertiary care centre and their use and maintenance care shared between different health care professionals and parents within the context of shared care (Bravery & Hannan 1997). Shared care has been described as a three-tiered model that encompasses primary, secondary and tertiary services (Hooker & Williams 1996). For this model of care of CVADs to be successful, it is essential that clear, written information, education and advice are available for both parents and PCNs. The onus for the provision of such education and information rests with the centre that places the device (Bravery & Hannan 1997).

Venous access

Peripheral venous access has been used for the home treatment of cystic fibrosis patients in the form of peripheral cannulae and percutaneously inserted silastic catheters (Ellis 1989, Sidey 1990, Williams et al 1988). A disadvantage of peripheral cannuale is that they require re-siting, necessitating a return trip to the hospital (Ellis 1989). A more permanent form of venous access is usually necessary to facilitate the long-term administration of i.v. therapies in the home setting, e.g. a tunnelled CVC or implantable port (Sidey 1990, Bisset et al 1992, Liesner et al 1995). However, parents and even children have been taught to cannulate to administer prophylactic factor concentrate (Liesner et al 1996).

Peripherally inserted central catheters (PICCs)

Despite the increasing popularity of the use of PICCs in adult populations, there has been no reference to the use of this device for home intravenous therapy administration for children in the UK. In comparison, the use of PICCs in the USA has extended to the area of home i.v. therapy (BeVier & Rice 1994, Frey 1995, Stovroff et al 1994). BeVier & Rice (1994) stated that the use of PICCs offers children a more positive overall experience of hospital and enables more patients the opportunity to continue or complete their course of therapy at home. Stovroff et al (1994) compared peripheral cannulae with PICCs for the administration of antibiotics in the home setting. They concluded that, as experience of the use of PICCs in home care increases, it may become the preferred method of treatment for a number of illnesses that currently require intermediate courses of i.v. therapy. Given the current interest in nurse placement of PICCs in the UK, it may well be that they do become the preferred means of central venous access in both adults and children and will ultimately be utilized in the home setting.

Long-term venous access

Children with a chronic disease should have a long-term venous access device placed to facilitate treatment. For further explanation of the criteria for device selection, Fig. 15.2.

Preparation of the child and family for home administration of intravenous therapy (HIVT)

Parental involvement in HIVT may vary in complexity from flushing a tunnelled catheter and changing an exit site dressing to administration of intravenous drugs or parenteral nutrition. Whatever the procedure to be taught, successful preparation for HIVT is dependent on:

- careful assessment of suitability of the child, family and home conditions for planned HIVT
- education of the child, family and paediatric community nurse teams involved in shared care
- meticulous discharge planning
- good communication between all staff involved in the care and support of families administering HIVT.

Assessment of the child, family and home conditions

The parents Assessment begins with the parents. Fundamental to paediatric nursing is the philosophy that the nurse and parents work in partnership in the care of a sick child (Casey 1988). Many paediatric nurses are increasingly concerned about the professional, ethical and legal consequences of parental involvement in care, in particular the administration of i.v. therapies by parents (Charles-Edwards & Casey 1992). Parents should be willing and able to learn home administration of i.v. drugs (Sidey 1994).

Parents should never be coerced to take on the responsibility for home administration of i.v. drugs. It should not be proffered as a means to early discharge or to relieve the pressure on hospital beds. Charles-Edwards & Casey (1992) suggested that the parents' willingness to learn about and perform care or treatment for their child and the potential coercion of parents to undertake this task raises ethical and legal issues.

Legal issues The legal context for consent to treatment applies when parents undertake nursing tasks in the home setting. To ensure that consent is legally valid, parents must be willing to undertake the proposed care of their child. Their consent must be given willingly without undue pressure and with sufficient information provided to inform consent (Charles-Edwards & Casey 1992).

Ethical issues Parents should have the freedom or autonomy to make their own decisions when offered home i.v. therapy. Whether parents choose to take on nursing care and treatment for their child may be limited by circumstances. Parental involvement in care can be either predicted and planned or unforeseen (Charles-Edwards & Casey 1992) (see Box 15.1).

If parents perform home administration of i.v. drugs, it is possible to keep some chronically sick children out of hospital and enable the family to achieve a more 'normal lifestyle'. This may, however, place a tremendous burden on the family to maintain this level of care over the years (Bisset et al 1992). Gill (1993) maintains that more research is needed to establish the full implications of setting up schemes for the administration of HIVT for children and their families. She also advocates that specialist centres join together with a view to developing common procedures for drug administration and forge better links with paediatric community nurses. Several studies in the USA, where home care is more established, have highlighted the tremendous stress and financial burdens experienced by families caring for technology-dependent children in the home setting (Fleming et al 1994, Leonard et al 1993, Patterson et al 1994, Teague et al 1993). Children receiving i.v. administration of drugs or nutritional substances at home are classified as technology-dependent in the USA (Fleming et al 1994). These studies emphasized the need for more community support services, and better education and information for these families. Specialist centres considering setting up HIVT schemes would be well advised to take these findings into account, especially in areas where there is limited or no paediatric community service available. Each request for HIVT should be individually assessed and support provided as a matter of routine.

■ **BOX 15.1**

Ethical issues in parental involvement in home care

Scenario 1

James, aged 18 months, is the first child of married parents. His father is a pharmacist and his mother a nurse. James has severe haemophilia and is admitted to the ward for insertion of an implantable port to enable home administration of prophylactic factor VIII. James's parents are keen to participate in a training programme for home administration of factor VIII run by the haemophilia nurse specialist.

Scenario 2

Lucy, aged 3 years, has been admitted to hospital with orbital cellulitis. She has been on the ward for 2 days. Lucy's mother is a single parent living in a bedsit. After four attempts to insert a cannula, it is decided to place a tunnelled central venous catheter to facilitate administration of i.v. antibiotics. Lucy's mother is distressed at the appearance of the catheter and is reluctant to cuddle Lucy for fear of the catheter falling out. The mother hates hospitals and is desperate to take Lucy home. The doctor tells Lucy's mother that she can take Lucy home if she agrees to give the antibiotics at home.

Think about the following:
- Is consent valid in both these situations?
- Are both families suitable candidates for home administration of i.v. drugs?
- What circumstances may limit discharge home in each case?

The child The child must be clinically stable (Ellis 1989) and assessed by the medical staff as suitable for home administration of i.v. drugs. If old enough, the child's wishes should be considered.

A means of venous access appropriate for the planned treatment and for the individual child and family should be established. In addition to the administration of i.v. drugs, the parents will need to learn the routine care and maintenance of the venous access device. This should be incorporated into the teaching plan. If a peripheral cannula is used, arrangements should be made for the re-siting of cannulae before discharge from hospital.

Suitability of the drug regimen Ideally, the drugs to be administered should be once or twice daily administration. Three times daily administration can be achieved in the home and is compatible with most families' lifestyles (Sidey 1994). However, multiple drug regimens that do not allow the parent time for rest and sleep are not suitable for HIVT. Drugs may be administered as a bolus dose via a syringe or as an intermittent infusion by means of a pump. To facilitate ease of administration, some private companies provide syringes pre-filled with the drug or the drug is supplied in a positive pressure closed pump that is portable. Electronic infusion devices can be used in the home setting. These may be more difficult for parents to learn to handle and use. Whether the hospital supplies the parents with the drugs and equipment or a private company is used is for the hospital/community to decide. Ease of use and availability of equipment must be considered before discharge.

Some antibiotics administered intravenously require blood levels to be taken. It should be established whether these can be taken from the venous access device or peripherally, as local policy varies. The child may need to attend a hospital for peripheral blood levels.

The first dose of an antibiotic should be administered under direct medical supervision, usually in hospital. If the child receives repeated courses of the same antibiotic(s), the first dose may be administered at home (Sidey 1994). Unless the child is receiving these i.v. drugs on a regular, planned basis, it is usual, in cases of parental administration of i.v. drugs, for the child to be in hospital for a period of stabilization prior to discharge home.

The home The family should have a telephone to allow access to medical and nursing advice and to summon help in an emergency, e.g. sudden deterioration of the child's condition or severe drug reaction.

There must be enough room in the house to store pumps, and a refrigerator, if necessary, to store drugs, parenteral feeds and other supplies (Bisset et al 1992). All this equipment must be stored safely out of reach of children. The house should be clean and a suitable area identified for preparation of drug and infusions. There should be access to hand washing facilities in the proximity of the drug/infusion preparation area. The child may need his own room if overnight infusions are planned, to allow enough room for the infusion pump. If the room is shared with a sibling who is mobile, there may be a temptation to interfere with the equipment.

A home visit may be required to assess the suitability of the home if long-term HIVT is planned. Provision should be made for the disposal of waste and sharps in accordance with local policy.

Support Drugs may be prescribed by the hospital or community-based medical staff (Sidey 1994). There is sometimes confusion, however, as to whether the GP or the hospital consultant is medically responsible when parents administer HIVT (Jennings 1994, Tatman et al 1992). The GP should be informed if parents are administering HIVT and the parents should have clear guidance as to who to contact for medical advice.

Nursing support for the parents may be via either a paediatric community nurse or a specialist nurse based in the hospital, or a combination of both. Not all health authorities have a paediatric community nursing service (Whiting 1990). Parents must be competent in the procedure before discharge if no PCN exists and support is provided by hospital-based outreach nurses.

Consideration should be given to the education needs of the community staff who support the family in the home setting. Sidey (1990) stated that paediatric community staff who do not possess the appropriate knowledge, skills or level of competence have the right to refuse to nurse a child receiving HIVT or be responsible for parents administering HIVT. Community staff may not have local access to specialist training in the care of CVADs. Gill (1993) urged specialist centres to provide training programmes for staff supporting families participating in HIVT schemes. Clear written information with step-by-step instructions for any procedure parents have been taught should be available from the specialist centre (Bravery & Hannan 1997).

Education of parents

There should be some form of formal training programme for parents. Various teaching programmes have been described (Bisset et al 1992, Cluroe 1989, Holden 1991, Stapleford 1990). These vary in content from supervised practice of drug administration to a formal written test. Demonstration of competence and safety in the administration of the drug should suffice (Gill 1993). Ideally, the programme should be carried out by one nurse experienced in both i.v. therapy and the education of parents in order to ensure consistency. Consideration should be given to training both parents and the child, if appropriate, in case one parent is ill (Ellis 1989).

The training programme must be supported by written guidelines specifically designed to include:

- step-by-step instructions of the procedures to follow
- side-effects of the drug
- hazards and complications of i.v. therapy, e.g. signs of infection of the cannula site or infiltration
- dose of drug(s) to be administered, and frequency and time of administration
- information on the reconstitution of drug(s) – volume of the reconstituted drug to be administered in ml and mg or mcg
- type of infusion fluid required with the amount specified in ml
- rate and duration of infusion clearly prescribed.

Documentation of parental education Written evidence of teaching should be documented in the care plan. Whether the parents and the nurse who taught them should sign some type of consent form is questionable (Dimond 1990). If the nurse has done all that can reasonably be expected in instructing the parents, has advised them of all foreseeable eventualities and provided written instructions and then if harm occurs to the child, the nurse will not be liable. The parents' signature will provide evidence of the information and instruction provided. However, if the nurse fails to give vital information or is negligent in her instruction of the parents, the consent form signed by the parents will not exempt her from liability for negligence (Dimond 1990).

Discharge planning

A discharge planning meeting should be convened, involving the parents, child and health care professionals who will provide continuing support and supervision for the family. The community staff should meet the family prior to discharge.

Communication

Successful home i.v. therapy is dependent on effective communication between all members of the team caring for the child and family, whether based in the hospital or in the community. Written communication may be facilitated by the use of a 'parent held record' containing all the relevant written guidelines, teaching record and contact numbers for advice (Hooker & Williams 1996).

METHODS TO REDUCE PAIN AND ANXIETY ASSOCIATED WITH INTRAVENOUS THERAPY PROCEDURES

Children may experience pain and anxiety during a number of procedures associated with i.v. therapy, e.g. venepuncture, cannulation and implantable port access. Venepuncture is one of the most common painful procedures experienced by children (Fowler-Kerry & Lander 1991). This procedure is distressing to the child, the parents and the nurse or doctor performing it. The nurse involved in paediatric i.v. therapy should be familiar with different methods and techniques designed to alleviate pain and anxiety in children undergoing painful procedures. An understanding of the developmental level is needed to initiate the most appropriate intervention (see Table 15.15).

Pain and venepuncture

Younger children experience more distress, anxiety and pain than older children when venepuncture is performed (Bennett Humphrey et al 1992, Lander et al 1992). 'Needle phobia' is a term that is often used to describe a child who cries and exhibits distress during venepuncture. However, most children do not have

Table 15.15 Interventions to reduce anxiety associated with intravenous therapy procedures (Collier & MacKinley 1993, Hansen & Evans 1981, Kachoyeanos & Friedhoff 1993, Lansdown 1987)

Age	Developmental stage	Intervention
0–1 years	Fears separation from parents, and strangers	Encourage parents' presence Provide physical comfort and warmth during procedure Wrap in a blanket; use dummy Distract with bright, noisy toys
0–3 years	Limited concept of time Prone to fantasies; bargains and stalls to avoid procedures Unable to comply with commands to sit still and not touch equipment Short attention span Limited language skills	Prepare immediately prior to procedure Provide simple explanations of what will happen Distract with blowing bubbles, 'pop up' books, books that make sounds Offer reward immediately after procedure, e.g. stickers Allow child to play with equipment used, e.g. syringes in the bath
4–6 years	Attention span 15 minutes Vivid imagination Fears bodily injury, loss of control, being alone and the dark May consider pain as a form of punishment	Prepare prior to procedure Use simple terminology in explanations Give control where possible, e.g. choice of plaster, help with cleaning site Use dolls to explain what is happening and how it will feel Use doll with CVC in situ. Use stories that involve the child or super hero Distract by getting child to blow away pain, blow feather off adult's hand, favourite video Praise cooperation. Reassure that it is okay to cry
6–12 years	Wants to participate in the procedure Grasps concept of time, including future and past Wants to understand what is happening Needs a sense of control Language skills improving Increasing awareness of body functions	Prepare hours in advance of procedure Offer choices Reassure that it is okay to cry Distract with games, counting, sums, telling jokes, favourite video Use dolls or models, photograph books or videos of procedure for explanations
12+ years	Fears loss of control, being different from peers, altered body image Peer group important to the child Able to think and reason in the abstract Understands how the body functions Increasing independence from parents	Prepare in advance Offer choices, e.g. site of cannula, method of fixation, time of procedure Explanations using adult terminology Promote independence Provide privacy during procedure Use another child of same age to explain procedure Use body diagrams and models to aid explanations Hypnosis, guided imagery Distract using Walkman and favourite music, videos or computer games

needle phobia in the sense of a psychiatric definition of a phobia (Rice 1993). Children simply dislike and fear needles and those who wield them. Young children frequently express their distress by crying and resisting attempts to site a cannula. The older child is more able to cope with the procedure (Bennett Humphrey et al 1992).

Topical anaesthetic agents

Topical anaesthetic agents have been effective in reducing the pain experienced during venepuncture in children (Robieux et al 1991, Woolfson et al 1990).

The pain of venepuncture has been found to be significantly lower with EMLA (eutectic mixture of local anaesthetics, lignocaine 2.5%, prilocaine 2.5%, 2 g) than with a placebo (Clarke & Radford 1986, Halperin et al 1989, Joyce 1993). Studies involving younger children are perhaps more inconclusive. Maunuksela & Korpela (1986) found EMLA to be no more effective than placebo in children aged 4–6 years (of all the children, those in this group exhibited the greatest amounts of pain and distress). Conversely, in children aged 7–10 years, all members of the EMLA group reported slight or no pain, compared with 43% of the placebo group ($P < 0.001$). This may reflect the fact that older children are more able to understand the meaning of medical procedures and display less overt distress. Robieux et al (1991) compared EMLA with placebo in children aged 3–36 months. Although EMLA was superior over placebo in alleviating pain associated with venepuncture, other behavioural concerns were highlighted by the study. The behavioural pain scale used demonstrated an increased score with both EMLA and placebo. However, the behavioural changes caused by venepuncture were statistically lower in the EMLA group. In addition, some of the children in this study exhibited signs of obvious distress before venepuncture. The children in this study were chronically sick and had previous experience of venepuncture, which may have contributed to this observed state of anxiety. When venepuncture was not achieved at the first attempt, the efficacy of EMLA was less certain. As previously discussed, younger children exhibit greater distress during venepuncture. The actual procedure, or even the application of topical anaesthetics, may cause more upset and anxiety than the pain of the venepuncture.

EMLA should not be used in children < 1 month, as it is associated with methaemoglobinaemia (Engberg et al 1987, Koren 1993). Other mild skin reactions of pallor and erythema have been reported with the use of EMLA (Clarke & Radford 1986, Joyce 1993, Maunuksela & Korpela 1986, Robieux et al 1991).

A more recent addition to the range of topical anaesthetic agents is Ametop gel (amethocaine 4% w/w, 1 g). This has been compared with EMLA in two studies (Lawson et al 1995, Morton 1996). Both studies report that Ametop is more effective in alleviating pain associated with venepuncture, but Ametop was associated significantly with a higher incidence of erythema than EMLA. The shorter application time of Ametop gel (30–45 minutes) may be advantageous to ward and clinic routines (Woolfson et al 1990).

Whatever topical anaesthetic agent is used it must be applied in accordance with the manufacturer's instructions for it to be effective.

Pain and implantable port access

Little research has been conducted into the pain and anxiety associated with implantable port access in children. Zappa & Nabors (1992) described the use of ethyl chloride spray to reduce the pain of port access. The children in the 7–12 year age group received the greatest benefit from use of the spray. Younger children in the study perceived the spray as painful due to the intense cold feeling.

Halperin et al (1989) compared EMLA with placebo for port access in children aged 6–14 years. Using a visual analogue scale, the pain scores were significantly lower ($P < 0.04$) when EMLA was used. The children in this study rated the pain of accessing a port as 3.9 with placebo, and 1.8 with EMLA on a scale of 1–10 (0 = no pain, 10 = the worst pain imaginable). Despite the lack of research into the efficacy of EMLA for the alleviation of the pain of port access, it is often used in paediatric practice. The effectiveness of Ametop in port access has yet to be determined.

Anecdotally, Ross et al (1988) maintained that the level of pain felt during port access is dependent on who inserts the needle. This has implications for nurses not experienced in this procedure.

Other techniques to reduce pain and anxiety

Both nurses and parents have an important role to play in employing various techniques to help children cope with painful procedures in i.v. therapy. The choice of technique is dependent on the child's age, developmental level and resources available.

The role of parents

Parents can help the child through painful procedures by their physical presence and by the provision of comfort. Not all parents are able to participate: some will prefer not to watch. The parent may have a fear of needles, and these fears may be transmitted to the child, increasing the distress (Sclare & Waring 1995). Parents in this situation will need help from staff to overcome their own fears in order to help their child. If parents choose not to participate, their wishes should be respected.

Distraction techniques

The aim of this technique is to capture the child's interest during the procedure. It will only be effective if the child's age, developmental level and interests are taken into account (Sclare & Waring 1995). Manne et al (1992) found distraction to be the only adult behaviour that had a beneficial effect on child coping during venepuncture. Some adult behaviours had a negative effect on child coping, e.g. praise and encouragement to cope. In addition, they found that explanations increased distress in the child. Manne et al (1994) found that the effectiveness of distraction and other coping behaviours increases with age. The short attention span of a young child makes it difficult to sustain the child's interest. If the child was upset at the outset, they were likely to reject the distraction technique employed.

Distraction should involve the child in an activity he enjoys. This may include singing, counting, story-telling, games, telling jokes or even the use of television, favourite videos and Walkman tapes. The school age child may enjoy a story that involves either themselves or a TV superhero, especially when they can add their own contribution to the story. The involvement of a play specialist to facilitate distraction is invaluable and allows the nurse or doctor to concentrate on the procedure.

Psychological interventions

Various psychological interventions have been used to reduce the anxiety and distress of painful procedures. These include relaxation techniques, guided imagery, hypnosis and deep breathing techniques (Broome 1990, May 1992, Sclare & Waring 1995). These methods require concentration on the part of the child and are more suitable for older children. Parents and staff need to be trained in these techniques for them to be effective. The technique should be rehearsed before the procedure takes place.

Play preparation

Play preparation is an invaluable tool for parents and nurses to help children cope with procedures associated with i.v. therapy. The language of play is understood by all children, whereas information conveyed verbally may be misunderstood or forgotten (Collier et al 1993). Dolls and puppets can be used to demonstrate, in a non-threatening manner, what will happen during a procedure. A doll with a central venous catheter in situ can be used to explain what will happen during a dressing change or drug administration. A puppet can tell the child what will happen during venepuncture, what it will feel like, how long it will last and how the child should respond.

Photographic books and videos that detail a child undergoing the planned procedure are useful for older children. These can convey information about the actual procedure and can be used by the adult as a focus for discussion. Story books centring on a child coping with the procedure have the advantage that they can be used in advance and repeatedly at the child's own pace.

CONCLUSION

There are many factors to consider when administering i.v. therapies to children. This chapter has highlighted the different physical and anatomical characteristics of children and how these relate to i.v. therapy in practice. The safe administration of i.v. therapy to children is paramount, but the child's developmental level and emotional needs must also be accounted for.

The nurse involved in the care of children receiving i.v. therapy should keep abreast of new developments in venous access devices and their after-care. In addition, the nurse must be cognizant of associated complications and the management of complications specific to children. The nurse also has a role to play in assisting families in their choice of a venous access device that is appropriate to the planned therapy, the child and the family's lifestyle. The continuing education of parents in how to care for these devices in both the hospital and home setting is an important and challenging role for nurses to undertake.

REFERENCES

Alfieris G M, Wing C W, Hoy G H 1987 Securing Broviac catheters in children. Journal of Pediatric Surgery 22(9): 825–826

Asquith J, Hicklin M, Griffiths C 1993 Care of the child with acute renal failure. In: Carter B (ed) Manual of paediatric intensive care nursing. Chapman and Hall, London, p 194–229

Axton S E, Fugate T 1987 A protocol for pediatric IV meds. American Journal of Nursing 87(7): 943A–946D

Axton S E, Hall B 1994 An innovative method of administering IV medications to children. Pediatric Nursing 20(4): 341–344

Bagnall H A, Gomperts E, Atkinson J B 1989 Continuous infusion of low-dose urokinase in the treatment of central venous catheter thrombosis in infants and children. Pediatrics 83(6): 963–966

Bagnall H, Ruccione K 1987 Experience with a totally implanted venous access device in children with malignant disease. Oncology Nursing Forum 14(4): 51–55

Bagnall-Reeb H A, Ruccione K 1990 Management of cutaneous reactions and mechanical complications of central venous access devices in pediatric patients with cancer: algorithms for decision making. Oncology Nursing Forum 17(5): 677–681

Banta C 1992 Hyaluronidase. Neonatal Network 11(6): 103–104

Baranowski L 1993 Central venous access devices: current technologies, uses, and management strategies. Journal of Intravenous Nursing 16(3): 167–194

Bard Access Systems 1994a Hickman, Leonard and Broviac catheters. Nursing procedure manual. Bard Access Systems, Utah

Bard Access Systems 1994b Bard implanted ports: use and maintenance. Bard Access Systems, Utah

Becton D L, Morris K, Golladay E S, Hathaway G, Berry D H 1988 An experience with an implanted port system in 66 children with cancer. Cancer 61: 376–378

Ben-Arush M, Berant M 1996 Retention of drugs in venous access port chamber: a note of caution. British Medical Journal 312: 496–497

Bennett Humphrey G, Boon C M J, Chiquit van Linden van den Heuvell G F E, van den Wiel H B M 1992 The occurrence of high levels of acute behavioral distress in children and adolescents undergoing routine venipunctures. Pediatrics 90(1): 87–91

BeVier P A, Rice C E 1994 Initiating a pediatric peripherally inserted central catheter and midline catheter program. Journal of Intravenous Nursing 17(4): 201–205

Bisset W M, Stapleford P, Long S, Chamberlain A, Sokel B, Milla P J 1992 Home parenteral nutrition in chronic intestinal failure. Archives of Disease in Childhood 67: 109–114

Bossert E, Beecroft P C 1994 Peripheral intravenous lock irrigation in children: current practice. Pediatric Nursing 20(4): 346–349

Bothe A, Piccione W, Ambrosino J J, Benotti P N, Lokich J J 1984 Implantable central venous access system. The American Journal of Surgery 147: 565–569

Bravery K 1998 Needle dislodgment and extravasation: a complication of implanted vascular access devices in paediatric oncology patients. Nursing Standard, accepted for publication

Bravery K, Hannan J 1997 The use of long term central venous access devices in children. Paediatric Nursing 9(10): 29–37

Broome M E 1990 Preparation of children for painful procedures. Pediatric Nursing 16(6): 537–541

Brothers T E, Niederhuber J E, Roberts J A, Ensminger W D 1988 Experience with subcutaneous infusion ports in three hundred patients. Surgery, Gynecology and Obstetrics 166(4): 295–301

Cameron G S 1987 Central venous catheters for children with malignant disease: surgical issues. Journal of Pediatric Surgery 22(8): 702–704

Camp-Sorrell D 1990 Advanced central venous access selection, catheters, devices and nursing management. Journal of Intravenous Nursing 13(6): 361–369

Casey A 1988 A partnership with child and family. Senior Nurse 8(4): 8–9

Charles-Edwards I, Casey A 1992 Parental involvement and voluntary consent. Paediatric Nursing 4(1): 16–18

Chathas M K, Paton J B 1996 Sepsis outcomes in infants and children with central venous catheters: percutaneous versus surgical insertion. Journal of Obstetric, Gynecologic and Neonatal Nursing 25(6): 500–506

Clarke S, Radford M 1986 Topical anaesthesia for venepuncture. Archives of Disease in Childhood 61: 1132–1134

Cluroe S 1989 Parental involvement in intravenous therapy. Nursing Times 85(9): 42–43

Collier J, MacKinlay D 1993 Play at work. Play preparation guidelines for the multidisciplinary team. Child Health 1(3): 123–125

Collier J, Mackinlay D, Watson A R 1993 Painful procedures: preparation and coping strategies for children. Maternal and Child Health 18(9): 282–286

Conn C 1993 The importance of syringe size when using implanted vascular access devices. Journal of Vascular Access Networks 3(1): 11–18

Cromwell P, Korones D, Robbins J 1997 Swimming and central venous catheter-related-infections in the child with cancer. Journal of Pediatric Oncology Nursing 14(2): 119–120

Cunningham R S, Bonam-Crawford D 1993 The role of fibrinolytic agents in the management of thrombotic complications associated with vascular access devices. Nursing Clinics of North America 28(4): 899–909

Danek G D, Noris E M 1992 Pediatric IV catheters: efficacy of saline flush. Pediatric Nursing 18(2): 111–113

Davenport M 1996 Paediatric fluid balance. Care of the Critically Ill 12(1): 26–31

De Backer A, Otten V J, Deconinck P 1993 Totally implantable central venous access devices in pediatric oncology – our experience in 46 patients. European Journal of Pediatric Surgery 3: 101–106

Decker M D, Edwards K M 1988 Central venous catheter infections. Pediatric Clinics of North America 35(3): 579–612

Denkler K A, Cohen B E 1989 Reversal of dopamine extravasation injury with topical nitroglycerin ointment. Plastic and Reconstructive Surgery 84(5): 811–813

Dimond B 1990 Parental acts and omissions. Paediatric Nursing 2(1): 23–24

Doran E M 1983 Care of the Hickman catheter in children. Nursing Clinics of North America 18(3): 579–583

Duck S 1997 Neonatal intravenous therapy. Journal of Intravenous Nursing 20(3): 121–128

Duffy L F, Kerzner B, Gebus V, Dice J 1989 Treatment of central venous catheter occlusions with hydrochloric acid. The Journal of Pediatrics 114(6): 1002–1004

Egan-Sansivero G 1995 Why pick a PICC? Nursing 25(7): 35–42

Ellis J 1995 Administering drugs. Paediatric Nursing 7(4): 29–39

Ellis J M 1989 Let parents give the care: IV therapy at home in cystic fibrosis. Professional Nurse 4(2): 589–592

Engberg G, Danielson S, Henneberg S, Nilsson A 1987 Plasma concentrations of prilocaine and lidocaine and methaemoglobin formation in infants after epicutaneous application of a 5% lidocaine-prilocaine cream (EMLA). Acta Anaesthesiology Scandinavica 31: 624–628

Essex-Carter A, Gilbert J, Robinson T, Littlewood J M 1989 Totally implantable venous access systems in paediatric practice. Archives of Disease in Childhood 64: 119–123

Few B J 1987 Hyaluronidase for treating intravenous extravasations. The American Journal of Maternal and Child Nursing 12(1): 23

Fleming J, Challela M, Eland J et al 1994 Impact on the family of children who are technology dependent and cared for in the home. Pediatric Nursing 20(4): 379–388

Flemmer L, Chan J S L 1993 A pediatric protocol for management of extravasation injuries. Pediatric Nursing 19(4): 355–358, 424

Fowler-Kerry S, Lander J 1991 Assessment of sex differences in children's and adolescents' self-reported pain from venipuncture. Journal of Pediatric Psychology 16(6): 783–793

Freedman S E, Bosserman G 1995 Tunneled catheters. Technologic advances and nursing care issues. Nursing Clinics of North America 28(4): 851–857

French J P 1995 Venous access. In: French J P (ed) Pediatric emergency skills. Mosby, St Louis, ch 1

Frey A M 1993 Pediatric intravenous therapy. In: Weinstein S M (ed) Principles and practice of intravenous therapy, 5th edn. JB Lippincott, Philadelphia, ch 25

Frey A M 1995 Pediatric peripherally inserted central catheter program report. Journal of Intravenous Nursing 18(6): 280–291

Fry B 1992 Intermittent heparin flushing protocols a standardization issue. Journal of Intravenous Nursing 15(3): 160–163

Gabriel J 1996 Peripherally inserted central catheters: expanding UK nurses' practice. British Journal of Nursing 5(2): 71–74

Gault D T 1993 Extravasation injuries. British Journal of Plastic Surgery 46: 91–96

Gill S 1993 Home administration of intravenous antibiotics to children with cystic fibrosis. British Journal of Nursing 2(15): 767–770

Goode C J, Titler M, Rakel B et al 1991 A meta-analysis of effects of heparin flush and saline flush: quality and cost implications. Nursing Research 40(6): 324–330

Goodinson S M 1990a The risks of IV therapy. Professional Nurse 5(5): 235–238

Goodinson S M 1990b Good practice ensures minimum risk factors. Complications of peripheral venous cannulation and infusion therapy. Professional Nurse 6(3): 175–177

Goolishan W, Konefal S 1989 An alternative method of securing Broviac catheters in children and infants. Journal of Parenteral and Enteral Nutrition 12(2): 218–219

Gullo S M 1993 Implanted ports: technologic advances and nursing care issues. Nursing Clinics of North America 29(4): 850–871

Gyr P, Smith K, Pontious S, Burroughs T, Mahl C, Swerczek L 1995 Double blind comparison of heparin and saline flush solutions in maintenance of peripheral infusion devices. Pediatric Nursing 21(4): 383–389

Hadaway L C 1995 Comparision of vascular access devices. Seminars in Oncology Nursing 11(3): 154–166

Halperin D L, Koren G, Attias D, Pellegrini E, Greenberg M L, Wyss M 1989 Topical skin anesthesia for venous, subcutaneous drug reservoir and lumbar punctures in children. Pediatrics 84(2): 281–284

Hanrahan K S, Kleiber C, Loebig Fagan C 1994 Evaluation of saline for IV locks in children. Pediatric Nursing 20(6): 549–552

Hansen B D, Evans M L 1981 Preparing a child for procedures. The American Journal of Maternal and Child Nursing 6: 392–397

Harris L C, Rushton C H, Hale S J 1987 Implantable infusion devices in the pediatric patient: a viable alternative. Journal of Pediatric Nursing 2(3): 174–183

Hazinski M F 1988 Understanding fluid balance in the seriously ill child. Pediatric Nursing 14(3): 231–236

Hazinski M F 1992 Children are different. In: Ladig D, Van Schaik T (eds) Nursing care of the critically ill child, 2nd edn. Mosby, St Louis, ch 1

Hecker J 1988 Improved technique in IV therapy. Nursing Times 84(34): 28–33

Hicks-Keen J 1995 Drug update. Slow down. Journal of Emergency Nursing 21(4): 323–326

Hindley M 1997 Reducing exit site infections and the risk of accidental removal of Hickman lines in children within the first month post insertion. Journal of Cancer Nursing 1(1): 54–55

Holcombe B J, Forloines-Lynn S, Garmhausen L W 1992 Restoring patency of long-term central venous access devices. Journal of Intravenous Nursing 15(1): 36–41

Holden C 1991 Home parenteral nutrition. Paediatric Nursing 3(3): 13–16

Hollis R 1992 Central venous access in children. Paediatric Nursing 4(2): 18–21

Hooker L, Williams J 1996 Parent-held shared care records: bridging the communication gaps. British Journal of Nursing 5(12): 738–741

Ingle R J 1995 Rare complications of vascular access devices. Seminars in Oncology Nursing 11(3): 184–193

Intravenous Nurses Society 1997 Position paper. Peripherally inserted central catheters. Journal of Intravenous Nursing 20(4): 172–174

Jennings P 1994 Learning through experience: an evaluation of 'hospital at home'. Journal of Advanced Nursing 19(5): 905–911

Joyce T H 1993 Topical anesthesia and pain management before venipuncture. The Journal of Pediatrics 122(5): S24–S29

Kachoyeanos M K, Friedoff M 1993 Cognitive and behavioral strategies to reduce children's pain. The American Journal of Maternal and Child Nursing 18: 14–19

Keller C A 1994 Methods of drawing blood samples through central venous catheters in pediatric patients undergoing bone marrow transplant: results of a national survey. Oncology Nursing Forum 21(5): 879–884

Kiely E 1988 Central venous catheters. In: Oakhill A (ed) The supportive care of the child with cancer. Wright, London, ch 10

Kleiber C, Hanrahan K, Loebig Fagan C, Zittergruen M A 1993 Heparin vs. saline for peripheral IV locks in children. Pediatric Nursing 19(4): 405–409

Koren G 1993 Use of the eutectic mixture of local anesthetics in young children for procedure-related pain. The Journal of Pediatrics 122(5): S30-S35

Lander J, Fowler-Kerry S, Oberle S 1992 Children's venipuncture pain: influence of technical factors. Journal of Pain and Symptom Management 7(6): 343–349

Lansdown R 1987 Helping children cope with needles. Department of Psychological Medicine, Great Ormond St Hospital, London

La Quaglia M P, Lucas A, Thaler H T, Friedlander-Klar H, Exelby P R, Groeger J S 1992 A prospective analysis of vascular access device-related infections in children. Journal of Pediatric Surgery 27(7): 840–842

Lawson R A, Smart N G, Gudgeon A C, Morton N S 1995 Evaluation of an amethocaine gel preparation for percutaneous analgesia before venous cannulation in children. British Journal of Anaesthesia 75: 282–285

Leese D 1989 My friend Wiggly. Paediatric Nursing 1(3): 12–13

Leonard B J, Dwyer Brust J, Nelson R P 1993 Parental distress: caring for medically fragile children at home. Journal of Pediatric Nursing 8(1): 22–30

Levy M, Benson L N, Bentur Y et al 1991 Tissue plasminogen activator for the treatment of thromboembolism in infants and children. The Journal of Pediatrics 118: 467–472

Liesner R J, Khair K, Hann I M 1996 The impact of prophylactic treatment on children with severe haemophilia. British Journal of Haematology 92(4): 973–978

Liesner R J, Vora A J, Hann I M, Lilleymann J S 1995 Use of central venous catheters in children with severe congenital coagulopathy. British Journal of Haematology 91: 203–207

Livesley J 1993 Reducing the risks: management of paediatric intravenous therapy. Child Health 1(2): 68–71

Livesley J 1996 Peripheral IV therapy in children. Paediatric Nursing 8(6): 29–33

Ljung R, Petrini P, Lindgren A K, Berntorp E 1992 Implantable central venous catheter facilitates prophylactic treatment in children with haemophilia. Acta Paediatrica Scandinavica 81: 918–920

Lokich J J, Bothe A, Benotti P, Moore C 1985 Complications and management of implanted venous access catheters. Journal of Clinical Oncology 3(5): 710–717

Lombardi T P, Gunderson B, Zammett L O, Walters K, Morris B A 1988 Efficacy of 0.9% sodium chloride injection with or without heparin sodium for maintaining patency of intravenous catheters in children. Clinical Pharmacy 7: 832–836

Long C A, Brynes K, Leclair J, Stashinko E E, Molchan E 1996 Central line associated bacteremia in the pediatric patient. Pediatric Nursing 22(3): 247–251

Lucas H, Attard-Montalto S 1996 Central line dressings: study of infection rates. Paediatric Nursing 8(6): 21–23

MacGeorge L, Steeves L, Steeves R H 1988 Comparison of the mixing and reinfusion methods of drawing blood from a Hickman catheter. Oncology Nursing Forum 15(3): 335–338

McGovern B, Solenberger K, Reed K 1985 A totally implantable venous access system for long-term chemotherapy in children. Journal of Pediatric Surgery 20: 725–727

McMullen A, Dutko Fioravanti I, Pollack V, Rideout K, Sciera M 1993 Heparinized saline or normal saline as a flush solution on intermittent intravenous lines in infants and children. The American Journal of Maternal and Child Nursing 18(2): 78–85

McVicar A, Clancy J 1992 Which infusate do I need? Physiological basis of fluid therapy. Professional Nurse 7(9): 587–591

Maki D G, Ringer M 1991 Risk factors for infusion-related phlebitis with small peripheral venous catheters. Annals of Internal Medicine 114: 845–854

Manley L 1988 Introsseous infusion: rapid vascular access for critically ill or injured infants and children. Journal of Emergency Nursing 14(2): 63–69

Manne S L, Bakeman R, Jacobsen P B, Gorfinkle K, Bernstein D, Redd W H 1992 Adult–child interaction during invasive medical procedures. Health Psychology 11(4): 241–249

Manne S L, Bakeman R, Jacobsen P B, Gorfinkle K, Redd W H 1994 An analysis of a behavioral intervention for children undergoing venipuncture. Health Psychology 13(6): 556–566

Marcoux C, Fisher S, Wong D 1990 Central venous access devices in children. Pediatric Nursing 16(2): 123–133

Marks M G 1994 Care of the hospitalized child. In: Marks M G (ed) Broadribb's introductory pediatric nursing, 4th edn. JB Lippincott, Philadelphia, ch 3

Maunuksela E L, Korpela R 1986 Double-blind evaluation of a lignocaine-prilocaine cream (EMLA) in children. British Journal of Anaesthesia 58: 1242–1245

May L 1992 Reducing pain and anxiety in children. Nursing Standard 6(44): 25–28

Mayo D J, Pearson D C 1995 Chemotherapy extravasation: a consequence of fibrin sheath formation around venous access devices. Oncology Nursing Forum 22(4): 675–680

Millam D A 1988 Managing complications of i.v. therapy. Nursing 18(3): 34–42

Miller K D, Dietrick C L 1997 Experience with PICC at a university medical center. Journal of Intravenous Nursing 20(3): 141–147

Mirro J, Rao B N, Kumar M et al 1990 A comparison of placement techniques and complications of externalized catheters and implantable port use in children with cancer. Journal of Pediatric Surgery 25(1): 120–124

Moore C L, Erikson K A, Yanes L B, Franklin M, Gonsalves L 1986 Nursing care and management of venous access ports. Oncology Nursing Forum 13(3): 35–39

Morton N S 1996 A comparison of ametop gel with EMLA cream in venous cannulation in children. In: Woolfson A D, McCafferty D F M (eds) Amethocaine gel, a new development in effective percutaneous local anaesthesia. Royal Society of Medicine Press, London, ch 3

Murdoch L, Bingham R 1990 Venous cannulation in infants and small children. British Journal of Hospital Medicine 44: 405–407

Nelson D, Garland J 1987 The natural history of teflon catheter associated phlebitis in children. American Journal of Diseases in Children 141: 1090–1092

Oakley C 1997 Peripherally inserted central venous catheters: the experience of a specialist oncology department. Journal of Cancer Nursing 1(1): 50–53

O'Brien R 1991 Starting intravenous lines in children. Journal of Emergency Nursing 17(4): 225–230

Oldman P 1991 A sticky situation? Microbiological study of adhesive tape used to secure IV cannulae. Professional Nurse 6(5): 265–269

O'Reilly C, McKay F M A, Duffy P, Lloyd D S 1988 Glyceryl trinitrate in skin necrosis caused by extravasation of parenteral nutrition. Lancet 8610(2): 565–566

Patterson J M, Jernell J, Leonard B J, Titus J C 1994 Caring for medically fragile children at home: the parent–professional relationship. Journal of Pediatric Nursing 9(2): 98–106

Pennington C R, Pithie A D 1987 Ethanol lock in the management of catheter occlusion. Journal of Parenteral and Enteral Nutrition 11(5): 507–508

Pettit J, Hughes K 1993 Intravenous extravasation: mechanisms, management, and prevention. The Journal of Perinatal and Neonatal Nursing 6(4): 69–79

Phelps S J, Helms R A 1987 Risk factors affecting infiltration of peripheral venous lines in infants. The Journal of Pediatrics 111: 384–389

Ramirez J M, Miguelena J M, Guemes A, Moncada E, Cabezali R, Sousa R 1993 Fully implantable venous access systems. British Journal of Surgery 80: 347–348

Reed T, Philips S 1996 Management of central venous catheter occlusions and repairs. Journal of Intravenous Nursing 19(6): 289–294

Reed W P, Newman K A, Applefeld M M, Sutton F J 1985 Drug extravasation as a complication of venous access ports. Annals of Internal Medicine 102(6): 788–789

Rice L J 1993 Needle phobia: an anesthesiologist's perspective. The Journal of Pediatrics 122(5): S9–S13

Robieux I, Kumar R, Radhakrishnan S, Koren G 1991 Assessing pain and analgesia with a lidocaine-prilocaine emulsion in infants and toddlers during venipuncture. The Journal of Pediatrics 118(6): 971–973

Ross M, Haase G M, Poole M A et al 1988 Comparision of totally implanted reservoirs with external catheters as venous access devices in pediatric oncology patients. Surgery, Gynecology and Obstetrics 167: 141–144

Rountree D 1991 The PIC catheter: a different approach. American Journal of Nursing 91(8): 22–28

Rutledge J C 1989 Pediatric specimen collection for chemical analysis. Pediatric Clinics of North America 36: 37–47

San Angel F 1995 Current controversies in chemotherapy administration. Journal of Intravenous Nursing 18(1): 16–23

Schulmeister L 1989 Needle dislodgement from implanted venous access devices: inpatient and outpatient experiences. Journal of Intravenous Nursing 12(2): 90–92

Schulmeister L 1992 An overview of continuous infusion chemotherapy. Journal of Intravenous Nursing 15(6): 315–321

Sclare I, Waring M 1995 Routine venepuncture: improving services. Paediatric Nursing 7(4): 23–27

Secola R 1997 Pediatric blood cell transplantation. Seminars in Oncology Nursing 13(3): 184–193

Sepion B 1990 Intravenous care for children. Paediatric Nursing 2(3): 14–16

Shulman R J, Reed T, Pitre D, Laine L 1988 Use of hydrochloric acid to clear obstructed central venous catheters. Journal of Parenteral and Enteral Nutrition 12(5): 509–510

Sidey A 1989 Intravenous home care. Paediatric Nursing 1(3): 14–15

Sidey A 1990 Co-operation in care. Paediatric Nursing 2(3): 10–12

Sidey A 1994 Administering intravenous antibiotics at home. In: Sidey A (ed) Administering intravenous therapy to children in the community, 2nd edn. Royal College of Nursing Paediatric Community Nurses Forum, London, ch 5

Sidey A 1995 Community nursing perspectives. In: Carter B, Dearmun A K (eds) Child health care nursing. Concepts, theory and practice. Blackwell Science, Oxford, ch 3

Soucy P 1987 Experiences with the use of the Port-a-Cath in children. Journal of Pediatric Surgery 22(8): 767–769

Southern D A, Read M S 1994 Overdosage of opiate from patient controlled analgesia devices. British Medical Journal 309: 1002

Stapleford P 1990 Parenteral nutrition in children. Paediatric Nursing 2(6): 18–20

Stovroff M C, Totten M, Glick P L 1994 PIC lines save money and hasten discharge in the care of children with ruptured appendicitis. Journal of Pediatric Surgery 29(2): 245–247

Strum S, McDermed J, Korn A, Joseph C 1986 Improved methods for venous access: the Port-a-Cath, a totally implanted catheter system. Journal of Clinical Oncology 4(4): 596–603

Styne D M 1994 Nephrology: fluids and electrolytes. In: Behrman R E, Kliegman R M (eds) Nelson's essentials of pediatrics, 2nd edn. WB Saunders, Philadelphia, ch 16

Tatman M A, Woodroffe C, Kelly P J, Harris R J 1992 Paediatric home care in Tower Hamlets: a working partnership with parents. Quality in Health Care 1: 98–103

Taylor D, Taylor S, Monarch K, Leon C, Hall J, Sibley Y 1996 Use of occlusive dressings on central venous catheter sites in hospitalized children. Journal of Pediatric Nursing 11(3): 169–174

Teague B R, Fleming J W, Castle A et al 1993 'High-tech' home care for children with chronic health conditions: a pilot study. Journal of Pediatric Nursing 8(4): 226–232

Testerman E J 1989 Current trends in pediatric total parenteral nutrition. Journal of Intravenous Nursing 12(3): 152–162

Tietjen S D 1990 Starting an infant's IV. American Journal of Nursing 90(5): 44–47

Vazquez R M, Racenstein M 1987 A method to prevent unintentional removal of a Hickman catheter. Journal of Parenteral and Enteral Nutrition 11(5): 509–510

Viall C D 1990 Your complete guide to central venous catheters. Nursing 20(2): 34–41

Vidler V 1994 Use of Port-a-Caths in the management of paediatric haemophilia. Professional Nurse 10(1): 48–50

Wachs T 1990 Urokinase administration in pediatric patients with occluded central venous catheters. Journal of Intravenous Nursing 13(2): 100–102

Weinstein S M 1993 Techniques of intravenous therapy. In: Weinstein S M (ed) Plumer's principles and practice of intravenous therapy, 5th edn. JB Lippincott, Philadelphia, ch 8

Wheeler C, Frey A M 1995 Intravenous therapy in children. In: Terry J (ed) Intravenous therapy. Clinical principles and practice. WB Saunders, Philadelphia, ch 27

Wheeler R A, Spalding T J W, Thomas J A, Carss G A 1991a The retrograde tunnel: a method for the fixation of central venous catheters in the military environment. Journal of the Royal Naval Medical Services 77: 75–77

Wheeler S, Stolz S, Maki D G 1991b A prospective, randomized, three-way clinical comparison of a novel, highly permeable, polyurethane dressing with 206 Swan-Ganz pulmonary artery catheters: Opsite IV 3000 vs Tegaderm vs gauze and tape. In: Maki D G (ed) Improving catheter site care. Royal Society of Medicine Services, London, p 67–72

Whiting M 1990 Home care for children. Nursing Standard 4(22): 52–54

Whitman M 1995 Delivering medications safely by I.V. bolus. Nursing 25(8): 52–54

Wickham R S 1990 Advances in venous access devices and nursing management strategies. Nursing Clinics of North America 25(2): 345–362

Wiener E S, McGuire P, Stolar C J H et al 1992 The CCSG prospective study of venous access devices: an analysis of insertions and causes for removal. Journal of Pediatric Surgery 27(2): 155–164

Williams J, Smith H L, Woods C G, Weller P H 1988 Silastic catheters for antibiotics in cystic fibrosis. Archives of Disease in Childhood 63: 658–659

Wilson D 1992 Neonatal IVs: practical tips. Neonatal Network 11(2): 49–53

Wiltgen-Trotter C 1996 Percutaneous central venous catheter-related sepsis in the neonate: an analysis of the literature from 1990 to 1994. Neonatal Network 15(3): 15–28

Wink D M 1991 Precision + caution = safety. The American Journal of Maternal and Child Nursing 16(6): 317–321

Winslow M N, Trammell L, Camp-Sorrell D 1995 Selection of vascular access devices and nursing care. Seminars in Oncology Nursing 11(3): 167–173

Wood L S, Gullo S M 1993 IV vesicants: how to avoid extravasation. American Journal of Nursing 93(4): 42–46

Woolfson A D, McCafferty D F, Boston V 1990 Clinical experiences with a novel percutaneous amethocaine preparation: prevention of pain due to venepuncture in children. British Journal of Clinical Pharmacology 30: 273–279

Wurzel C L, Halom K, Feldman J G, Rubin L G 1988 Infection rates of Broviac-Hickman catheters and implantable venous devices. American Journal of Diseases of Children 142: 536–540

Zappa S C, Nabors S B 1992 Use of ethyl chloride topical anesthetic to reduce procedural pain in pediatric oncology patients. Cancer Nursing 15(2): 130–136

Zenk K E, Dungy C I, Greene G R 1981 Nafcillin extravasation injury. Use of hyaluronidase as an antidote. The American Journal of Diseases in Children 135(12): 1113–1114

Safe handling and administration of intravenous cytotoxic drugs

CHAPTER 16

Lisa Dougherty

INTRODUCTION

The word cytotoxic means 'toxic to cells'. It refers to a group of drugs used mainly in the treatment of cancer to prevent proliferation and destroy abnormal cells, although some cytotoxic drugs have been administered for non-malignant conditions such as psoriasis.

The primary action of a cytotoxic drug is in destroying as many dividing cells as possible and preventing cells from further division. Since cancer cells exhibit uncontrolled cell division, they are very receptive to the action of cytotoxic drugs (Robinson 1993). However, certain organs, such as bone marrow, are also areas of rapidly dividing cells and as a result are also affected by the cytotoxic action of the drugs. This often results in the problems of toxicity which are associated with cancer therapy. The drugs can be administered via a variety of routes, e.g. oral, intramuscular, subcutaneous and intracavity, but the main route is intravenous, administered as bolus injection, or intermittent or continuous infusion.

This chapter will focus mainly on how the practitioner manages intravenous cytotoxic therapy, focusing on the handling, administration and prevention of specific complications such as extravasation.

CLASSIFICATION AND TYPES OF DRUGS

Cytotoxic drugs are grouped according to their specific effects on the cell and the phase of the cell cycle upon which they are active. The cell cycle describes a sequence of steps through which all cells grow and replicate. This process of growth and replication consists of five phases (Tortorice 1997; Fig. 16.1). Cell cycle phase

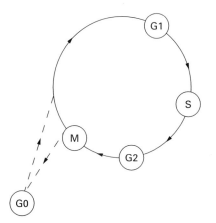

G1 Initial resting phase
(RNA and protein synthesis)

S Synthetic phase
(doubling of DNA)

G2 Premitotic phase
(also known as second
resting phase)

M Actual process of mitosis

G0 Phase where cells are not
actively dividing and enter
G1 phase when suitably
stimulated

Fig. 16.1 The five phases of the cell cycle: G_0, G_1, S, G_2 and M.

specific drugs are active only during a particular phase of the cell cycle. These give the greatest tumour kill when administered in divided doses or as a continuous infusion with a short cycle time. Cell cycle phase non-specific drugs are active at any point in the cell cycle, including the G_0 resting phase. They are effective in the treatment of slow-growing tumours, and cell kill is directly proportional to the amount of drug given. Ninety per cent of human tumour cells have cell cycle times within the range of 15–120 hours, with an average of 48 hours (Priestman 1989, Robinson 1993).

Cytotoxic drugs are further classified according to their chemical structure, e.g. vinca alkaloids, antimetabolites, alkylating agents (Table 16.1).

RATIONALE FOR METHOD OF DELIVERY OF CYTOTOXIC THERAPY

Continuous infusional chemotherapy

By administering a single drug or combination of drugs as a continuous infusion, regardless of the length of cell cycle of individual tumour cells, the cytotoxic drugs would always be present when a sensitive phase of the cycle was reached. The transport of cytotoxic drugs across a tumour cell membrane may depend not only on drug concentration, but also on the time the drug is available to the cell membrane. As many cytotoxic drugs have short pharmacological half-lives, such agents may be more effective if exposed to tumour cells for prolonged periods rather than given by intermittent bolus injections. When given continuously, the concentration of the drug in the plasma is far lower than levels seen immediately after bolus injections or short infusions. Many of the acute toxicities of the drug may therefore be avoided (Priestman 1989).

Intermittent chemotherapy

The normal cell population is diminished by treatment but recovers initially far more rapidly than malignant cells. Restoration is achieved more quickly in normal tissue than malignant tissue; therefore, if a series of treatments is given with an interval for recovery of normal tissue between each treatment, it is possible to eradicate the tumour without jeopardizing the normal cell population. The time of the treatment is very important. If the interval is too short, normal stem cells will not have recovered sufficiently and cumulative toxicity will result, preventing adequate treatment. If, on the other hand, the interval between courses is too long, tumour cell recovery will be complete, allowing the tumour to remain static or even increase in size between treatments. The splitting of chemotherapy into short intensive intervals is known as intermittent chemotherapy and it has allowed multiple drug combinations to be used without causing irreversible toxicity and with a consequent increase in response rates (Priestman 1989).

Combination chemotherapy

Cytotoxic drugs have a variety of actions on the dividing cell. Therefore, a tumour cell which may be resistant to one drug with a particular mode of action might well be susceptible to a different agent with an alternative form of cytotoxicity. Combining drugs with different mechanisms of cell kill reduces the risk of encountering resistant cells and toxicity and increases fractional cell kill, thereby improving response rates (Tortorice 1997). The choice of drugs for combination chemotherapy is based on the following:

- All drugs in the combination should be of proven value against the disease they are intended to treat.

Table 16.1 Classification of cytotoxic drugs

Group of drugs	Mechanism of action	Names of drugs in category	Administration methods	Common side-effects
Cell cycle specific Antimetabolites	Class II S phase action	Methatrexate	Intravenous bolus or infusion	Stomatitis, anorexia, malaise, eye irritation, bone marrow depression (BMD), renal failure, photosensitivity, pulmonary changes, fever, chills
		Fluorouracil	Bolus, infusion, continuous infusion	Diarrhoea, stomatitis, anorexia, palmar/plantar syndrome, hyperpigmentation, mild alopecia with high doses
		Raltitrexed	Intravenous infusion	Mucositis, nausea and vomiting, anorexia, diarrhoea, rash, fatigue
		Cytarabine	Intravenous infusion	Nausea and vomiting, flu-like syndrome, BMD, stomatitis, lethargy
		Cladrabine Pentostatin	Intravenous bolus	Abdo pain, flushing, rash, pruritus, nausea and vomiting, BMD thrombophlebitis, dysuria, constipation
		Fludarabine	Intravenous bolus, short infusion	Mild nausea and vomiting, fatigue, anorexia
		Gemcitabine	Intravenous infusion over 30 minutes	Rash, injection site reaction, flu-like syndrome, mild peripheral oedema, bronchospasm
		Hydroxyurea 6-Mercaptapurine 6-Thioguanine	Oral	Stomatitis Nausea Diarrhoea
Vinca alkaloids	Class II phase-specific Occurs in S phase and shows in M phase, binds to tuberlin	Vincristine	Intravenous bolus or infusion (central venous route only)	Cold sensation along vein during injection, jaw or tumour pain, neurotoxicity – peripheral neuropathy, constipation, alopecia (high doses only), BMD
		Vinblastine Vindesine Vinorelbine		As above and phlebitis As above As above, severe injection site pain, in arm and back during injection, venous discoloration and phlebitis
Antitumour antibiotics	Class III Binds with DNA, active in S phase	Bleomycin	Intravenous bolus or infusion	Tumour pain, allergic reactions, fever, chills, skin reactions, nail ridging, stomatitis, pulmonary fibrosis
		Actinomycin D	Slow i.v. bolus into side arm of saline infusion	Nausea and vomiting, anorexia, stomatitis, skin changes, BMD, reactivation of radiation sites, alopecia

(cont'd)

Table 16.1 (cont'd)

Group of drugs	Mechanism of action	Names of drugs in category	Administration methods	Common side-effects
		Mitomycin C	Slow i.v. bolus	Pain on injection, nausea and vomiting, diarrhoea, anorexia, BMD, fatigue, nephrotoxic, phlebitis, stomatitis'
Epipodophyllotoxins	Inhibits at metaphase, G_2 and S phase also affected	Etoposide	Intravenous infusion over 30 minutes	Severe hypotension if infused rapidly, nausea and vomiting, alopecia, BMD
Taxanes	Effective in G_2 and M phase, inhibits cell division	Paclitaxel	Intravenous infusion	Severe anaphylaxis, nausea and vomiting, diarrhoea, stomatitis, alopecia, BMD, hypotension, sensory perception loss, neuropathy
		Docetaxel	Intravenous infusion	Mild skin reaction, phlebitis, allergic reaction, nausea and vomiting, fluid retention, diarrhoea, stomatitis, rash, BMD, alopecia, myalgia, paraesthesia
Anthracyclines		Daunorubicin	Slow i.v. bolus into side arm of a fast-running infusion	Red venous flush, nausea and vomiting, fever, red discoloured urine, BMD, diarrhoea, alopecia, phlebitis, stomatitis, congestive cardiac failure
		Doxorubicin	Intravenous bolus or infusion (central venous route only)	Red flush 'flare reaction', aching along veins, nausea and vomiting, alopecia, stomatitis, red discoloured urine, BMD, thrombophlebitis, cardiotoxic
		Epirubicin	Slow i.v. bolus into side arm of a fast-running infusion	As above
		Idarubicin	Slow i.v. bolus	Venous pain, rash, nausea and vomiting, stomatitis, diarrhoea, BMD, alopecia, cardiotoxicity
		Mitozantrone	Slow i.v. bolus or infusion	Green discoloration of urine, anorexia, mild nausea and vomiting, blue discoloration of vein, minimal alopecia, fever, amenorrhoea
		Adarubicin	Intravenous bolus into fast running infusion	Mild phlebitis, nausea and vomiting, stomatitis, red urine, BMD, mild alopecia, cardiotoxicity
Miscellaneous	Inhibits intracellular protein synthesis	Asparaginase	Intravenous bolus	Severe anaphylaxis, malaise, anorexia, hepatotoxic, central toxicity, pancreatic dysfunction
Nitrosurea (alkylating)	Cell cycle non-specific	Carmustine	Intravenous infusion over 1–2 hours	Intense venous pain when given rapidly, facial flushing, BMD, nausea and vomiting, gynaecomastia

Table 16.1 (cont'd)

Group of drugs	Mechanism of action	Names of drugs in category	Administration methods	Common side-effects
		Lomustine	Oral	Anorexia, nausea and vomiting, BMD
		Streptocozin	Intravenous infusion over 30–60 minutes	Burning along the vein, hypoglycaemia if infused too rapidly, nausea and vomiting, hepatotoxicity, renal toxicity, anaemia
Alkylating	Class III, cell cycle non-specific. Interferes with DNA replication	Cyclophosphamide	Intravenous bolus or infusion	Hot flush, dizziness, metallic taste, nasal stuffiness – all during injection, nausea and vomiting, anorexia, BMD, alopecia, chemical haemorrhagic cystitis, sterility
		Busulphan	Oral	BMD, skin pigmentation, hyperuricaemia
		Chlorambucil	Oral	Nausea and vomiting in high doses, BMD, sterility, secondary malignancy
		Dacarbazine	Intravenous infusion	Pain along the vein if infusion too rapid, facial flushing, flu-like syndrome, anorexia, BMD, alopecia
		Ifosfamide	Slow i.v. bolus or infusion	Nausea and vomiting, haematuria, anorexia, chemical thrombophlebitis, alopecia, nephrotoxicity, haemorrhagic cystitis, lethargy, confusion
		Melphalan	Slow i.v. bolus, oral	Anaphylaxis, nausea and vomiting, BMD, alopecia, dermatitis, pulmonary fibrosis
		Thiotepa	Slow i.v. bolus or infusion	Pain at injection site, rare nausea, allergy, alopecia, BMD, amenorrhoea
		Treosulfan	Slow i.v. bolus	Nausea and vomiting, mild allergic reaction, BMD, alopecia
		Cisplatin	Infusion over 1–6 hours	Rare anaphylaxis, metallic taste, nausea and vomiting, nephrotoxic, BMD, otological and neurological toxicity
		Procarbazine	Oral	Nausea and vomiting, flu-like syndrome, diarrhoea, CNS toxicity, BMD, reacts with alcohol and certain foods
		Carboplatin	Intravenous infusion over 30–60 minutes	Rare allergic reaction, nausea and vomiting, BMD, nephrotoxicity

● The drugs should have different modes of cytotoxic action.

● If possible, the dose-limiting toxicities of the chosen agents should be different, so that the additive toxicity does not limit the dose intensity of treatment (Holmes 1990, Priestman 1989).

High-dose chemotherapy

A few drugs (those for which the major toxicity is to the bone marrow) may be used in very high doses if bone marrow/stem cells are taken from the patient prior to treatment and returned later. In this way, doses of the drug which are severely toxic to the bone marrow may be given safely, as the bone marrow autograft is not exposed to the drug. When it is returned to the patient, the autograft will restore the blood count to normal within a few weeks. However, a bone marrow/stem cell autograft will not reduce the other toxicities that may result from high-dose chemotherapy (Robinson 1993).

OCCUPATIONAL HAZARDS

Cytotoxic drug handling by nursing and pharmacy personnel is an acknowledged occupational hazard (Valanis et al 1993), but concerns have increased over the last 10–15 years as more scientific evidence has come to light regarding the potential and actual hazards of exposure to cytotoxic drugs (Falck et al 1979, Selevan et al 1985, Valanis et al 1993, Vennit et al 1984, Waksvik et al 1981). This is because these drugs are mutagenic, teratogenic and/or carcinogenic (Allwood et al 1997, Mallett & Bailey 1996, Reymann 1993).

The health risk associated with exposure to cytotoxic drugs is measured by the time, dose and route of exposure (Powell 1996). Primary routes for exposure include absorption through the skin, inhalation or ingestion. Exposure can occur during drug preparation and reconstitution, administration and handling. This can be as a result of aerosolization of powder or liquid during reconstitution, contact with contaminated equipment used in preparing or administering the drugs, or contamination of food leading to oral ingestion (Valanis et al 1993). Patients may excrete some drugs in their urine or faeces, and therefore staff are exposed when handling and disposing of waste. Exposure has been reported to result in local effects, caused by direct contact with the skin, eyes and mucous membranes, and systemic complaints from handling (see Box 16.1) (Mallett & Bailey 1996, Speechley 1984, Valanis et al 1993, Weinstein 1997).

A number of studies have suggested that there are serious long-term effects of exposure. For example, some nurses exposed to cytotoxic agents have suffered spon-taneous abortion or given birth to children with malformations, while others have shown increased mutagenic activity in their urine and serum (Behamou 1986, Falck et al 1979, Hemminki et al 1985, Selevan et al 1985, Taskinan 1990). As a result of these studies, a number of safety measures have been introduced in order to protect all per-sonnel who prepare, administer or handle cytotoxic drugs or waste products. In 1988, the Heath and Safety Executive introduced the Control of Substances Hazardous to Health (COSHH) regulations and these were updated in 1996. Whilst these regula-tions cover a wide range of hazardous substances, they include guidelines on the safe handling of cytotoxic drugs. Employers are now obliged to identify hazardous sub-stances, the people who may be exposed to them, how they should be handled and what to do in the event of accidental exposure. The literature supports the theory that the use of proper protective practices and equipment when handling cytotoxic drugs will provide adequate protection from their effects (Wiseman & Wachs 1990). Since such measures have been introduced, studies have focused on how the use of protec-tive clothing can substantially reduce staff exposure levels, including levels and

■ **BOX 16.1**

Effects of cytotoxic drugs (from Mallett & Bailey 1996)

Local effects
- Dermatitis
- Inflammation of mucous membranes
- Excessive lacrimation
- Pigmentation
- Blistering
- Other miscellaneous, allergic reactions

Systemic effects
- Light-headedness
- Dizziness
- Nausea
- Headache
- Alopecia
- Coughing
- Pruritus
- General malaise

changes found in urine and serum (Allwood et al 1997). Other studies have looked at the issue of compliance with protective measures in practice.

Nieweg et al (1994) carried out a survey of Dutch nurses who were involved in caring for patients receiving cytotoxic drugs on a regular basis. They wanted to discover how many of these nurses utilized the protective measures provided. The majority of nurses wore gloves (91%) when preparing and administering drugs, but few wore masks, gowns or goggles, and this use was even lower in those handling excreta. The study concluded that although not all guidelines were up to date, the nurses still did not always follow the established guidelines. This was also the case in a survey carried out by Wiseman & Wachs (1990), who concluded that health care workers still did not use available protective equipment and procedures.

However, it is expected that all institutions should develop and implement reasonable policies and procedures that will lower the risk to practitioners and the environment (Mayer 1992). Christensen et al (1990) found that the existence of a formal hospital policy for handling of cytotoxics positively influenced the use of personal protective equipment. The aim of such a policy should be to recognize the hazards of cytotoxic drugs and to prevent, or reduce to a minimum, exposure to these hazards in the workplace. This would be achieved by the provision of adequate protective equipment and clothing, regular staff monitoring, and effective written procedures and guidelines for dealing with preparation, administration, disposal and handling of spillage. It would also require ongoing staff training to ensure that these drugs are only administered by skilled, knowledgeable and experienced health care professionals (Allwood et al 1997, Mallett & Bailey 1996, Mayer 1992).

SAFE HANDLING

Environment

All reconstitution of cytotoxic drugs must be conducted within a suitable safety cabinet or isolator such as a biological safety cabinet class II vertical laminar air flow. This equipment should meet national standards and be inspected appropriately and serviced regularly according to the manufacturer's recommendations. Cabinets should ideally be situated within a specified or dedicated area with the access restricted to supervised personnel. This is in order to prevent the possible contamination of other personnel or work areas. Standard operating procedures should be in place and strictly adhered to for maximum operator protection (Allwood et al 1997, Doyle 1995, Reymann 1993, RCN 1989, Weinstein 1997).

Protective clothing

Allwood et al (1997) suggested that 'protective clothing should be worn at all times when handling cytotoxics'. There are minimum requirements for the degree of protective clothing to be worn and these are often based upon the amount of possible exposure and the situation in which the practitioner is handling the drug, e.g. controlled or uncontrolled preparation environment, administration or transportation. The requirements are usually based on local or nationally agreed guidelines.

Gowns This category includes gowns, suits, armlets and aprons. It has been suggested that gowns be made of a lightweight, low-linting, low-permeability material with a solid front and long cuffed sleeves; these may be either disposable or made of conventional fabric (Allwood et al 1997, Powell 1996, Reymann 1993, Weinstein 1997). There are many commercially available gowns and suits and these are commonly used by personnel who are reconstituting cytotoxic drugs. Allwood et al (1997) suggested that disposable gowns made of polyurethane-coated Tyvek and Saranex-laminated Tyvek offered the maximum protection. In studies, the non-porous Tyvek did allow some drug penetration, but when used with armlets it is suitable for all administration and waste disposal procedures, along with the use of plastic aprons. The practitioner should be provided with a protective water-resistant barrier to accidental spills or sprays. Tyvek aprons provide added protection in an uncontrolled environment.

Both Doyle (1995) and Powell (1996) highlighted the negative effect that all this protective clothing could have on the patient and suggested that the degree of use during administration should be based on personal preference. However, Reymann (1995) suggested that patient education regarding cytotoxic drug handling was the answer, in order that patients and family members understand why gloves and gowns are being worn and do not feel alienated by the practice.

Masks It appears that standard surgeons' masks are suitable for most procedures carried out in a contained environment (Allwood et al 1997). The risk of inhalation should be reduced by use of a correct and safe technique when reconstituting drugs and by the use of equipment such as 0.2 mm filtered venting needles. If there is a possibility of inhalation, a suitable dust mask should be worn, e.g. BS 6016 (Allwood et al 1997).

Eye protection Goggles are used to protect the eyes from splashes and any dust particles and so should fully enclose the eye, e.g. BS 2092C. Goggles should be worn whenever reconstituting or dealing with a spillage.

Gloves There is little doubt that disposable gloves should be worn at all times when reconstituting, administering and handling cytotoxic drugs or when handling the excreta of patients receiving the drugs. It is the one piece of protective clothing that most practitioners wear when dealing with any aspect of cytotoxic therapy. However, there is some debate as to which gloves are the most suitable and which offer the best protection – as yet there is no consensus. Studies carried out have attempted to determine glove thickness, particularly the variation in thickness within batches, and the permeability of the gloves (Kotilainen 1989, Laidlaw 1984, Thomas & Fenton-May 1987). Allwood et al (1997) concluded that no glove material is completely impermeable to every cytotoxic agent. The major factors affecting penetration rates include glove thickness, molecular weight of the drug, lipophilicity, the nature of the solvent in which the drug is dissolved and glove material composition (Allwood et al 1997).

When selecting gloves, the material should be of a suitable thickness and integrity to maximize the protection whilst maintaining manual dexterity (Laidlaw 1984). Certainly, the use of poor-quality, low-cost gloves is neither safe nor cost-effective (Allwood et al 1997). Some authors recommend the use of unpowdered latex gloves, suggesting that latex affords a superior protection to polyvinyl chloride and is less permeable (Doyle 1995, Powell 1996, Reymann 1993, Weinstein 1997); the thickness should be between 0.007 and 0.009 inches.

Some experts recommend the practice of double-gloving during reconstitution (Doyle 1995, Powell 1996, Weinstein 1997). However, this may be unnecessary if gloves are of good quality and is usually only required when cleaning up large spills (Reymann 1993). Regular changing of gloves is common, although the frequency varies from changing them every 30–60 minutes to changing them at each work session; they should also be changed immediately following known contact with a cytotoxic agent or following puncture (Allwood et al 1997, Gibbs 1991, Mallett & Bailey 1996, Powell 1996, Weinstein 1997).

RECONSTITUTION

There are a number of possible options when choosing the environment in which to reconstitute cytotoxic drugs (see Table 16.2):

- A pharmacy-controlled centralized unit where reconstitution of cytotoxic drugs is only performed by specially trained individuals (Allwood et al 1997, RCN 1989).
- A pharmacy-controlled satellite unit where work is centralized in designated hospital areas.
- A ward/clinic based in a controlled environment but operated by a nurse/doctor.
- A ward/clinic based in an uncontrolled environment, such as a clinical room, where nurses or doctors prepare drugs using certain techniques and procedures to reduce exposure to the drugs. Whilst this is not ideal, occasionally it may be necessary. In these circumstances, a room which is well ventilated and which has a sink with running water as well as impermeable work surfaces should be utilized (Mallett & Bailey 1996) to enable cleaning of surfaces in the event of a spillage. It is important to have minimal traffic of staff in the area in order to minimize interruptions and reduce the risk of contamination (Mallett & Bailey 1996, Weinstein 1997).
- A commercial service where the drugs are bought in already prepared.

The use of a plastic absorbent pad or liner on the work surface or the use of a plastic or stainless steel tray is recommended, to contain and minimize contamination (Powell 1996, Reymann 1993, Weinstein 1997). Protective clothing should be worn, i.e. gown/apron, gloves, goggles, mask, armlets. Aseptic technique should be used throughout the reconstitution procedure. Ampoules should be handled carefully and the neck of the ampoule covered with a gauze swab and held away from

Table 16.2 Advantages and disadvantages of the different environments in which cytotoxic drugs are reconstituted (adapted from Allwood et al 1997)

Environment	Advantages	Disadvantages
Pharmacy-controlled cytotoxic unit	• High sterility assurance • Standardization of presentation • Trained and skilled staff	• Potential cost • Out of hours may not be provided • Potential long-term exposure of pharmacy staff • Loss of expertise at ward level
Pharmacy-controlled satellite unit	• Workload centralized in designated areas • Increased interprofessional contact • Potential for access by non-pharmacy staff out of hours • Ability to respond more quickly to requests	• Deployment of staff from pharmacy • Potential for greater wastage • Negotiating space within other departments • Increased stock holdings
Ward/clinic-based (uncontrolled)	• Status quo	• High level of wastage and stock holdings • Possibility of untrained staff preparing doses • No product protection
Ward/clinic-based (controlled)	• Reduced pharmacy labour costs • Rapid response 24-hour service	• High nursing and medical staff turnover, leading to increased training • Less time for patient care • Hard to maintain standard of quality assurance • Reduced assurance of sterility and increased wastage and stock holdings
Commercial	• No added capital or staff costs • Full range of ready-to-use drugs • Minimal stock holdings and reduced wastage • Comprehensive documentation	• Increased revenue expenditure • Delivery and communication problems if not on site

the face when broken. This will prevent contamination of the skin and liberation of powder or the formation of aerosol (Mallett & Bailey 1996, Powell 1996, Reymann 1993, Weinstein 1997).

When reconstituting drugs in powder form, care should be taken when adding diluents to vials or ampoules. The drug should be added slowly, 'dribbled' down the side of the container so it gradually mixes with the powder and prevents the formation of an aerosol (Mallett & Bailey 1996, Powell 1996). The use of filtered venting systems and large-bore needles will help to reduce the risk of aerosol formation by creating a negative pressure in the vial and filtering the air released (Allwood et al 1997, Powell 1996, Reymann 1993, Weinstein 1997). Some authors have suggested that needles should be capped before the expulsion of air, the tip covered with a sterile swab or the air expelled into the vial in order to prevent contamination and the risk of splashing (Mallett & Bailey 1996). Reymann (1993), however, suggested that air should not be expelled. If air is present in the syringe, it should be held in such a way that the air is near the plunger and the practitioner should simply stop pushing on the plunger when all the drug is expelled and the air is reached. Luer-lock syringes should always be used to ensure that there is no risk of disconnection during the procedure (Mallett & Bailey 1996). Ideally, administration sets should be primed in the reconstitution unit (Powell 1996). However, where accidental spillage is possible, infusion bags should be connected to i.v. administration sets and primed before adding cytotoxic drug to the infusion solution. If this is not possible then the bag should be laid flat and the administration set spike pushed firmly into it, as it may be unsafe to spike a hanging bag because of the risk of splashing or puncturing the side of the bag.

Once reconstituted, the syringe or infusion bag must be labelled according to institutional policy – this usually includes the patient's name, hospital number, name and dose of drug, volume of drug, expiration date and diluent fluid.

ADMINISTRATION

Cytotoxic drugs must be administered by specially trained nurses (Powell 1996, RCN 1989, Weinstein 1997). The nurse must be satisfied that the patient has given informed consent and has been given a full explanation regarding the side-effects that may occur during or following administration. Appropriate laboratory results, e.g. full blood count and renal function tests, should be within acceptable levels and the prescription should be dated, legible and signed. Protocols and dosage should also be checked and the appropriate premedication administered, e.g. prehydration or anti-emetics (Mallett & Bailey 1996, Powell 1996, Weinstein 1997).

Patients who are commencing cytotoxic therapy often have a lack of knowledge about what it involves and the possible side-effects. Many may have gleaned inappropriate information from the media or friends and family. Moreover, patients receiving therapy are repeatedly exposed to venepuncture and cannulation unless they have had a central venous catheter inserted at the beginning of treatment. All this can be stressful for patients and provoke a good deal of anxiety. In addition, practitioners should be aware that aspects of cytotoxic drug administration which they may dismiss as unimportant can also be causes of concern to patients (Colbourne 1995; see Box 16.2).

A change in a patient's routine can also be upsetting. As Kaplan (1983) reported:

'One patient became anxious when her chemotherapy was administered in a different manner than it had been previously. The first time the drug was given by i.v., the nurse was at her side. The second time, the i.v. was begun and the patient was left unattended; she mistakenly assumed she was receiving the wrong drug.'

These concerns and worries must be addressed prior to starting treatment and an adequate explanation should be given, along with written information in the form of booklets or videotapes; cassettes or other teaching aids should be available to support verbal information.

Protective clothing should be worn and its necessity explained to the patient. Aseptic technique should be followed throughout the administration procedure. All syringes and infusion bags should be checked for any leakage or contamination and the details on the labels should correspond with the prescription chart and the patient. Use only i.v. administration sets with luer-lock fittings to ensure that there is no risk of accidental disconnection during administration.

Drugs may be administered via a winged infusion device, a peripheral cannula or

■ **BOX 16.2**

Examples of patient anxiety

'The roots of my anxiety stemmed from the knowledge of the inevitable side-effects of nausea and vomiting, pain on starting i.v.s and foley catheters, isolation, dependency versus independency issues and hospitalisation itself.' (Buckalew 1982)

'Other stressful situations include i.v.s that stop dripping or run dry before a nurse appears. Infusion pumps that continue to beep after the nurse resets them are also worrisome.' (Kaplan 1983)

'During my second treatment, the i.v. infiltrated. After this experience, my anxiety skyrocketed prior to having an i.v. started or blood drawn ... having my husband or family member watch the i.v. alleviated my fear of infiltration. ... The oncology nurse practitioner periodically checked the i.v. on her rounds. Her presence during my treatment was emotionally supportive and helped to relieve my anxiety.' (Buckalew 1982)

■ **BOX 16.3**

Needle size

Favouring use of larger gauges

● Irritants reach general circulation faster, with a less irritating effect on peripheral veins
● Administration time is decreased which reduces patients' exposure

Favouring use of smaller gauges

● Less likely to puncture posterior wall of small vein
● Less scar tissue formation
● Less pain on insertion
● Increased blood flow around the needle, increasing dilution of the drug
● Reduced risk of mechanical phlebitis

a central venous access device. A winged infusion device is used for bolus injections of non-vesicant drugs and is associated with an increased risk of infiltration (Tully et al 1981). Cannulae may be used for both bolus and short-term infusions, and the size of the needle chosen is often based on the type of outcome the practitioner wishes to achieve (Box 16.3). Central venous access is preferred for patients who require long-term therapy or who are at risk of extravasation caused by vein inaccessibility or fragility (Weinstein 1997). The suggested order for site selection of winged infusion devices or cannulae is the forearm, the dorsum of the hand and the wrist, with the antecubital fossa as a last resort (Doyle 1995) (see Fig. 16.2). If the patient has an established peripheral cannula in situ, the dressing should be removed and the site assessed for redness, pain or tenderness. Patency of the cannula must be checked by withdrawing blood and then flushing using 5–10 ml of sodium chloride 0.9% to ensure there is no resistance to the flow of fluid. This also allows the practitioner to observe for any swelling or signs of pain or discomfort from the patient.

Cytotoxic drugs may be administered:

● by bolus injection
● via the side arm of a fast running infusion of sodium chloride 0.9%
● as a continuous infusion.

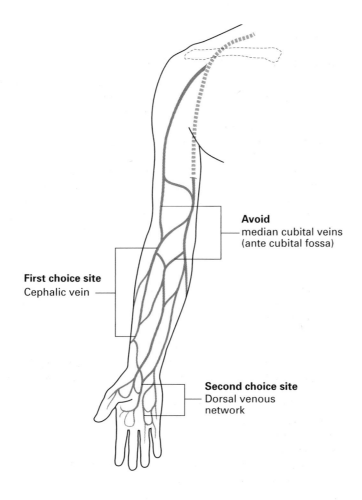

Fig. 16.2 Sites for cannulation and administration of chemotherapy.

Avoid
median cubital veins
(ante cubital fossa)

First choice site
Cephalic vein

Second choice site
Dorsal venous
network

The choice is often dependent upon the type of drug, the pharmacological considerations (such as stability or the need for dilution in a certain volume of fluid), the degree of potential venous irritation, whether the drug is a vesicant or not, and the type of device in situ.

Bolus injection

By administering a drug as a bolus injection, the integrity of the vein can be assessed and the early signs of extravasation can be noted more easily. Any observation of signs or symptoms of infiltration or extravasation will ensure the immediate discontinuation of the injection, investigation and the appropriate management. However, bolus injection can increase the risk of venous irritation due to the constant contact of the drug with the vein, and this could result in pain and make it difficult to distinguish between venous spasm and extravasation.

Via a side arm

Bolus injections can also be administered via the side arm of a free flowing infusion of sodium chloride 0.9%. This ensures maximum dilution of the potentially irritant drugs and aids rapid circulation away from the insertion site. It can also allow the practitioner to observe for early signs of infiltration or extravasation. However, if the veins are small or the cannula is too small, there will still not be a brisk flow of the infusate, the drug may come back up the tubing and the practitioner is still required to clamp off the tubing to check for blood return and continually check flow of the infusate, interrupting constant observation of the site.

Continuous infusion

Infusions allow increased dilution of the drug, thereby reducing the chemical irritation that can occur if drugs are given as a bolus injection, and may be necessary depending on the side-effects, e.g. hypotension or hypoglycaemia. However, vesicants given as a continuous infusion into a peripheral vein should be avoided where possible, as the risk of extravasation is great (Weinstein 1997). Blood return cannot be assessed frequently with infusions, and the longer the infusion, the greater is the possibility of needle dislodgement. Infiltration and extravasation may be subtle and difficult to detect until a large volume has infiltrated, and the patient may be sedated and unable to report any sensations associated with extravasation. The practitioner should not rely on the pump to alarm if an infusion begins to infiltrate. Initially, the flow is free and it is only when the pressure builds up in the tissues that the pump will alarm 'occlusion'. When vesicants are given as infusions via a central venous access device, it is recommended that an external catheter, e.g. a tunnelled catheter, is used instead of an implantable port, where extravasation is well documented, especially with long infusion times. Where necessary, the patient can be taught to check the port needle site at least three times a day.

The drugs should be administered in the correct order, e.g. vesicants first (Mallett & Bailey 1996, Speechley 1987, Weinstein 1997) (Table 16.3). At least 5–10 ml of sodium chloride 0.9% should be used to flush in between each drug, to avoid mixing and chemical interactions. Blood return should be checked regularly, especially when administering a vesicant, i.e. every 2–5 ml (Doyle 1995, McCaffrey et al 1995, Weinstein 1997). If attaching an infusion, ensure that all the connections are secure and the giving set is taped so that the tubing cannot be pulled or the cannula dislodged. Monitor the site throughout the bolus injection to check for signs of infiltration, extravasation or leakage at the site. This will ensure the prompt recognition and management of any complication, thus minimizing local damage and preserving venous access for future treatment (Mallett & Bailey 1996). A gauze swab should be kept at connecting points in case of droplets (Reymann 1993). After all the drugs have been administered, a final flush of 5–10 ml of sodium chloride 0.9% should be given to ensure clearing of the device, the tubing and the vein. On completion,

Table 16.3 When to give vesicants

When?	For	Against
First	Vascular integrity decreases over time Initially, practitioner observation is more accurate Patient may be sedated if anti-emetic given first and less able to report pain	Vesicant is irritating and compromises integrity Venospasm may occur early, altering assessment of patency
Last	Venous spasm occurs early; less likely to be confused with pain of extravasation if vesicant given last Assumed that if vein can tolerate non-vesicant, it can tolerate vesicant	Vein may be irritated and not remain patent for vesicants
Between two non-vesicants	Cytotoxics are irritating to veins and non-vesicants are less irritant than vesicants	

waste should be disposed of according to the institution's policy. Documentation must be carried out immediately after completion of administration, including any adverse reactions, to prevent duplication of treatment.

DISPOSAL OF WASTE

Each institution should have a clear and concise procedure for the safe handling and disposal of cytotoxic drugs and material contaminated by them (Allwood et al 1997) – the recommended method is incineration. Sharps should be placed in designated sharps containers as complete needle–syringe units to prevent the risk of needlestick or splashing during disconnection. Protective clothing, administration sets and other contaminated material should be placed in leakproof waste disposal bags and sealed and labelled according to the institution's policies. Contaminated linen should be bagged and labelled as contaminated to ensure that it is handled correctly by laundry staff. All re-usable equipment such as goggles or trays should be washed with soap and water and dried thoroughly. Disposal via domestic sewerage systems should not be used for large quantities of pharmaceutical waste (Allwood et al 1997), but may be acceptable for small quantities (Mallett & Bailey 1996). Cytotoxic drugs can be excreted as unchanged drug or active metabolites in urine, faeces, blood, vomit and even saliva. In order to comply with safe technique and practice, universal precautions should be used and gloves worn whenever disposing of any excreta of patients receiving cytotoxic therapy (Doyle 1995, Mallett & Bailey 1996, Weinstein 1997).

DEALING WITH A SPILL

It is recommended that, wherever cytotoxic drugs are being reconstituted, administered or handled, a spill kit is available and that staff are trained in its use (Doyle 1995, Mallett & Bailey 1996, Powell 1996). This enables the practitioner to have immediate access to all the necessary equipment which will help to prevent further contamination of the environment and aid prompt cleaning. The contents of spill kits vary but there are some basic requirements (Box 16.4).

In the event of a spill, the immediate area should be cleared where possible and the necessary protective clothing worn, i.e. two pairs of latex gloves, gown or

---

■ **BOX 16.4**

Contents of a spill kit

- Plastic apron
- Plastic overshoes
- Disposable armlets
- Latex gloves (two pairs)
- Face masks
- Goggles
- Disposable clinical waste bags
- Paper towels
- Eye irrigation kit
- Instruction/documentation sheet
- All contained within a large plastic bucket

apron, armlets, overshoes, goggles and, in the event of a powder spill, a good-quality surgical face mask or particulate respirator face mask. Powder spills should be contained with dampened paper towels to prevent dispersal of powder. All spills should be wiped up with absorbent towels, starting from the outside edge and working towards the centre to prevent spread of contamination to a larger area (Doyle 1995). All contaminated surfaces should be cleaned with cold soapy water at least three times, and dried to remove residual contamination (Doyle 1995, Powell 1996, Weinstein 1997).

The ONS (Powell 1996) does not recommend the use of chemical inactivation (with the exception of sodium thiosulphate) to absorb drug spills because of the potentially dangerous by-products which may be produced.

Accidental exposure of patient or practitioner

If a cytotoxic drug is spilled onto the clothing of staff or the patient, the piece of clothing should be removed as soon as possible and treated as contaminated linen. If the spill has penetrated clothing and come into contact with the skin of the person, the area must be thoroughly cleansed with soap and large amounts of water (Doyle 1995). In the case of exposure or splashing into the eye, the eye should be flooded with water or an isotonic eye wash solution for at least 5 minutes (Mallett & Bailey 1996, Reymann 1993, Weinstein 1997). In the event of any direct exposure of the practitioner, the incident should be reported to the occupational health department and documented.

STAFF MONITORING/SURVEILLANCE

It is essential that a system of health surveillance is provided for staff directly involved in handling cytotoxic drugs. What this consists of is more controversial. Allwood et al (1997) recommended a programme which contains a medical history, physical examination, laboratory tests (FBC) and biological monitoring (although the value of monitoring levels of drugs and their metabolites is limited due to the wide range of drugs and the test methods available), reliability of sensitivity and validation. Reymann (1993) suggested that there are no data to support a cause and effect relationship between precautionary cytotoxic drug handling and abnormal physical and laboratory findings, and it is therefore less common for staff to undergo extensive testing. In general, staff who are pregnant, planning a pregnancy or breast-feeding may elect to refrain from preparation or administration of cytotoxics and most institutions would support this (Powell 1996, Reymann 1993).

SIDE-EFFECTS

Most side-effects are temporary and usually result from the action of the cytotoxic drug on the rapidly dividing cells, e.g. stomatitis, nausea and vomiting, alopecia and bone marrow suppression. Some toxicity may be permanent, such as when an organ is affected, e.g. cardiac myopathy, pulmonary fibrosis or sterility. Side-effects can be further categorized in relation to their onset, as follows (Speechley 1987; see also Table 16.4):

- immediate – occur within 30 minutes of commencing treatment
- short-term – occur between 3 and 7 days after treatment
- long-term – manifested later than 7 days; many are cumulative in nature.

The practitioner administering i.v. cytotoxic therapy will need to be aware of the immediate effects or those that may affect the choice of veins when establishing

Table 16.4 Side-effects of cytotoxic drugs

Immediate effects	Short-term effects	Long-term effects
Cold sensation along vein	Anorexia	Bone marrow depression
Pain at insertion site	Nausea and vomiting	Alopecia
Red flush along vein	Stomatitis	Skin reactions
Metallic taste	Potentiation of radiation	Nail ridging
Nasal stuffiness	skin reactions	Thrombophlebitis
Anticipatory nausea	Pain at tumour site/jaw	Pulmonary fibrosis
and vomiting	Malaise	Congestive cardiac failure
Allergic reaction	Flu-like syndrome	Renal toxicity
Hot flush	Chemical cystitis	Liver dysfunction
Dizziness	Haematuria	Neurological problems
Hypotension	Discoloration of urine	CNS toxicity
Hypoglycaemia	Constipation	Sexual dysfunction
	Diarrhoea	

venous access. He must be able to recognize and differentiate the side-effects of more serious complications and respond appropriately (Box 16.5).

Pain at the insertion site

A number of cytotoxic drugs are irritants or vesicants. During administration, chemical irritation by the drug can lead to venous spasm, resulting in an ache or pain at the insertion site. It is important that the practitioner can distinguish between this venous spasm and extravasation. Knowledge of the drugs which are likely to cause pain is vital, as well as methods to prevent and relieve the pain. Drugs which are known to cause pain include:

- doxorubicin
- epirubicin
- dacarbazine
- cytosine
- vinorelbine
- thiotepa
- streptocozin
- BCNU (Powell 1996, Reymann 1993, Rittenberg et al 1995, Eli Lilley 1997, Weinstein 1997).

Where possible, the drug should be diluted and either given as an infusion, preferably via a central venous catheter, or administered slowly via the side arm of a fast running infusion of sodium chloride 0.9%. Heat can be applied above the peripheral cannula to relieve the spasm. The application of a glyceryl trinitrate (GTN) patch below the cannula encourages vasodilation and results in better dilution and more rapid circulation away from the insertion site (Hecker 1988).

Local allergic reaction or 'flare reaction'

Some drugs cause a red streak or flush from the insertion site along the vein. This is known as a flare reaction and it is caused by a venous inflammatory response to subsequent histamine release (Curran et al 1990). This reaction is characterized by redness and blotchiness, and may result in the formation of small wheals, having a similar appearance to a nettle rash. It is usually associated with red-coloured drugs, such as doxorubicin and epirubicin, and occurs in about 3% of cases (ONS 1996). It does not cause pain, although the area may feel itchy, and it usually subsides within 30–45 minutes with or without treatment (Mallett & Bailey 1996); however, it responds well within a few minutes to the application of a topical steroid or an i.v. injection of hydrocortisone (Weinstein 1997). Prevention includes dilution of the drug or administering via the side arm of an infusion.

■ **BOX 16.5**

Side-effects and nursing interventions (adapted from Eli Lilley 1997)

1. Dermatological

Venous sensations, e.g. cold or pain
- Distinguish from extravasation
- Explain to patients the possibility of it occurring
- Administer drug slowly with fast running infusion of sodium chloride 0.9%
- Use local heat to aid vasodilation
- Dilute drugs where possible

Skin pigmentation/venous discolouration
- Explain to patients the possibility of it occurring
- Reassure that it is only temporary
- Advise against prolonged exposure to sunlight

Dermatitis/rash
- Explain to patients the possibility of it occurring
- Administer antihistamine where appropriate
- Seek dermatology opinion

Flushing along the vein
- Advise patients of the possibility at the time of administration
- Apply local steroid cream when necessary

Body and facial flushing
- Administer drug slowly
- Reassure patients that the effect is short-lived

Alopecia
- Explain to patients the possibility of it occurring
- Reassure that it will grow back
- Advise on hair care and order wig before hair loss
- Use scalp cooling where appropriate

2. Gastrointestinal

Taste aberration
- Advise patients that it may occur during injection or at any time during the course of treatment
- Encourage sipping of drinks and sucking of sweets
- Concentrate on foods that taste good

Anorexia
- Encourage small, frequent meals
- Refer to dietician for advice and food supplements where necessary   *(cont'd)*

■ BOX 16.5 *(cont'd)*

Stomatitis

- Regular observation of mouth
- Teach patients good mouth care and to avoid hot, spicy and citrus foods, alcohol and smoking
- Administer analgesics and/or antifungals

Nausea and vomiting

- Administer effective anti-emetics and encourage patients to take them regularly
- Encourage patients to utilize distraction, meditation, relaxation and other therapies such as acupuncture or aromatherapy
- Observe for symptoms of fluid and electrolyte imbalance and treat as required

Diarrhoea

- Encourage low roughage diet and good perianal care
- Observe for symptoms of dehydration and electrolyte imbalance, and treat as required
- Administer antidiarrhoeal agents

Constipation

- Inform patients of the possibility of it occurring and encourage high-roughage diet with plenty of fluids
- Administer prophylactic aperients

3. Haematological

Anaemia

- Observe for pallor, dizziness and shortness of breath
- Check full blood count on regular basis
- Encourage high-iron dietary intake, e.g. liver, dark green vegetables
- Administer blood transfusions as required

Leucopenia

- Prevent exposure of patients to known infections
- Teach patients to perform meticulous hygiene and recognize early symptoms of infection such as fever or cough
- Check full blood count on a regular basis
- Administer antibiotics and GCSF as required (either prophylactically or for treatment)

Thrombocytopenia

- Inform patients of the necessity to avoid physical injury (while shaving, brushing teeth, gardening, etc.)
- Avoid drugs which further interfere with platelet function, e.g. aspirin
- Observe for signs of bleeding, including petechiae and haematoma
- Check full blood count on regular basis
- Administer platelet transfusions

4. Organs

Hepatic

- Observe for signs of jaundice
- Monitor liver function tests and report abnormalities
(cont'd)

■ **BOX 16.5** (*cont'd*)

Cardiac
- Ensure baseline ECG before treatment
- Observe for cumulative effects

Pulmonary
- Ensure baseline chest X-ray
- Observe for onset of symptoms, e.g. shortness of breath, wheezing and report

Renal
- Monitor renal dysfunction
- Record all intake and output
- Test urine for pH and blood
- Administer mesna for protection of bladder
- Inform and reassure patients of the possibility of discolouration of urine

CNS
- Observe for signs and symptoms
- Reassure patients re. peripheral neuropathy and report – drug may be changed

Sexual dysfunction
- Warn female patients of amenorrhoea, early menopause and possible sterility
- Discuss pretreatment sperm banking with male patients
- Advise both sexes on contraception

5. Miscellaneous

Malaise / fatigue
- Inform patients of the possibility of it occurring, when it may occur and for how long
- Advise patients to plan actions and have regular rest periods

Flu-like syndrome
- Inform patients of the possibility of fever, chills and headache and that it is only temporary
- Administer prophylactic steroids

Allergic reactions
- Be prepared if anaphylaxis is a possibility
- Carry out regular observations
- Administer drugs as required

Pain, e.g. tumour, jaw
- Reassure patients that it is only temporary
- Administer analgesics as required

Hyperglycaemia / hypotension
- Observe for signs and symptoms
- Administer infusion slowly

Discolouration of the veins/hyperpigmentation

This is not an immediate side-effect but one which can progressively become evident and may influence the practitioner's choice of veins. There is an increased incidence in dark-skinned patients, and it may be associated with exogenous trauma/post-inflammatory changes or areas of increased vasodilation (Powell 1996). This side-effect is associated with many cytotoxic drugs, but the incidence is highest with alkylating and antitumour antibiotics, e.g. 5FU, vinblastine, mustine and dactinomycin. The exact mechanism is unknown, but it may result in direct stimulation of the melanocytes. It usually disappears 2–3 months after completion of treatment and causes no other adverse effects. It has been suggested that the use of heating pads or warm compresses to aid vasodilation should be avoided during the administration of the causative drugs (Powell 1996).

Cold sensation

The patient may complain of a cold sensation along the vein. This is often related to the difference between the temperature of the drug and that of the patient. However, some drugs specifically cause a cold sensation, e.g. vinca alkaloids, and the patient should be informed and reassured that this is normal.

Chemical phlebitis and thrombophlebitis

This can result from repeated administration of irritant drugs and can make it more difficult for the practitioners when locating suitable veins for subsequent cannulation and cytotoxic drug administration. The incidence is increased when combinations of drugs are administered. Early signs include pain, erythema, oedema, a sensation of warmth and protracted discolouration of the venous pathway. The patient will suffer discomfort, and in some extreme cases the skin becomes taut and stretched, the vein becomes cord-like and, depending on the location, it can lead to restricted use of the limb. Knowing which drugs have the potential for this will enable the nurse to apply all preventative measures at the time of administration. Diluting the drugs (if pharmaceutically acceptable), administering the drug slowly with frequent flushing with sodium chloride 0.9%, and application of heat to the area to aid vasodilation may all reduce the incidence. The use of a small-gauge cannula in a large vein with good blood flow can also help, but if the veins are deep, difficult to visualize or extremely small, it may be necessary to reassess the patient's venous access and opt for a central venous access device.

Anaphylactic reaction

According to Weinstein (1997): 'the practitioner should be prepared for any anaphylactic reaction at any time with any drug'. Some cytotoxic drugs are known to cause anaphylaxis, e.g. bleomycin and asparaginase, and the practitioner should be aware of which drugs are more likely to cause the reaction, how to administer the drugs safely and what to do in the event of a reaction. The patient should be monitored for signs of flushing, shaking, sudden agitation, nausea, urticaria, hypotension, generalized pruritus or wheezing and shortness of breath. If undetected, this reaction can progress to cardiac arrest.

EXTRAVASATION

Extravasation comes from the Latin word *vesicare*, meaning 'to blister', and is defined as the inadvertent administration of a vesicant drug into the surrounding tissues (infiltration is the inadvertent administration of a non-vesicant drug into the tissues). A vesicant is a drug which has the potential to cause blistering, severe tissue damage and even necrosis if extravasated and usually requires some form of management. An irritant drug can cause local sensitivity and if it infiltrates can cause local inflammation and discomfort but no long-term damage (How & Brown 1998).

Extravasation is one of the most serious complications associated with the administration of i.v. drugs (Beason 1990). The incidence of cytotoxic drug extravasation has been estimated to range from 0.1 to 6% in patients receiving peripheral chemotherapy, but it is difficult to be accurate and this may not reflect the true rate, as incidents of extravasation may not be recognized or reported (Cox et al 1988, Powell 1996). The incidence appears to be higher in children than in adults (Doyle 1995), and in central venous catheters it appears to occur mostly in the implantable port devices, often as a result of needle dislodgement (Powell 1996).

Risk factors

Risk factors for extravasation are as follows:

- Patient-related risk factors – the inability to communicate appropriately, e.g. neonates, infants, young children, comatose or sedated patients, confused patients, very restless patients. In children with smaller veins, there is a blunt perception of pain (Rudolph & Larson 1987).
- Vascular impairment and reduced vascular integrity, e.g. the elderly, Raynaud's disease, radiation areas, multiple attempts at venepuncture, cardiac disease, obstructed venous drainage and lymphoedema, superior vena cava syndrome (Banerjee et al 1987), fragile, sclerosed, thrombosed and small veins
- Skill level of the person performing cannulation and administering the drugs (Beason 1990).

Selection of vein and device

Veins on the dorsum of the hand are unsatisfactory due to the lack of subcutaneous tissue and the proximity of tendons and joints to the skin, which could be damaged if extravasation occurs. Severe problems have been reported with ulceration in this area (Banerjee et al 1987, Wood & Gullo 1993, Rudolph & Larson 1987). Veins in the antecubital fossa are in close proximity to nerves and arteries, and manufacturers of doxorubicin originally recommended against the administration of the drug in this area. Extravasation is often difficult to detect in this region and it is best left for venepuncture and collection of blood samples (Table 16.5).

Table 16.5 Use of antecubital fossa

For	Against
Larger veins permit rapid infusion of drug	Mobility is restricted
Larger veins allow irritant drugs to reach general circulation more quickly and with less irritation than small veins	Risk of extravasation increased if patient tends to be mobile
Easier to palpate and therefore increases successful insertion of device	Early recognition of extravasation is difficult due to the deeper veins – less chance of observing swelling and could go undetected; delayed response to pain Damage can result in loss of structure and function; ulceration and fibrosis

Perhaps the most reasonable location is the proximal forearm over the flexor and extensor muscle bulk, but these veins are often not available or have already been used extensively (Wood & Gullo 1993, Rudolph & Larson 1987). Weinstein (1997) advocated that a large straight vein in the dorsum of the hand is preferable to a smaller vein in the forearm. Veins which have been previously used for blood sampling or which have multiple punctures are not suitable due to the risk of leakage of the drug from the old sites. If a cannulation has been unsuccessful, then a different vein, and if possible one in the opposite limb, should be used. If none is available, then a site in the same vein may be selected, but it should be proximal to the previous puncture (Wood & Gullo 1993).

A vesicant drug should never be administered via a winged infusion device, as it has been shown that the incidence of extravasation is greater when steel needles are used than with plastic cannulae (Tully et al 1981).

The cannula must be securely fixed and it is essential that the insertion site is visible throughout the administration. Venous patency must always be checked with at least 5–10 ml of sodium chloride 0.9% prior to administration of a vesicant and the area assessed for pain and swelling. Should the patency be in any doubt, the device should be removed and resited.

Use of an existing device

Weinstein (1997) recommended that a pre-existing peripheral device should not be used for vesicant drug administration in the following circumstances:

- the i.v. cannula was placed more than 12–24 hours earlier
- the area or insertion site is red, swollen or painful or there is evidence of infiltration
- the site is over or around the wrist (or over a joint)
- blood return is sluggish or absent
- the infusion fluid is flowing erratically and seems positional.

However, if the fluid runs freely, there is a good and consistent blood return and the site is free of swelling, pain and redness, then it is up to the practitioner to make the decision to use the device if he feels confident and wishes to avoid the need for the patient to undergo another cannulation.

Skill of the practitioner

The key to preventing extravasation is good venous assessment and using methods to improve venous access. The practitioner should be proficient at performing cannulation (Beason 1990) before attempting to cannulate for vesicant drug administration, as well as being knowledgeable about the signs and symptoms of extravasation. Multiple attempts after failure to cannulate a vein should be discouraged and inexperienced practitioners should not attempt to cannulate difficult veins (Cox et al 1988). If the practitioner does not feel confident in his ability or is unsuccessful after one or two attempts at cannulation, he should seek the assistance of an experienced colleague. Any patient who consistently requires frequent attempts to successfully obtain vascular access should be considered for a central venous access device.

Preparation of the patient

Patients should be informed about the drugs being given, any anticipated side-effects and the risks of extravasation (How & Brown 1998). They should be advised not to move the limb that has the cannula in situ during the bolus drug administration and should be instructed to report immediately any pain, burning or unusual sensations. If patients cannot verbalize the discomfort, the practitioner should observe them closely for any non-verbal signs of pain, e.g. facial expressions. The dressing must be removed if not transparent, to ensure adequate visualization of the site. The device should then be checked for patency.

Signs and symptoms

Pain

Pain and stinging are usually the first signs of an extravasation. However, extravasation can occur in the absence of pain and the sensation must be distinguished from venous spasm or a feeling of cold that can occur with some cytotoxic drugs. Pain is indicative of both peripheral and central venous extravasation. Patients may complain of pain along the catheter tunnel or around the port site. This may be a result of needle dislodgement from the port, poor needle placement or a split catheter. It is rare that extravasation results from the disconnection of the catheter from the portal body (Wood & Gullo 1993, Schulmeister 1992).

Leaking, swelling or induration

The practitioner should be constantly assessing the i.v. site for signs of swelling. Observation of this may be delayed if the patient has a cannula sited in an area of subcutaneous fat or if the leak is via the posterior wall, deep into subcutaneous tissue.

Redness

Redness is not usually present at the time of extravasation and often occurs later. Redness at the site may indicate flare.

Blood return

The return of blood should be checked at regular intervals, although blood return does not guarantee vein patency and any change should be investigated. If the lack of blood return is the only sign, it should not be regarded as an indication of a non-patent vein. A vein may not bleed back for a number of reasons, e.g. if the device is situated in a small vein which collapses when the syringe plunger is pulled back, or if excess fluid from an infusion has prevented blood from pooling at the tip of the cannula.

Other signs

Other signs of extravasation include a reduction or absence of flow rate during an infusion and any resistance felt on the plunger of the syringe when administering a bolus injection. If any signs or symptoms are present or if there is any doubt in the practitioner's mind that the drug is being administered correctly, administration should be discontinued immediately (Powell 1996, Weinstein 1997). If unsure of an extravasation, the practitioner may check with a solution of sodium chloride 0.9%; however, if an extravasation has occurred, this may cause the drug to spread further into the tissues.

Pathogenesis of extravasation

When an extravasation occurs:

1. Fluid leaks into the tissue.
2. The tissue is compressed due to the restricted blood flow.
3. This in turn reduces the amount of oxygen to the site and lowers the cellular pH.

4. There is loss of capillary wall integrity, an increase in oedema and eventual cellular death.

This is further compounded by the chemistry of an extravasation and by whether or not the drug binds to DNA.

Drugs which do not bind to DNA These drugs tend to inhibit mitosis and often cause immediate damage. However, they are quickly metabolized and inactivated. The type of injury which occurs is similar to a burn and ulceration can result. These drugs tend not to erode down to deeper structures and healing occurs within 3–5 weeks. These injuries rarely require any surgical intervention. Examples of drugs in this group are the vinca alkaloids.

Drugs which bind to DNA These drugs do not always cause any immediate damage but lodge in the tissues, binding to the DNA, preventing the fibrostem cells from replicating and reproducing, and resulting in the cells losing their ability to heal spontaneously, which explains the prolonged effect. Drugs in this group include mustine (nitrogen mustard), which tends to bind rapidly to the tissues and cause immediate injury, and the drugs in the antibiotic family, e.g. doxorubicin, daunorubicin and mitomycin C.

Clinically, most experience has been gained from doxorubicin, the most widely used of the cytotoxic drugs, and most studies have been carried out on this drug. A correlation has been found between the degree of concentration of doxorubicin and the degree of ulceration. Active drug has been isolated from wounds between 3 and 5 months after a doxorubicin extravasation (Banerjee et al 1987, Doyle 1995, Rudolph & Larson 1987). Under ultraviolet light, tissue containing doxorubicin glows a dull red and this helps to identify the area of injured tissue (Rudolph & Larson 1987).

Stages of damage

The first suggestion of an extravasation of doxorubicin may be a burning sensation, although local discomfort does not always occur. This pain can be quite severe and last minutes, hours or even days but will eventually subside.

In the following weeks, the tissue will become reddened and firm (see Fig. 16.3). The skin may blanch when pressure is applied and necrosis may become obvious as early as a few days depending on the size of the area of extravasation (Fig. 16.4). If the area is small, the redness gradually reduces over a few weeks. If the extravasa-

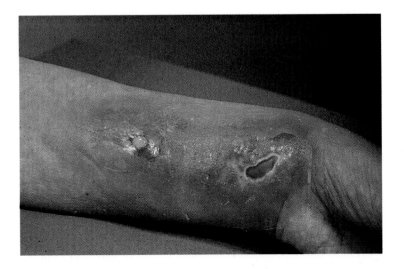

Fig. 16.3 Blistering following vincristine extravasation.

Fig. 16.4 Extensive damage following an extravasation of doxorubicin.

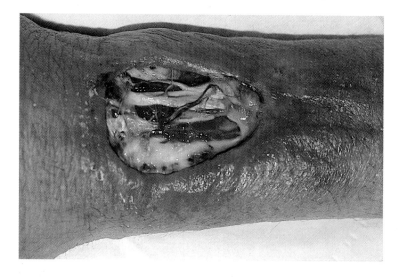

tion is large, a small necrotic area will appear in the centre of the red, painful skin and once necrosis occurs then surgical debridement is indicated. If this is not performed, a thick black eschar will result, surrounded by a rim of red painful skin. When this is removed, deep subcutaneous necrosis is found. The key feature of doxorubicin ulceration is that it is often progressive and may lead to extensive joint stiffness and neuropathy (Rudolph & Larson 1987).

Extravasation syndrome

Allwood et al (1997) have suggested that there is a three-part syndrome of extravasation, although the management of types I and II is the same:

- *Pre-extravasation syndrome* often involves little or no leakage of vesicants, but particularly severe phlebitis and/or local hypersensitivity, together with a number of other local risk factors such as difficulty cannulating. This is an indication that patients may be more susceptible to extravasation and may be candidates for early central venous access.
- *Type I extravasation* injuries cause a blister and have a defined area of firmness around the site of injury. They are usually associated with bolus injections where pressure is applied by the person administering the drugs.
- *Type II extravasations* are differentiated by a diffuse, 'soggy' type of tissue injury, where dispersal into intracellular space has occurred. These injuries are associated with gravity-fed infusions or bolus injections through the side arm of an infusion.

Management of extravasation

One of the main aims when administering vesicant cytotoxic drugs is to prevent extravasation. However, despite the skill of the practitioner, extravasations do occur and the emphasis should be on immediate recognition and prompt management. It is these two factors which will prevent the serious consequences of an extravasation injury. Sometimes it is difficult to detect whether an extravasation has actually occurred, but the literature stresses that in the event of a suspected extravastion it is better to assume it has occurred and act accordingly (Weinstein 1997).

Comprehensive treatment and expert advice must be available as early as possible following an extravasation. Ideally, this should occur within 10 minutes of the event, certainly within 1 hour and definitely within 24 hours (Allwood et al

1997). After 24 hours, the management will no longer be aimed at preventing injury, but will be more an exercise in damage limitation. Whatever form of treatment is chosen, it should not cause further damage or, in the case of misdiagnosis of an extravasation, any damage at all (Allwood et al 1997).

The issues related to the management and treatment of extravasation are complex and controversial. There has been a lack of controlled clinical trials, for a number of reasons. First, while there are serious implications for untreated extravasations, the incidence is relatively small and thus the number of patients available for entry into studies is low (Cox et al 1988, Reymann 1995). Secondly, there are moral and ethical considerations with having a treatment arm and a control arm where patients sustaining injuries are offered no treatment. Some studies performed on animals have demonstrated both effective and ineffective antidotes, but extrapolation from animals to humans has its limitations (Powell 1996).

Once an extravasation is suspected, clinicians agree that the infusion or administration should be stopped immediately, followed by aspiration of any remaining drug in order to reduce the size of the lesion (Allwood et al 1997, Cox et al 1988, Doyle 1995, Rudolph & Larson 1987, Weinstein 1997).

Ignoffo & Friedman (1980) described a protocol where, following cessation of the injection, an attempt to aspirate 3–5 ml of blood was carried out. However, in the majority of cases the device is displaced or the vein damaged and the likelihood of withdrawing any blood is small, and the practitioner may waste valuable time attempting to achieve this.

It is here that the first dilemma arises: should the peripheral device be removed or remain in place? Cox et al (1988) advocated that the device be left in situ in order to instil the antidote through it and into the surrounding tissues, thus infiltrating the area where the extravasation has occurred; this view is supported by Ignoffo & Friedman (1980), Powell (1996) and Weinstein (1997). However, Rudolph & Larson (1987) recommended that the device be removed and felt that the evidence for leaving it in situ is anecdotal, a view supported by Doyle (1995) and Mallett & Bailey (1996).

Hot packs or cold packs?

There appear to be two main courses of treatment (Allwood et al 1997):

- localize and neutralize
- spread and dilute.

Localize and neutralize In order to localize the extravasated drug, the recommended course would be to apply a cold pack to the area. This would result in vasoconstriction, which reduces the locally destructive effects by reducing the local uptake of the drug by the tissues, decreasing local oedema and slowing the metabolic rate of the cells. It has also been suggested that the reduced blood supply and the cooling effect may help to reduce local pain (Beason 1990, Doyle 1995, Weinstein 1997). There is still no decision as to how long the pack should be left in situ, although some suggest periods of 15 minutes (Rudolph & Larson 1987) or 20–40 minutes (Cox et al 1988) four times a day for up to 24–48 hours. The use of cold packs is recommended for a number of vesicant drugs, but in the treatment of vinca alkaloid extravasation the use of heat packs has been particularly advocated. However, it is important that heat is not used inappropriately – Dorr et al (1983) found experimentally that, while cooling could be helpful in preventing ulcers due to doxorubicin extravasation, heat could be harmful. Doyle (1995) found that ulcers were four times larger in the presence of hot packs than untreated controls.

Spread and dilute It appears that heat is beneficial in non-DNA-binding vesicant drugs and it is used once the antidote is given with the aim of increasing blood supply and therefore increasing dispersion and absorption of the antidote into the subcutaneous tissues. Also, the increased blood supply may help to promote healing by increasing metabolic demands and reducing cellular destruction (Weinstein 1997). The use of heat is recommended for vinca alkaloid extravasation by Reymann (1993), Mallett & Bailey (1996) and Powell (1996) – the pack should be applied for 15–20 minutes four times a day for 24–48 hours.

Elevation of the extremity

The elevation of the extremity is recommended, the aim being to minimize swelling. Both Rudolph & Larson (1987) and Powell (1996) stress the importance of elevation, following the application of an ice pack, for up to 48 hours. Movement should also be encouraged to prevent adhesion of damaged areas to underlying tissue, which could result in restriction of future movement (Mallett & Bailey 1996).

'Antidotes'

There are two main types of 'antidote':

- those with the aim of diluting the drug, e.g. sodium chloride 0.9% and hyaluronidase
- those with the aim of neutralizing the drug and reducing subsequent local inflammation, such as steroid injections and/or cream, e.g. dexamethasone or hydrocortisone.

Some centres have a list of antidotes for each vesicant drug. For example, sodium bicarbonate 8.4% can be used in carmustine extravasations (however, Allwood et al (1997) pointed out the documented risks associated with using sodium bicarbonate 8.4% which itself can be a causative agent of extravasation injuries). Sodium theosulphate (useful with mustine or cisplatinum) was evaluated in a study by Tsavaris et al (1992). They found that by using sodium theosulphate with hydrocortisone and dexamethasone in extravasated drugs such as doxorubicin, epirubicin, vincristine and mitomycin-c, healing time was reduced; they concluded that this may reduce the need for extensive surgery. Topical antidotes aim to minimize skin inflammation and erythematous reactions. Application of dimethyl sulphoxide (DMSO) 99% has been found to be beneficial in treating doxorubicin and mitomycin C extravasations (Hammond & Bachur 1987). The recommended application is 1–2 ml applied to the site every 6 hours (Powell 1996), although this could delay healing. Vasodilators (e.g. GTN patches) have been used in neonates following the infiltration of PN with high concentrations of dextrose and calcium and show promise as a treatment, but they are not advocated for vesicant cytotoxic extravasation.

Hyaluronidase is an enzyme that destroys tissue cement, aiding in the reduction or prevention of tissue damage by allowing rapid diffusion of the extravasated fluid and promoting drug absorption. The usual dose is 1500 IU administered following vinca alkaloid extravasations. However, sodium chloride 0.9% has also been used successfully to limit the effects of vinca alkaloid extravasation, by diluting the concentration of the drug, and a combination of both of these drugs has been reported to be effective in the reduction of local ulceration (Cox et al 1988, Heckler 1989).

Surgery

When is surgical intervention necessary? Some centres suggest that a plastic surgery consultation be performed as part of the management procedure (Weinstein 1997). Early surgical intervention with excision of the area (particularly with doxorubicin) helps to stop progression of cellular destruction, thereby minimizing damage (Heckler 1989). However, the requirement for surgery is probably related to the size and location of the extravasation as well as the type of drug that has been extravasated. The use of sodium chloride 0.9% flushing conducted within the first 24 hours following an extravasation has been suggested as a less traumatic and cheaper procedure. This technique involves four small stab incisions, which facilitates the cleansing of any drug from the subcutaneous tissues, and is advocated for use with drugs, such as doxorubicin (How & Brown 1998).

Rudolph & Larson (1987) felt that once ulceration and pain occurred, surgery was often indicated. However, if pain, erythema and swelling persist, it may be necessary to intervene before ulceration occurs. Linder et al (1981) found a high incidence of residual joint stiffness and sympathetic dystrophy related to delay in excision of necrotic tissue. Excision should include removal of all indurated, reddened, oedematous and pale tissue with a margin of normal appearing tissue (Banerjee et al 1987). Identification and demarcation of the area can be achieved by the use of fluorescence microscopic analysis (Dahlstrom et al 1990). Photographs are also useful, as is marking the area of extravasation with a pen to observe for an increase or decrease in swelling and redness.

Patient feedback

Patients should always be informed when an extravasation has occurred and an explanation should be provided of what has happened as well as what is required in order to manage the situation. Following the management of the extravasation, the patient should be instructed as to what signs and symptoms to observe for and when to contact the hospital during the follow-up period.

Consequences of poor or no treatment

The consequences of an untreated or poorly managed extravasation can be extensive, but such occurrences can be greatly minimized through careful preparation, administration and monitoring by the practitioner experienced in cannulation and chemotherapy administration.

Physical defect (Fig. 16.5)

Patients may already have undergone surgery (e.g. a mastectomy or stoma forma-

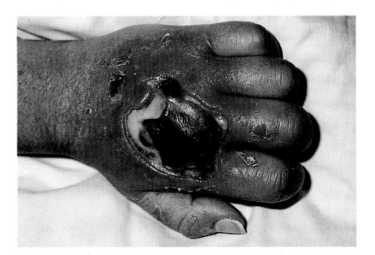

Fig. 16.5 Necrotic area as a result of a doxorubicin extravasation.

tion) and may have suffered side-effects from treatment (e.g. loss of hair), all of which will have had an impact on body image and self-esteem. A necrotic ulcerated injury left as a result of extravasation could therefore be devastating and have an additional impact on the patient's ability to work and function normally, both socially and emotionally. This is particularly difficult if the extravasation has occurred over a joint, limiting mobility and even resulting in permanent disability. As a result of the injury the patient may suffer from pain, which in turn may lead to problems with working, sleeping and generally coping with treatment.

Disease control

Various aspects of an extravasation injury may affect the patient's long-term prognosis. A patient may not be able to continue treatment as the wound may need time to heal, and if she becomes myelosuppressed during treatment, the wound is a potential area for infection. This is also the case for patients waiting to undergo intensive or high-dose chemotherapy. If the patient is debilitated through the injury, this could lead to secondary medical problems, which may also impact on the patient's ability to receive and cope with further treatment.

Cost

There are costs in time and money and to the patient's overall health and quality of life. If a patient cannot resume work due to disability or the need to take time off for plastic surgery, then it may impact on both the patient and her family. There may be costs involved in surgery both to treat the injury and to repair the damage cosmetically, and repeated hospitalization may be necessary (Weinstein 1997).

The use of extravasation kits

The use of an extravasation kit and policy is recommended (Allwood et al 1997, Beason 1990, Mallett & Bailey 1996). An extravasation kit is particularly useful in areas where staff routinely administer vesicant cytotoxic drugs as it gives them immediate access to a step-by-step guide to management, as well as having all the required equipment to hand (see Box 16.6).

The kit should remain simple in order to avoid confusion (especially as the practitioner will be anxious), but comprehensive enough to meet all reasonable needs (Allwood et al 1997). The instructions should be clear and easy to follow and the use of a flow chart is an easy way to help staff follow the management procedure (see Fig. 16.6). Kits will be assembled according to the particular needs of the individual institution.

■ **BOX 16.6**

Contents of an extravasation kit
- Hot/cold packs
- Injectable antidotes, e.g. steroids/hyaluronidase
- Steroid cream
- Syringes
- Needles
- Alcohol swabs
- Copy of extravasation management procedure
- Documentation forms

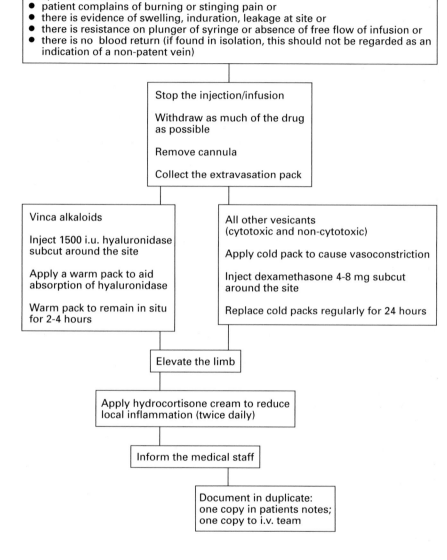

Fig. 16.6 An example of a flowchart for the treatment of extravasation.

Treatment of extravasation

Suspect an extravasation if:
- patient complains of burning or stinging pain or
- there is evidence of swelling, induration, leakage at site or
- there is resistance on plunger of syringe or absence of free flow of infusion or
- there is no blood return (if found in isolation, this should not be regarded as an indication of a non-patent vein)

Stop the injection/infusion

Withdraw as much of the drug as possible

Remove cannula

Collect the extravasation pack

Vinca alkaloids

Inject 1500 i.u. hyaluronidase subcut around the site

Apply a warm pack to aid absorption of hyaluronidase

Warm pack to remain in situ for 2-4 hours

All other vesicants (cytotoxic and non-cytotoxic)

Apply cold pack to cause vasoconstriction

Inject dexamethasone 4-8 mg subcut around the site

Replace cold packs regularly for 24 hours

Elevate the limb

Apply hydrocortisone cream to reduce local inflammation (twice daily)

Inform the medical staff

Document in duplicate:
one copy in patients notes;
one copy to i.v. team

Documentation and reporting

Documentation of an extravasation is vital for a number of reasons:

- An extravasation is an accident and must be reported and fully documented.
- The patient will require follow-up care and the documentation must be available to all practitioners involved in the follow-up.
- The information will be used for statistical purposes.
- It may be required in the case of litigation.

The documentation should contain the following aspects:

- patient details
- the drug given
- the method used, e.g. bolus or infusion
- type of device, e.g. cannula, CVC
- a diagram to indicate the location and size of the area
- the appearance of the area
- any signs and symptoms felt by the patient/observed by the practitioner
- procedure performed step by step
- if photographs were ordered
- any referrals to plastic surgeons
- section for follow-up documentation
- date and signature of practitioner.

There is a scheme for the collation and analysis of extravasation events called the 'green card scheme', which is organized by St Chad's Hospital, Birmingham. The aim is to obtain accurate statistics of the number of incidents, the treatment methods and the outcome.

CONCLUSION

The preparation and administration of cytotoxic drugs is a procedure which must be undertaken by specially trained practitioners, as it is associated with hazards for both patient and staff. Knowledge of protective measures and of the immediate, short- and long-term side-effects of the drugs to be administered will enable the practitioner to handle the drugs safely, as well as provide the necessary teaching and support for the patient.

REFERENCES

Allwood M, Stanley A, Wright P 1997 The cytotoxic handbook, 3rd edn. Radcliffe Medical Press, Oxford

Banerjee A, Brotherson T M, Lamberty B G H, Campbell R C 1987 Cancer chemotherapy agent induced perivenous extravasation injuries. Postgraduate Medical Journal 63: 5–9

Beason R 1990 Antineoplastic vesicant extravasation. Journal of Intravenous Nursing 13(92): 111–114

Behamou S 1986 Mutagenicity in urine from nurses handling cytotoxic drugs. European Journal of Cancer Clinical Oncology 22: 1489–1493

Buckalew P G 1982 On the opposite side of the bed: a nurse clinician's experience of anxiety during chemotherapy. Cancer Nursing 5(6): 435–439

Christensen C J, Le Masters G K, Wakeman M A 1990 Work practices and policies pharmacists preparing antineoplastic agents. Journal of Occupational Medicine 32(6): 508–511

Colbourne L 1995 Patients' experiences on chemotherapy treatment. Professional Nurse 10(7): 439–442

Cox K, Stuart-Harris R A, Addini G, Grygiel J, Raghavan D 1988 The management of cytotoxic drug extravasation: guidelines drawn up by a working party for the Clinical Oncological Society of Australia. The Medical Journal of Australia 148: 185–189

Curran C F, Luce J K, Page J A 1990 Doxorubicin associated flare reactions. Oncology Nursing Forum 17: 387–389

Dahlstrom K K, Chenoufi H L, Daugaard S 1990 Fluorescence microscopic demonstration and demarcation of doxorubicin extravasation. Cancer 65: 1722–1726

Dorr R T, Alberts A S, Salmons S E 1983 Cold protection from intradermal doxorubicin ulceration in the mouse. Proceedings of the Annual Meeting of the American Association Cancer Residents 24: 255

Doyle A 1995 Oncologic therapy. In: Terry J, Baranowski L, Lonsway R A, Hedrick C (eds) Intravenous therapy: clinical principles and practices. WB Saunders, Philadelphia, ch 13, p 249–274

Eli Lilley 1997 Cytotoxic chemotherapy, 5th edn. Lilley Oncology, Hampshire

Falck G, Rohn P, Sorsa M, Vainio H, Heinenon E, Holsti L 1979 Mutagenicity in urine of nurse handling cytotoxic agents. The Lancet 1: 1250

Gibbs J 1991 Handling cytotoxic drugs. Nursing Times 87(11): 54–55

Hammond K, Bachur N 1987 Evaluation of dimethyl sulfoxide and local cooling as antidotes for doxorubicin extravasation in a pig model. Oncology Nursing Forum 14(1): 39–44

Health and Safety Executive 1988 The control of substances hazardous to health regulations. HMSO, London

Hecker J 1988 Improved techniques in IV therapy. Nursing Times 84(34): 28–33

Heckler F R 1989 Current thoughts on extravasation injuries. Clinics in Plastic Surgery 16(3): 557–563

Hemminki K, Kyyronen P, Linbohm M 1985 Spontaneous abortions and malformations in the offspring of nurses exposed to anaesthetic gases, cytostatic drugs and other potential hazards in hospitals based on registered information of outcome. Journal of Epidemiological Community Health 39: 141–147

Holmes S 1990 Cancer chemotherapy. Austin Cornish, London

How C, Brown J 1998 Extravasation of cytotoxic chemotherapy from peripheral veins. European Jounal of Oncology Nursing 2(1): 51–58

Ignoffo R J, Friedman M A 1980 Therapy of local toxicities caused by extravasation of cancer chemotherapeutic drugs. Cancer Treatments Review 7: 17–27

Kaplan M 1983 Viewpoint: the cancer patient. Cancer Nursing 6: 103–107

Kotilainen H R 1989 Latex and vinyl examination gloves – quality control procedures and implications for health care workers. Archives of Internal Medicine 149: 2749–2753

Laidlaw J L 1984 Permeability of latex and polyvinyl chloride gloves to 20 antineoplastic agents. American Journal of Hospital Pharmacy 41: 2018–2023

Linder R M, Upton J, Osteen R 1981 Management of extensive doxorubicin hydrochloride extravasation injuries. Journal of Hand Surgery 8: 32–38

McCaffrey Boyle D, Engleking C 1995 Vesicant extravasation: myths and realities. Oncology Nursing Forum 22(1): 57–65

Mallett J, Bailey C (eds) 1996 Cytotoxic drugs: handling and administration. In: The Royal Marsden NHS Trust manual of clinical nursing procedures, 4th edn. Blackwell Scientific, London, Ch. 13, 191–212

Mayer D K 1992 Hazards of chemotherapy – implementing safe handling practices. Cancer 70: 988–992

Nieweg R M, De Boer M, Dubbleman R C et al 1994 Safe handling of antineoplastic drugs: results of a survey. Cancer Nursing 17(6): 501–511

Powell L L (ed) 1996 Cancer chemotherapy guidelines and recommendations for practice. Oncology Nursing Press, Pittsburgh

Priestman T J 1989 Cancer chemotherapy: an introduction, 3rd edn. Springer-Verlag, Berlin

Reymann P E 1993 Chemotherapy: principles of administration. In: Groenwald S L, Goodman M, Frogge M H, Henke Yarbro C (eds) Cancer nursing – principles and practice. Jones, Bartlett, Boston, ch 15, p 293–330

Rittenberg C N, Gralla R J, Rehmeyer T A 1995 Assessing and managing venous irritation with vinorelbine tartrate. Oncology Nursing Forum 22(4): 707–710

Robinson S 1993 Principles of chemotherapy. European Journal of Cancer Care 2: 55–65

Royal College of Nursing Oncology Society 1989 Safe practices with cytotoxics. Scutari Projects, Middlesex

Rudolph R, Larson D L 1987 Etiology and treatment of chemotherapeutic agent extravasation injuries: a review. Journal of Clinical Oncology 5(7): 1116–1126

Schulmeister L 1992 An overview of continuous infusion chemotherapy. Journal of Intravenous Nursing 15(6): 315–321

Selevan S G, Lindbohm M, Horning R, Hemminki K 1985 A study of occupational exposure to antineoplastic drugs and foetal loss in nurses. New England Journal of Medicine 19: 1173–1178

Speechley V 1984 Administration of cytotoxic drugs. Nursing Mirror 158(2): 22–25

Speechley V 1987 Nursing patients having chemotherapy. In: Tiffany R (ed) Oncology for nurses and health care professionals, 2nd edn. Harper & Row, London, Ch. 13, 74–121

Taskinen H K 1990 Effects of parental occupational exposures on spontaneous abortion and congenital malformation. Scandinavian Journal of Work and Environmental Health 16: 297–314

Thomas P H, Fenton May V 1987 Protection offered by gloves to carmustine exposure. Pharmaceutical Journal 238: 775–777

Tortorice P V 1997 Chemotherapy: principles of therapy. In: Groenwald S L, Frogge M H, Goodman M, Henke Yarbro C (eds) Cancer nursing – principles and practice. Jones & Bartlett, Boston, ch 14, p 283–316

Tsavaris N B, Komitsopoulou P, Karagiaouris P, Loukatou P, Tzannou I, Mylonakis N,

Kosnidis P 1992 Prevention of tissue necrosis due to accidental extravasation of cytostatic drugs by a conservative approach. Cancer Chemotherapy Pharmacology 30: 330–333

Tully J L, Friedland G H, Baldrini L M, Goldmann D A 1981 Complications of intravenous therapy with steel needles and teflon catheters: a comparative study. The American Journal of Medicine 70: 702–706

Valanis B G, Vollmer W M, Labuhn K T, Glass A G 1993 Acute symptoms associated with antineoplastic drug handling among nurses. Cancer Nursing 16(4): 288–295

Vennit S, Crofton-Sleigh C, Speechley V, Briggs K 1984 Monitoring exposure of nursing and pharmacy personnel to cytotoxic drugs: urinary mutation assays and urinary platinum as markers of absorption. The Lancet 1: 74–76

Waksvik H, Klepp O, Brogger A 1981 Chromosome analysis of nurse handling cytostatic agents. Cancer Treatment Reports 65: 607–610

Weinstein S M 1997 Antineoplastic therapy. In: Plumer's principles and practice of IV therapy, 5th edn. JB Lippincott, Philadelphia, ch 20, p 463–530

Wiseman K C, Wachs J E 1990 Policies and practices used for the safe handling of antineoplastic drugs. American Association of Occupational Health Nursing Journal 38(11): 517–523

Wood L S, Gullo S M 1993 IV vesicants: how to avoid extravasation. American Journal of Nursing 4: 42–45

Appendix: British Intravenous Therapy Association Guidelines: a response for today

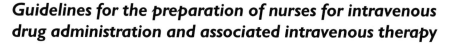

Guidelines for the preparation of nurses for intravenous drug administration and associated intravenous therapy

PURPOSE OF THE GUIDELINES

- To identify factors for consideration when generating policies related to i.v. therapy and nurse role extension.
- To provide the profession with a positive forward path for the education of nurses who undertake role extensions within i.v. therapy.
- To provide a standardized educational format which will achieve inter-district acceptability of educational preparation.
- To identify the key concepts within i.v. therapy on which educational programmes may be based.
- To provide guidance on the assessment of individuals who have undertaken such a programme.

PART I

Policy making

The health service of today demands a cost-effective and efficient utilization of resources. Accountability by managers, clinicians and educators for the way resources are utilized is required. In the light of these factors, it is recommended that policy makers should consider these following questions when formulating policy and/or procedures in the administration of intravenous medication:

- Why should nurses administer intravenous drugs?
- Which nurses should administer intravenous drugs?
- In which clinical areas may nurses administer intravenous drugs?
- Under what conditions may nurses administer intravenous drugs?
- Which drugs should the nurse administer intravenously?
- How should nurses be educationally prepared to administer intravenous medication?

Why should nurses administer i.v. drugs?

The philosophy of care today is holistic in emphasis. The concept of holistic care embraces the administration by the nurse of intravenous medication to the patient in his/her charge.

Who should administer i.v. drugs?

All registered general nurses can administer intravenous drugs in their own specialist clinical area, provided they have been educationally prepared, follow health authority guidelines and are willing to do so.

Enrolled nurses can administer intravenous drugs in the speciality in which they have a specialist qualification, provided they have undergone a specific educational programme for the administration of intravenous drugs, follow health authority guidelines and are willing to do so.

This applies also to enrolled nurses who have extensive experience and are regarded by clinical colleagues (i.e. ward sisters) to be expert practitioners, provided they have undergone a specific educational programme for the administration of intravenous drugs, follow health authority guidelines and are willing to do so.

Only nurses with a Registered Sick Children's Nursing Certificate or registered general nurses with a post-basic paediatric qualification or extensive experience in paediatric nursing should be permitted to administer intravenous drugs to children, provided they have been educationally prepared, follow health authority guidelines and are willing to do so.

Where nurses should move from one speciality to another speciality, specialist education for the administration of drugs for the new area should be available.

In which clinical areas may nurses administer i.v. drugs?

Suitably qualified nurses should only administer intravenous drugs in the area in which they are practising.

Safe standards of practice cannot be maintained if the nurse moves from ward to ward with the sole responsibility of administering intravenous drugs.

Clearly, it is necessary for the nurse administering the medication to be familiar with both the patient and the drug. He/she must be able to administer the appropriate care to the patient should any complications develop throughout the administration of the intravenous drug.

Under what conditions may nurses administer i.v. drugs?

The decision to administer intravenous drugs remains the sole responsibility of the individual nurse practitioner. Provided the nurse is satisfied that the prescription of the drug meets with the health authority policy and the manufacturer's instructions and provided the nurse him/herself has been adequately prepared for this role, then he/she may proceed to administer the drug.

When generating the policies the health authority should consider the following points:

- The nurse is under an obligation to the patient to administer safe, competent care. He/she is accountable to the United Kingdom Central Council for his/her practice through the *Code of Conduct*.
- Policy statements should leave the decision whether or not to administer intravenous drugs to the nurse him/herself.
- If the health authority decides that it is part of the nurse's role to administer intravenous drugs, then the manpower implications of this statement must be examined at a local level.
- Should the health authority, in its policies, indicate that the nurse may only undertake the extended role when basic role requirements have been met then it must be aware that this places the nurse in a difficult position with regards to who decides what is a basic care requirement.

Which drugs should the nurse administer intravenously?

A clearly defined list of which drugs the nurse may administer should be drawn up by the Drugs and Therapeutics Committees of individual districts. This list will require periodic review.

New drugs appear on the market at an ever increasing rate. To maintain safe and competent practice, the nurse should only administer drugs on which pharmacological and pharmaceutical data are available and with which he/she is familiar. Ideally, the pharmacy will provide clinical nurses with a service for this information.

How should nurses be prepared to administer i.v. drugs?

Following registration as a nurse, a period of consolidation is required in which the nurse gains competence and confidence. Once this period (which should be a minimum of 3 months) is completed, then role extension may be considered.

It is the responsibility of each individual nurse to decide when to take on role extension.

Preparation required needs to comply with the recommendations issued by the DHSS: DHSS circulars *HC(76)9*, 'Addition of drugs to intravenous fluids', and *HC(77)22*, 'The extended role of the clinical nurse – legal implications and training' requirements.

The guidelines compiled by the BITA Working Party meet these recommendations.

PART 2

Educational programme

This programme is designed to enable the nurse to develop his/her knowledge, skills and attitudes further so that he/she may competently administer intravenous medication.

The programme is based on the belief that each nurse is responsible and accountable for his/her own practice and the educational preparation required for that practice.

It will therefore provide a framework for further learning and professional development as well as meeting the educational requirements outlined in *HC(77)22*, 'The extended role of the clinical nurse – legal implications and training requirements'.

Aims of the educational study days

- To review the role of the nurse within the practice of intravenous therapy.
- To identify the professional/legal/moral implications within the practice of intravenous therapy and i.v. drug administration.
- To identify the pharmaceutical principles implicit in i.v. drug administration and the implications for nursing practice.
- To explore the practical aspects of i.v. drug administration.
- To provide an environment where free discussion is encouraged and personal views valued.

Pre-course work

Prior to attending the educational preparation programme, staff should be sent a package of material containing:

- district drugs policy

- district drugs handbook
- suggested reading list
- study day programme
- study day aims and objectives
- district intravenous therapy procedures.

Pre-course self-assessment to aid the identification of specific learning needs

Should the nurse have access to this material through other channels (i.e. on the ward) then the package may be modified. The educator should, however, bear in mind that the aim of this material is to familiarize the nurse with as much of the course information as possible prior to attending the study days. Only then will it be possible to facilitate learning on the study day without information overload and the consequent learning difficulties.

Suggested study day programme

This is a 2-day programme:

- *Day 1*

9.00–10.00	Introduction to the programme
10.00–10.30	Coffee
10.30–12.30	Legal, professional and moral aspects of i.v. therapy
12.30–1.30	Lunch
1.30–4.30	Fundamental review of i.v. therapy
4.30	Close

- *Day 2*

9.00–10.00	Pharmaceutical aspects of i.v. therapy
10.00–10.30	Coffee
10.30–11.30	Mathematical aspects of i.v. therapy
11.30–12.30	Theoretical aspects of i.v. therapy
12.30–1.30	Lunch
1.30–4.00	Practical aspects of i.v. drug administration
4.00–4.30	Conclusion to programme
4.30	Close

PART 3

Assessment strategy

Assessment, both practical and theoretical, is a requirement of both the statutory body (see UKCC *Code of Conduct*) and the DHSS recommendations related to i.v. therapy. Guidelines are offered for both aspects.

Practical assessment

Following the educational study programme the nurse returns to the clinical area and fulfils the following procedure chronologically:

- *Observation* – the nurse observes administrating medication by the accepted routes/procedures practised in his/her own clinical area.
- *Supervised practice* – a period of supervised practice is undertaken for each method practised. Supervision is given by any nurse who is competent to administer intravenous medication.
- *Assessment* – when the nurse assesses him/herself to be competent to administer

intravenous medication without supervision, he/she arranges to be assessed by a nurse assessor.

An assessor is:

- a practising senior nurse, i.e. staff nurse/ward sister/clinical nursing officer/teacher, who regularly administers intravenous drugs him/herself
- chosen by the nurse to be assessed
- able to assess utilizing the suggested guidelines
- ideally one who has undertaken a course in assessment skills, e.g. ENB Course 998 or GNC Assessors' Course.

The observations/practice/assessment should be undertaken in the clinical area in which the nurse works.

The senior manager, to whom the nurse is accountable, should review at regular intervals the nurse's progress through the process. This will highlight any difficulties the nurse is experiencing and allow for a speedy resolution to be achieved. This will prevent nurses attending the study programme and then being unable to undertake the role extension because of difficulty in being assessed.

Guidelines for the assessor

Prior to undertaking the procedure the nurse must demonstrate his/her understanding of:

- the present condition of the patient and his/her relevant medical/nursing history
- the district policy and intravenous drug checking procedure
- the patency and suitability of the i.v. infusion site
- drug:
  — according to manufacturer's instructions
  — reconstitution of the drug
  — rate of administration
  — action and possible side-effects
  — normal dosage range
  — storage
  — compatibility
- equipment required
- potential complications of the procedure.

The following aspects must be considered in assessing the practical skills which will fulfil the need for patient comfort, patient safety and maintenance of asepsis:

- preparation:
  — patient
  — equipment
  — environment
- procedure:
  — checking of the i.v. site
  — aseptic technique
  — correct administration of drug
  — re-establishment of i.v. infusion to previous state
  — correct disposal of equipment
  — post-administration patient monitoring.

Assessment of competence must incorporate the following communication skills:

- verbal:
  — explanation of procedure to patient

    — explanation of procedure to other members of care plan
    — clear delivery of instructions to any assistant
    — demonstration of a caring sensitive manner in dealing with the patient
- written:
    — correct completion of drug record
    — correct completion of drug additive label.

Failure of the assessment

Should competence not be reached in the assessment, then further periods of supervised practice with specific guidance for improvement in practice should be given.

Theoretical assessment

Theoretical assessment is undertaken as a self-assessment process. Responsibility for the successful completion of this assessment rests with the individual nurse.

The continuing education unit should provide each nurse with the assessment and guidelines for him/her to decide if he/she has a satisfactory knowledge base with which to practise.

Index

Page references in **bold** indicate main discussions; those in *italics* indicate tables, boxes or figures.